“Tosquelles had genius. This remarkable edition at last makes his thought available in English. Its importance cannot be overstated.”
—Jean Khalfa

“‘Physicians, heal thyselves’ might be the best epigraph for this revolutionary and revelatory book. Grounded in the assumption that madness, not rationality, is the essence of man, Tosquelles sought to transform psychiatry from a cure for sick minds into a practice of humanization at every level, from the clinic to the community. This book is a landmark achievement.”
—W.J.T. Mitchell

“From the bordellos-turned-annexes of the Almodóvar clinic for the Catalan militia, to a psychiatric barrack at a refugee camp that was also a means of flight, Tosquelles consistently unsettled demarcations of inside and out across the nosological, the analytic couch, the state, and the enclosed hospital—endlessly actualizing, instead, asylum-villages and therapeutic communities. Joana Masó’s careful work maps Tosquelles’s predecessors, inheritors, and legacies to come. This book presents us with existing vectors of escape and the responsibility of proliferating and mutating these at the level of the spatial, the social, and desire.”
—Perwana Nazif

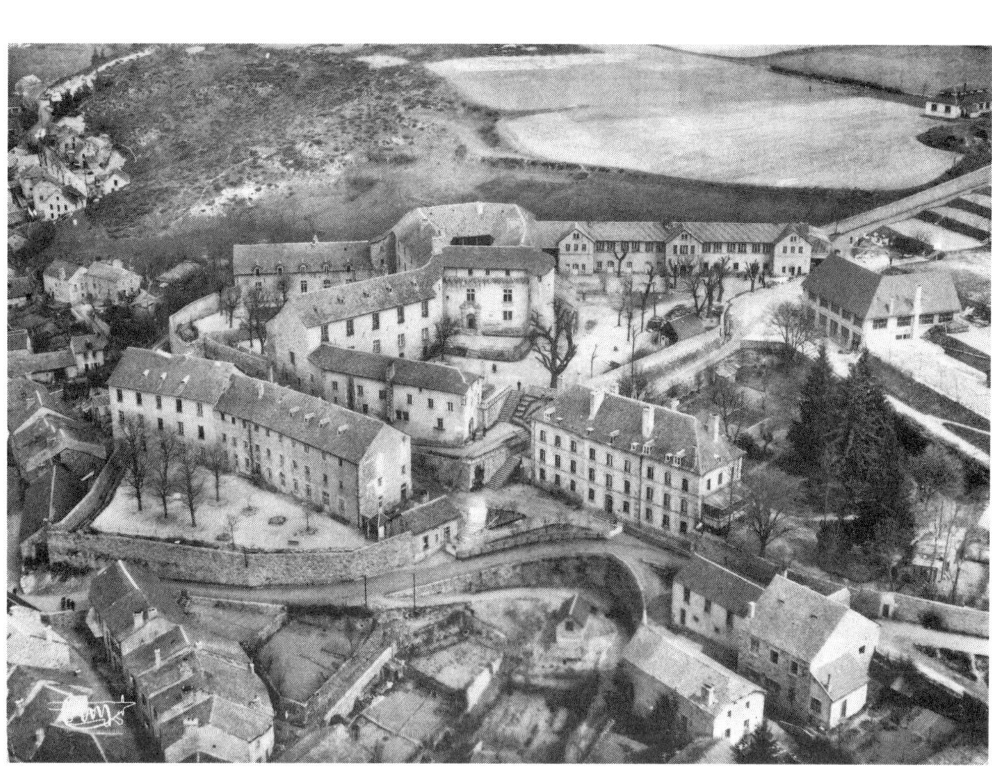

This book is copublished by Arcàdia, Divided, and Semiotext(e) in 2026. First published in Barcelona, Spain, in 2021 by Arcàdia as *Tosquelles: Curar les institucions*. First published in the United States by Semiotext(e). First published in the United Kingdom by Divided Publishing.

All rights reserved. No part of this book may be reproduced, stored in a retrieval system, or transmitted by any means, electronic, mechanical, photocopying, recording, or otherwise, without prior permission of the publisher.

Published by Semiotext(e)
PO Box 629, South Pasadena, CA 91031
www.semiotexte.com

This book was translated with the help of a grant from the Institut Ramon Llull.

institut
ramon llull

Cover Design: Hedi El Kholti

Cover: Francesc Tosquelles in the garden of the house of the medical director of the Saint-Alban hospital, 1944 or 1945. Source: Tosquelles family archives (photographic reproduction by Roberto Ruiz).

ISBN: 978-1-63590-255-6

10 9 8 7 6 5 4 3 2 1
Distributed by the MIT Press, Cambridge, MA, and London, England
Printed in the United States of America

Tosquelles: Healing Institutions

Joana Masó

With Texts by Francesc Tosquelles

Translated by Robert Hurley and Mara Faye Lethem

Semiotext(e)

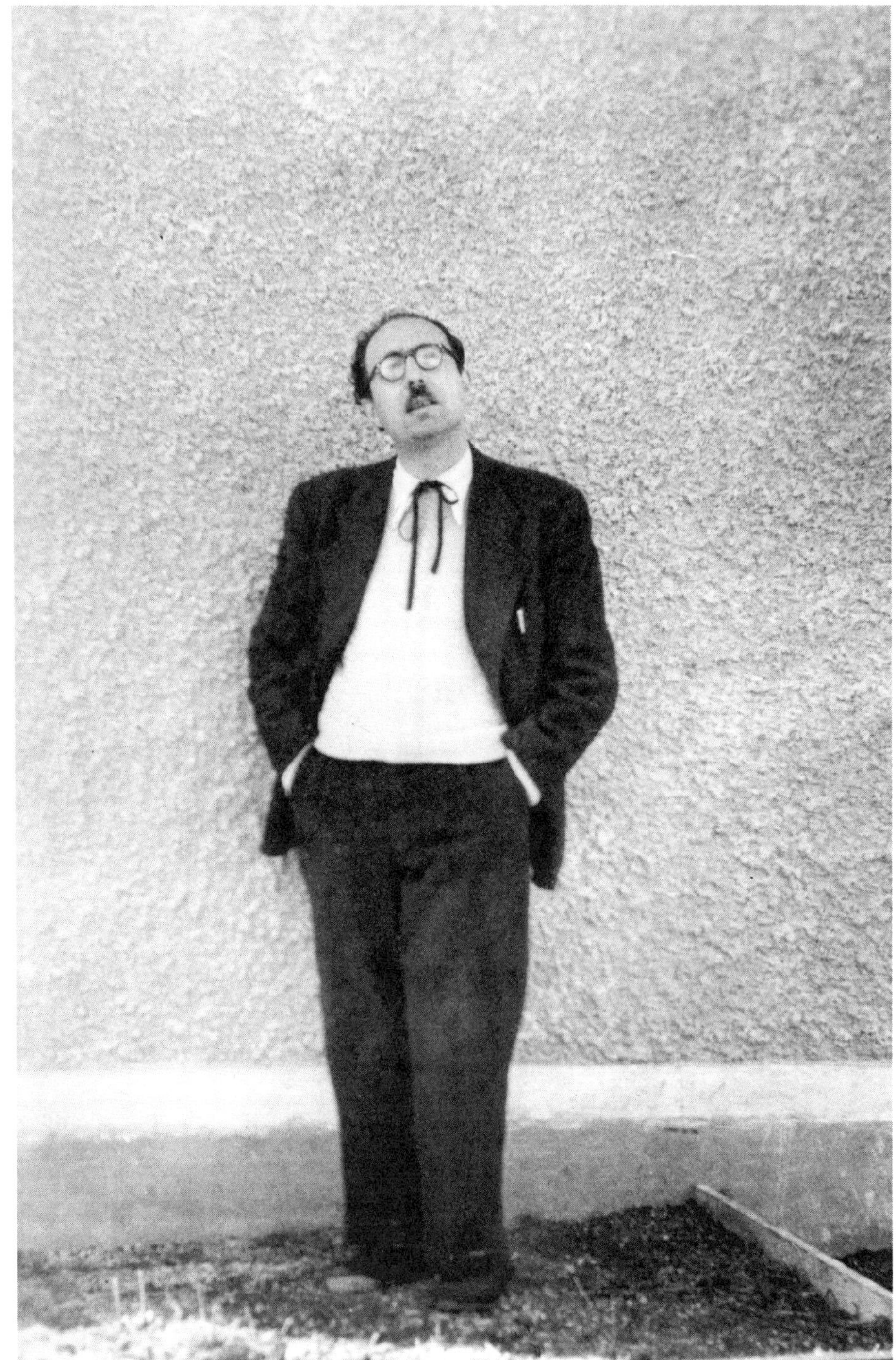

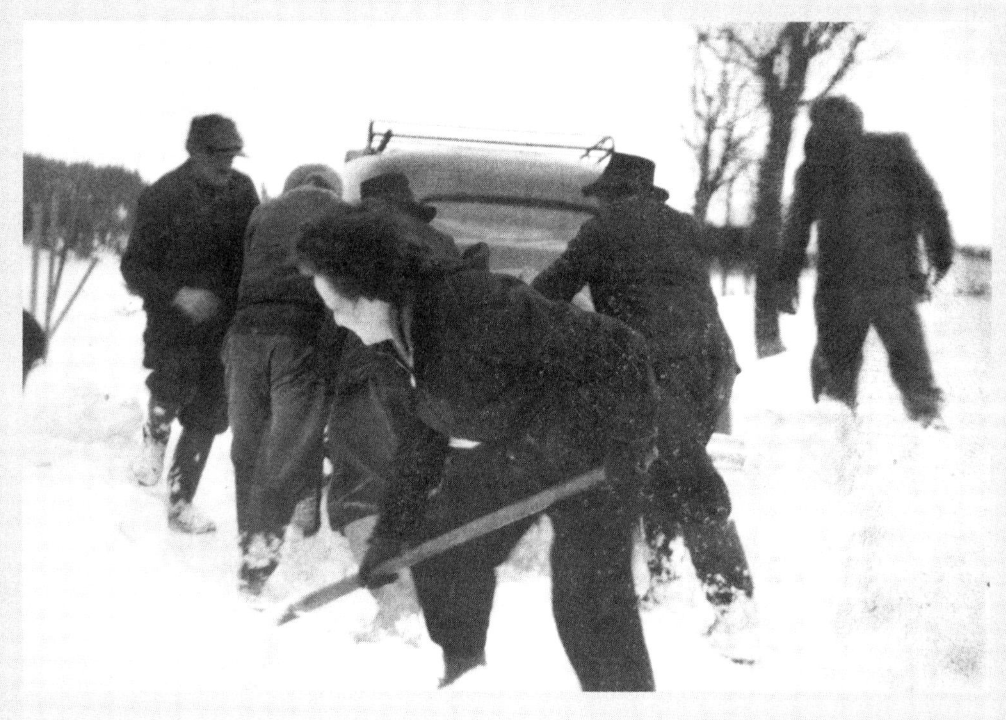

PRESENTATION

In the autumn of 2012, Barcelona's Museum of Contemporary Art was showing *Déconnage*, the video-essay by Angela Melitopoulos and Maurizio Lazzarato on the Catalan psychiatrist Francesc Tosquelles, who was born in Reus in 1912 and exiled to France, where he died in Granges-sur-Lot in 1994. Throughout the film, Tosquelles spoke of collective experiences of transformation within institutions, during the Second Republic, the Spanish Civil War, and the Nazi occupation of France.

Curing sick institutions: that was the surprising experience Tosquelles carried out in unexpected places, such as psychiatric hospitals forged in the nineteenth century. Following the contributions of the psychiatrist Hermann Simon, Tosquelles thought that patients could only be cured by curing the hospitals. The entire hospital had to be treated as ill: without curing its administrative foundations, its associations and contexts, everything that makes us sick would remain unchanged. Tosquelles also wanted to transform other institutions in crisis, such as those that dealt with work, through professional training institutes; with childcare, through pediatric institutions; and with politics, through the anarcho-communist Workers and Peasants' Group (BOC), the Workers' Party of Marxist Unification (POUM), and through collaboration with the Resistance networks of occupied France.

In *Déconnage*, Tosquelles spoke about psychiatry and about the cooperatives and unions that, during the Second Republic, had been organized to heal the lack of public social health care. And he spoke of amateur psychiatric experiences during the Civil War as a moment of experimentation and urgency, when the world was ending and at the same time being born. He spoke of an institutional psychoanalysis within the institution, far from private therapy or "clientele." He spoke about the link between psychoanalytic practice and foreign languages: about the unconscious, about accents and intonation. About the voice as matter. About posture, body and gait. About mothers who tickle their children's feet because our feet are what lead us places. And about a way of understanding psychiatry as a form of anti-culture and at the same time a practice radically located in a landscape.

However, some of us knew nothing of what *Déconnage* was explaining. We had never heard of Tosquelles, or of the experiences—amateur, political, and clinical—referred to in the video-essay. This book and the research informing it were born of that lack of knowledge. Born of the absence of Tosquelles in our collective imaginary. We knew nothing about him and we wanted to know more, to listen to him, to read him. We wanted the forgotten legacy of Tosquelles to illuminate an unknown past and, at the same time, a collective adventure that could speak to us in the present: of our sick institutions and our sick people; of experimental institutional practices that would allow us to imagine, today, other ways of experiencing and reshaping our institutions, ways that didn't involve perpetual conflict.

A concatenation of collective experiences led Francesc Tosquelles to imagine open institutions. Institutions open to the psychiatric vanguard, in order to convert spaces of reclusion into inhabitable environments and to humanize discounted lives. These institutions were informed by the political practices that had fought against the fascisms of the 1930s and '40s, and against the new faces of depoliticization of the second half of the twentieth century. They were spaces of artistic, literary, and pedagogical experimentation centered in antiauthoritarianism.

Above all, they were institutions open to their surroundings, because they wanted to live and put down roots in them while transforming them. This openness allowed for a reconsideration of the private asylum, the campaign hospital, the refugee camp, and the public psychiatric hospital. It redrew their walls and perimeters, their centers and their margins. It strengthened bonds between political, medical, and creative practices, and connected them with material life in the rural homes, the fields, and the outskirts through geopsychiatry; with the work of self-management, with patient cooperatives and constant mutual education by everyone; with allowing patients to have a voice in meetings, the community theater and cinema; in the creation of wall newspapers, internal dailies and the press; with the legal dispute over the art brut market and cultural appropriation.

This group history that, starting in the fifties, was referred to as "institutional psychotherapy" sought to transform all that which Erving Goffman had labeled "total institutions": places of isolation in which individuals were stripped of social contact and enclosed within a bureaucratic management of their lives and needs. Tosquelles associated the possibility of this transformation with war. Both with his commitment as a psychiatrist during conflict—

the Spanish Civil War, the Francoist dictatorship, the Second World War and the Nazi occupation of France—and with the general state of war as an experience of the world. Years later, in the seventies and eighties, he himself wrote that there should be a war or two each generation. If it weren't for all the casualties, if it weren't for all the damage, it would be a coveted experience. Because there are less neuroses than in the so-called times of peace; because it situates you, roots you, allows you to embody, confront, and act; because it leads us to question what struggle is and which battles are meaningful.

Tosquelles's provocative words warned of the looming depoliticization that continues to threaten our institutional culture. He pointed out the dangers of a depoliticized relationship to our institutions and their normalized ways of defining health and madness—from primary schools to universities, from places of work to places of leisure, from convalescence to old age. If we are unable to identify the wars affecting our institutions, along with the contemporary forms of authoritarianism, paternalism, and lack of freedom, the sick institutions are hurting us in ways we cannot name nor transform. As such, these historical experiences are not only history, since they are not in the past. They do not only address fascist Europe. They are experiences that continue to resonate in the neoliberal malaise of our institutions. The collective practices promoted by Tosquelles introduced the question of lived experience—which is so often absent in our contemporary understanding of institutions—into the clinical and therapeutic field, into the political field, and into the literary field.

Francesc Tosquelles's trajectory is usually recounted as an adventure whose maximum political expression and collective transformation began in January 1940, when Tosquelles began working at the psychiatric hospital of Saint-Alban-sur-Limagnole, in the *département* of Lozère in southern France. It comes to us as a mythical tale of a group of men who met during the Nazi occupation. Men who came together at Saint-Alban to remake their lives within the Resistance, in a France that allowed forty thousand mental patients to die in its psychiatric hospitals over those years. The psychiatrist Max Lafont deemed that the "soft extermination": years of deaths from abandonment, starvation, cold, and general neglect in French hospitals, while at Saint-Alban they organized ways to collaborate with the local community in order to survive.

During the first half of the 1940s, thanks to psychiatrist Lucien Bonnafé's ties to the avant-garde, the Resistance, and French communism, renowned figures arrived at the Saint-Alban hospital. They included the poet Paul Éluard, the painter Gérard Vulliamy, the philosopher, teacher, and science historian Georges Canguilhem, the film historian Georges Sadoul, the photographer Jacques Matarasso, and the poet and Dada theorist Tristan Tzara. After the Second World War, and through Paul Éluard, the artist and art brut theorist Jean Dubuffet would also arrive to Saint-Alban and find one of his privileged interlocutors in the psychiatrist Jean Oury, a colleague of Tosquelles's there and, later, of Félix Guattari's at the La Borde clinic. The psychiatrist, writer, and critic of colonialism Frantz Fanon worked with Tosquelles at Saint-Alban as a resident in 1952 and 1953, after writing *Black Skin, White Masks* and before he joined the Algerian Independence movement.

These big names and their cultural output have overshadowed many others' contributions. Most of all, the names and lives of the women in the hospital: the psychiatrist Agnès Masson, director of Saint-Alban during the 1930s, who introduced geopsychiatry; or the psychiatrist Germaine Balvet, author of a thesis on insulin treatments and the initiator of homeopathic practice with medicinal herbs at the hospital, where her husband Dr. Balvet was the director when Tosquelles arrived; or Nusch, an artist and Éluard's wife, who accompanied him during his stay at Saint-Alban, where she was involved in establishing a theater. Nusch Éluard's name is too often left out of this story, along with Cécile Éluard's, the daughter he'd had with Gala and who was a contributor to the communist newspaper *Les Étoiles* under the pseudonym Cécile Agay. Tosquelles remembers Nusch and Cécile Éluard taking part in the psychotherapy of the schizophrenic inpatients. The silencing of these women is a betrayal of the hospital's collective history, and in order to recover that history and comprehend Saint-Alban's survival, we cannot leave out Tosquelles's wife, Elena Álvarez, nor the nuns of the order of Saint-Régis and their mother superior, Théophile, as well as the nurses, caregivers and trainers, and the patients both male and female. Francesc Tosquelles had a life in Saint-Alban with Elena that was simultaneously personal and professional. They and their four children lived in the hospital—and their children had been born there, with the exception of Marie-Rose, who was born in Reus in 1936—as did the children of the other doctors and administrators.

This book aspires to redraw the outlines of this collective history and its material life, imbuing it with another genealogy of proper names, bodies, and lived experiences. It strives to unlearn some of the iconic, mythical moments of that history and instead follow the red thread that links Saint-Alban with other experiences of cultural, political, and psychiatric transformation that Tosquelles had been taking part in over more than a decade before arriving in France. In Catalonia, between Reus and Barcelona. In Spain, between Sariñena, Benabarre, Bujaraloz, and Almodóvar del Campo. In France, at the Judes internment camp in Septfonds.

Most of the essays Tosquelles wrote in French have never been translated, and many of the texts he wrote in Catalan and in Spanish were unavailable. As such, this book brings together a series of new translations and obscure texts published in journals, newspapers, and scientific editions. This first anthology of texts by Tosquelles in English presents a selection of excerpts from his vast intellectual, clinical, and political production in the decades from 1930 to 1980, and complements the project of Francesc Tosquelles's complete works in French, which is being carried out by Jacques Tosquellas from the *Archives complètes* with Éditions d'une publishing house, run by Sophie Legrain.

I hope this book allows for both remembering and learning, inheriting and creating, at the meeting point there between the memory we do not yet have and the imagination we lack, in order to tackle the problems and maladies within our contemporary institutions.

Joana Masó, Barcelona, June 2021

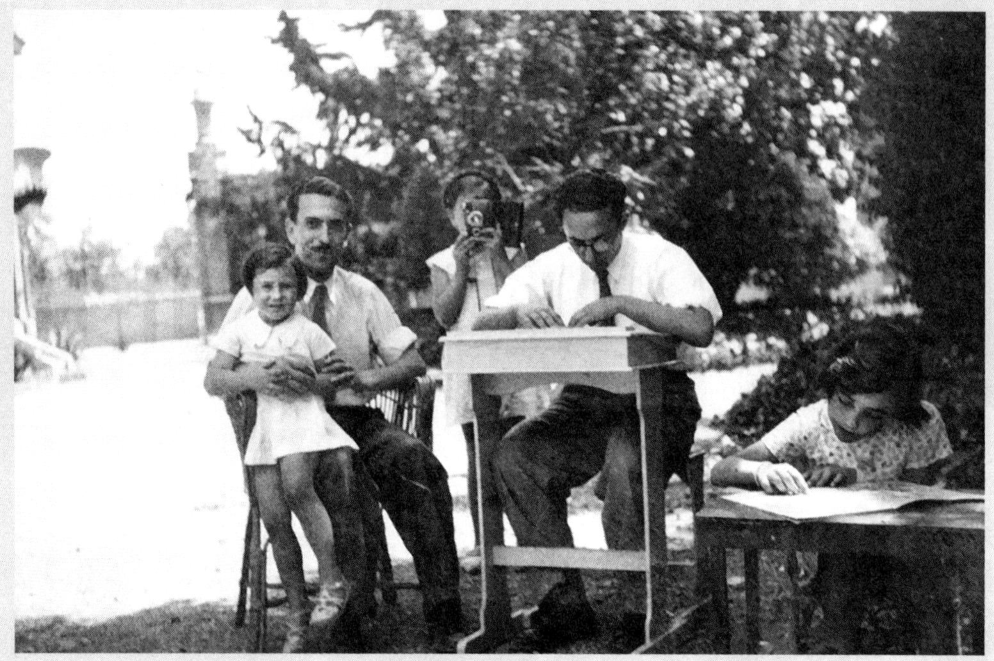

"I've always had a theory that to be a good psychiatrist, one needs to be a foreigner or pretend to be a foreigner. For example, it's a mannerism and it's not a mannerism on my part to speak French poorly. It's necessary for the patient, or even a normal person, who doesn't understand … to make a special effort to understand. They're obliged to translate. And they take an active position towards me."

THE LIVES OF FRANCESC TOSQUELLES

1912 Francesc Tosquelles i Llauradó is born in Reus on August 22. His family home is on Carrer Major, where his parents have a notions store called La Chic, right across from the Centre de Lectura, founded in 1859 by artisans and working-class activists.

1913 Francesc Llauradó, philanthropic doctor and maternal uncle of Francesc Tosquelles, publishes a commentary about Sigmund Freud's *The Interpretation of Dreams* (1899) in the journal *Archivos de Terapéutica y de las Enfermedades Nerviosas y Mentales: Eco Científico del Manicomio de Reus*, stating that Freud's work will effect change in psychiatric hospitals.

1914 The Mancomunitat of Catalonia is established on April 6. This new government makes the first attempts to decentralize psychiatric institutions, an effort that is interrupted in 1923 by the dictatorship of Miguel Primo de Rivera.

1917 Spurred on by José Ortega y Gasset, the Biblioteca Nueva publishing house starts publishing the *Complete Works* of Sigmund Freud in Spanish, with a translation by the Germanist Luis López Ballesteros. The first volume appears in 1922.

1922 The German psychiatrist and art historian Hans Prinzhorn publishes *Bildnerei der Geisteskranken: Ein Beitrag zur Psychologie und Psychopathologie der Gestaltung* (*Artistry of the Mentally Ill: A Contribution to the Psychology and Psychopathology of Configuration*), which reproduces part of his own collection, primarily acquired during his time at the psychiatric hospital in the University of Heidelberg between 1919 and 1921, continuing an initiative begun by the psychiatrist Karl Wilmanns.

1927 During the academic year 1927–1928, Tosquelles completes his baccalaureate degree with a specialization in sciences and studies two years of German between 1925 and 1928 at the Institut Nacional de Segon Ensenyament in Reus. On April 8, 1929, he will receive his degree.

He begins to study medicine under Dr. Salvador Vilaseca and specializes in psychiatry. He collaborates informally with the Institut Pere Mata in Reus. He is familiar with the hospital, founded in 1900 by the doctor and politician

Emili Briansó and designed by the architect Lluís Domènech i Montaner, because of the relationship his uncle and godfather had with Dr. Briansó.

1928 Tosquelles, under the byline Tosquellas, writes two short articles for the monthly school magazine *Letras*: "Vides adelerades" (Accelerated lives) and "L'afer de Glozel" (The case of Glozel).

Between May and September, he takes his final exams for his baccalaureate degree, which include both oral and written exercises, as well as a foreign language, German in his case. Tosquelles's knowledge of German will play a fundamental role in allowing him to access the pioneering contributions of Central European psychiatry.

He begins his formal study of medicine at the Universitat de Barcelona. His classes include Descriptive and Topographical Anatomy I, Histology and Micrographic Technology, and Anatomical Technique I. He will finish his studies at the age of twenty-two, in the academic year 1932–1933, with Medical Pathology III, Surgical Pathology III, and Legal Medicine.

1929 In the framework of the International Exposition, the 33rd Congrès des médecins et neurologistes de France et des pays de langue française is held in Barcelona—and travels to Reus for one day. The French psychiatrist and psychoanalyst Henry Ey participates. The presence of Hungarian psychoanalyst refugees in Catalonia allows Tosquelles to familiarize himself with such authors as Sándor Ferenczi, Michael Balint, and Leopold Szondi.

Hermann Simon publishes his *Aktivere Krankenbehandlung in der Irrenanstalt*, which is translated into Spanish by the psychiatrist Ramon Sarró as *Tratamiento ocupacional de los enfermos mentales* (1937). In Saint-Alban, Tosquelles will prompt the French translation of the book, still today unpublished in France, by Eugénie Balvet, the sister of the hospital's director Paul Balvet, in collaboration with the medical community there.

1930 The Workers and Peasants' Group (BOC) is created by the fusion of the Catalan Communist Party (PCC) and the Catalan-Balearic Communist Federation (FCCB).

On February 11, at a gathering in honor of the student Antoni Maria Sbert, leader of the University Federation, Tosquelles reveals, in the name of the university section of the Centro de Reus, Sbert's role in toppling the dictatorship of Primo de Rivera.

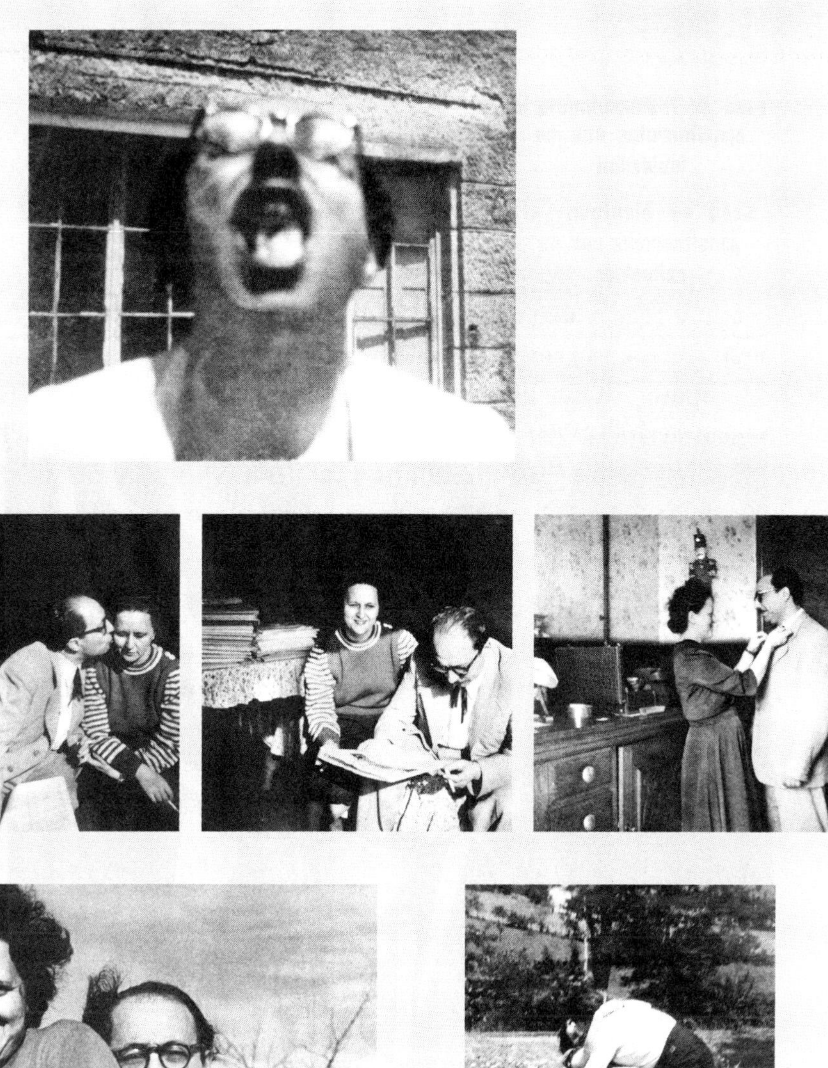

"The unconscious is a thing that doesn't exist, it insists but doesn't exist."

1931 On April 14, the Second Republic is proclaimed. Tosquelles attends the proclamation ceremony at the Palau de la Generalitat when President Francesc Macià declares the Catalan Republic within an Iberian Federation. A period begins in which Barcelona becomes known as "Little Vienna" due to the considerable number of Central European psychoanalysts exiled there, including Sándor Eiminder, Werner Wolff (who was part of the Gestalt school), Adlerian psychoanalyst Ferenc Olivér Brachfeld, and Alfred Strauss, professor of child psychiatry.

On May 27, Tosquelles gives the lecture "L'estructuració de la societat i de la follia" (The structuring of society and madness) at the Ateneu Enciclopèdic Popular, gathering place of anarchist and socialist workers where they program courses that couldn't be taught at the university because of the general strike. On the list of speakers in 1931 there are politicians like Joaquín Maurín, who discusses Leninism and Trotskyism and the Spanish political moment, and Andreu Nin, who speaks on the government and the problems of the Spanish revolution.

Salvador Dalí gives the lecture "El Surrealisme al servei de la revolució," (Surrealism in the service of the revolution) followed by a lecture by the French surrealist writer René Crevel, "L'esprit contre la raison" (Spirit versus reason), in an event organized by the BOC weekly *L'Hora* (The time), on September 18 in the Sala Capsir in Barcelona.

Tosquelles begins his own psychoanalysis at the Ateneu Barcelonès with Sándor Eiminder, a Jewish Hungarian teacher and psychoanalyst who is a refugee in Barcelona. Eiminder was a colleague of the educator and psychoanalyst August Aichhorn, a member of Freud's Viennese circle, and an associate of Sándor Ferenczi's.

1932 On the recommendation of Dr. Emili Mira y López, Tosquelles reads the thesis that French psychoanalyst Jacques Lacan has just defended in Paris that same year, *De la psychose paranoïaque dans ses rapports avec la personnalité* (On paranoid psychosis in its relations with personality), and months later, uses it as material for training doctors and nurses at the Institut Pere Mata.

Emili Mira gives a seminar on Freud and Marx at the Ateneu Enciclopèdic Popular that includes a criticism of abstract psychology that will mark Tosquelles's trajectory. He serves as secretary for the seminar, which is given as a show of gratitude for the Ateneu's offering its space in solidarity with the 1930 Universitat de Barcelona strike.

Until November of 1933, Tosquelles is a member in the Moral Sciences section of the Ateneu Barcelonès, where a large part of the period's psychoanalytical, cultural, and sociopolitical debate takes place. That membership allows him access to the Ateneu's library when he begins studying medicine. From there he maintains a correspondence with his friend Josep Solanes, a doctor at the Institut Pere Mata.

On the invitation of Emili Mira, he becomes a collaborator at Mira's newly founded Psychotechnical Institute of the School of Work in Barcelona, where he continues until 1936.

1933 In October, Emili Mira occupies the Experimental Psychiatry chair at the Universitat Autònoma de Barcelona.

In December the journal *Estudis: Revista de l'Associació Cultural* begins publishing in Reus. Tosquelles is its editor through its final issue in June of 1936. There he publishes, along with other collaborators, articles on cooperativism, feminism, unionism, ecology, motherhood, poetry, war, and psychoanalysis.

From 1933 to 1936, Tosquelles works officially for the Institut Pere Mata. He also collaborates with Dr. Strauss at the Institute of Psychological Observation La Sageta, a child psychiatry clinic founded by Strauss and Mira inspired in the child guidance clinics in the United States and England; with Dr. Subirana at the Hospital Clínic in Barcelona; and at the Reus Childcare Institute La Gota de Llet (The Drop of Milk), founded by Dr. Alexandre Frias in 1919.

The German psychologist Werner Wolff, persecuted by the Nazis, is given refuge by Emili Mira at La Sageta.

1934 The newspaper *La Publicitat* announces, on April 21, that Tosquelles has been awarded his official medical degree in a ceremony at the Universitat Autònoma de Barcelona.

The Catalan government passes the law establishing the bases of their public health system, which defines a new concept of health care regions that allows more autonomy in therapeutic treatments.

In these years, the staff at the Institut Pere Mata is already actively participating in the institutional life of the hospital. On March 18, 1934, doctors, administrators, caregiver, and patients, along with the director Emili Briansó's daughters, perform

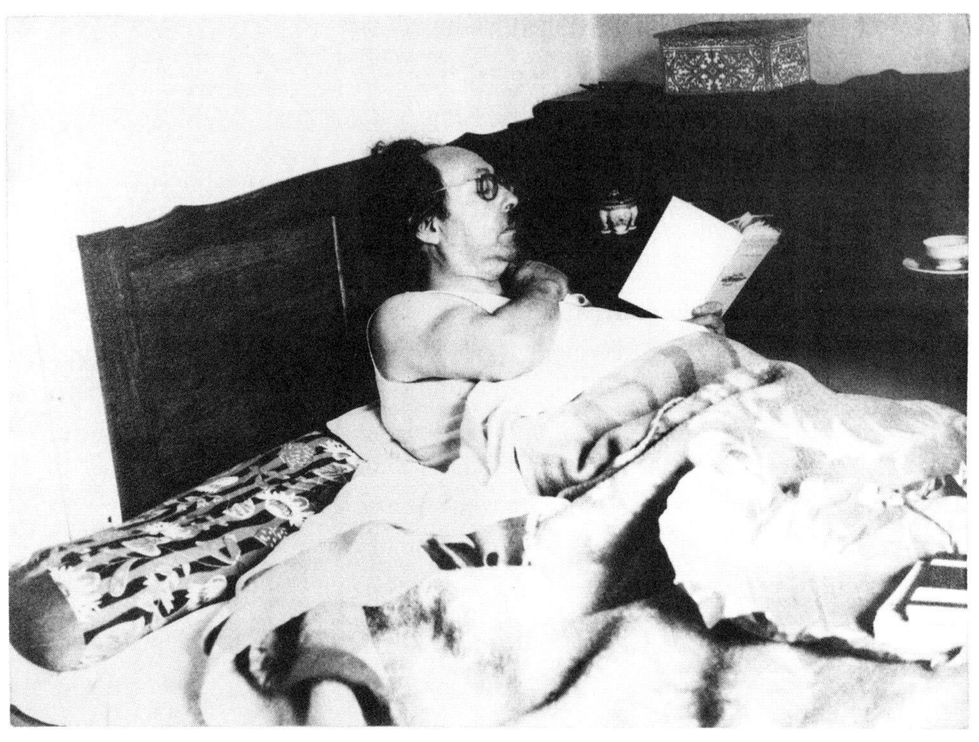

"My father and my uncle had a definite political ideology—left-wing, let's say, or rather cooperativist. They were militants of Catalan cooperation. And my father was perhaps even more rooted in that, because somewhat by chance, up to his death, his coming to France before dying, he was treasurer of the cooperative of health workers, because at the time there was no public health program and people formed cooperatives to be able to pay the doctor or for their prescriptions. That was called *la humanitat*. My father was the treasurer of humanity. Not bad, I think."

Shakespeare's *The Taming of the Shrew* at the Institut's theater. Tosquelles plays the role of Baptista and is also the master of ceremonies.

In December, Tosquelles publishes an article with Dr. Antoni Subirana in the *Revue neurologique* entitled "Un nouveau cas de calcification intracérébrale visible radiologiquement chez une hémiplégique de l'enfance avec crises épileptiques jacksoniennes: Aspects encéphalographiques." This article will make a name for Tosquelles in France, which is crucial to his later being able to leave the Septfonts refugee camp and begin working at the Saint-Alban hospital.

1935 On February 12, Francesc Tosquelles marries Elena Álvarez Fernández in the parish of Santa Maria de Gràcia in Barcelona. They had met on a streetcar five years earlier.

The Workers' Party of Marxist Unification (POUM) is founded as a result of the unification of Andreu Nin's Communist Left of Spain (ICE) with Joaquín Maurín's Workers and Peasants' Group (BOC).

In the Reus journal *Fulls clínics*, Tosquelles publishes "A propòsit de l'anàlisi d'una personalitat anormal," a reflection on a case study of a patient, in dialogue with German psychiatry, where he begins to formulate his institutional critique.

Mira publishes his *Manual de Psiquiatría*, which not only includes numerous photographs from the Institut Pere Mata, but stems from his collaboration with the psychiatrists there, including Tosquelles.

1936 On February 16, the Second Republic's third general elections are held, and won by the Popular Front. On May 10, Manuel Azaña is chosen as president.

Tosquelles, a member of the Iberian Communist Youth (JCI) party in Reus, enters into the orbit of the POUM, a Trotskyist party distanced from the official Communist line.

On May 17, Maria Rosa, the Tosquelles family's first child, is born in Reus, on Carrer Jesús.

The military uprising against the Republic takes place between July 17 and 20. Following Franco's coup in August, the Generalitat de Catalunya nationalizes—with the leadership of the anarchist psychiatrist Fèlix Martí Ibáñez—all the Catalan hospitals, including the Institut Pere Mata. The

Catalan process of psychiatric regionalization is interrupted when the military uprising breaks out, changing Tosquelles's plans to go to Tortosa.

On August 7, the POUM holds its first meeting at the Teatre Fortuny in Reus, with speeches by prominent POUM members, including Tosquelles.

On November 21, Tosquelles participates as a speaker at an event organized by the JCI and the Aleixar POUM that sought to consolidate the party guidelines. His talk focuses on the political history of the workers' movement. The following year he publishes, in the January 30 issue of *La Torxa: Portantveu del POUM i de les JCI de Reus i el Baix Camp*, an article titled "Sentit de les consignes del POUM."

During the first months of the war, the head of health in Reus, Josep Hortoneda, a member of the POUM, requisitions the Mas del Quer (Mas d'en Boule) farmhouse on the road to Salou, where Tosquelles develops the bases of his child and adolescent psychotherapy. The farmhouse will be demolished in 1968.

1937 On June 16, the POUM is made illegal. Andreu Nin, along with many party members, is arrested and killed by Stalin for his anarcho-Trotskyist affiliation.

Deployed on the Aragon front, Tosquelles organizes the evacuation of patients from the psychiatric hospital of Huesca, then in the hands of the fascists. He is in charge of restructuring the Sariñena sanitarium and, later, the hospital in Almodóvar del Campo.

On November 21, Tosquelles is named provisional medical lieutenant under the head of health care of the XI Unit of the Republican Army.

Between 1937 and 1938, the German sexologist Max Hodann volunteers as a medic in the International Brigades and sets up a therapeutic practice for the soldiers' sexual healing in the convalescent house of Cueva de la Potita in Albacete. As a result, he will write several articles on "sexual problems in the army" for the journal *La Voz de la Sanidad*.

1938 In May, Tosquelles is appointed head of psychiatric services of the Extremaduran Army and director of the hospital of Almodóvar del Campo (province of Ciudad Real), where he works in particular with prostitutes.

1939 Tosquelles, who has held the rank of lieutenant, is promoted on January 6 to acting captain of the Military Health Corps of the psychiatric services of the Extremaduran Army (official state bulletin of January 13, 1939).

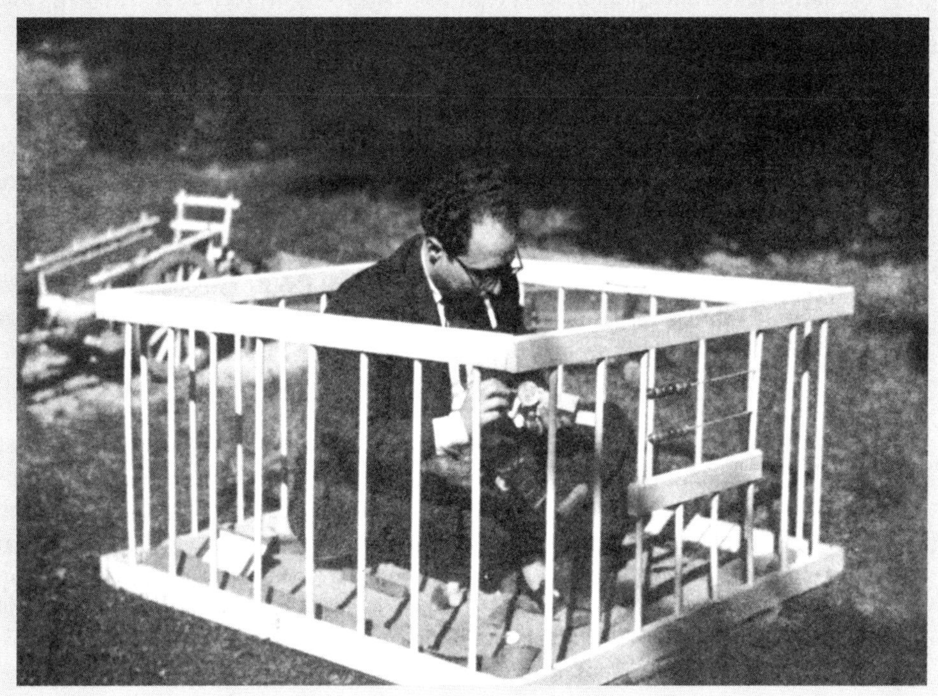

"Freud's first teacher, the first teacher he had, was his hysterical patient. The patients are our teachers. Our only teachers. The other ones are merely elaborating theories."

Barcelona is occupied on January 26.

The Spanish Civil War ends on April 1, with the victory of the Francoist troops.

After the fall of Almodóvar del Campo, Tosquelles must protect himself from the fascists and the pro-Soviet forces.

He continues working as a "fascist" doctor, both to help the patients and to allow himself the chance to plan his escape. Fleeing Francoism, on September 1, Tosquelles crosses the Pyrenees on foot and spends three months in the Septfonts refugee camp, where he runs a psychiatric unit.

1940 Starting in January, he begins working at the Saint-Alban-sur-Limagnole psychiatric hospital in the French *département* of Lozère, at the request of Dr. Paul Balvet, director of the hospital between 1936 and 1943. At that same hospital, between 1933 and 1936, Balvet's predecessor, Agnès Masson, had begun the practice of geopsychiatry, now considered the start of French sector psychiatry.

In June, France is occupied by Hitler's troops. From then until the 1945 liberation, between thirty-five and forty thousand patients will die in French psychiatric hospitals in what Max Lafont will later deem the "soft extermination."

Between December 6 and 8, Tosquelles travels to Prats de Molló to collect his wife Elena and his daughter Maria Rosa, who have spent the war in Reus.

1941 In January, André Chaurand arrives at Saint-Alban; there, the club begun by Paul Balvet becomes the tool through which the hospital's collective life takes shape, managed by the patients themselves.

1942 On February 11, Elena and Francesc's second daughter, Germaine, is born; Tosquelles calls her Montserrat, a Catalan name.

In August, the Bonneval Symposium takes place, and Henri Ey, the organizer, presents his book project *Une Histoire naturelle de la folie* (A natural history of madness).

In December, Dr. Lucien Bonnafé becomes the director of Saint-Alban, a position he will hold until 1944. His grandfather, Dr. Maxime Dubuisson, had been named director of the hospital in 1914, the year they began collecting the artwork of patients such as Auguste Forestier.

1943 From November through February of 1944, Nusch and Paul Éluard (under his birth name Eugène Grindel) take refuge at the Saint-Alban hospital, in Bonnafé's apartments. There Éluard writes *Les Sept Poèmes d'amour en guerre* (1943), *Le Lit la table* (1944), *Lingères légères* (1945), and *Souvenirs de la maison des fous* (1945). In an autobiographical text, film critic Georges Sadoul will recount his time at the hospital during the period that Nusch and Éluard were there, when Éluard read to him from *Les Sept Poèmes d'amour en guerre* and other poems inspired by Goya's titles, such as *El sueño de la razón produce monstruos*. The hospital becomes a refuge for many other members of the Resistance and Jews, like Gaston Baissette, who led the medical front for the Resistance, and Denise Glaser who, once the war is over, will become a well-known producer, journalist, and host on French television with the musical show *Discorama*.

The CEMÉA (Centres d'Entraînement aux Méthodes d'Éducation Active) is created, a movement and association that practices new forms of education to transform environments and institutions through various types of group action.

1944 In January, the third issue of the magazine *Nuit et Jour: Le grand hebdomadaire illustré* publishes a photo-essay on Septfonds by the Russian photographer Isaac Kitrosser, who sought refuge in Puget-Théniers and was interned at Septfonds during the Second World War.

On June 12, Tosquelles's third child and first son, Jacques, is born.

Between June 23 and July 5, the doctor, philosopher, and science historian Georges Canguilhem takes refuge in Saint-Alban, where he takes part, with Tosquelles, in the Société du Gévaudan, a debate group comprised of the medical collective at Saint-Alban in dialogue with the intellectuals, poets, and political dissidents at the hospital. A few months before arriving at Saint-Alban, Canguilhem had defended his thesis *Essai sur quelques problèmes concernant le normal et le pathologique* (Essay on some problems concerning the normal and the pathological), which he would publish in 1966 with the title *Le normal et le pathologique* (*The Normal and the Pathological*); in this book he elaborates the concept of pathology as a socially determined construct.

As part of a POUM conference held in Toulouse on November 11 and 12, Josep Rovira launches the creation of the Socialist Movement of Catalonia (MSC), which strives to be, in Rovira's words, an "organic front of Catalan socialism." Shortly after, in the June and October 1945 issues of *Endavant: Òrgan del Moviment Socialista de Catalunya*, Tosquelles publishes the articles "Invalidesa i treball: A propòsit dels mutilats de guerra" (with Dr. Jaume Sauret) and "Perspectives i Miratges."

1945 The poet and essayist Tristan Tzara and his son spend the summer at Saint-Alban along with the painter Gérard Vulliamy and his wife, Cécile (Éluard's daughter). Tzara writes the poem *Parler seul*, which Joan Miró will illustrate in 1948.

During Tzara's stay, the artist Jean Dubuffet spends twenty-four hours at Saint-Alban in order to get a look at the artwork of the inpatient Auguste Forestier, although he doesn't get to meet him because the hospital denies him access. Dubuffet's first mention of art brut is on August 9 of that same year, in a letter to the psychiatrist Charles Ladame.

Tosquelles, together with the doctors Sauret, Llambies, and Josep Martí Feced, gives the talk "Medicina social" at the second gathering of the Association of Catalan Doctors for the Renewal of Medicine, which takes place in Toulouse on April 21 and 22.

France is liberated and the Nazi occupation ends.

1946 Between 1946 and 1947, Tosquelles visits Antonin Artaud and Dr. Gaston Ferdière at the Rodez hospital. He corresponds with Ferdière in 1946 and 1957; some of their letters are saved, and in them we see such names as Artaud, Hans Bellmer, Paul Éluard, Gerard de Nerval, and Ilarie Voronca mentioned.

The psychiatrists Julián de Ajuriaguerra and Georges Daumézon and the sociologist Georges Gusdorf organize a series of lectures at the École Normale Supérieure de París, as a way to extend the Bonneval conference.

In Paris, from February 16 to 28, the Sainte-Anne psychiatric center holds an exhibition of artwork by patients, conceived as a response to the show of degenerate art (*Entartete Kunst*) that the Nazis had presented for the first time in 1937, which included both modern art and works by psychiatric patients. On February 15, Dr. Gaston Ferdière gives a lecture in the context of the exhibition.

In May, the English psychiatrist Thomas Main coins the term "therapeutic community" in an article published in the third issue of the journal *Bulletin of the Menninger Clinic*; Main details the working processes of a therapeutic environment at Northfield Military Hospital.

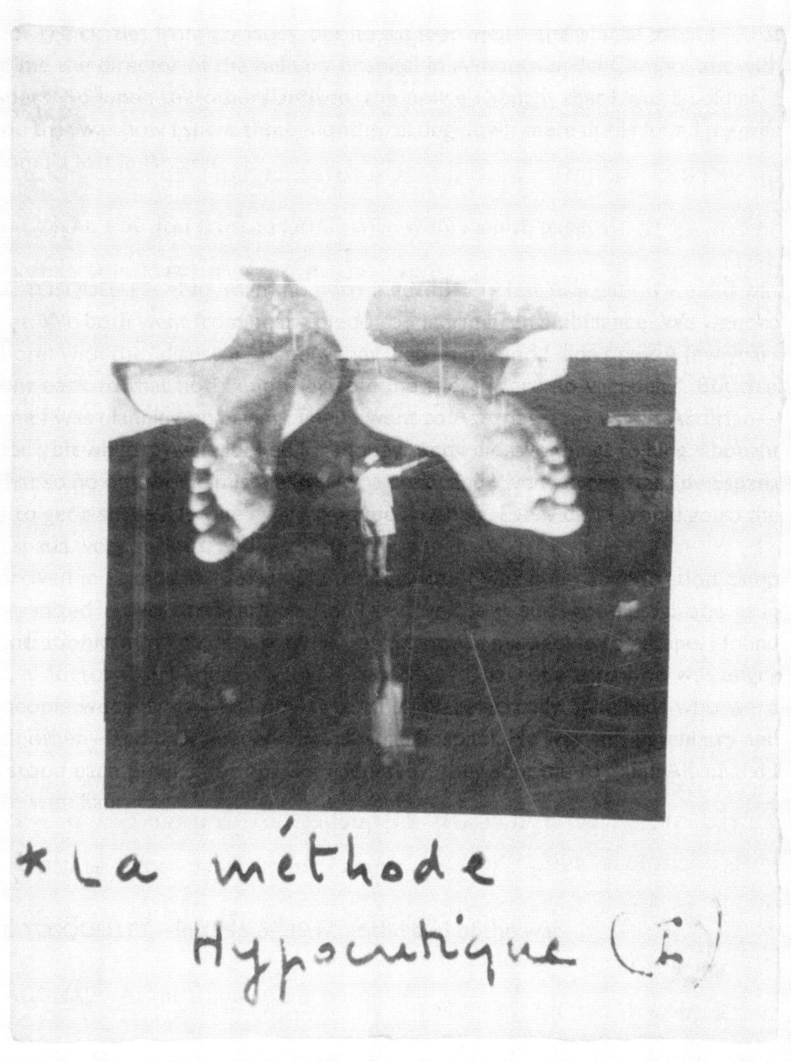

"When one goes about in the world, what counts is not the head, it's the feet. Knowing where you put the feet. It's the foot that is the great reader of the world, of the geography. Walking is not with the head, I have to know where I place the foot, you understand? That's all. The foot is the apparatus, the locus of reception, of what will become the dynamic. That is why a mother, the first thing she does is to tickle the feet. Because it's a matter of standing up."

1947 Psychiatrist Jean Oury is in residence at Saint-Alban until 1949.

On February 6, Tosquelles delivers a lecture titled "La médecine face à l'homme actuel" at the Hôtel des sociétés savantes in Paris as part of a series on social medicine organized by Cultura Catalana, an exile group.

In April, Tosquelles gives the lecture "Psychopathologie et materialisme dialectique" in a series of conferences on modern psychology organized by the École Normale Supérieure de Paris.

From July 7 through September 30, the International Exhibition of Surrealism presented by Marcel Duchamp and Frederick Kiesler at the Maeght Gallery in Paris displays the work of numerous avant-garde artists alongside objects and works by mental patients loaned by the psychiatrist Gaston Ferdière.

The educator, writer, and filmmaker Fernand Deligny publishes *Les Vagabonds efficaces.*

On September 2, Michel, the final child of Elena and Francesc Tosquelles, is born.

1948 Tosquelles defends his thesis titled *Essai sur le sens du vécu en psychopathologie: Le témoignage de Gérard de Nerval* at the Faculté de médecine de Paris. Paul Éluard encourages and assists Tosquelles in this project by providing him with documents about Nerval.

Le Chemin, the Saint-Alban newspaper—a precursor to the internal newspaper *Trait d'union*—is published.

In October, Jean Dubuffet creates the Compagnie de l'Art Brut, which will eventually include work by Benjamin Arneval, Auguste Forestier, Clément Fraisse, Aimable Jayet, and Marguerite Sirvins, all Saint-Alban patients.

In the autumn, André Breton publishes "L'Art des fous, la clé des champs."

In November, in issue 214 of the magazine *Action: Hebdomadaire de l' indépendance française*, Tosquelles concludes his research into psychoanalysis, "La Psychanalyse: Science ou mystification" with the text "Les Conflits humains sont toujours sociaux."

1949 In the autumn, Jean Dubuffet publishes "L'Art brut préféré aux arts culturels" ("Art Brut Preferred to Cultural Art") in the catalog accompanying the first exhibition of the collection of the Compagnie de l'Art Brut at the René Drouin Gallery.

1950 In December, Jean Oury defends his doctoral thesis *Essai sur la conation esthétique*, which studies the work of Benjamin Arneval, Auguste Forestier, and Aimable Jayet. His analysis will be central to Dubuffet's construction of the story of art brut at Saint-Alban.

On July 14, Saint-Alban's internal newspaper *Trait d'union* begins publication; it will continue to feature work by patients, doctors, and nurses until 1981.

The first international exhibition of psychopathological art opens at the Hospital Sainte-Anne in Paris to accompany the first international psychiatry conference held in the French capital.

1951 Jacques Lacan begins to deliver his seminars, which will continue until 1980, the year prior to his death.

1952 In April, Frantz Fanon, who has recently published his book *Black Skin, White Masks*, starts his residency at Saint-Alban, during which he works and writes with Tosquelles. He will be there until August 1953.

After various obstacles relating to the recognition of his doctoral degree, in 1952 Tosquelles passes an examination that allows him to be officially named director of Saint-Alban in 1953.

Georges Daumézon and Philippe Koechlin coin the term *institutional psychotherapy* in the article "La Psychothérapie institutionnelle française," published in *Anais portugueses de psiquiatria*.

Tosquelles takes part in the creation of the Fédération d'Aide à la Santé Mentale Croix-Marine, which works to foster mental health.

In December, the magazine *Esprit* publishes the volume *Misère de la psychiatrie*, with texts by Francesc Tosquelles, Lucien Bonnafé, Louis Le Guillant, Georges Daumézon, Philippe Koechlin, Henri Ey, Albert Béguin, and André Bazin, and a chronicle by the nurse Marius Bonnet.

1953 La Borde clinic is founded by Jean Oury; among those who will work there are Félix Guattari, Ginette Michaud, Jean-Claude Polack, and Nicole Guillet. Oury will live and work for more than six decades with the patients at La Borde, where his practice is linked to the spoken word with his seminars and to writing, to questions of the collective and the ties between the institutional and the political, and between listening and schizophrenia.

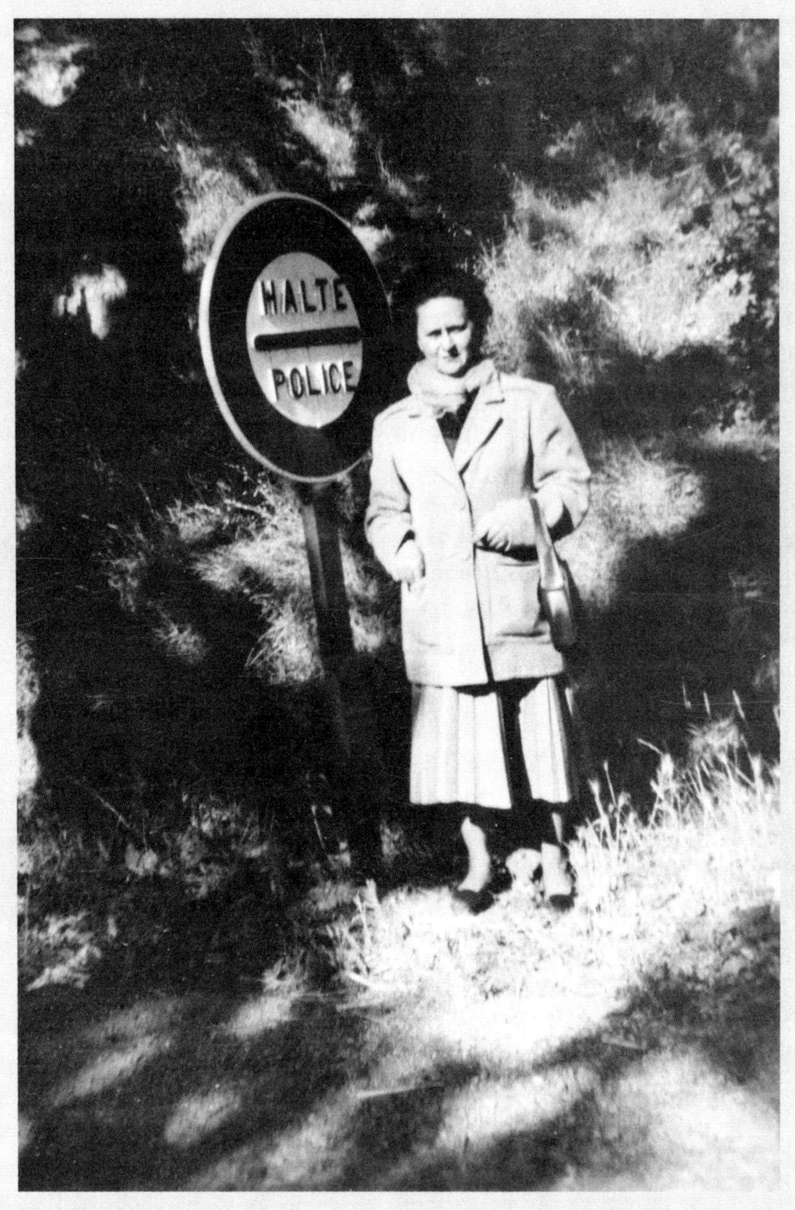

"I got in the habit of offering care to the doctors. [...] I chose lawyers who were afraid to go to war, who had never treated a mad person, painters, men of letters, priests, prostitutes—I mean, seriously."

On July 20 through 26, Tosquelles and Fanon present three lectures on the practice of electroshock treatment and institutional psychotherapy at Saint-Alban, as part of the 51st Congrès de médecins aliénistes et neurologues de France et des pays de langue française, held in the town of Pau.

Fanon arrives in Algeria to work at the Blida-Joinville hospital, where he will be the director until his resignation in July 1956, before being deported in January of 1957.

Gilles Deleuze edits the anthology *Instincts et institutions*, which gathers texts that reflect on institutions, written by Sigmund Freud, Claude Lévi-Strauss, Bronisław Malinowski, Immanuel Kant, David Hume, and Honoré de Balzac, among other authors.

1955 Inspired by Francesc Tosquelles's work, Lucien Oziol decides to take in disabled children and help their families, and on December 16, Le Clos du Nid association—a pioneer in aiding people with disabilities who are overlooked by the state government—is created in Marvejols.

1956 Roger Gentis arrives at Saint-Alban. With the departure of Tosquelles in 1962, he will be named temporary physician in charge for three months.

Dr. Jean Oury publishes the first essay on the work of Auguste Forestier, in issue 6 of the magazine *Bizarre*.

1957 Félix Guattari spends time in residence at Saint-Alban.

1958 Tosquelles briefly returns to Barcelona, which he left in 1939, for the 4th International Congress of Psychotherapy. On September 5, at 6 p.m., Tosquelles shows a film there that was made at Saint-Alban in collaboration with his wife Elena, also present.

Jacques Lacan visits Spain for the first time for the congress, where he delivers the lecture "True and False Psychoanalysis."

1959 Tosquelles meets with the educator Fernand Deligny in Curières, in Thoiras, in the southern Cévennes. Josée Manenti will recount their meeting in Patrick Faugeras's book *L'Ombre portée de François Tosquelles*.

In the April 25 edition of *France-Soir*, as part of the feature story "Le tour d'Europe de la folie," the novelist Hervé Bazin quotes Tosquelles speaking about the experience of demolishing a hospital wing with the patients.

1960 David Cooper, Aaron Esterson, and Ronald Laing develop anti-psychiatric therapeutic communities in England.

On March 15, a text by the French Ministry of Health recognizes the sector psychiatry practiced by Tosquelles, Bonnafé, Daumézon, and Oury at Saint-Alban.

On June 4 and 5, the first meetings of the Groupe de Travail de Psychothérapie et de Sociothérapie Institutionnelles (GTPSI) are held at Saint-Alban with Tosquelles, Jean Oury, Roger Gentis, Horace Torrubia, Jean Ayme, Yves Racine, Jean Colmin, Maurice Paillot, and Hélène Chaigneau, who are joined by Félix Guattari, Ginette Michaud, Claude Poncin, Henri Vermorel, Michel Baudry, Nicole Guillet, Robert Millon, Jean-Claude Polack, Gisela Pankow, and Jacques Schotte.

1961 The philosopher Michel Foucault publishes *Madness and Civilization: A History of Insanity in the Age of Reason* in France, and the sociologist Erving Goffman publishes *Asylums: Essays on the Social Situation of Mental Patients and Other Inmates* in the United States.

Tosquelles meets the documentary fimmaker and writer Mario Ruspoli through Gilbert de Chambrun, the mayor of Marvejols and Ruspoli's uncle.

Shortly before his death, Frantz Fanon writes *The Wretched of the Earth.*

1962 Mario Ruspoli premieres his films on the rural life of Lozère, *Les Inconnus de la terre,* and on the Saint-Alban hospital, *Regard sur la folie* and *La Fête prisonnière*, created in collaboration with Tosquelles and Roger Gentis. *Regard sur la folie* was filmed in May and June of 1961 and not shown in theaters until the fall of 1962. On June 2, 1961, in the movie theater in Saint-Chély d'Apcher, very nearby to the Saint-Alban hospital, *Les Maîtres fous*, by Jean Rouch, and *Chronique d'un été*, by Edgar Morin and Jean Rouch, are screened at the initiative of Tosquelles, who is an admirer of Rouch. Some twenty-odd patients, hospital medical staff, and townspeople attend the screening. In the case of *Chronique d'un été*, it was a preview. *Les Inconnus de la terre* and *Regard sur la folie* are shown for six weeks at the La Pagode cinema in Paris during the autumn of 1962. *Les Inconnus de la terre* garners better reviews than *Regard sur la folie*, which is received less enthusiastically in general.

Ruspoli's films document Tosquelles's final period at Saint-Alban, which concludes when he is named director of the Timone hospital in Marseille.

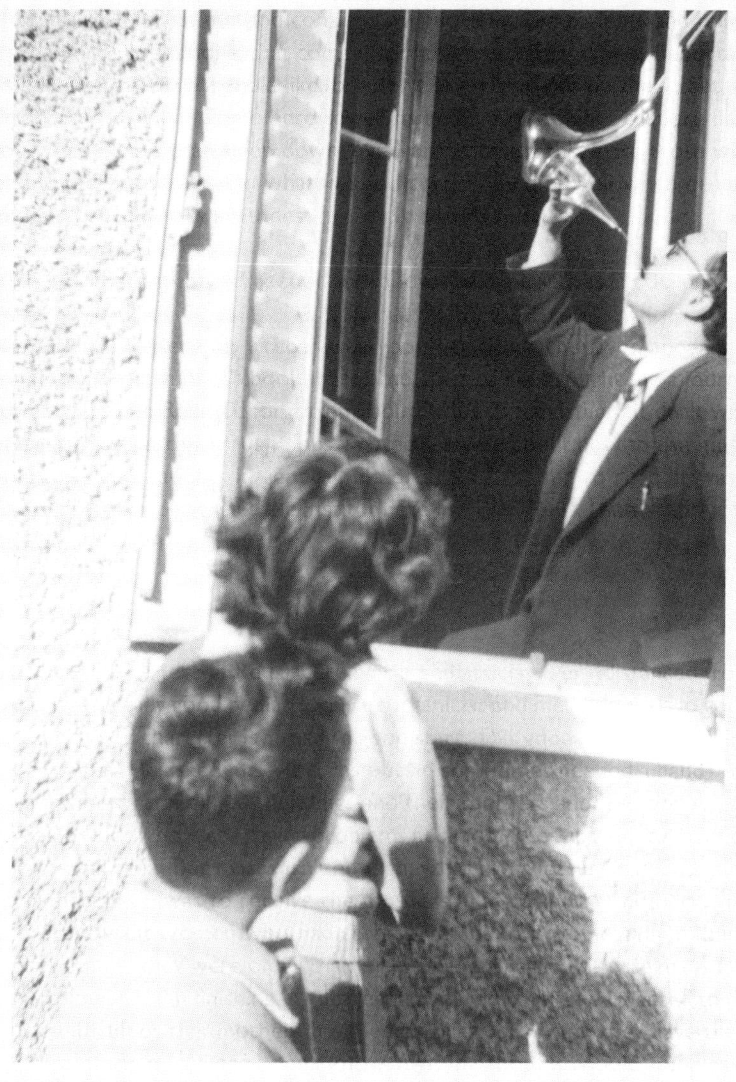

"I also spoke in Castilian. But almost just as badly or maybe worse than I now speak French. Like the Arabs. When you are an occupied country, you naturally speak the language of the oppressors, but you deform it. One speaks *petit nègre*, as people here say. So over there we would call it speaking *municipal*, because there were collaborators, Catalans who were employees of the Spanish state, and of course they would speak Castilian, but very badly, and we would imitate that in speaking Castilian; we would imitate those imbeciles who spoke Castilian so miserably."

Between 1962 and 1964, Fernand Deligny shoots, in the Cévennes and far from medical and penitentiary institutions, the film *Le Moindre Geste* with a psychotic teenager, Yves G., in the lead role. The camera operator is Josée Manenti, a member of the La Grande Cordée association, founded by Deligny in Paris in 1947. The crew is entirely nonprofessional.

Roman Jakobson and Claude Lévi-Strauss publish the book *"Les Chats" de Baudelaire*, which influences Tosquelles's reading of and writing on the poetry of Ferrater in *Funció poètica i psicoteràpia: Una lectura de "In memoriam" de Gabriel Ferrater.*

Maxwell Jones returns to Scotland to head up the Dingleton Hospital in Melrose, where he implements a therapeutic community in the psychiatric hospital and expands it to the surrounding area, creating an open system that includes general practitioners, families, and social services. That same year he publishes the monograph *Social Psychiatry in Practice: The Idea of a Therapeutic Community.*

1963 Clément Fraisse's wall panels and Marguerite Sirvins's wedding dress (they are both resident patients at Saint-Alban) are acquired, via Dr. Roger Gentis, for Dubuffet's art brut collection.

1964 Jacques Lacan establishes the École Française de Psychanalyse.

Jean Dubuffet publishes the first of the twenty-six *Fascicules de L'Art Brut* with an essay by Jean Oury on the work of Benjamin Arneval, a patient at Saint-Alban. This volume also includes a detailed study of *Lambris* by Clément Fraisse, based on notes by Dr. Roger Gentis.

1965 In February, after the filming of *Le Moindre Geste*, Fernand Deligny and his crew begin a two-year stay at the La Borde clinic at the invitation of Jean Oury and Félix Guattari.

1966 The Institut Pere Mata incorporates a group of young doctors from Zaragoza: Antonio Labad, Jesús Otín, and José García Ibáñez, with whom Tosquelles will carry out a new transformative phase of the institution.

Psychopathology of Everyday Life, the first translation of Sigmund Freud's work into Catalan, is published. In the eighties it will be followed by the translations of *Civilization and Its Discontents* (1984), *The Interpretation of Dreams* (1984–1985), *A General Introduction to Psychoanalysis* (1986), and *Beyond the Pleasure Principle* (1989).

The Oviedo hospital begins a project of sectorization inspired by the experiences of Hermann Simon, Francesc Tosquelles, and Maxwell Jones, among others. The project will be unsuccessful.

Félix Guattari creates the self-managed research collective Centre d'Etudes, de Recherches et de Formation Institutionnelles (CERFI).

1967 Tosquelles works as head of psychiatry at the general hospital in Melun until 1970.

Tosquelles's gradual return to the Institut Pere Mata begins, followed by the incorporation of other doctors, including some from Zaragoza such as Antonio Virgós and Eduardo González.

1968 On April 7 and 8, the first psychiatric conference launched by Tosquelles at the Institut Pere Mata takes place in Reus with the title *Aspectes legals de la rehabilitació laboral del malalt mental intra i extrahospitalari*. Celebrated annually during Easter week, the final conference, *Qualitat de la vida en psiquiatria: Malalt, família i equip assistencial*, will take place between March 28 and 30, 1996, and be dedicated to psychiatric quality of life.

The events of May 1968 lead to much criticism of psychoanalysis and psychiatry as privileged disciplines.

Franco Basaglia publishes *The Negated Institution: Report from a Psychiatric Hospital*, which describes the anti-psychiatric experience at the hospital in Gorizia.

1970 Tosquelles is named director of children's psychiatry at Nouvelle Forge in the *département* of L'Oise, where he will work until 1975.

Weekly meetings called "cassette groups" begin to be held at the Institut Pere Mata and will continue until Tosquelles's death in 1994. These groups analyze therapeutic countertransference and attitude; all the doctors and psychologists at the Institut, as well as some caregivers, take part in them.

Roger Gentis publishes *Les Murs de l'asile*, where he proposes expanding the limits of the concept of institution, which will be understood within the concept of anti-psychiatry, although Gentis will set his ideas apart.

1972 *Outsider Art*, a UK introduction to Jean Dubuffet's "art brut" by Roger Cardinal, is published in London.

Gilles Deleuze and Félix Guattari publish *Anti-Oedipus: Capitalism and Schizophrenia.*

Tosquelles's work *La pràctica del maternatge terapèutic en els deficients mentals profunds*, originally published in French in 1966, is published in Catalan translation. The Spanish-language edition will come out a year later, simultaneous with another of his books, *Estructura y reeducación terapèutica.*

The psychiatric sectorization of the province of Tarragona begins, propelled by the Institut Pere Mata with Tosquelles's consultation.

1973 Michel Foucault publishes the case of parricide *I, Pierre Rivière, Having Slaughtered My Mother, My Sister, and My Brother* . . . , the result of a collaboration with Blandine Barret-Kriegel, Gilbert Burlet-Torvic, Robert Castel, Jeanne Fauret, Alexandre Fontana, Georgette Legée, Patricia Moulin, Jean-Pierre Peter, Philippe Riot, and Maryvonne Saison in the working group at the Collège de France in Paris. Pierre Rivière's confession allows Foucault to muse on the modern border between mental illness and criminality as the limit on which the new power of medicine in the nineteenth century was established.

1974 The Club Emili Briansó is founded at the Institut Pere Mata, continuing on the Club Paul-Balvet at Saint-Alban.

1975 Tosquelles becomes head of psychiatry at the hospital of La Candélie, in Agen, where he works until his retirement in 1979.

The translation of his "Frantz Fanon à Saint-Alban" is published in issue 9 of the journal *Teoría y críticia de la psicología.*

1977 The Argentine intellectual and psychoanalyst Oscar Masotta, considered one of the main introducers of the teachings and practice of Jacques Lacan to Spanish-language readers, establishes the Biblioteca Freudiana de Barcelona, which will become a key space in Catalonia for research on Freud and psychoanalysis.

1978 On March 7, Tosquelles delivers a lecture, as part of a colloquium at the Círcol de Reus organized by that city's Jove Cambra, on the poem "In memoriam," by Gabriel Ferrater, titled "Qüestions de lògica de la vida i de la psicopatologia a propòsit de certes estances, errances i estampes poètiques de Gabriel Ferrater." Following a suggestion by translator and linguist Joaquim Mallafré, Tosquelles develops the content of his lecture, with linguistic and psychoanalytic aspects, into the book *Funció poètica i* *psicoteràpia: Una lectura de "In memoriam" de Gabriel Ferrater*, which will be published in 1985.

1980 Gilles Deleuze and Félix Guattari publish *A Thousand Plateaus: Capitalism and Schizophrenia.*

1983 The journal *Clínica y análisis grupal* begins the Spanish recuperation of Tosquelles with the publication of a translation of his article "Encore quelques précisions sur la psychothérapie institutionnelle." In the same journal they will also publish "A propósito del narcisismo en sus relaciones con la formación de la personalidad" (1985) and "El padre" (1987).

1984 On January 7, the city of Reus approves naming Francesc Tosquelles an Illustrious Son. He is awarded the medal on April 15 as part of the opening ceremony of the 17th Jornades d'Interès Psiquiàtric.

1985 Jean Oury writes the prologue to the reedition of *Le Vécu de la fin du monde dans la folie: Le témoignage de Gérard de Nerval*, in which he describes the "Tosquelles method" as a practice that defies "constructivism" and "decisionism."

In October, the first journal of Lacanian psychoanalysis written in Catalan, *L'Acudit: Publicació de psicoanàlisi*, begins publishing, edited by Miquel Bassols and Elvira Guilañá; the inaugural issue includes an interview with Tosquelles.

Tosquelles delivers the academic year's opening lecture, titled "La patologia psiquiàtrica a la cruïlla de les funcions del sistema nerviós, de la formació de la personalitat i la problemàtica sociològica," at the newly inaugurated Medicine Faculty in Reus.

1986 Francesc Tosquelles presides over the Perpignan Symposium on the history of psychoanalysis in the Catalan countries. Over the course of these meetings, he declares that this history has been sabotaged by other, better-known developments in other parts of Spain expressed in the Spanish language.

Between April 1986 and December 1987, Tosquelles directs a series of seminars at the Institut Pere Mata on various topics including child psychiatry, the creation of "clubs," and the importance of language in the therapeutic environment.

On June 20 and 21, the first Rencontres de Saint-Alban are held.

1990 The Catalan translation of Jacques Lacan's *The Four Fundamental Concepts of Psychoanalysis* is published; it was originally published in French in 1973, and in English translation in 1978.

1994 Catalan President Francesc Macià awards the Presidential Medal to Tosquelles shortly before his death. Antonio Labad, then professor of psychiatry at the Universitat Rovira i Virgili and one of the main supporters of Tosquelles's return to Catalonia, reads Tosquelles's acceptance speech for him.

Francesc Tosquelles dies on September 25 in Granges-sur-Lot, France.

I

THE INSTITUTIONS IN LITTLE VIENNA

REUS AND BARCELONA 1929–1936

> What role do foreigners play in the concrete history of psychoanalytic practice? [...] We are filled and permeated by the foreigner we carry within us, and then the analytical process works much better. When those who only spoke German or Czech or Hungarian came to Barcelona, there began to be a concrete analysis with lived experience, because they were foreigners. I wanted to say that to underscore an association with borders.
>
> FRANCESC TOSQUELLES

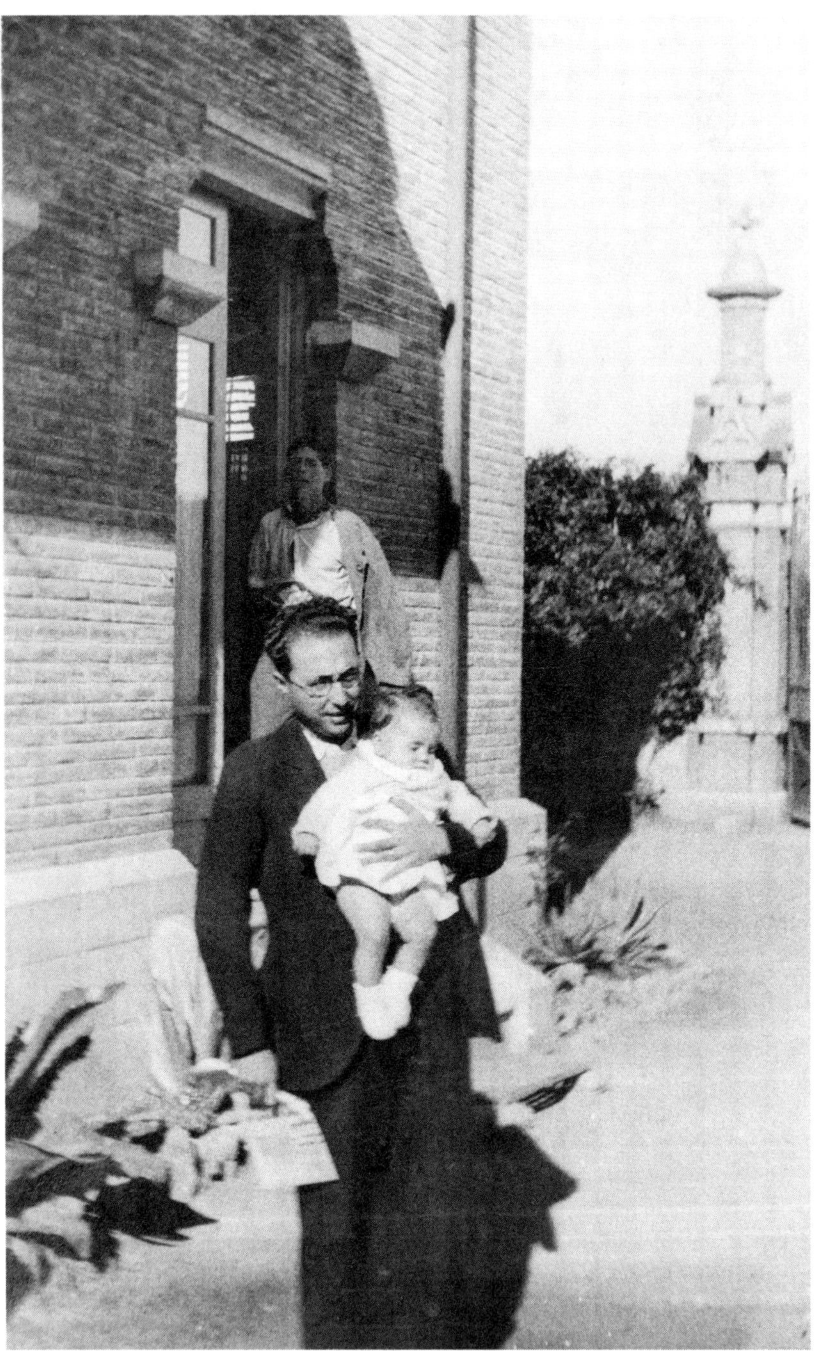

Francesc Tosquelles with his daughter Marie-Rose at the Institut Pere Mata, Reus, circa 1936–1937

At right, Jacques Lacan's thesis, printed by the patients of Saint-Alban circa 1960, preserved today in the library of the Institut Pere Mata

Transforming Establishments into Institutions

Tosquelles's first institutional experience was at the Institut Pere Mata, the Reus asylum. It was there, in the late 1920s, where he began to elaborate the project that would bring together his clinical work with his political work: the transformation of establishments into institutions. In a text of 1969, entitled "What Is to Be Understood by Institutional Psychotherapy?," he writes: "But speech can never be simply an event of me and you, isolated from the social context and from any preformation ex nihilo. In the field of speech, one is never just a duo; there is at least a reference to a third, to a mediator, and ultimately to something that must be given the name of *institution* by contrast precisely with all the institutional qualities that are stifled for the sake of the established, be it the establishment or the state: nothing less than the subjectivity of desire."[1] Gathering the writings and experience of the psychiatrist Ginette Michaud—who worked at the La Borde clinic beginning in 1955, inspired by the Saint-Alban project—Tosquelles imagined the policies of the institution as a process of constant institutionalization, mediation, and circulation of desire that strives to distance itself from the bureaucratic establishment and its inertias (reification and enclosure). What the establishments needed to become true institutions was the working material from the experience carried out at the Institut Pere Mata. A new practice of institutionality and of the group condition was required, one which allowed desire to exist, as well as other ways of moving, of working, of being together and being alone.

German psychoanalysis and the doctoral thesis that Jacques Lacan had defended in 1932, *De la psychose paranoïaque dans ses rapports avec la personnalité* (On paranoid psychosis in its relations with personality), were the tools for these new institutional and relational practices. In 1932, Tosquelles prepared a six-month training course, based in the transformative function of Lacan's text, for the doctors at the Institut. Not long after, in 1935, in the local Reus journal *Fulls clínics*, he published the case study of a patient using a dialogue with the new formulations of German psychoanalysis that he had found in the complete works of Freud, in Helen Deutsch's reflections on female homosexuality, in the essays of Alfred Adler, Otto Rank, Theodor Reik,

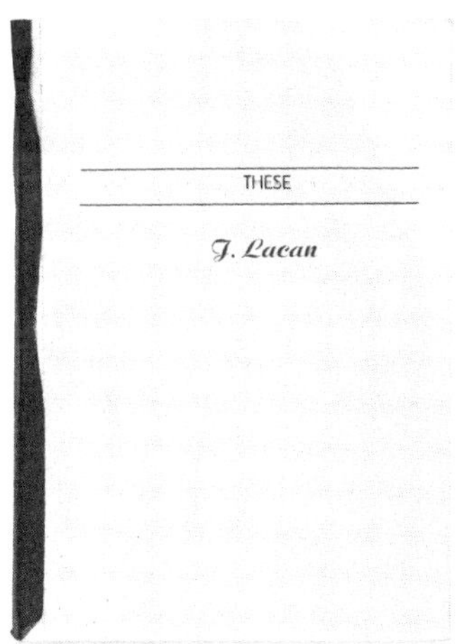

and Wilhelm Reich.[2] Those German texts and Lacan's thesis in French circulated as working materials in the hospital community. Lacan's text was read by doctors, nuns, nurses, and caregivers, but also by patients of the Institut, just as, years later at Saint-Alban, everyone had access to it in volumes that were printed and bound by the hospital press and sold within the small local economy that financed the material life of the institution.

This distribution promoted the reading of psychoanalytic texts and modified the reception of psychoanalysis's legacy. Tosquelles shifted individual-focused practice, which he called "clientele psychoanalysis," and transformed it into an institutional practice. In 1913, Francesc Llauradó, Tosquelles's uncle on his mother's side, published a review of Sigmund Freud's *The Interpretation of Dreams* in the journal *Archivos de terapéutica y de las enfermedades nerviosas y mentales: Eco científico del manicomio de Reus*, in which he pointed out how the book would change the course of psychiatric institutions. Tosquelles's work is organized around this psychoanalysis that is not private or focused on the individual, but rather that of an individual in relationship with the practices of institutional transformation: an extensive psychoanalysis that links disciplinary frontiers, places, and limits of meaning, from clinical practice to anthropology, critical sociology, and linguistics. An image, that of the institutional field that exceeds its own limits, traveled with Tosquelles from Reus to Saint-Alban. But his real work with collectives and collectively, from the moment in which, in the early thirties, this extensive psychoanalysis became common practice at the Institut, is a story that is still missing from the history of psychoanalysis in Spain, which is so often explained as the story of Argentine exiles from the military dictatorship in the 1970s bringing psychoanalysis to Spain as it was beginning to emerge from Francoism.

> I think in particular of the American anthropologists whose areas of research have oscillated between the study of primitive peoples and the experience of psychiatric activities, more or less. There are a good many of them … Bateson of course and the bunch at Palo Alto, or Yale … etc., notably Erikson and his *Childhood and Society.* All of them also influenced to some extent by psychoanalysis, which they have worked into their own sauce. Keeping to France, how could one not take the work of Mauss into account, precisely on the corporeal technique, which marked my activities at the Clos du Nid in a fundamental way, or the work of his anthropological disciple, Lévi-Strauss, on the *Elementary Structures of Kinship*, and I won't go on, while not forgetting the others, including Kristeva's observations on signifying practices or rather on the operation of signs in the human being, always in an anthropological situation of praxis.[3]
>
> A letter by Francesc Tosquelles to an unknown addressee, 1979

Forgotten Paths

As Andrés García Siso wrote, today this Catalan history of psychiatry can only be a political history: because the Spanish Civil War and Franco's dictatorship played a role of interruption, censorship, and collective oblivion. The entry of psychoanalysis into Catalonia and its use and experimentation in such crucial institutions as the Institut Pere Mata has been erased from the collective accounts, like so many other enduring experiences of the Republican project. Although Tosquelles had begun frequenting the Institut Pere Mata in the late 1920s, it wasn't until July of 1934 that he formalized his link with that medical community. He worked there until June 1937, when he went to the Aragon front. As such, his time at the Institut took place primarily during the Second Republic's project of psychiatric transformation. When Tosquelles arrived at the psychiatric hospital, he was determined to transform the old asylum regime with its cloistered economy and geographic isolation.

From the 1931 proclamation of the Republic and until Franco's defeat of the leftist forces in 1939, the Republican Generalitat (Catalan government) tried to reshape public mental health in a continuation of the project begun by the Mancomunitat of Catalonia. In 1934, in the context of the discussion around the legal framework for the organization of health care and social services, the health care region was defined. Abandoning the previous territorial demarcation, new health care regions were projected based on economic and social needs, limiting them to no more than eighty thousand people, and ensuring they were equidistant from health care hubs. The goal was to break up the uniformity of health care and make it more local. The Republican government worked on planning a municipal and regional network of caretaking and therapeutic work designed to create local social ties that the centralized Spanish system—inherited from the nineteenth century—had not wanted to create. This planning incorporated experiences from the German psychiatric vanguard (Hermann Simon and Emil Bratz) that allowed for a system of care spread out through territories and cities that built on the concept of health care regions that the Mancomunitat had imagined.

Josep Maria Comelles has studied how, a few years earlier, the Mancomunitat of Catalonia (1914–1925) had begun a project of decentralizing psychiatric treatment, allowing patients who did not need to be hospitalized to continue being seen at home, favoring nonhospital environments for those patients. In 1911, at the Society of Neurology and Psychiatry of Barcelona, the psychiatrist and politician Domènec Martí i Julià declared the contents of the institutional transformation program in these terms: to work on creating a corps of nurses and social workers, university professors, museums and laboratories to carry out contemporary research in psychiatry and neurology; and to elaborate new legislation regarding the confinement and release of patients, which allowed for the creation of a support network—through economic and social assistance—for when they left the hospital, and included a reflection on the work and means of remuneration. In the context of this program, they envisioned a project that didn't come to fruition: the clinic in Santa Coloma de Gramenet for patients who no longer needed to be institutionalized, organized around a system of farmhouse-shelters and sewing- shelters.[4] This program became more radicalized during the Civil War, from 1936, when, under the influence of the anarchist psychiatrist Fèlix Martí Ibáñez, the Generalitat nationalized all of the Catalan hospitals, including the Institut Pere Mata.[5] From his post at the health ministry, Martí Ibáñez promoted measures in response to the concerns of the unions, such as social aid, and endorsed the legalization of abortion between 1936 and 1937, which Federica Montseny would expand to encompass Republican Spain.

The 1910s and 1930s were decades that allowed for ideas to move into actions, for forms of reflection to become forms of activity, for grand public policies to transform the collective image of madness.

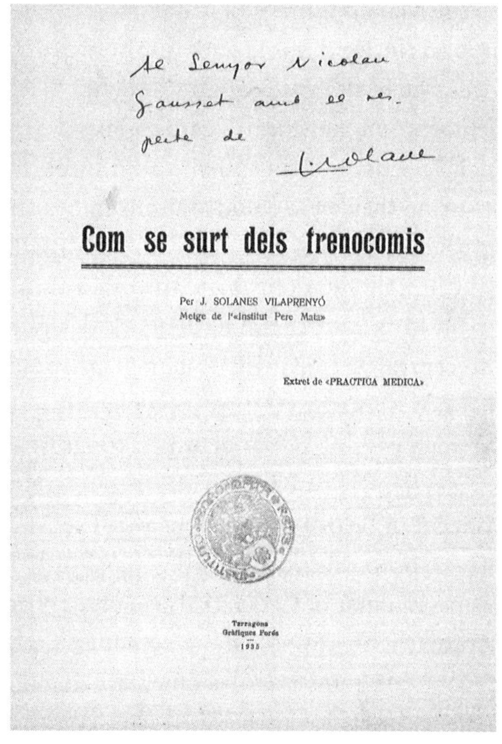
Com se surt dels frenocomis

Per J. SOLANES VILAPRENYÓ
Metge de l'«Institut Pere Mata»

Extret de «PRACTICA MEDICA»

Tarragona
Gràfiques Forés
1935

Cover of the book by Josep Solanes, Tarragona, Gràfiques Forés 1935

The July 3, 1931, decree, with which the Republic organized psychiatric aid along rational bases, just as it notably simplifies admittance of patients into the phrenopathic establishment, it makes their release easier as well. The *permanent reclusion cases* are now nearly relegated to history. No one is now forced to remain forever in a sanitorium. As Roller stated, *only curable mental patients should be assisted in asylums, and of the incurable ones, only those who are dangerous or defenseless.* The modern psychiatric concept, which puts the asylum service at the center of a spectrum that ranges from the dispensary to open homo-familiar and hetero-familiar psychiatric assistance, should be universally known. Not all the patients who leave the sanatorium are cured, but they are all improved; furthermore, the percentage of those who are cured is higher than in the past.

Therefore, keeping this fact in mind, if the closed sanatorium is not the only means of treating patients, and if, furthermore, the old idea of the incurability of psychiatric affectations must be modified in more optimistic terms, there is no possible way that the statistics on phrenopathic establishments can coincide with the popular conception of all institutionalization as irreparable. Many people leave bedlams. [...]

Medicine has branches that require more pressing public attention than that required by mental medicine. Yet we mustn't forget that the attention devoted to the therapies of psychiatric affectations cannot be eliminated. The pessimistic appraisals that could arise from considering a single patient would necessarily become almost optimistic when studying a large number of patients over a long period of time. The efficacy of current therapeutic measures has been demonstrated in the comparison of two statistics and two dates: 1904 and 1934. Mental illness is, therefore, a vast problem, but not overwhelmingly terrifying. It would be even less terrifying if the attention of official organisms and popular support were applied to it.

Public support has a long road ahead. It is evident, for example, that the mixed type of psychiatric establishment, still today almost the only sort that exists in Catalonia, is not the most appropriate for the extinction of mental maladies. We will not insist on the comments we've made about the burden of invalids. The tendency, currently in process of concretion here, of offering—unlike in the former asylums—a whole continuum of services ranging from the dispensary to the colony for the tranquil chronically ill should soon give practical results. Notwithstanding, we must also procure the expansion of open services, especially in regard to making voluntary internment accessible to poor neurotics. It is also evident that we mustn't prolong the current manner of understanding the released patient. The rapid creation of a group of visiting nurses is essential, along with the systematization of hetero-familiar, and trained, and homo-familiar assistance ...[6]

Josep Solanes, *Com se surt dels frenocomis* [How one gets released from phrenopathic institutions] 1935

The lives of Josep Solanes and Francesc Tosquelles crossed several times over the years. They both worked at the Institut Pere Mata, as protégés of Emili Mira, and were both supporters of the POUM and the Republican army in Aragon, and both went into French exile in 1939. Solanes worked at the psychiatric hospital in Rodez, headed by Gaston Ferdière, where he met Antonin Artaud; and in the Sainte-Anne hospital, with Eugène Minkowski and Paul Guirard, when he was living in southern France, where he wrote about the pain of exile before emigrating to Venezuela in 1949, where he lived until his death in 1991.

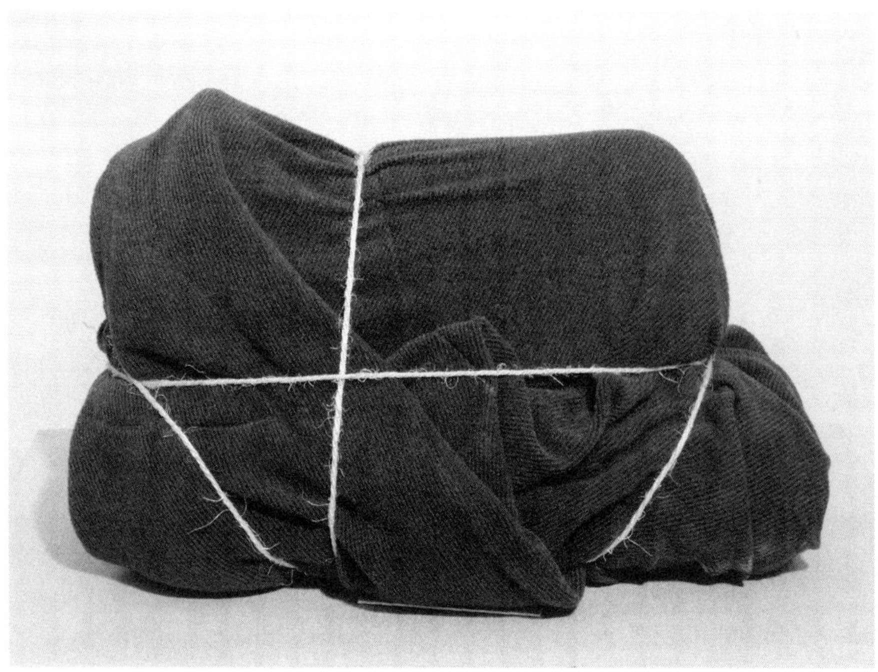

Man Ray, *The Enigma of Isidore Ducasse*, 1920

Like a Sewing Machine in a Wheat Field

The health care network traced through the regional sphere, which was elaborated between the two dictatorships, was interrupted and left unfinished, like so many other projects of that period. Tosquelles recalled it as one of the first failures of what in France was called, beginning in 1960, "psychiatrie de secteur," or sectorization. He also remembered his involvement in the Psychiatric Council of the Generalitat, the local Catalan invention of the concept of region that would be equivalent to the French sector, and the link between the psychiatric avant-garde and surrealism. In the seventies, Tosquelles associated the experience he began in Catalonia with a phrase by Lautréamont, from *The Songs of Maldoror*, which the surrealists made famous as prophetic of their new forms of creation and random beauty: "As beautiful as the fortuitous encounter of a sewing machine and an umbrella on a dissection table." But when Tosquelles evoked the Catalan psychiatric vanguard, he shifted the meaning of that phrase to give it a new materiality. According to him, what had been done in Catalonia during the 1910s and 1930s was to

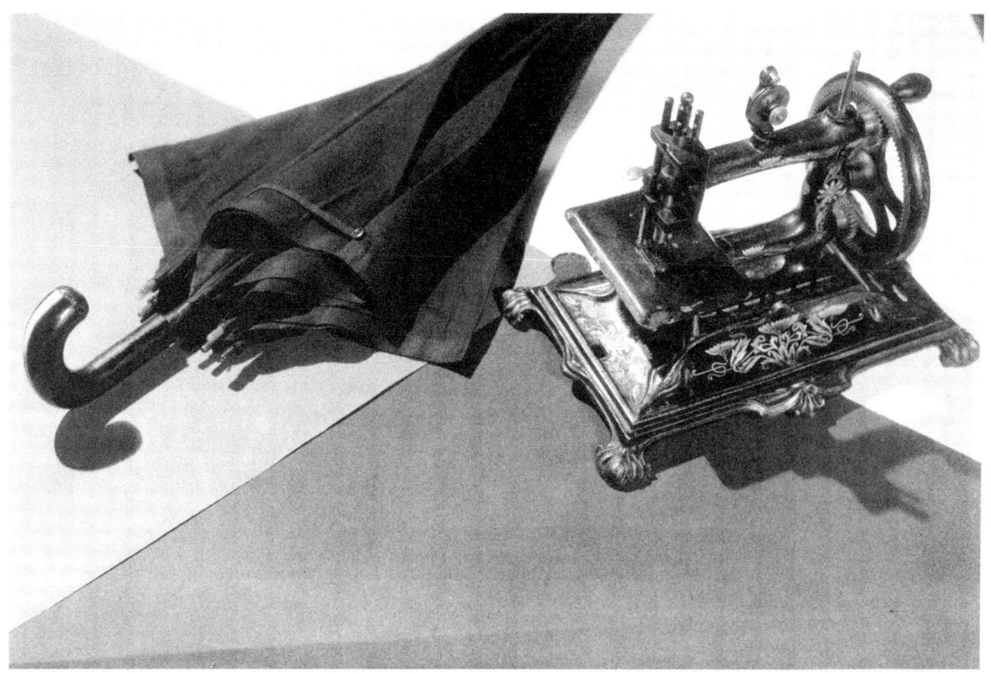

Man Ray, *Homage to Lautréamont*, 1933

The Enigma of Isidore Ducasse (a sewing machine wrapped in a blanket and tied with cord) and *Homage to Lautréamont* (in the photograph above) are two works by Man Ray that reference Lautréamont through surrealism. They were created, respectively, during the Mancomunitat and the Second Republic. Francesc Tosquelles referred, in various ways, to this surrealist legacy through language, when speaking of drift, navigation, transport, transference, and skidding, which allow one to leave the previously drawn paths and shift direction, including controlled slippage, derailings, and delirium; misunderstandings, impasses, and the unsaid.[7]

"place a sewing machine in a wheat field." With this expression he preserved the memory of the Mancomunitat and the Republic's attempts to organize therapeutic cures in close conjunction with the towns, with the countryside and manual labor, as had been imagined in the project of the farmhouse-shelters and sewing-shelters. By resituating Lautréamont's surrealist quote, Tosquelles produced a true "fortuitous encounter" between an unfinished political experience and one of the formal icons of the surrealist avant-garde.

These attempts to make a situated and transformed psychiatry possible were the backdrop of Francesc Tosquelles's trajectory at the Institut Pere Mata, which he experienced as "an almost delusional project, namely: that

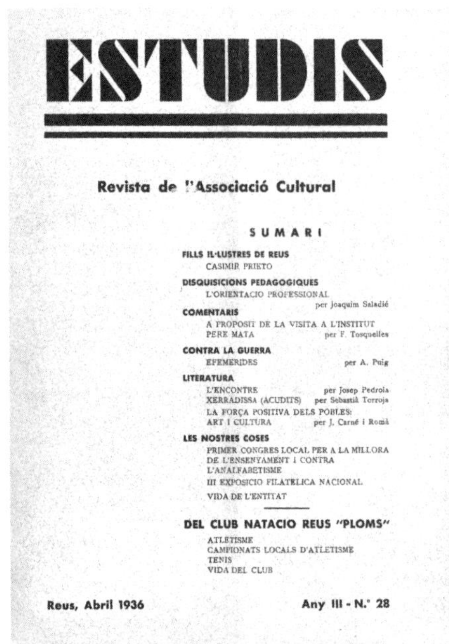

ESTUDIS

Revista de l'Associació Cultural

SUMARI

FILLS IL·LUSTRES DE REUS
CASIMIR PRIETO

DISQUISICIONS PEDAGOGIQUES
L'ORIENTACIO PROFESSIONAL per Joaquim Saladié

COMENTARIS
A PROPOSIT DE LA VISITA A L'INSTITUT PERE MATA per F. Tosquelles

CONTRA LA GUERRA
EFEMERIDES per A. Puig

LITERATURA
L'ENCONTRE per Josep Pedrola
XERRADISSA (ACUDITS) per Sebastià Torroja
LA FORÇA POSITIVA DELS POBLES: ART I CULTURA per J. Carné i Romà

LES NOSTRES COSES
PRIMER CONGRES LOCAL PER A LA MILLORA DE L'ENSENYAMENT I CONTRA L'ANALFABETISME
III EXPOSICIO FILATELICA NACIONAL
VIDA DE L'ENTITAT

DEL CLUB NATACIO REUS "PLOMS"
ATLETISME
CAMPIONATS LOCALS D'ATLETISME
TENIS
VIDA DEL CLUB

Reus, Abril 1936 Any III - N.° 28

The human condition of madness and malaise is an idea taken up again in the journal *Estudis* (1933–1936), which Francesc Tosquelles edited and in which he published texts by various contributors on cooperativism, feminism, unionism, ecology, maternity, poetry, war, work, and psychoanalysis. He wrote several articles himself, including one about the Institut Pere Mata in which he recommended reading *In Praise of Folly* by Erasmus because, in his view, it did not describe madness as torture but rather as a form of grace associated with escapes and voyages.

people—doctors and non-doctors—believe that 'crazy' people could be cured if they were treated well." Humanizing the treatment of patients coincided with his own conception of madness in the human dimension. As he puts it in the heading of one of his genealogical drawings: "la folie phénomène humain" (madness, a human phenomenon) and "essais de réintégration du fou dans son humanité, dans la cité" (efforts to integrate the mad, with all their humanity, back into society).[8]

Antonio Labad described the Institut's "humanistic project," begun in 1896 by Dr. Emili Briansó, as a revolution of both the era's medicine and urban development. Financed by the bourgeoisie of Reus, the architectural project designed by Lluís Domènech i Montaner prioritized open spaces and natural light, wooded and landscaped areas, vegetation separating the various buildings, and creating an environment that favored gatherings and physical contact inspired by the experiences of the nonrestraint system introduced in 1829 by Dr. Charlesworth at the Lincoln Lunatic Asylum. The system of wings housed in different buildings created a kind of township of patients with eighteen wings, organized by pathology and social class. This design was the model for the Hospital de la Santa Creu i Sant Pau in Barcelona, where Dòmenech i Montaner would soon develop this same architectural plan on a larger scale.

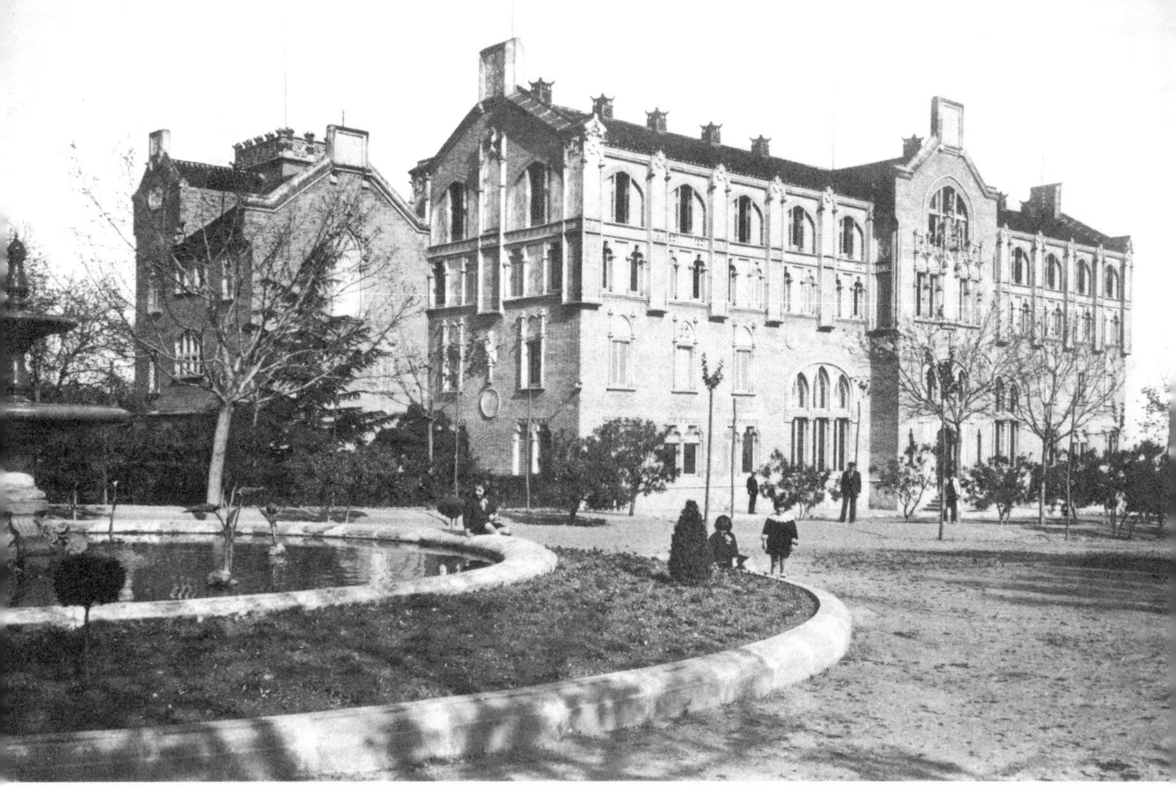

Above, view of the landmarked Pavilion of the Distinguished (reserved for guests from polite society) at the Institut Pere Mata.
Below, a room for gathering in that same building.

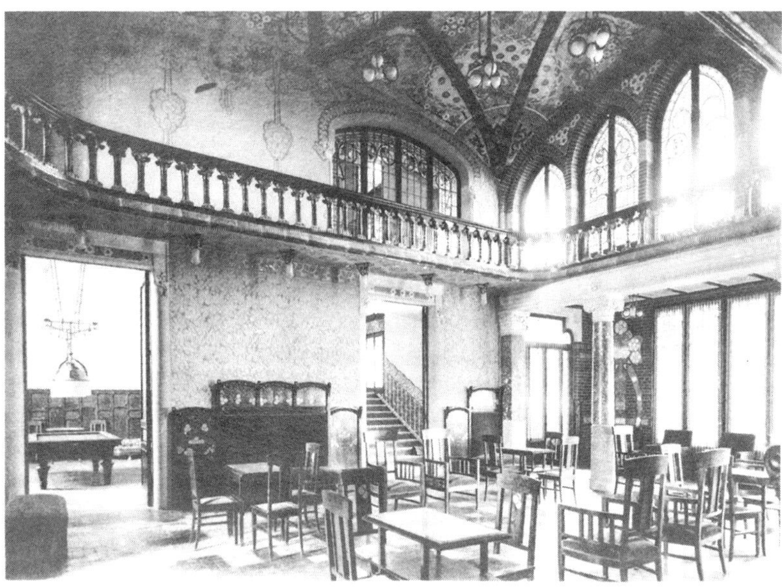

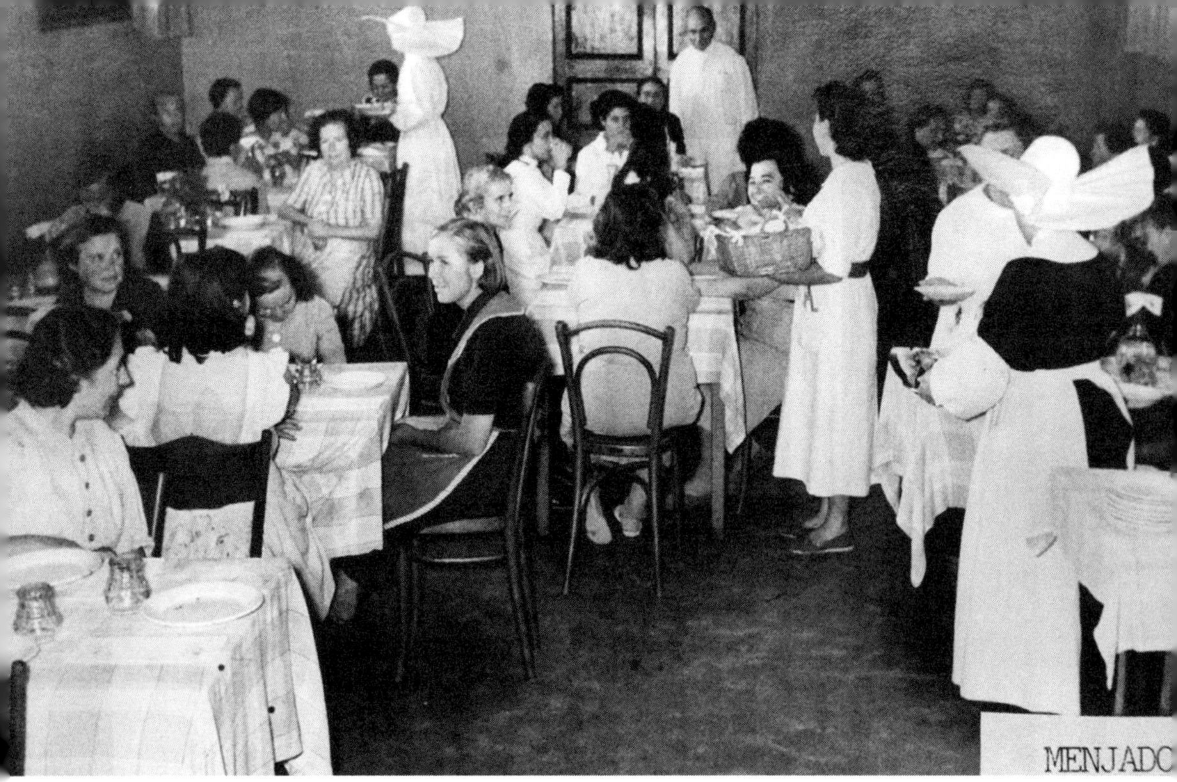

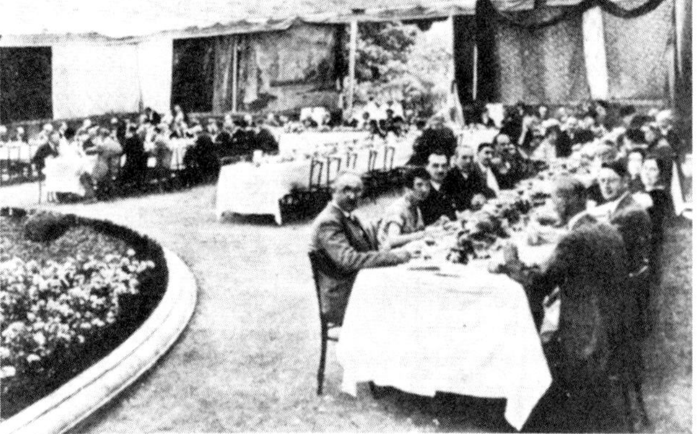

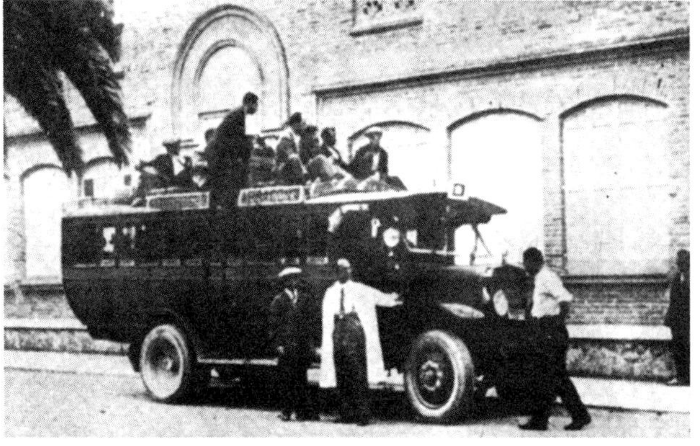

Above, women's dining hall at the Institut Pere Mata

Middle, an image from Pere Anguera, Albert Arnavat, and Xavier Amorós's *La història gràfica del Reus contemporani, 1803–1939* (A graphic history of contemporary Reus, 1803–1939), of the 33rd Congress of Psychiatrists and Neurologists of France and French-speaking Countries, held in Barcelona with two hundred attendees, who spent the day of May 24, 1929, in Reus at the Institut Pere Mata

Bottom, a group of inpatients going on a field trip, accompanied by members of the Institut's medical community

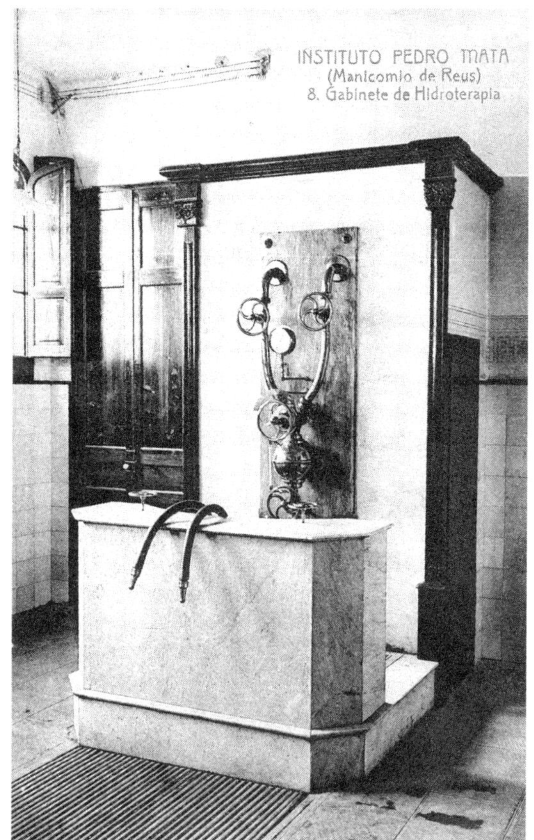

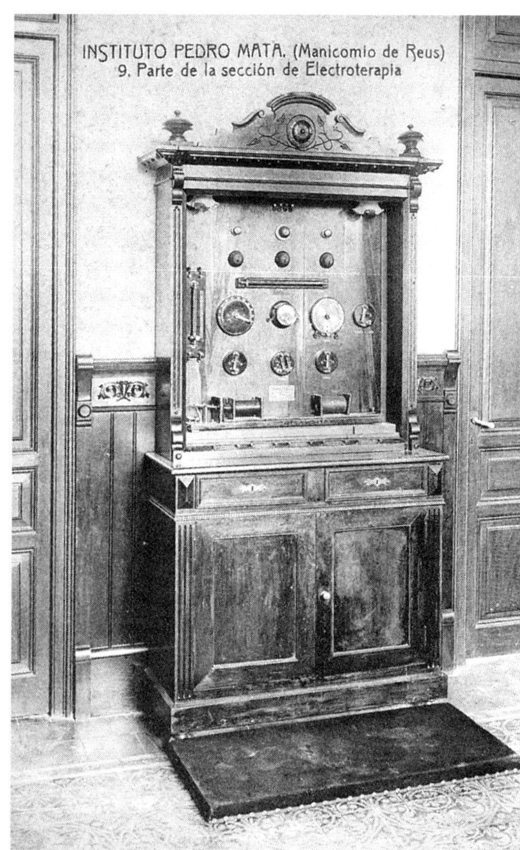

INSTITUTO PEDRO MATA
(Manicomio de Reus)
8. Gabinete de Hidroterapia

INSTITUTO PEDRO MATA. (Manicomio de Reus)
9. Parte de la sección de Electroterapia
Postcards of the hydrotherapy room and the electrotherapy machine

This urbanistic modernity found an equivalent in the contemporary treatments of hydrotherapy and electrotherapy, as well as in the system of doctors and consultants, a context which allowed Tosquelles to work with Emili Mira i López, a consulting doctor at the Institut and the first full professor of psychiatry in Spain (Barcelona), who would become Tosquelles's mentor. He also worked with Salvador Vilaseca, director of the Biological Analysis Laboratory at the Institut, scholar of the work of Carl Gustav Jung and an archeology enthusiast, and with Josep Solanes, Jaume Sauret, and Joaquim Alier, among others.[9]

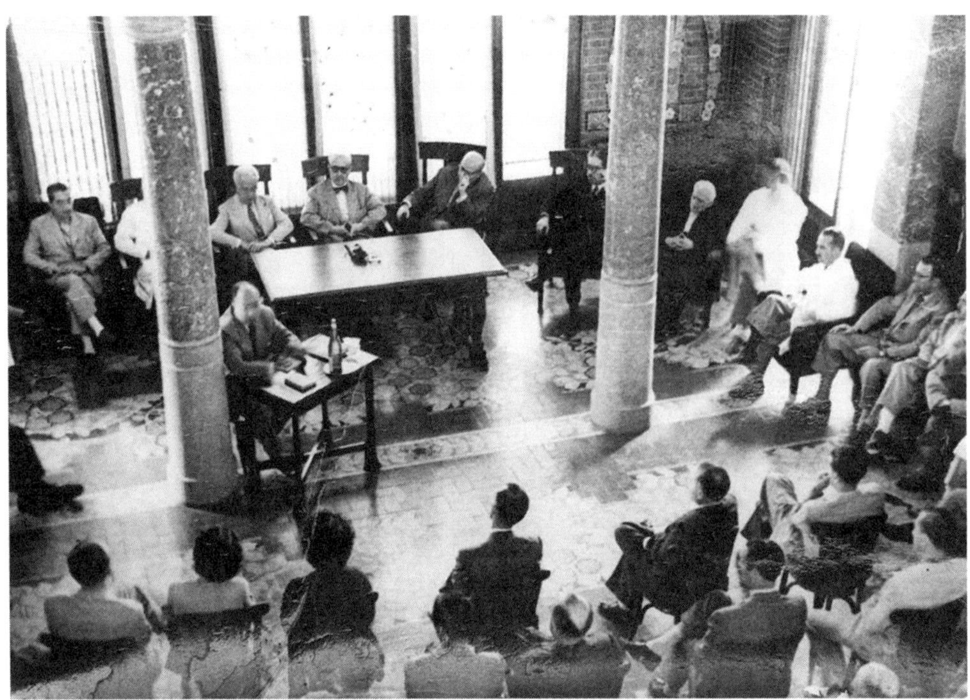

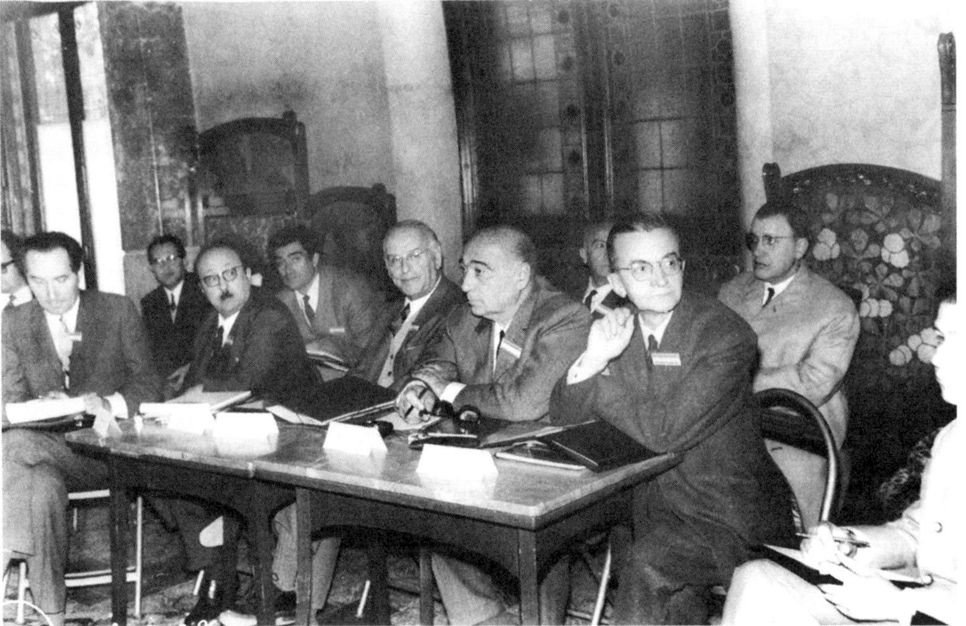

Top, a meeting of the hospital's medical staff in the Pavilion of the Distinguished

Bottom, Francesc Tosquelles with other speakers

Therapeutic Work: An Action Itself

In the early 1930s, Emili Mira and Francesc Tosquelles discovered the German psychiatrist Hermann Simon's work undertaken at the Gütersloh hospital, which had been published in 1929. Simon's book was translated into Spanish by Ramon Sarró in 1937, with the title *Tratamiento ocupacional de los enfermos mentales*, and some years later, at Saint-Alban, a collective translation into French was created, *Une thérapeutique plus active à l'hôpital psychiatrique*. Tosquelles adopted the two pillars of Simon's experience at Gütersloh: the idea that patients would be cured by curing the institution; and the conviction that, by situating activity at the center, they could avoid the immobility, bed rest, and constant baths typical of old asylum life. Practices geared toward curing the institution in order to cure the mad are precursors to institutional psychotherapy as understood by Tosquelles. And the centrality of work gave rise to ergotherapy, sociotherapy, and occupational therapy being used at the Institut Pere Mata and at Saint-Alban.

More active therapeutic treatments, like those of Hermann Simon, led Tosquelles to experiment with his own patient activities, which were integrated into the life of the hospital. These trials were being developed at the same time that Simon veered toward Nazism and suggested envisioning work as a cog in their social Darwinism and eugenics apparatus. In Simon's fascist evolution, occupational therapy that originally seemed designed to shorten long hospital stays, reduce patient costs, and improve relationships in the institutional context became a mechanism for selecting the patients more useful for the workforce from the expendable ones: a process that divided the patients' lives into necessary or superfluous; the superfluous could die.[10] In his writings, Tosquelles doesn't make much mention of the National Socialist reality of Simon's occupational therapy, which transcended the German borders without his ideas on racial hygiene affecting the general understanding of his "work therapy." In 1984, in an essay titled "A propósito de los modelos de asistencia en psiquiatría," Tosquelles references his reading of Simon whose practices, in the hands of disciples in thrall to Nazi ideology, would become authoritarian. Tosquelles expresses his radical rejection of fascist uses of therapeutic work, although not necessarily explicitly. For Tosquelles, this work cannot be just any sort of activity. It can only be "personal and personalized" work that is not imposed, and that is implicit in the overall therapeutic context. The Hermann Simon we find in Tosquelles's writings seems to be his own interpretation of Simon's ideas, because Tosquelles consistently refers to his own experiences of using work in the institutional setting.

> In citing the title of H. Simon's book here, I've stressed that it should be understood as a proposal to do psychiatry that's not just active but as active as possible. And I draw attention to the trap which the notion of activity might constitute for French ears. What was connoted in the notion of activity—placed in circulation by German psychiatry—was radically contrary to restless movement or even movement at the behest of, imposed or proposed, by someone other than oneself. Here the notion signifies a free, personal and personalizing activity, one that originates and takes root in each individual. I took this to be the operative justification of what came to be called therapeutic communities. [...]
>
> Currently, one speaks in this regard of ergotherapy, occupational therapy, praxotherapy, ludotherapy, and even sociotherapy.
>
> Medical jargon employs and often combines Latin or Greek words to christen and frame new concepts that everyone would understand if they were described with ordinary words. [...]
>
> Such is the case with work (*ergo*), occupations, activities of every sort (*praxis*), games and pastimes (*ludo*), or even the relatively artificial and limited concrete social milieu in which the patients live, if need be, when they are cared for (*therapy*) in certain institutions. This is what justifies these scientific words, composed of a first particle (*praxo, ludo, ergo, socio, occupational,* etc.), to which is added the word *therapy*. What gives weight to the whole word is this second term, which qualifies the act or behavior which the first particle announces. The accent and the sense of the thing in question, banal in itself, are given to it only by therapeutic effects that it aims for subsequently. It is on the basis of the therapeutic goal that the structure and unfolding of such apparently mundane actions will be reconsidered, modified, and articulated. [...]
>
> Consequently, it's clear that in order to speak of ergotherapy correctly and without mystification, it's not enough that some or even all the patients of a psychiatric center engage in work. To speak of ergotherapy, a particular kind of work, based in science, must be put in place; I mean a systematic and analytic knowledge of the structure of one's object (the structure of the work), of the mechanisms that such activities bring into play, of the effects produced, and even of the conditions necessary to those effects—for healthy people and patients alike. It must not be a matter of simply offering patients any old activities to be done any old way.
>
> So one can see that this will almost never involve the organization of a type of work that's regulated by a labor code such as might exist in a given society, contemporary with the therapeutic action that's underway. I mean that it's never a matter of copying or miniaturizing a labor code that, in the society in question, assembles the legislative texts defining the rights and obligations of workers. By the same token, the therapeutic activities must not be conceived simply as an occupation to pass the time or to distract oneself while waiting for a discharge or a cure. Nor will it be a matter of working "to make a living."

These two models of work, which may be employed in this way in everyday life in society, do not have any therapeutic aim in themselves, and the absence of such an aim makes their whole internal structure different from that of ergotherapy, even if in many cases ergotherapy assumes a similar or identical form.

By definition, the perspective of ergotherapy can only be a medical perspective. [...]

Neither the patient nor the nurse can be reduced here to an obedient passivity, to a passive wait for medical indications and prescriptions, organized with rigor, precision, and detail, as when it's a matter of administering a purge or thirty drops of X every three hours. [...]

Activity cannot mean just any movement nor a special movement. Activity means self-motivated activity: an activity that originates and is rooted in the active subject and is capable of opening up in a social context, in the right circumstance.

A second point that H. Simon insists on, where he's concerned with choosing the type of work that's suited to the patient, is of great importance, despite its somewhat anecdotal appearance: the choice of work doesn't just depend on "the upper limit of the patient's work capacity," and most often following an ascending progression with stages that last a certain time. It is made "within a certain aspect of occupational organization," which in the institution needs to be "unitary and clear."

Doubtless in a Germanic style that finds our own Mediterranean style to be unsatisfactory, with good reason, Simon places meetings of caregivers before a set of possible work activities. This set comprises various groups classed according to "progress in independence," with certain of these groups, moreover, being under the sole responsibility of the patients themselves. This shows that Simon not only had the good sense to envision the work only within the concrete limits announced by the set, but also that he wanted to make sure that this set of possibilities could be clearly grasped, and potentially modified, by the group of caregivers first of all, then by the group of patients. Ultimately it was a matter of making it easy for each patient to have a clear idea of their work as situated in a set of projects that by themselves defined what was most active in this veritable "institutional therapeutics." [...]

There are still ergotherapy groups pretty much everywhere in France but nowhere has ergotherapy been maintained as a problematic of the hospital as a whole. The most coherent organizations still seem to be those of Saint-Alban—outlying and in a poor region—and the La Borde clinic. One of the last bastions of overall organization of ergotherapy, aligning itself overtly with Simon while emphasizing "pedagogical" and social "reconditioning" aspects, supported by the author one imagines, was the hospital of Lannemezan. One fears that it is undergoing serious modifications that will not necessarily be favorable, its inspirer and principal actor, Dr. Ueberschlag, having had to take another post.

This kind of crisis is not just a French development. One thinks of the evolution of the Júlio de Matos Hospital in Lisbon, where Barahona Fernandes was able to implement one of the most complete and pertinent projects of ergotherapy, one that was integrated, moreover, into biological therapeutics. All that's left of it is the buildings and the patients.[11]

François Tosquelles, "Essence et place du travail thérapeutique dans le dispositif de soins psychiatriques" [Essence and place of therapeutic work in the organization of psychiatric care], 1967

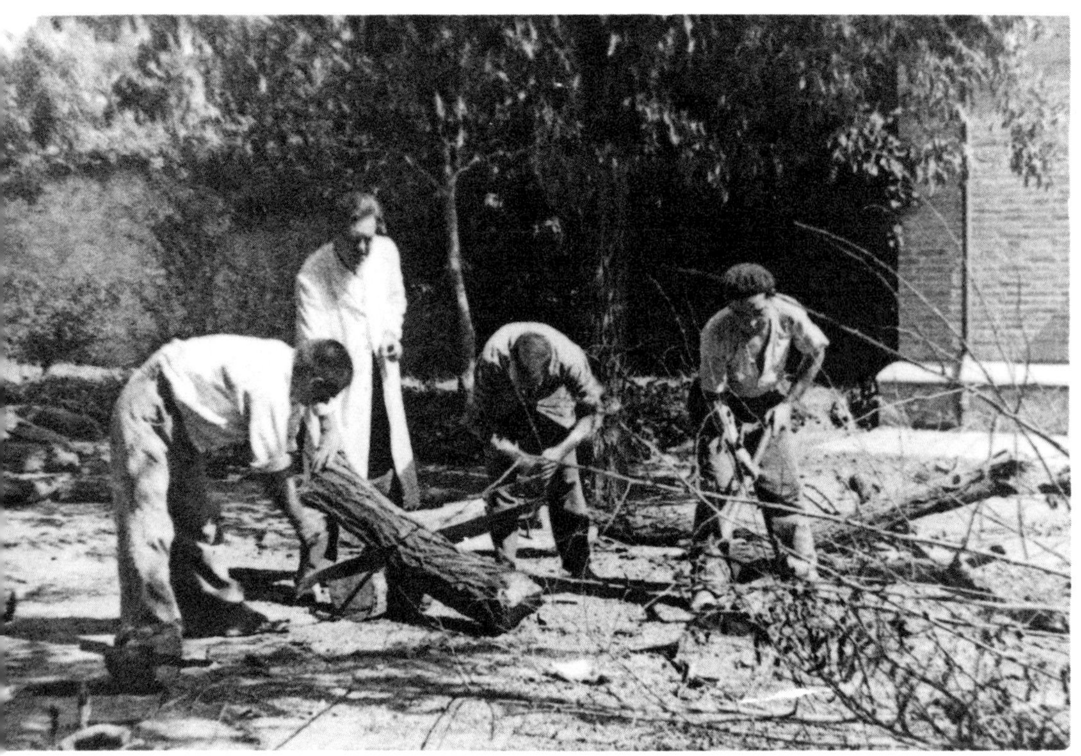

Above and at right, peasants sawing wood and raking hay at the Institut Pere Mata, in the presence of a hospital doctor

If I mentioned what goes on here in our discussion, it was to highlight a very important notion in ergotherapy, which is the notion of gymnastic exercice, of functional games, as [Henri] Wallon would say, a notion that includes identification with the aggressor [for the] analysts. When something is not going well, one rehearses it more or less alone, often by playing, till one has mastered it. To clarify this idea, its impact on ergotherapy, I'll adduce, for example, the case of memory troubles, carbon monoxide–poisoning patients with memory impairments, or the case of pseudo-schizophrenic reactions. It is evident that such patients should do memory exercises; but when you try to get a carbon monoxide patient to do such exercises like at school, they'll show you the door! All the more so if it's a patient who conceals or compensates for their memory troubles through a regressive activity with a schizophrenic look to it; but, if one can get them to do the same exercises in a spontaneous way, for example by making them the bartender, for a certain time and just as stealthily, they will make notes on little scraps of paper, for example the prices. Every time they sell a coffee, they will repeat these prices as a mental exercise, and in two weeks' time, they won't make any more notes, they will remember. One supposes that they have done the exercises in secret.

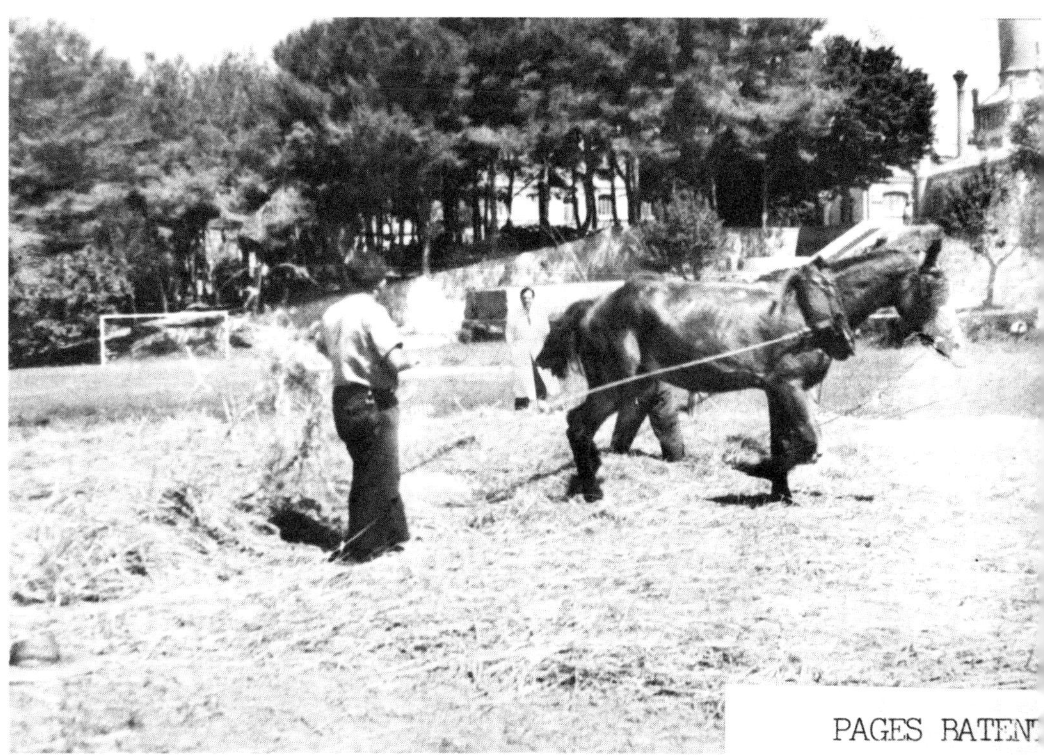

I'm reminded of a completely delirious patient like that, with a delirium that hid memory troubles of a toxic origin and who, thanks to work in the hospital canteen, was able to do memory exercises; she no longer needed to rave. She was even able to say spontaneously, "Well then, maybe a few more exercises wouldn't hurt," because she noticed, as Goldstein would say, that she got something out of them as such, and instead of telling her doctor that the Holy Virgin had horns and that she had appeared one Good Friday over the Eiffel Tower, she said to him, "Monsieur, I have memory troubles, maybe you could suggest something that might help me further?" With this overdrawn example, one sees that ergotherapy has nothing to do with production.[12]

François Tosquelles in discussion with Jean Oury, Roger Gentis, Georges Daumézon (*et al.*), "Les échanges matériels et affectifs dans le travail thérapeutique" [Material and affective exchanges in therapeutic work], *Bulletin technique du personnel soignant*, December 1961

Gateway Institutions

The collective organization of work forms part of the new world that began with the twentieth century. Taylorism and new forms of professionalization marked the character of these new institutions. In 1908, the first professional training was created for the High School Teachers Association of New York, and in 1915—a few years before Madrid—Barcelona already had an Institut d'Orientació Profesional within the Escola del Treball, which was public and in which both Tosquelles and Mira took part. Its training in primary schools involved the study of all aspects of choosing a trade, market studies, managing apprentices, the discussion of remuneration, and the elaboration of aptitude testing. The Career Guidance Institute published the journal *Psicologia i pedagogia*, directed by Emili Mira, head of the psychology section, and by Joaquim Xirau. Recognized by psychologists, teachers, and counselors of the era, the journal was in dialogue with the international community. In addition to its training programs, the Escola de Treball conducted research and hosted important conferences. With the advent of the Republic in 1932, Emili Mira managed to create the Institut Psicotècnic, which would develop real studies on the psychology of work; in addition to organizing the teaching of various branches of experimental psychology, he created a library of experimental psychology and supported doctoral studies on the subject.

Mira advised Tosquelles to work at an institution that dealt with "the lives of normal people," so he collaborated in the selection of bus drivers for the Barcelona General Bus Company.[13] Thus, he simultaneously combined two institutional practices, in Reus and in Barcelona. Tosquelles understood that his own training and exercise of his profession as a doctor of mental suffering were inseparable from the collective functioning of normality, and he associated the world of productive work and its forms of organization with the excluded members of society. This way of comprehending the links between institutions facilitated gateways between two stagnant worlds: the world of professionalization and the therapeutic world; the world of normality and the world stigmatized by illness.

Throughout the 1930s, Tosquelles sought out other gateway institutions, such as childcare institutions, that allowed him to experience psychiatry without dissociating it from child psychiatry and psychology, as was the norm in that period. His desire to overcome such separations of disciplines led him, beginning in 1935, to link the therapeutic activity of the patients

INSTITUT PSICOTÈCNIC
DE LA GENERALITAT

CONSULTORI MEDICO - PEDAGÒGIC

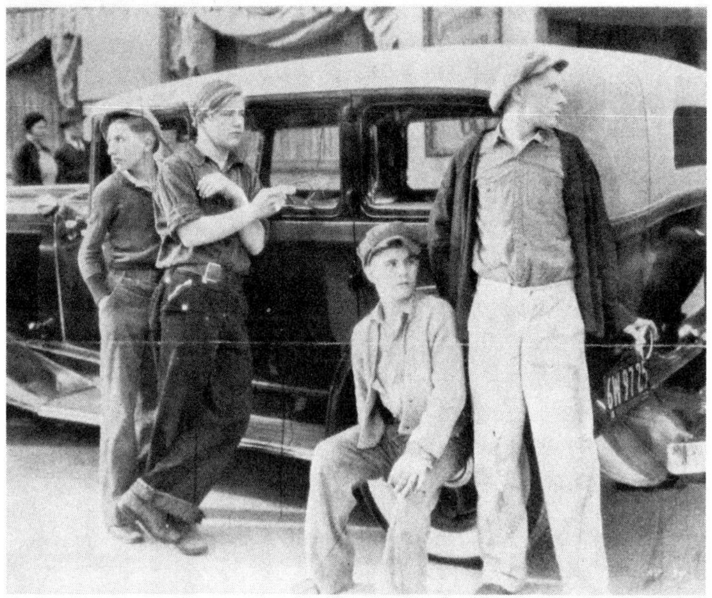

CICLE DE CONFERÈNCIES
SOBRE PSICOPATOLOGIA INFANTIL

CURS 1934 - 35

Advertisement of the activities at the Psychotechnical Institute of the Barcelona School of Work, in the early 1930s

The setting was the gardens of the Institut Pere Mata, when I had only just begun my medical studies in Barcelona. One day, with youthful enthusiasm, I commented to Mira—my friend—on a work by Dr. Vilaseca that discussed Cotard's delusion and the legendary poem of Count Arnau. I got tangled up in pretentious musings on guilt, tinged with a marked Dostoyevskian accent. Mira seemed to be scarcely listening to me, but afterward he said something along these lines: "Kid, if you want to be a psychiatrist, don't get dazzled by the aesthetics of delirium and other pathological creations. I believe that a psychiatrist should, above all, take an interest in the process of normal production, he should be interested in normal man. If you'd like, come to the School of Work, whenever. I'm at your disposal."

That anecdote, however, could be misconstrued if not completed by two other bits of "boost/advice" that I received from Mira.

The first: "If you want to be a psychiatrist you should work hard to be a good doctor. A general practitioner, like the old town doctors, located in an environment, a town they know well and where psychopathologies emerge. The danger of the town doctor is if he allows himself to be swept up in the demand for magic, in believing in his own charismatic power, getting involved in vanity and politicking."

The second "boost/advice" I received from Mira in this regard was his suggestion that I work with Dr. Subirana. "The brain—he told me—is a mystery and, undoubtedly, many aspects of neurological practice have little relationship to psychiatric practice. But Professor Barré—from whom Subirana learned his style—focuses on something that is of great interest to us in psychiatry: the eyes (seeing, perception), the ears (listening and speaking, which are interrelated activities), and body posture and attitude, the coordination of movements—in other words, the vestibular and cerebellar systems, etc. 'Fine' neurological exploration—à la Barré—is undoubtedly fundamental for psychiatry."[14]

Francesc Tosquelles, "Maestro y amigo," 1973

BARCELONA GENERAL BUS COMPANY,

CORP. (C.G.A.)

SAFETY IS OUR PRIORITY

According to the results obtained in the examinations by the "Professional Orientation Institute," aspiring drivers of the C.G.A. are classified into four groups: good, normal, medium, and unacceptable.

The final group is rejected and those ranked medium are subject to certain restrictions.

Five years of experience have proven that those drivers qualified as good had four times less accidents than those ranked medium, under identical conditions. As such, currently our services only employ drivers ranked normal or good.

Every two years a general review is carried out, with similar tests, and when the drivers reach 50 years of age, this review is carried out annually. Any driver who has frequent accidents is also subject to a new assessment.

Once the aspiring drivers have passed the initial tests, they must study an instruction course in the C.G.A. Driving School and pass the corresponding exam in order to be officially hired.

Thanks to this selection process, the C.G.A. can offer its services to the public with the utmost safety.

C.G.A.

N.º 4 1929

COMPAÑIA GENERAL DE AVTOBVSES DE BARCELONA S.A.

SEGURIDAD ANTE TODO

Segun los resultados obtenidos en las pruebas del "Instituto de Orientación Profesional", **los aspirantes a conductores de la** C.G.A. **se clasifican en cuatro grupos:** buenos, normales, medianos e inaceptables.

El último grupo no es admitido **y los medianos lo han sido con determinadas restricciones.**

La experiencia de cinco años ha demostrado que los clasificados como buenos han ocasionado cuatro veces menos de accidentes que los medianos **en igualdad de condiciones.** Por ello actualmente en nuestros servicios solo actúan los normales y buenos.

Cada dos años se procede a una revisión general, con iguales pruebas, y cuando los conductores alcanzan los 50 años la revisión se efectúa anualmente. También es sometido a nuevo exámen todo conductor que ocasione accidentes con frecuencia.

Pasadas estas pruebas, los aspirantes deben seguir un curso de instrucción en la Escuela de Conductores de la C.G.A. **y sufrir el exámen correspondiente para quedar difinitivamente admitidos.**

Gracias a esta selección la C.G.A. puede ofrecer al público la máxima seguridad en sus servicios.

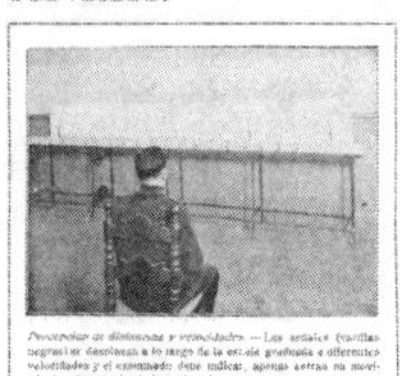

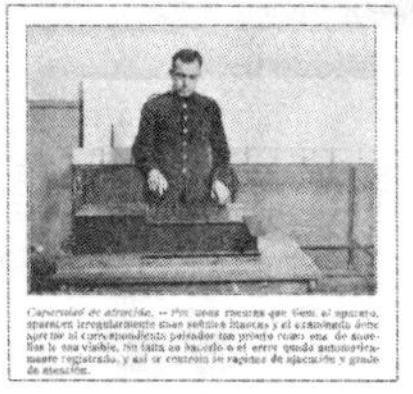

C.G.A. significa SEGURIDAD

in the Institut Pere Mata with the work in the child psychiatry clinic of the Institut d'Observació Psicològica de Barcelona La Sageta, which was inspired by institutions such as the British and American child guidance clinics, as well as by the work of Reus child-rearing center La Gota de Llet. At La Sageta, Tosquelles familiarized himself with the patients' cultural and domestic context, as well as with home visits, which would become central to sector psychiatry, and a series of practices that were designed to maintain links with families, who could even come and live in the clinic for a while. The director of La Sageta was the psychiatrist and Heidelberg University professor Alfred Strauss, who had come to Barcelona fleeing anti-semitism and Nazi repression. The German psychiatrist Werner Wolff was also welcomed by Emili Mira to work at the Psychotechnical Institute between 1933 and 1936.[15]

Tosquelles refered to Barcelona as "Little Vienna" during those years when the Republic was a place that welcomed Jewish psychiatrists from Central Europe, including Sándor Eiminder, a Hungarian refugee who was Tosquelles's analyst; their sessions were held at the Ateneu Barcelonès, even though Eiminder barely spoke Catalan. That meant that Tosquelles experienced foreignness in two ways: through the therapeutic practices that came from abroad (distancing him from the nineteenth-century Spanish tradition and bringing him closer to the Central European tradition) and through his listening to other languages—Hungarian, Czech, German ...—with their accents, their tones, inflections and cadences, that denatured his own relationship to language.

The Ateneu Barcelonès and the Ateneu Enciclopèdic Popular also fulfilled the function of gateway institutions, since they were two important centers in the sociopolitical and psychoanalytical debate of the period. Tosquelles trained and taught courses in both. Although there are no remaining documentary traces of Tosquelles's lectures and activities at the Ateneu Barcelonès, there is a record of his time at that institution. Tosquelles joined the Ateneu in 1932 as a "temporary member," in the Moral Sciences section, surely allowing him access to the library and the books he couldn't then afford, until he canceled his membership in November 1933. While the Ateneu Barcelonès is bourgeois, the Ateneu Enciclopèdic Popular was an anarchist and socialist institution. In the early 1930s, Tosquelles was the secretary for the lectures on Freud and Marx that were given there by Emili Mira, as part of programming that offered language classes (Catalan, French, English, and Esperanto), seminars on economy, Marxism, and sexology, and

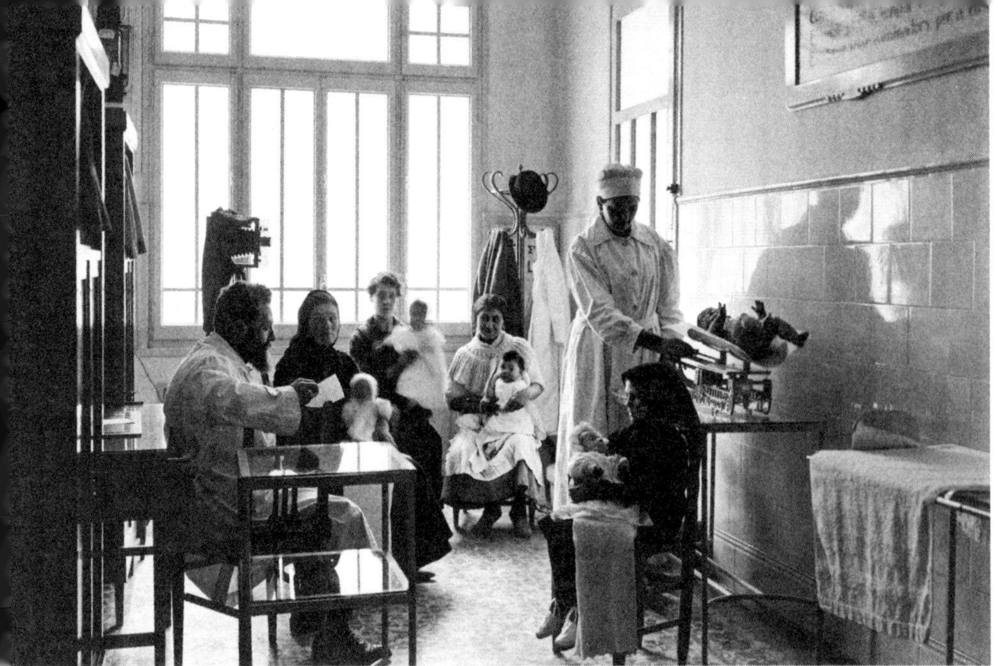

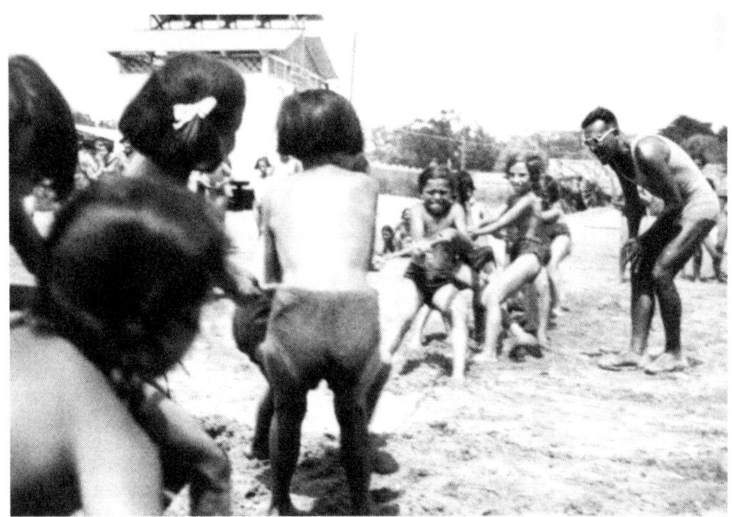

Above, Dr. Alexandre Frias in the office he opened at Reus in 1919. Here he's seen consulting with working-class mothers with limited resources, whose care he took on after an earlier trip through Europe.

Right, one of the first summer camps organized during the Republic, in 1935

In 1934, when I returned to Reus—my activity didn't stop, no—Dr. Frias himself, at La Gota de Llet—the first of its kind on the peninsula—helped me organize a mental hygiene office for children with difficulties and above all for their mothers. And with Prof. Ganigué we began working in the same miserable moral and physical conditions of the Casa de la Caritat with "mental weaklings" to achieve better possibilities and ambitions—possibilities and ambitions that would soon vanish, at least for me, in 1937.[16]

Francesc Tosquelles, *La pratique du maternage thérapeutique chez les débiles mentaux profonds*, 1966 colloquia like the one organized by Catalan workers in homage to the poet Federico García Lorca, in which Lorca himself and the actress Margarida Xirgu recited several of his poems.

> Emili Mira had made important studies on psychomotricity. Unfortunately, Mira was accused of collaborating with the Bolsheviks, and his colleagues refused to accept him as their representative. Things like this were revealed in an article by Sarró, published by *La Vanguardia* in 1966: I've saved the article and can show it to you. The silence surrounding Mira in Spain has been a true attack on psychiatry and its possibilities of development. I remember that around 1932 there was a seminar on Marx and Freud, for which I was secretary. In it, Mira said that the phenomenology of Husserl and Heidegger was an overture to fascism. That behind phenomenology was the emphasis of death. In 1931, Sarró made a grand entrance into the Psychiatry Congress in Granada, speaking on Heidegger's theories and existentialism in general. He was aware, like Heidegger, that they led to fascism. However, there was an open struggle to conceal all that. Mira also realized this opening toward fascism. He said that the basis of existentialism was apragmatism. When there was a hiring call for the post of director at Santa Coloma, Sarró's name was bandied about. Seven or eight days after Sarró surveyed the services there, he said there was nothing that could be done. As a result, he wasn't named as director. Apragmatism is the gateway to fascism, which makes speeches and insists all others are silent. I say all this because we must make a commitment to child psychiatry in order to be able to practice psychiatry of adults and the elderly.[17]
>
> Francesc Tosquelles, "Seminari per a metges i psicòlegs," December 14, 1987

Unfinished Revolutions

L'Ateneu Enciclopèdic was one of the sites of transmission and experimentation of ideas for the BOC (Bloc Obrer i Camperol, or the Workers and Peasants' Group) and the POUM (Partido obrero de unificación Marxista, or the Workers' Party of Marxist Unification), in both of which Tosquelles was an active member. The BOC, established in 1930 following the merging of the Catalan Communist Party and the Catalan-Balear Communist Federation, was dissolved into the POUM in the merger with the Spanish Communist left in 1935, since both shared their criticism of Soviet authoritarianism and their defense of political plurality against Communist bureaucratic centralism. In January of 1935, the BOC published a manifesto that called for the creation of a revolutionary party that could combine the different existing socialist/Marxist organizations and proposed a common front of the working-class vanguard. The BOC had rehearsed forms of political plurality: discussions in local assemblies combined with decision-making from the bottom up and from the top down; the defense of the Estatut de Catalunya and the compatibility of an independent Catalonia with internationalism, a question that, in a

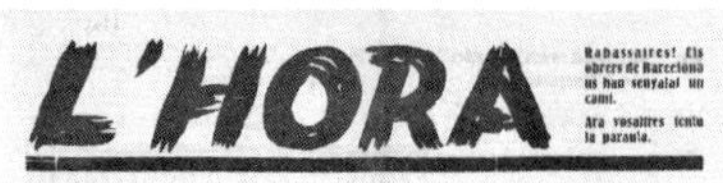

L'HORA

Rabassaires! Els obrers de Barcelona us han senyalat un camí.

Ara vosaltres teniu la paraula.

Al crit de "Visca el Bloc Obrer i Camperol!" i "Visca l'Aliança Obrera!" equips de combat dels treballadors de Barcelona, assaltaren i cremaren, dimecres al vespre, el niu dels provocadors reaccionaris de l'Institut Agrícola Català de Sant Isidre

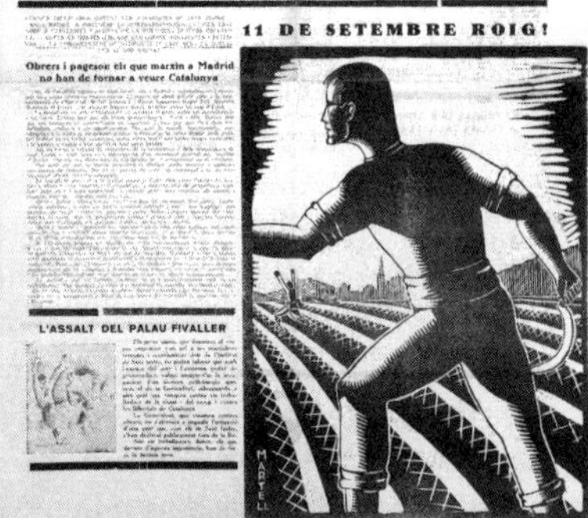

11 DE SETEMBRE ROIG!

Obrers i pagesos els que marxin a Madrid no han de tornar a veure Catalunya

L'ASSALT DEL PALAU FIVALLER

federal Spain, radically challenged the structure of Communist centralism, as evidenced in journals such as *L'Hora* and *La Torxa*.[18]

In any case, what I can tell you about Helios Gómez is very little. From the beginning he was already legendary and mythical (in the sense that the subject and style of his drawings was unlike anything being published at the time). I believe I only saw and spoke with him twice. The first was in a spectacle of "revolutionary" magic. I don't know if it was 1928 or 1929, or perhaps it was 1930. One day we "stormed" the rectorate of the Universitat de Barcelona. A banner we [hung] in the windows announced "to the people" that we had proclaimed a republic of "students, farmers, and workers." There was a real shoot-out for a few hours; nobody was hurt. A few horses did receive some blows, horses of the "security" forces, the ones with the "coffeepot" [drawing] inscribed on their helmets.

He was there, an older young person than me; I found him elegantly dressed, he did take part in the shooting. He seemed to me like something out of a musical vignette with tango airs or, even better, like an Andalusian with grace and flair. I don't think I'm exaggerating when I say that his voice was the finishing touch of that somewhat fascinating aesthetic impression. Yet what he said, what we said, could fit inside a walnut; it was merely mundane "niceties."

Another time, with some "political" friends—who included a "Venezuelan" of Valencian origin, Simón Gómez Malaret, also with a lot of flair but a true poet, despite the fat that rounded out his figure—we went to the home of Juanito el Dorado, where they sang and danced flamenco. I think we went there with Helios, or we met him there. There was talk of the relationship between dance, spontaneous poetry (with less narcissistic popular styles), and "revolutionary projection." Perhaps I've retained some of those ideas and they've insinuated themselves into my practice of psychiatry rooted in humanity and social expression. In that sense, Helios Gómez's memory has persisted within me, although in "reality" the concrete biographical encounters prevailed, offering subjects for a grammar or a "realist" novel in the style of Zola or Pérez Galdós. So I don't know anything concrete of "anecdotal" value about your father, neither about his "precedents" or historical ["paths"]. Therefore, I don't think my testimony can be useful for your historical research. His drawings, like him, seemed to me to reveal the rhythmic contrast of life itself. If other anecdotes or events brought us together, I have no memory of them. Only the transcendence of art—of communicative actions—endures. I haven't forgotten him, and I'm pleased to be able to answer your letter.

Letter from Francesc Tosquelles to Gabriel Gómez Plana, son of Helios Gómez, November 28, 1986

Above, cover of *L'Hora*, a Barcelona publication with an irregular publishing schedule, mouthpiece of the BOC and the FCE (Federació Comunista Catalana, or the Catalan Communist Federation) between 1930 and 1931

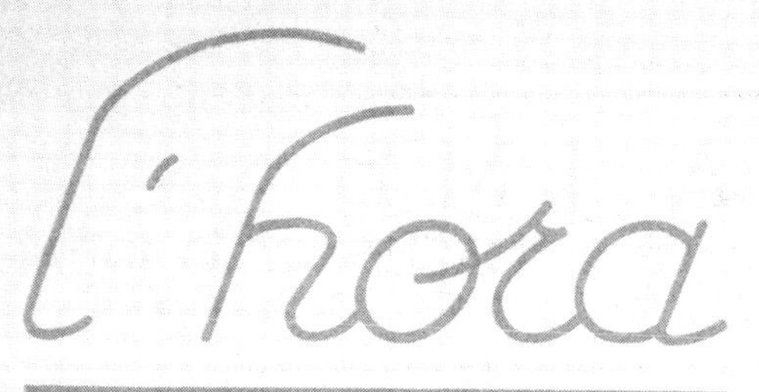

el pronunciament es basa
en una autoconfiança
individual

la revolució es basa
en una autoconfiança
col·lectiva

any I barcelona, 10 de desembre de 1930 n.º 1

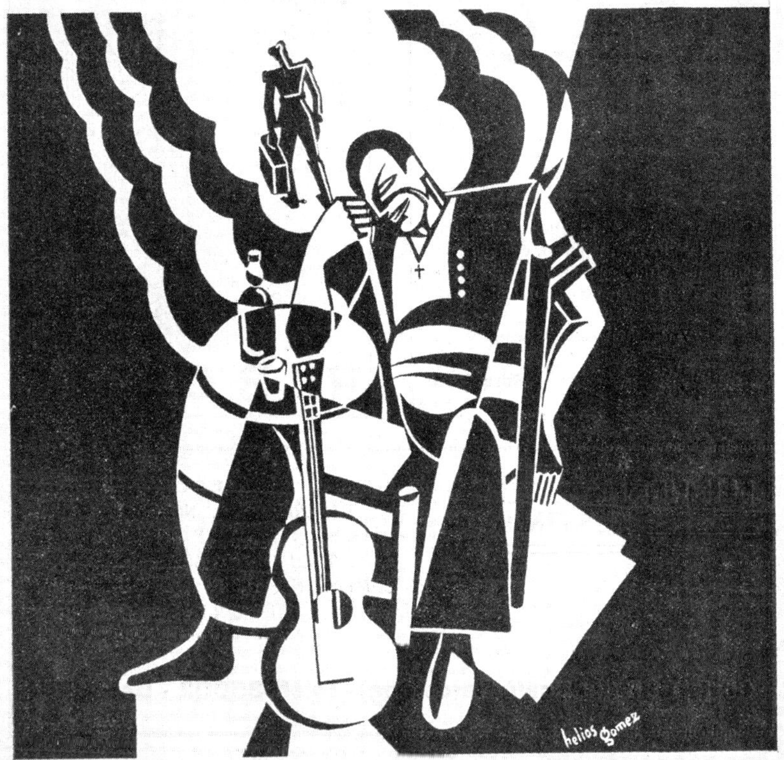

Somni

20 cts.

Above, an advertisement for the first issue of *L'Hora*, with a reproduction of *Somni* (Dream) by Helios Gómez

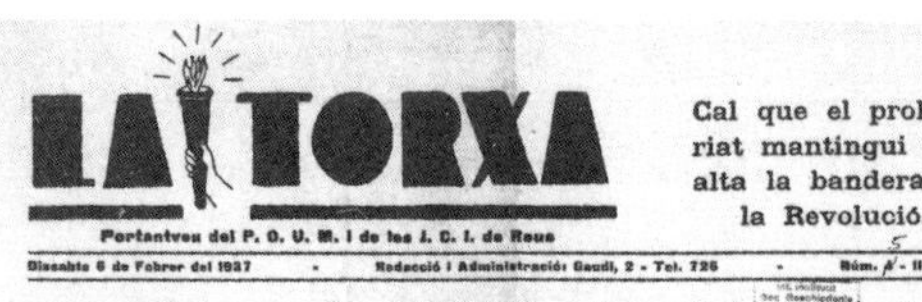

Cal que el proletariat mantingui ben alta la bandera de la Revolució.

Dissabte 6 de Febrer del 1937 · Redacció i Administració: Gaudí, 2 - Tel. 726 · Núm. 5 - II Època

Contra el confusionisme del P. S. U. C. nosaltres exigim la Dictadura del Proletariat

EDITORIAL

Assemblees

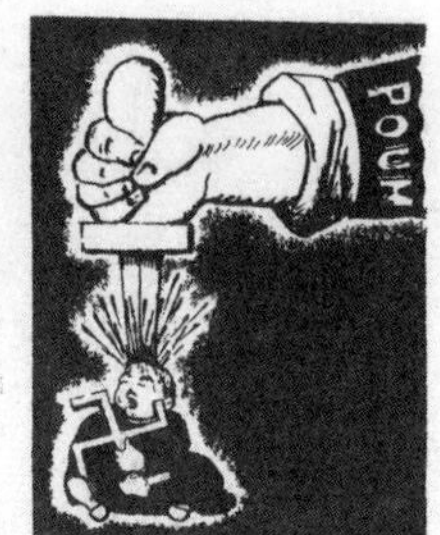

La Torxa: Portantveu dels BOC del Baix Camp was a monthly magazine published in Catalan that contained strategic articles on anti-fascism, unionism, and gender equality. In its first period there is only one known issue, published in 1933. It was restarted in 1937 with the title *La Torxa: Portantveu del POUM i de les JCI de Reus.*

It was in 1930 maybe, or 1931, during the crisis that set Stalin and his people against the small core group that had struggled mightily during the first dictatorship to clandestinely form the Federació Comunista Catalano-Balear, a debate group I was part of as a student in Barcelona. My colleagues in the Bloc Obrer i Camperol, which emerged from that political crisis, asked me—since I was heading to Reus on vacation—to bring some texts and information to some militants there: Oliva, Hortoneda, and some others I can't recall as clearly. In Barcelona they believed that the militants in Reus, with the legitimate illusions that gave rise to the Russian Revolution, might follow the instructions decided by the agents of the "party," which according to Stalin had to come from Moscow or Madrid, and had to go against the Republicans, against the socialists, and against the anarchists, as much or more as against the monarchists and the right wing. It was necessary, they said, to defend a single tactic that could be summed up as "all power to the Soviets." Someone joked that in any case, in Catalonia, that would have to be translated to "all power to the debate groups," because there wasn't a single Soviet in all the towns on the Iberian Peninsula. [...] I remember that he suggested I tell Quim (Joaquín Maurín) that here in Reus, in any case, if things went very badly, that the people of the BOC would keep their own quacks to themselves. "The Reus group will not be a trolley for Stalin's Russia nor for the branch offices of Hitler's bragging idiots."[19]

Francesc Tosquelles, *Funció poètica i psicoteràpia: Una lectura de "In memoriam" de Gabriel Ferrater*, 1985

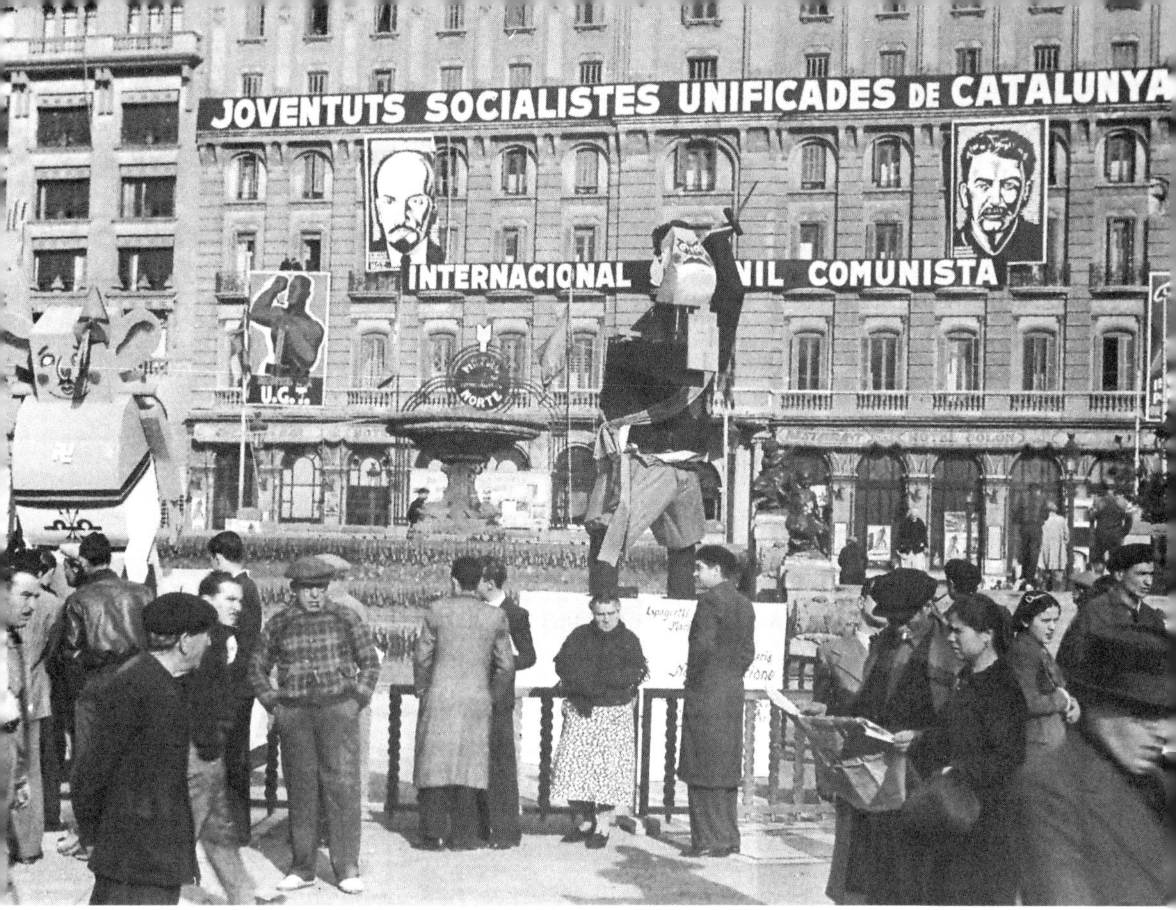

Above, headquarters of the Joventuts Socialistes Unificades de Catalunya at the Hotel Colon in Barcelona's Plaça de Catalunya, February 28, 1937

Right, the Casal Carles Marx (formerly the Jockey Club) headquarters of the central committee of the PSUC (Unified Socialist Party of Catalonia), on the Passeig de Gràcia in Barcelona, January 17, 1937. Photographs taken by Alec Wainman, a member of the International Brigades. Wainman drove ambulances and served as an interpreter and a volunteer administrative medical officer in the British Medical Unit during the Spanish Civil War.

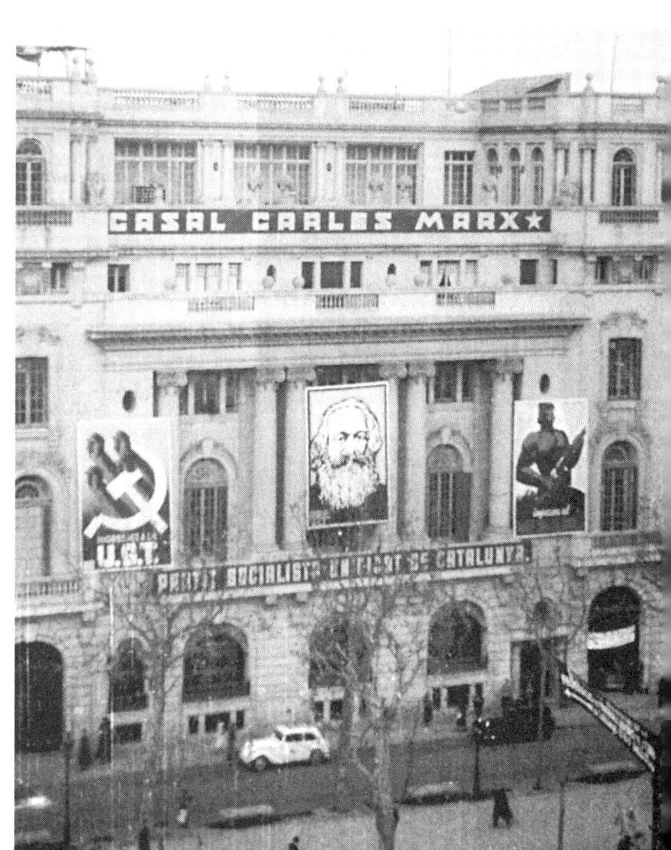

There was an important group of doctors among the membership of the BOC, which included Dr. Solanes and Dr. Sauret, colleagues of Tosquelles's at the Institut Pere Mata. Like them, Tosquelles moved from the BOC to the POUM, and back and forth between Reus and Barcelona. Highly critical of the Stalinist centralism that ended up making the POUM illegal, in a legendary letter addressed to Stalin, Tosquelles wrote that far from handing over all power to the Soviets, in Catalonia the power could only possibly be given to the already existing social groups that were linked to particular places: conversational debate groups that formed part of the models of local socializing in cafés, sharing current events and leisure time. In various writings from the seventies and eighties, he reiterated that neither in Catalonia nor in Spain had reproducing the Soviets' hierarchy nor their workers' councils ever been feasible. This "communism without communism" with libertarian roots, in a historical context marked by anarchy, situated his experience of the thirties in a world that was not yet the world of communist politics in the forties at Saint-Alban. There, French residents linked to the surrealist movement associated anarchy with individualism and aspired to build the avant-garde cultural program of official communism: an ambition that made them turn a blind eye to Stalinism in order to be able to win their own battle for French cultural hegemony. Some French surrealists, such as Benjamin Péret, joined the ranks of the POUM and the Durruti Column; and René Crevel, in 1931, delivered the lecture "L'Esprit contre la raison" in a conference organized by the magazine *L'Hora*, at the Sala Capsir in Barcelona, rented by the BOC, along with Salvador Dalí, whose speech was titled "El surrealisme al servei de la revolució" (Surrealism in the service of the revolution). Dalí published three drawings, *Crucifixió*, *El pobre*, and *Lectors de "La Veu de Catalunya" et de "La Publicitat,"* in *L'Hora* on October 30, 1931.[20]

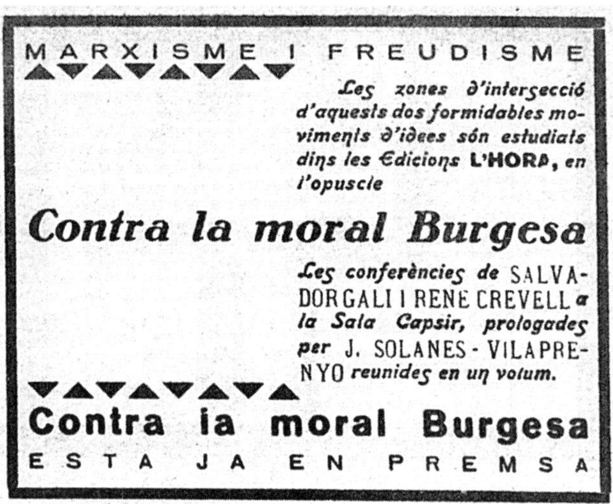

Announcement of talks given by Salvador Dalí and René Crevel, published in *L'Hora*, no. 43, October 30, 1931

It was precisely from these positions of antiauthoritarian and anti-Stalinist communism, and from within groups that suffered reprisals and illegalization, that Tosquelles rehearsed forms of "therapeutic community" both in Reus, in farmhouses requisitioned by the POUM, during the Civil War, and in the refugee camp upon his arrival in France. As Jean Oury would write following Tosquelles's death, this improbable experience left an intermittent and unfinished legacy, a political legacy that Oury, along with Félix Guattari, wanted to recoup and continue at the La Borde clinic.

> Of course, if one is to understand something at La Borde, there is the history of the POUM and a lot of things about the POUM, because the POUM was enmeshed in a whole context. The proceedings against Andreu Nin, for example ... The horror ...
>
> What was dominant in Spain was not the anarchist movement, marked by the naivety of believing that by changing the economy things would go better. Those people got crushed by the Stalinists. After all, it was the period of the Moscow trials. People disappeared, or were tortured. Trials without end, even post-mortem. But already a libertarian movement had been crushed in Oviedo in 1934 by Franco, coming from Morocco ... One would also have to talk about the Trotskyists. [...]
>
> That today's history, our present time, is tied to History writ large, where the Spanish Civil War sits in its proper place, is something that we need to reflect on in general, but it seems that this also concerns the development of psy concepts and practices. The question could be the following: What is the function of the Spanish Civil War, of what played out there, of what failed, of what is still dogging us? You see, it's like an unconscious political function that would be at work at the geographic level of our history ... What is that blind spot that marks the history of Europe and on which, moreover, La Borde is sustained?[21]
>
> Jean Oury, "Psychothérapie institutionnelle et guerre d'Espagne" [Institutional psychotherapy and the Spanish Civil War] 2010

THE FUNCTION OF THE STATE IS TO AVOID INSTITUTIONS

OTIUM DIAGONAL—In Spain we are familiar with your publications and activities in the field of psychoanalysis and in psychiatric and pedagogical institutions. Some of them have been translated from the French. However, you had an important role in the earliest psychiatric movements in Catalonia, which led you to this work on psychoanalysis and institutions. What can you tell us about this trajectory?

FRANCESC TOSQUELLES—Well, in order to explain that I'll have to mention some things about my history. There is an article I wrote for the Reus journal *Fulls clínics*[1] based on a conversation with my uncle, who didn't participate in the asylum because of a political and economic problem—they didn't want to, as he had proposed, have everyone in the town pay a part and so no capital accumulated—and my uncle, my mother's brother, stepped down. But many friends remained there. When I was a small child, at home we always said that my uncle was a psychiatrist who acted as the town doctor. And he was the one who had Freud's book on dreams and *Psychopathology of Everyday Life*, and we would discuss them with him. So, at ten years old, I already knew, because of the ego ideal—or the ideal ego, I don't know, whatever—I already knew what I would do. I would inject psychoanalysis in asylums. And I received a lot of support in that from Emili Mira.[2] I also had another bit of extraordinary luck: Mr. Hitler—well, really, all that fascist absurdity. I can't complain about it because it led to something extraordinary, which is that beginning in 1931 Jewish refugees began arriving in Barcelona, mostly from Austria.

In 1931, there was a conference on *contre-transfert* with Folch and others from the Institut,[3] and I took part because I was a bit pissed off that everything we'd done there had passed into oblivion. Because, in the end, the only Spaniard who's talked about is Ángel Garma, when he was in Argentina. And in Madrid Garma had started doing some things, but he was in Madrid. And in Barcelona they were doing things at La Sageta[4] with children, I did some things here. And not only that but in 1932 or 1933, I worked there as a secretary. They had closed the university in 1931, before the Republic, and then we created a university outside of the university with a group of professors—Trias, Bellido, Mira—at the Ateneu Obrer. Speaking of which, the Ateneu Barcelonès wouldn't allow us to do it there because it was controlled by the Lliga. I was the secretary. Every four or five days, at the Ateneu Enciclopèdic Popular, on Carrer del Carme, there were gatherings about Freud and Marx. Perhaps Jaume Miravitlles and Jordi Arquer, of the POUM [Workers' Party of Marxist Unification], were the most active. I was also with the POUM. Anyway, all this is to say that there's a through line here.

Excerpt from Miquel Bassols and Rosa Maria Calvet's interview with Francesc Tosquelles. Originally published in *Otium Diagonal*, no. 4–5, 1982, pp. 14–22.

Miquel Bassols revised the interview in August 2020, maintaining the colloquial and unacademic tone of the conversation.

OTIUM DIAGONAL—And what written sources can we consult to trace that through line?

FRANCESC TOSQUELLES—If you have the chance to read the summary of the Barcelona Congress, you'll find those things. Because Ramon Sarró and Santiago Montserrat spoke about Vienna. They'd traveled to Vienna. But, hell, I prefer that Vienna be here. Vienna was here in Barcelona.

OTIUM DIAGONAL—And why was it that you decided to go to France?

FRANCESC TOSQUELLES—Oh, that's very important! What I wanted to say is this: here, the events of 1936 happened. At that time, Josep Solanes, Jaume Sauret, Josep Capella, Borrell—a young guy who hadn't finished his degree—and I were a group of doctors affiliated with the POUM. The day the war started we were in the medical zones in Aragon. Solanes and I saw the need and we suggested organizing psychiatric posts in the army, and we set up a few "sectors": Sariñena, Benabarre, Bujaraloz ... It's the same idea as the sector: avoiding separating people too much from the place they are, the place where they live, because if people who go nuts in a war are just marginalized, that's it, there's no coming back from that. They have to be cured right there where things are happening. That was what we did and it went pretty well.

But, to be blunt, those in Madrid—I mean the Russians, the Communist Party—well, they didn't want to have anything to do with it. First of all, because we were from the POUM and, secondly, because we were dealing with psychiatry. There was one group in particular who showed up to organize a repression, which was not only directed against the POUM, because in the Russian army there was no psychiatry. Not like in the next war, when the British organized psychiatric units influenced by Wilfred Bion and Wilhelm Reich, who played an important role in the discussions of morale in the troops and things of that sort.

OTIUM DIAGONAL—That was the practice based on the study of war neurosis ...

FRANCESC TOSQUELLES—No, it was with the normal troops. And the communists didn't want to hear about that, of course, because there are no crazy soldiers on the front.

OTIUM DIAGONAL—Emili Mira has a book on war neurosis where he discusses all that.

FRANCESC TOSQUELLES—I think so. He wrote it from the Americas. I haven't seen that book, but I understand it mentions me. Well, anyway, those people prevailed. There was to be no psychiatry in the organization of the people's army. Thank goodness they didn't kick out Mira, who came from the Socialist Union of Catalonia—when the PSUC [Unified Socialist Party of Catalonia] was formed, it was under communist control. They needed someone well known, a big name, so they kept him. He'd already had conflicts with the communists, even in Russia, because—I'll never forget this—they held a psychology conference and he presented the work he was doing here with employee selection. And then they published it saying that he was a bourgeois professor psychiatrist. Yet Mira stayed and managed—even after they'd tried to kill us, physically, especially me—to get them to recognize that we were doing things.

There was one man, a doctor named Taberner—I'll never forget—who came as a psychiatrist of the army corps. He kicked me out of Sariñena. Then I took refuge in Monzón. Since I was the head of the Health Service, they once asked me to study people's moods for organizing leaves. From there I went to Madrid. I saw that recognizing psychiatry during wartime wasn't simply a question—like normal psychiatry—of dealing with those labeled as crazy. Because clearly we were all facing some problem or another …

OTIUM DIAGONAL—Clearly, otherwise, you wouldn't be here …

FRANCESC TOSQUELLES —Exactly, I say that because, despite my friendship with Lacan, thanks to my training I've always been more Kleinian than Lacanian. That's because with children I've seen, here in Reus, when working in the child psychiatry service, at the Institut de Puericultura, between 1932 and 1936, I would meet with their mothers and talk to them in the waiting room, that sort of thing. I was very Kleinian, because Klein has the advantage over Freud in that she really worked with children and with psychotics—in other words, with people you can't ask to lie down on a couch, and as such you have to intervene, you have to activate them. It's much more similar to what we could do in a psychiatric hospital simply with the discourse of the talking cure.

OTIUM DIAGONAL—That's something I wanted to ask you about. I've worked with deficients for quite a few years and one of the selection tests we used with them was from your book on therapeutic mothering. And now I was surprised, when rereading your contributions to the book *Infancia alienada*, to see a large theoretic gap between that therapeutic mothering and what you propose here.[5]

FRANCESC TOSQUELLES—*El maternatge terapèutic*[6] is a book I wrote but it's aimed at educators, for their training. There are anecdotes, but it is related to what could be said or what could be done. Well, let's move on. Let's return to the war. Then, just as they were about to finish me off, a young guy had me come through the front lines to see the political commissar who, coincidentally, recognized my name and where I was from. "Holy hell! Aren't you Tosquelles?" "Hell, yes!" It turns out we'd gone to school together at five years old. He was shocked. I told him, "How could someone like you turn into a fascist?" Instead of returning to Sariñena, I stayed for seven or eight days with the young soldier and the commissar. Meanwhile, Mira finally got a psychiatric service set up and they were selecting staff. I sent in a text and I ended up officially named as the head of the psychiatric organization in Spain—not here, because Franco had stopped the offensive. The truth is I've never again worked as well as I did with the Spanish Communist Party. I left Bergman in Madrid and I didn't have to worry about it anymore. I was in charge in Toledo, at the Hospital de Consuegra. Emili Mira had told me that during the war in Austria, Lang—a psychiatrist, also forgotten—had organized a therapeutic community with the soldiers. So I, thanks to Mira, what I did was organize, in Almodóvar del Campo, a therapeutic community for the war mutes and schizophrenics; that lasted about two years. They had to be mute for me to accept them into the community. That, for me, was a "psychic inflation." Everyone who took care of the crazy people was chosen by me: one was a lawyer, another was a priest ... people who'd never treated crazies before. And anyone who's not stupid can become the best of psychologists, with a month of training.

Sauret was at the asylum here and took care of President Companys's son—his son was a schizophrenic. He wasn't part of the hospital staff and he was constantly dealing with the administration—like a good Catalan—of the therapeutic community. What I did was prepare ambulances, and when there was fighting going on we had ambulances for the people going through hysterical crises or whatever ... And I also organized—again, something anyone could do—welcoming the injured and those with head surgeries. So the focus was always psychoanalysis, but I never rejected either classic psychiatry or neurology.

By the way, when Lacan published his thesis in 1932 on paranoiac psychosis as it relates to the personality, we did a six-month course for the doctors because we thought that Lacan's thesis was the way to introduce, based on classic psychiatry, something that up until then hadn't worked. Lacan's thesis was extraordinarily transformative. By the way, in France it was not very well known and that is one of the few things my wife was able to save when we fled. And later Lacan's thesis was published clandestinely at Saint-Alban.

OTIUM DIAGONAL—Was that the first time you read Lacan's text? It was published here?

FRANCESC TOSQUELLES—Yes, that was my first encounter with Lacan's thesis, but the edition was the French one. You know that we're quite Frenchified here. I was upset about having to take care of anything in Madrid, having to go to Madrid to be the boss, I didn't want to get involved. I met Bergman and he seemed to me to be a man with a vision that was a bit of an Olivier salad, by that I mean he knew how to ride the fence, he must have been a radical socialist. [...]

OTIUM DIAGONAL—When the norms of the International Psychoanalytical Association place psychoanalysis in the realm of medicine—rather than psychiatry—they are excluding both psychology on one hand and psychiatry on the other, and it creates the situation we see in the International. But psychoanalysis, as it's established in Spain, is quite removed from those problems.

FRANCESC TOSQUELLES—What you do is clientele psychoanalysis. Look, I have quite a lot of experience with didactic psychoanalysis. Since 1943, I haven't accepted a single guy who tells me he wants to be a psychoanalyst. I say: "Go to an analyst." I do didactic psychoanalysis with people who want to join the field, who will do public psychoanalysis. I'm not interested in the others, because, what do you want me to do? If you lie down with dogs, you'll wake up with fleas. I'm not saying that private clientele shouldn't exist, but that's not my calling. As such, let's leave it at that it doesn't interest me.

Let's go back to the situation in Reus, even today. There were some folks who were already receiving psychoanalysis, but in Reus the progress that was made began once I'd started doing psychoanalysis with didactic doctors who were my patients. That began in 1933, with the book Mira published in 1934, which was done at Pere Mata and has one chapter written entirely by me, with the version of some drawings of the *expressive circle* or some such shit. And Mira summarized some things that I was doing in institutional analysis. I saw the problem inherent in becoming a psychoanalyst but I was lucky, because I started to do psychoanalysis with institutionalized patients and, of course, failed miserably. I published it in a journal here without explaining much about why I had failed—that was in *Fulls clínics*, a journal from Reus, in 1934. For me that was the end—well, actually it was the beginning. I began that psychoanalysis and it was my fault I failed. Because, for example, I had a patient who was a kleptomaniac and I sent him packing after three days because he stole my watch and I couldn't stand it. But I didn't explain that. What I wrote about was the other failure that led me to decide to introduce psychoanalysis very slowly into the institution. I was following a treatment with a girl who was a borderline obsessive but she could lie on a couch, and it went well for about six months or something like that. Very well! She was talking, I wasn't doing anything, and it seemed like it was going well. And suddenly one day she stopped talking. I was following the control with Sándor Eiminder and Sándor gave me a speech about mutism and such things. Well, there was a German refugee, Werner Wolff—he also worked at La Sageta—at that control too and he told me: "I know why that woman isn't speaking, and if you were more inside the institution, you would know why too." Because that woman, before coming to her analysis sessions, would lie down on the floor and another patient got behind her and listened to her. Somewhere Wolff said: "The institution is a totality."

Sándor stayed in Barcelona. By the way, for almost a year of my analysis I didn't pay, thanks to the Ateneu Barcelonès, because there was a guy there named Francisco who brought the coffee to the dining area. You would meet up with everyone there, the library was open all night, it was a fabulous place to work. I met Dalí there and a lot of other interesting people. I not only ate there every once in a while without paying, because the waiter extended me credit, but my psychoanalyst also ate there without paying, on my line of credit. Sometimes I would go to eat on Carrer Tallers, but he liked eating at the Ateneu more. Then, after the war, I paid the bill at the Ateneu for my analyst's meals.

OTIUM DIAGONAL—What was the end of the war like for you?

FRANCESC TOSQUELLES—For me the war ended on April 1. Thanks to an acquaintance and thanks to the mutes. Because, in the town I was in, I had a General Staff officer's helmet and a raincoat to go from one sector to the other, even though in my practice I always dressed as a civilian. They said I was a Catalan, and Catalans are always bustling about nervously, and that I worked miracles, because I could make the mute speak, people considered that a miracle. Every Thursday four or five got "miracled." So I was very well known in that region. And when the North African troops came in, thanks to some small maneuvers, I stayed there because officially I was already in France. But I stayed there with documents from the Spanish army and I took care of buying food for the crazies, because in that situation normal people pretended to be crazy and I had to feed them. And then I suggested to the new fascist mayor of the town that the crazies be evacuated and he didn't understand a thing. He gave me some papers so I could go get food for the crazies from Logistics, but he did it so well—the official papers—that he named me the director of the military hospital in Almodóvar del Campo, but with fascist papers. So when the others arrived, the police thought that I was a soldier, a fascist. And that was how I spent three months resting down there until I found my wife again, whom I'd lost in Aragon.

OTIUM DIAGONAL—So you crossed into France with Spanish papers?

FRANCESC TOSQUELLES—No, man, no, into Madrid! The last evacuation we did was with Sauret. We both went from near Toledo to Madrid in an ambulance. We went to the best hotel with the "director" papers they'd given me and I didn't pay. A few years later I went back to that hotel and they told me there were no vacancies. But that second time I was planning on paying. Then I went to Asturias—my wife is Asturian—and I hid for a bit while my wife looked for money. And I did two things to hide: I bought a bowler hat so no one would mistake me for a crazy and I went to the Casa de España every day to get a shave. No one ever asked me anything. Every day, I would go to the Casa de España, very serious, and read the newspaper.

I arrived in France in 1939, in September, and I was in a concentration camp where I organized a psychiatric service. And I've never done such good psychiatry as in the concentration camp. That also made it possible for some people to escape. I found an officer, a doctor from Andalusia and a relative of Charcot's son, who was angry because people were dying—well, dying ... they were actually Spaniards who were killing each other—and they needed a psychiatric hospital. He was anti-psychiatry and we understood each other right off. Coincidentally, they sent me to Saint-Alban and I went there with Sauret.

OTIUM DIAGONAL—When did you meet Lacan?

FRANCESC TOSQUELLES—In 1946 or 1947, at the end of the war.

OTIUM DIAGONAL—At the Sainte-Anne hospital?

FRANCESC TOSQUELLES—No, I didn't meet him in a hospital. I met him because I went to Paris every month to get my baccalaureate. I was the director of a hospital but I was working on my baccalaureate! I had to become French and start my studies. And, of course, I met Julián Ajuriaguerra. I'd already known him in Barcelona, because during the war he took part in taking Majorca. The Spanish socialists, along with the fascists, kicked us out because you should never let Catalans take Majorca or Valencia. But Axurria—as they called Ajurriaguerra—understood it right away, and when he came back from Majorca he went to Paris to take part in what the group of psychiatry students from Sainte-Anne were doing, in 1936; it was mostly Lacan, Ajuriaguerra, Henri Ey, and many others. [...]

Another advantage is that we were in the middle of nowhere, in a hospital with nothing and with the psychiatric tradition of the previous century shut down. Because that hospital—Saint-Alban[7]—had been created in 1820 by an anti-psychiatrist, a guy from the order of Saint-Jean-de-Dieu named Hilarion Tissot who created the first free asylum. He founded twenty-five in France and Belgium before the 1838 law. The French government was able to pass the 1838 law because of this man who'd provoked all this agitation around the creative work with the townspeople. In Montauban I met two guys who were the sons of the sons of the sons of the first psychiatric nurses in France, who were caregivers at Saint-Alban.

So, all I had to do was restart the already existing tradition, which had been forgotten. The hospital was so poorly organized, it was magnificent. Some people say that I invented the theory of vouchers and things like that. In classic hospitals, the patients were tied down. There the caregivers would bring a little cask of wine into the room and drink with the patients and they also made some money. And the patients' going out was very well organized by the caregivers, since the hospital was surrounded by a lot of forests and the patients could go out. Then the caregivers would say: They've escaped. And they would pay them five francs. They had them "escape" and the patients would spend two or three days in the caregivers' homes and then they'd split the money. So it was a magnificent hospital. I didn't have to invent anything, it was all there, I just had to give it a theoretic shape. At the same time, there was a war going on, and the Maquis were there. We were so independent that between December 1939 and 1941 Jews and Christians started arriving from all over, from the Institut Pasteur, and poets, like Paul Éluard, Tristan Tzara, the daughter of that Catalan ... Dalí, Gala's daughter. All those people lived with us. And meanwhile we had a restaurant and we had to wait for the machine guns to fall from the sky. What could we do except psychiatry and discussion? ... Because of all that France recognized me as a national hero of the Resistance over three years.

And then came the occupation of Paris, and the French couldn't live anywhere—especially if they were civil servants—if it wasn't thinking of working in Paris. I always said that we shouldn't go to Paris, that Paris would be taken by surrounding it with Maquis. They had to train twenty-five Maquis like in Saint-Alban, and with that theory I stayed in the Maquis for twenty-five years until, because of Lacan, I couldn't resist going to Paris. And thank goodness I was only there for eight years. By then they'd already opened up the borders and I could occasionally come down to the Institut Pere Mata.

OTIUM DIAGONAL—What was your link with Emili Mira?

FRANCESC TOSQUELLES—When I began studying medicine I went to Barcelona and I said to Mira: I have to work to continue with psychiatry. And he recommended I go to the Psychotechnical Institute on Carrer Urgell, because he said that to be a psychiatrist one has to study normal people. Until you understand normal people you can't learn the first thing about psychiatry. I'm talking about the Mira I met when I was six or seven years old, a relatable man, like a comfy old slipper.

OTIUM DIAGONAL—You used to say, or that was my impression, that Mira was a very eclectic person.

FRANCESC TOSQUELLES—No, not eclectic. Mira knew exactly what he was doing, he was a very practical man. As seen, for example, in his opposition to Sarró and

Montserrat. Sarró was a psychiatrist who knew a lot of things. In 1931, at the congress of the Sociedad Española de Psiquiatría in Granada, Sarró spoke on Heidegger and existentialism in psychiatry. Mira would never have tolerated that. He always said: There are the crazies, but be careful with masturbation, with fleeing the clinic, with entering the philosophers' field.

OTIUM DIAGONAL—Would you say that Mira was a clinician?

FRANCESC TOSQUELLES—Not really, because Mira's only clinic was here, in Reus. What he did have was good experience working with children, normal people, workers. I don't know if you know that the Psychotechnical Institute, on Carrer Urgell, was practically in the hands of the Socialist Union of Catalonia. There were about twenty-five of them who worked with Capdelans and Mira, with Comorera even, who came from the Socialist Party of Catalonia, and he was a teacher there and he didn't deal with psychiatric problems. The first two institutes of professional training were founded in Barcelona and Chicago, and that was Mira's doing. In that sense, when I asked him about studying the mad in Barcelona, Mira told me: Go study normal people.

OTIUM DIAGONAL—Mira worked on tests to choose bus drivers, right?

FRANCESC TOSQUELLES—Yes, for the Roca company. I was involved too and I had a ton of fun. We tried to do psychodramatic things—not Moreno's psychodrama, not that. That was the first time I cured a guy from Cotard's delusion. I was interested in that syndrome because Dr. Vilaseca had published an article about it. Coincidentally, a Valencian painter showed up with Cotard's delusion,[8] and of course what always happens happened. With Rusiñol's nephew—because everybody came to the Institut Pere Mata to be with us—we'd made some attempts at psychodrama to cure a hysterical girl. We had him act out *The Taming of the Shrew*. Well, Rusiñol took it seriously. That must have been around 1929, because around 1931 he was already somewhat better. We did theater every Sunday, and one day he had the balls to organize a trial with the patients—the "lawyers" were drug addicts—and we found the stage set up like a courtroom. Suddenly, two civil guards showed up and grabbed the guy with Cotard's delusion, who was in the audience, and the trial began. Solanes and I were worried, we didn't know what to do. After a little while they suspended the trial and the hearing continued a few days later. Then we interceded. The psychotherapy continued and the guy was cured. We still have a couple of his paintings hanging at the Institut. He was a pretty good painter. He was a plagiarist, but the real plagiarism wasn't the paintings, it was his son. The day he was able to make a painting of his son as the plagiarism of a son, his Cotard's delusion abated!

OTIUM DIAGONAL—You've had experiences in hospitals, were you able to confirm what Lacan proposes about the relationship between psychosis and the Name-of-the-Father?

FRANCESC TOSQUELLES—Cotard's delusion is perhaps easier to cure because, as Klein would say, it is post-depressive, it is manic-depressive psychosis. And for that, not even contemporary psychiatry maintains anti-Abrahamic attitudes. To alarm you I'll say that classic psychoanalysis can only cure normal people, the so-called normal people. Of course, "the normal" have a lot of nerve …

OTIUM DIAGONAL—The question was whether you believe that paternity is the nodal point in psychosis, as put forth by Lacan.

FRANCESC TOSQUELLES—That wasn't what I understood, because you mentioned the Name-of-the-Father. That said, which father are we talking about? It's a mythical name. Sometimes it's God, or it doesn't matter whom it refers to. In any case, I think it is important. Once a melancholic period ends, the patient might enter into a hypomanic phase. To enter into Oedipus, one must kill the father. One of the aspects of law—as the Jews rightly said—is not the law of the father, but rather the interdiction on killing the father or mother. And this very law of not killing is as important or more than the prohibition of incest, mostly because it is a law that everyone transgresses. People kill each other like lice and nothing happens—well, or it seems as if nothing happens.

These ideas are more indebted to Mira than to my own analysis, because Mira was very clear on this point: it is not about a real father. On the other hand, the Lacanian basis in language I owe to Sarró. He had theorized about the language of schizophrenics and that which is called "the change" or the destruction, the way words lose their connotations and become only denotive, becoming purely denotational without any connotations.

Four years ago I finished writing a book on the poetic function of language in the poetry of Gabriel Ferrater. The Centre de Cultura[9] is due to publish it. These books are of interest to everyone, even poets, as long as they don't mention psychiatry. It's the same in France.

Going back to what we were saying about the father. In relating with my mother, all I had to do was eat, shit, smile, and so on … But one day I discovered that there were people who could mobilize my mother more easily than I, who got her to speak. Because there is no maternal language, maternal language is this [*he points to his mouth*], like dogs licking you. Language is always paternal, it's the language that is collective. And access to language is access to the language of a collective community. And the father is not just a guy who fucks, it doesn't matter, anyone can be the father.

OTIUM DIAGONAL—That's what Freud proposes in *Totem and Taboo*. The father is anyone who holds that function, not necessarily the progenitor.

FRANCESC TOSQUELLES—Of course. There are always several fathers. Any guy who comes by and talks to the mother is a father, even if it's a woman. I mention that because there are women who are much more paternal than any father. Just as people say: What a woman! But it's not about whether they have a penis or not, it's because they talk to the mother instead of just saying "waah-waah." Pissing, shitting, and waah-waahing is enough to be able to relate to the mother. Well, on a basic level …

OTIUM DIAGONAL—That is related to hypochondria, the mortified body.

FRANCESC TOSQUELLES—Of course. Especially when the mother says, "Does it hurt you here? Don't eat that, it'll hurt your tummy. Are your lips hurting? Is your foot hurting?" Medea's passion is that of the mothers who eat their own children—half the things mothers say are about headaches, tummy aches, about all the nasty bodily things. Luckily there are fathers who work outside the home, go out dancing, brothers, neighbors, things like that, things that separate you from hypochondria. If by some miracle the mother speaks to her son, he's probably a hypochondriac, he has no choice.

Then, you can see how, arriving in France with such clear, sibylline, anti-psychiatric ideas, Lacan waited until I left Saint-Alban to visit there. I was always inviting him and he never dared come. That is due to the articulation of castration with the country's geography and history, because to get to Saint-Alban, you had to pass through "Lacan de la Roche" where there was a Roman *castrum*. *Castrum*, or castle—in other words, the limits that cannot be passed.

Okay, let's go back to the institutions. When I lived in Reus, on one corner there was the secondary school I studied at and on the other was the Institut Pere Mata. As you can see my childhood was very institutional! All that made me consider the problem of what the hell the institution meant. And what they call institutions is precisely the lack of institution. They are "establishments," or as we say in French, *établissements*. And what psychiatrists did is convert establishments into institutions. It also happens with marriage, because getting married is adopting a state, and the problem becomes turning this "adopting a state" into an institution, because if you get married and fuck because it's Friday, that's not an institution, that's an *établissement*. So it has to go from an establishment to a permanent state. Which is why I've always been in favor of the permanent nation and not the permanent state.

OTIUM DIAGONAL—Do you believe the state is always maternal?

FRANCESC TOSQUELLES—The state is always fascist, they are the people who hinder institutions, and that's from the very invention of things, be they Telefónica or the LOAPA [Ley Orgánica de Armonización del Proceso Autonómico, a 1982 law designed to facilitate the establishment of Spain's autonomous regions], it doesn't matter. It's the same when they're right-wing, left-wing, or center. The function of the state is to impede institutions, even marriage. It's right there in the word: adopt a state. And the same thing happens if we think about an asylum or a clinic: "We've placed her there, we've got the girl placed." There are people who become like states, in analysis too. And look, they do their little state song and dance, they live in the analytic state.

OTIUM DIAGONAL—It's the ritualization, the state of grace …

FRANCESC TOSQUELLES—What state of grace? State of disgrace! Grace is a way of leaving the state. Just look at Barcelona, it would've been a disaster if not for Sants on one side, Sant Andreu on the other, and above it all the Passeig de Gràcia. Gràcia is what saves Barcelona.

OTIUM DIAGONAL—Dr. Tosquelles, *moltes gràcies* [thanks a lot] for this conversation!

PSYCHOANALYSIS IN CHURCH, SCHOOL, OR THE CIVIL GUARD

FRANCESC TOSQUELLES—The Institut Pere Mata came about in a very unique way, compared to the psychiatric assistance in Catalonia and Spain at the start of the twentieth century. From the beginning it was organized around two or three "original" ideas. There is a project, which I can't call mythic, because that's not what myth is, an almost outrageous project: namely, that people, both doctors and not, believe that "crazy" people would be cured by being treated well. Even if they were isolated. Yes, as the philanthropists said, they would put them in a luxurious cage, with all the accommodations, air—that was a French idea, so the patients could breathe, they would have the right to eat calmly and breathe calmly, and also to clean themselves, to purify themselves with water ... Then, if they were treated well, with all the ambiguity implied in that term, the patients would find the peace, the calm, the tranquility and as the Institut Pere Mata motto says, their intelligence would be reignited—*Flammabo Iterum*. Intelligence, the fire of the soul, the spirit would be aflame again ... It's a simple idea, repeated throughout the history of psychiatry, even now ...

If only it were accompanied by another that was characteristic of the previous century: people who guard over the insane in a prison, in a total institution—in Goffman's definition—contribute to their madness, or at the very least maintain it.

After all, who made them go crazy? I will give a common answer and say: society or family. Now it is also said—it's been said since the start of the century, but they gave another response: if it is family who makes them crazy, separating them from their family will bring them calm. The asylum—the ideas that built asylums in the last century are not what Foucault says—exists to protect the patients from their families, first of all, and, secondly, from society. Protect them, at least, from their family and society.

Tranquility, air, good water, calm, and perhaps friendship to cure the crazy. That was the philanthropists' project and ideology. And that was basically what the Institut Pere Mata organized with a certain atmosphere of freedom, openness. The patients could leave, work, do theater, dance. [...]

FRANCESC VILÀ—Maybe we should mention the beginning of the Mira period.

FRANCESC TOSQUELLES—Yes, it gained some new momentum when Mira took over. In 1929, with the Barcelona International Exhibition, a congress was organized with the French doctors at the Institut. There was a new energy and I was involved from the very start. Projects by old Briansó were carried out and by Mira, no longer about how to organize work and leisure time, but about group psychotherapy, the class method, Kaplan's.

FRANCESC VILÀ—The class method?

Excerpt from Francesc Vilà's interview of Francesc Tosquelles, *L'Acudit: Publicació de psicoanàlisi*, no. 1, October 1985, pp. 38–45.

FRANCESC TOSQUELLES—That method consisted of gathering the patients and telling them: "You speak of hallucinations, that comes from the brain. That is very important for you, let's talk about it here if you'd like, but don't bring it up out on the street, or with the mayor, or your wife. Come here to tell us about those things that are happening to you." The idea is that, deep down, everyone is crazy, there are those who conceal it and those who don't. Do what we do. It worked quite well when dealing with delirious and hallucinatory attitudes.

FRANCESC VILÀ —Other psychotherapeutic and innovative experiences for the period?

FRANCESC TOSQUELLES—Recently I received a young music teacher who appears in the photograph of a choir in Mira's book. His name is Tous. He brought me a journal that I used to edit, here in Reus. I'd forgotten about it. It's called *Estudis*. It dealt with a little bit of everything [in the 1930s]. Tous wrote an article about how to use music with schizophrenics and patients in general. He brought it for me to read. It was a journal that was also tied to those at the Institut Pere Mata, to Reus. I spoke about La Gota de Llet, too …

FRANCESC VILÀ—Can you explain more?

FRANCESC TOSQUELLES—Here in Reus there was a pediatrician, very distanced from Winnicott, who was a really good pediatrician, an organicist and meticulous. Two good characteristics, and good character is already a good start. This good man was teaching mothers how to nurse. He asked me—it turns out he sometimes needed a hand—to take care of two things: attending to nurslings and their mothers and, additionally, to the somewhat older kids who were having problems at school. I set up a doctor's office to do tests on the children. But that wasn't enough: what I was looking to do, and he authorized it straightaway, was to receive the mothers in a group, the mothers with babies, even the pregnant women who hadn't yet given birth. I would gather them. Since I was very young—they were older than me—I never played the wise man. The excuse was the following: "I'm finishing my degree, I'm still studying and I wanted to do a project on the difficulties that mothers have, when pregnant, when they have their babies, taking care of them … Since I don't know anything about it, would you please tell me? That way I can do this research project." That shifted the attention from me to them: "I don't know anything about it, explain it to me."

For me, it was research that would enrage Lacan, that concern for mothers' behavior and their babies; that's more Kleinian, even Freud's daughter ended up doing it, sending people to the maternity ward.

FRANCESC VILÀ—You insisted they explain things to you. You were listening to what the mothers were saying …

FRANCESC TOSQUELLES—You cannot start analyzing someone because he tells you "I want to be analyzed." There is a pretransference that means, if you don't take it into consideration, that much classical analysis won't work. It won't work for the following reason: because the client has a false idea of what he has to do and, most of all, because he doesn't want to do it. There are many people who say "I want to do analysis" but, actually, they don't want to. For a while you have to use tricks, not to seduce the patient but so the analysis can begin. After coming for a year, two years, three years, they say now they understand it differently. I tell them: Fine, start all over again. There are clients who start their analysis two, three times … Before that happens, you have to reach the end of a part that while it isn't entirely a waste because it always has some effect, it's a waste in terms of the trajectory toward a successful ending of the analysis.

I still have two didactic-analysis patients who've been coming and paying for four and six years, and they still haven't begun. When I say "begin," I mean never systematically—Freud never did it; it's called the fundamental rule and, okay, the analyst starts listening like a chump for the red thread that ties together the *acudits* (jokes) that make no sense, they come out as jokes. I love the title of your magazine because if you say "witticisms" it doesn't mean anything, if you say "free association" it sounds very intellectual … I really like the use of *acudit* because it's like a mash-up of *orella* (ear)—"acoustic"—and *dit* (said). I've used that many times with Oury. I explain things to him in Catalan, I think that if you don't speak Catalan you can't understand any language. If Freud had known Catalan instead of Spanish, he would've done better. He would've spoken about the *acudit*, the way I do in my book: *ear* and *said* coming together. That's better than "joke," which sounds like mocking: an *acudit* can be very serious, but what's important is not that but the red thread, as Freud said, the link with something that might be related to the poetic function of language I study in my book.

If Freud had identified as Jewish and Catalan, instead of wanting to conceal the fact that he was Czech and Jewish! Some of his colleagues from Budapest had problems with him because they were separatists and didn't want to have anything to do with Austrians, while Freud was pro-Austrian, he would say he was an Austrian. He wrote German very well, but he didn't know Czech, and when he writes in Jewish, it's a mess. […] If Freud knew a little bit of the history of the Jews, and particularly the Jews in Catalan lands … Or another Aragonese who wrote in Catalan, Arnau de Vilanova. He wrote the best work on dreams—it's almost as good as Freud's and, in some aspects, better—but, of course, Freud only knew the Spanish horses that paraded with soldiers through Vienna … He read *Life is a Dream* by Calderón …

I discovered Arnau de Vilanova through the *Monografies Mèdiques* that in those days was run by the mayor of Barcelona, Jaume Aiguader. I talk about that in an article.[1]

His difference from Freud is clear. In that period they would hire him because they wanted to know what their dreams meant so they could predict the future … He did that work because of the social demand of the time. He follows a method similar to the one Freud used for cocaine, which was a scientific method, of methodical application and explanation. Freud is exemplary in the study of cocaine, both in terms of research and in exposition.

FRANCESC VILÀ—Can you talk a little bit about your experience in analysis?

FRANCESC TOSQUELLES—It's good if one starts analysis working, doing ergotherapy … or as a bricklayer or even at school working on spelling errors, for example. One has to wait for the opportunity—otherwise it doesn't function, the analysts can see that clearly, it's something else, it's not psychoanalyzing the child because of spelling errors.

The first analysis I did here, in Reus, people came the way they visit doctors, Adlerian doctors. I would ask them: "Is your father dead? Is he alive? Did he die of a hernia? ... Tell me what you remember about your father ... your mother ..." etc. Instead of looking for germs, we were looking for memories of the elements of the family constellation, and then, of course, he would work on it himself in an Adlerian fashion. And often, maybe ten out of every forty times, the client would say, "Oh, I think there are other things, sexual problems." Finally, more or less secretly, he would end up saying that there were sex problems. Then my moment would come and I would say, "That can't be treated like this, for that you need to be lying on a couch, with a different method. Say whatever you want as long as it's not about sex. But I can't tolerate us discussing your sexual conflicts when you're seated, it's useless." I had a dozen private psychoanalysis clients here in Reus. Turning the Adlerian relationship into psychoanalysis. I say that because in analysis what is most difficult is how to introduce the analytical relationship. That's not simple. That's also important for what we've been discussing during these days of the conference, about the analytic work at the Centre Balmes. How to sell psychoanalysis at the Plaça Prim or at the Civil Guard station.

I recall a French experience that I didn't organize. Many years ago—around 1953 or 1954—I went to a conference in Bordeaux. An analyst brought me to Cambo—a small town in the mountains—where there were ten Spanish priests and a dozen French ones. They all had sexual problems, they brought them to that institution in Cambo to live in an analytic community and this guy was in charge of the group analysis sessions for the priests. I really enjoyed it, because it was surprising to talk to Spanish priests who were being psychoanalyzed. While it might seem foolish, it made me think about how one introduces analysis. And why not into a group of priests, or in the army, just as into a school? It's the same thing. There are the same difficulties in introducing psychoanalysis in the Catholic church, in a school, or in the Civil Guard headquarters. Or, as you know firsthand, into families, when things go differently than they'd ideally hoped for.

IT'S THE DESTINY OF MADNESS THAT IS MAN'S ESSENCE

CÉCILE HAMSY—You're of Spanish origin—

FRANÇOIS TOSQUELLES—I am Catalan. I've tried to communicate with the Spaniards, since I'm married to a Spanish woman. I've also made civil war against the Spaniards, but I haven't managed to communicate. I do still have …

CÉCILE HAMSY—You mean to say that there are things that are blocked, and it makes more sense to look at what is not possible, to face that instead of trying right away—

FRANÇOIS TOSQUELLES—That's it, I think you've found an expression I can use. It's more pragmatic to try and see what is not possible, than to think in a silly way that everything is possible … to think that what I desire is possible, to confuse the vagaries and sometimes the absolute of my desire with what is possible. I've never understood what Lacan calls the *petit a*, but in the end I think it must be that. When one can't go on thinking like a dimwit that my desire is possible, as an absoluteness, one lets the capitalized "Other," *l'Autre*, drop—it remains *a*, and perhaps that is sort of a little sign, a little indication of the absolute. The *petit a* is a little indication of the absolute … But anyway, I say these things to warm us up. People are a bit surprised, especially when the talk is centered around my reading of, my acquaintance or my work with, Lacan, in parentheses. Because when you come down to it, I've had very few direct relations with Lacan. The first was almost imaginary … That is, I was going about my business at the psychiatric hospital of Reus, in 1934 it seems to me … Reus, in Spain, at the Institut Pere Mata. Wait, I have a photo here. In that same office we held a meeting, you would call it a seminar now, but with no more than five or six persons, to read and comment on Lacan's dissertation that was given to me and explained somewhat by my mentor and friend, Professor Mira, who was an extraordinary figure, not eclectic but he could make it possible to know all the directions and diverse forms that psychiatry was taking in the world. He wasn't an enthusiast reduced to a single system …

CÉCILE HAMSY—He was open.

FRANÇOIS TOSQUELLES—He was open. He didn't know how to tell stories, but though he believed he should play the professor role, and introduce his students to all types of psychiatrists or psychiatry, he reserved the things that seemed useful to him for his practice, jetissoning all the nonsense that might be talked about or encountered in the history of psychiatry, although he would explain everything. Obviously, Lacan, his theory, reached us at the right moment … because in Catalonia in those days we were already very aware,

---

Radio interview with François Tosquelles by Cécile Hamsy and Jean Guir, *France Culture*, October 4, 1985, published in *L'Interdit*, no. 14 (1987), pp. 54–61. Revised transcription.

I was very aware, of where I was headed professionally. My orientation, my professional destiny was to see how one could introduce, in a practical way, psychoanalytic theories and practice into the psychiatric hospitals. I don't mean hiring a psychoanalyst who would come and pretend to do psychoanalysis in their bureau, but I had the notion, along with Freud I believe, that psychiatry, if it was anything serious, could only be the history of the various forms that the dialectic of drives could take in the defense system that every person, every group, will marshal in facing the libidinal flux. So it was necessary to bring into a field of action, of practice, this postulate, this a priori view of man's malaise, of man's existence, of which the deranged are only a sort of caricature, only one example among others. The notion of biological illness is rather cheap, really. I'm not saying that biological illness doesn't exist, but even if it does in certain cases it's obvious that if you go into the street and a roof tile falls on your head you will get a brain hemorrhage, you will have an organic lesion. But for that to make you crazy, all your being will have to be engaged, perhaps on the occasion of the tile striking its blow. So as Freud would say, it's a question that concerns the future of the drives and your system of defense. Now all this is still very abstract, because one doesn't learn anything about your drives and your defense system if it's not through the act of speaking, through what you may say, and all the more readily if you're bullshitting, if you're fooling around, instead of speaking too seriously, so that nothing is revealed. This is the sense in which culture is a cover, a mask for not knowing anything about oneself or others.

Already when I was very little, around the age of ten or eleven, I decided on psychiatry as a serious path for myself. I more or less knew then that what it was about was the problems that had been touched upon in the study of human beings through the practice of psychoanalysis, through Freud's practice. Everything I was told about people, about human psychology, stuff that circulated at school, the foolish stuff of the lycées—human will, intelligence, memory, I don't know what, the workings of the soul—all of that seemed perfectly stupid to me. And it was even starting then that Mira's teaching, which I was already acquainted with when I was ten years old, seemed right, since he rejected the whole of classical psychology, with two curious bridges: on the one hand, the value that an experimental psychology might have, the testing business, not IQ tests, but all the tests of behavior, all the experimental psychology, which is an activity full of consequences and on the other hand, that experimental situation which is psychoanalysis, which is the experience of the birth of speech, the rebirth of memory. And for that, for knowing something about your way of being and how you put yourself together, about your construction as a subject, there is only one path. It's by way of the lies and errors and the obfuscations of memory, what you can recreate once more about yourself, that something of your truth will appear. That's what psychoanalysis is. No psychoanalysis without speech, and not speech as a dialogue: I speak, you reply to me, you speak, I reply to you, to see who wins and who conceals themselves the best. Freud's discovery, a gradual one moreover, was to abandon dialogue, leaving only the evocations, the instantiations of speech, the *evocare* of the client—I don't say the patient—of anyone—which the analyst tries to follow ... not even a monologue, because in the analytic situation one doesn't expect the person stretched out on the couch to be forced to respond toc and toc like in a tennis match ... I ask you, you answer back, and so on. Finally, then, on that basis there may be a sort of shift and one witnesses the creation of the subject, the creation of oneself. So it's all of this that is thwarted, or placed in check, one might say, in so-called mental illness, or at least in what is at the origin of people's distress.

CÉCILE HAMSY—You spoke of Lacan's doctoral thesis.

FRANÇOIS TOSQUELLES—It was a chance awareness, deliberately occasioned, let's say, by Mira, who was behind a seminar we did over a period of three months to read Lacan's material, but the true goal of which was not just familiarization with what Lacan was saying—it was more of a ploy to interest some aging classical psychiatrists in problems of the complexity of personhood, of the personality, with a kind of mélange of poetry and politics, from a Freudian orientation, already, or love in any case—the case of Aimée—*poetry and politics*.

CÉCILE HAMSY—And you spoke of surrealism?

FRANÇOIS TOSQUELLES—Yes. We were all a bit surrealist at the time. You mustn't forget that we're from the land of Dalí and that when I was little I knew Dalí and we laughed a lot together. It was the avant-garde social service, you see, and perhaps even the site of avant-garde political activities ... For that matter, Catalans are avant-gardist by definition. One had to be at the forefront. And there is another important story perhaps, which Lacan fits right into. It's that Lacan was largely the student of Gatian de Clérambault. French psychiatry had a big impact in the last nineteenth century, let's say in Catalonia rather than in Spain. In the last century in Catalonia, French psychiatry was cutting-edge. It was what interested everybody, and services were created that were oriented essentially in the French perspective. When French psychiatry disappeared, at the turn of the century, there floated up valuable pieces of French psychiatry, known not only in Catalonia but here and there and everywhere: Minkowski, the phenomenologist, on the one hand, and de Clérambault on the other. It's a thing that surprised me greatly that when I arrived in France and was asked what I thought of current French psychiatry, I'm talking 1939–1940, I would say "Minkowski, de Clérambault," and the average French psychiatrist had no awareness at all of de Clérambault nor of Minkowski. It was guys who were not fully of the profession, or not at all of the medical profession, civil servants, so those two were not known, and on the other hand they appeared by way of a contrast. Especially de Clérambault, who had already entered into crisis, one could say, against the medico-psychological cohort, which had created a separate society, by showing the human being's complexity from various perspectives ... So we had become very interested in de Clérambault, because of the matter of complexity ... A statement by de Clérambault spoke of "self-constructive delirium." One needs to take that literally. You are an impersonal delirium, you have constructed yourself. You are an architecture, you have pinched stories from your father, from your mother, from your first cousin, from the dog that passed by in the street, and even from Monsieur de Gaulle. But with these pieces, these bricks, you have constructed your swell architecture, using several levels of logic. There are several levels of logic in yourself, I don't say several persons, but in washing your suit of clothes, one sees the logic of your skin with its holes, and before the skin one finds another logic, and you are the outcome of the overlapping and interferences between these several logics.

CÉCILE HAMSY—Who is the psychiatrizable subject here? Is it someone who's not succeeded in this work?

FRANÇOIS TOSQUELLES—Ah, precisely. It's someone poorly constructed, or someone who's swallowed a dose of de Gaulle and been thrown into a state that has blocked their whole heart, or their whole liver, both their balls, as you like. Because this movement of the human being that I call self-constructive is not an operation upon stable matter, it's a mobile impetus. You are Calder's mobile. As soon as you try to move in your core material, that's when it gets too heavy. Maybe you can manage a Rodin-type thing, with a monument of I don't know how many kilos, but you're fucked, you're dead. Those Rodin monuments are for dead people … I say that to contrast them with the mobiles of Calder.

So in any case, for us what was useful was to produce a kind of subversion of the psychiatrists who risked nodding off peacefully into the generalized psychiatric idiocies … And so Lacan came to pick up on a couple of items in classical psychiatry, especially in his course on the delirium of being loved … and who doesn't have an interest in the delirium of being loved? Madame, you yourself know, though I don't know anything about you, but in this monumentally mobile construction of you, it is love that counts, even the love of de Gaulle, you understand? If you take a piece of de Gaulle and you stand it up straight, it's out of love of de Gaulle. This is always a sort … a way of being … At the time they called it, along with de Clérambault, erotomania, which doesn't mean … It's the delirium of being loved. Who loves me and what are my loves? What my loves are, that's what my being is. It's everything. So it was very good for perverting the psychiatrists who wanted to do a purely biological psychiatry, or a psychiatry of notation. Someone shows up and says: "Last night the Chinese came and scratched my brain from inside, and nearly killed me." The psychiatrist listens to them, and he writes, "A delusion of Chinese persecution." That introduces nothing from the point of view of construction, of what this signified, how the dreamer placed these Chinese within their history, if you like.

The utility of Lacan, for us, was the subversive effect, the psychoanalytic introduction of an opening, of saying, "Gallant psychiatrists, if you close the house to every psychoanalytic problem you're screwed." It's not that they're cops like the anti-psychiatrists say—that they're persecutors, cops, which doesn't serve any fucking purpose … because their theory, their theory of practice is a story that goes nowhere, because it's radically false.

CÉCILE HAMSY—What is it that's false exactly?

FRANÇOIS TOSQUELLES—The whole concept of man. On that exact subject at liberation, in 1947 it seems to me, there was a series of lectures in Paris at the École normale, rue d'Ulm. A whole series of lectures was organized on the notions of man in psychiatry and contemporary neurology, and a lot of people participated. Minkowski and Lacan, obviously me. In my case, it was curious, because obviously, since I was not in the Communist Party … but still I knew Marxism rather well …

CÉCILE HAMSY—Yes, I saw that you gave a seminar on the relations between Marx and Freud.

FRANÇOIS TOSQUELLES—That's right. So in 1947 or 1946, rue d'Ulm, it was my assignment to elaborate on the understanding of man in Marxism, the psychiatric conception of man, I mean. And as you can imagine, the judgment of the Communist Party was on the angry side, because what I said mattered to me, obviously. Wallon was there, incidentally ... Henri Wallon, who was the minister of national education at the time. I considered that it was a clearly Marxist approach to man, as to the beginnings and development of children. However, I had gotten back into a rather big fight there with Zazzo for example ... He was a protégé of Wallon, but it was national education, you see what I'm saying? He understood nothing about man's evolution, I mean man whose essential quality—and on this point I'm in agreement with Lacan—is to be crazy. If man isn't crazy, then he is nothing. The problem is determining how he deals with his madness. If you are not crazy, how do expect someone to be in love with you? Not even yourself, you see. Which doesn't mean that if you don't know how to be crazy, then they will stick you in the psychiatric hospital, because the crazies that are put in the psychiatric hospitals are folks who make a hash of their madness. What is crucial for humans is to carry their madness off successfully. Lacan speaks seriously about the matter, he says it better, he talks about a "limit situation," about *liberté*, which is very smooth, but in reality, this is how it is. So finally, madame, I will tell you, "If you're not crazy, you're lost," because you won't have any access to yourself and you won't be able to give any of yourself to the other, to the other that you love. Everybody knows that love is a madness. It's madness that's not just pleasurable, but ... that discovers, precisely. Love is not getting naked in order to see your meat, it's to discover your being! You can discover your being only in madness, and in the madness that is for the other—that is, if you're not crazy in love with some fool, like me or somebody else, you will never know what you are. That's clear, no? It's the destiny of madness that is the essence of man. If an individual makes a mess of their own madness, if everyone, and they first of all, denies their madness—it's the function of denial, as in Lacan's dénégation or Freud's—from that moment, everything is hopeless, it's zero, really.

CÉCILE HAMSY—But you yourself have tried to treat what are called the mentally ill?

FRANÇOIS TOSQUELLES—Yes, I've done nothing but that all my life. I began at the age of seven.

CÉCILE HAMSY—So how did you do that?

FRANÇOIS TOSQUELLES—As best I could with what I had. That is—

CÉCILE HAMSY—With your own madness?

FRANÇOIS TOSQUELLES—Ha, yes, with my madness!

II

THERAPEUTIC EXPERIENCES IN WARTIME

REUS, THE ARAGON FRONT, THE EXTREMADURAN ARMY, AND THE SEPTFONDS CAMP

1936–1939

In Aragon, first of all, we suggested they listen to Schubert's *Unfinished Symphony*. I don't know if it was the music itself or the title that suggested that life never ended and didn't stop at the first obstacle. We all felt the fear of dying with our boots on. Lying down and with the music playing, they loosened up and relaxed a little. In any case, then they managed to say something about their lives without any explicit questioning on our part. *Interrogating someone increases their fear.*

FRANCESC TOSQUELLES

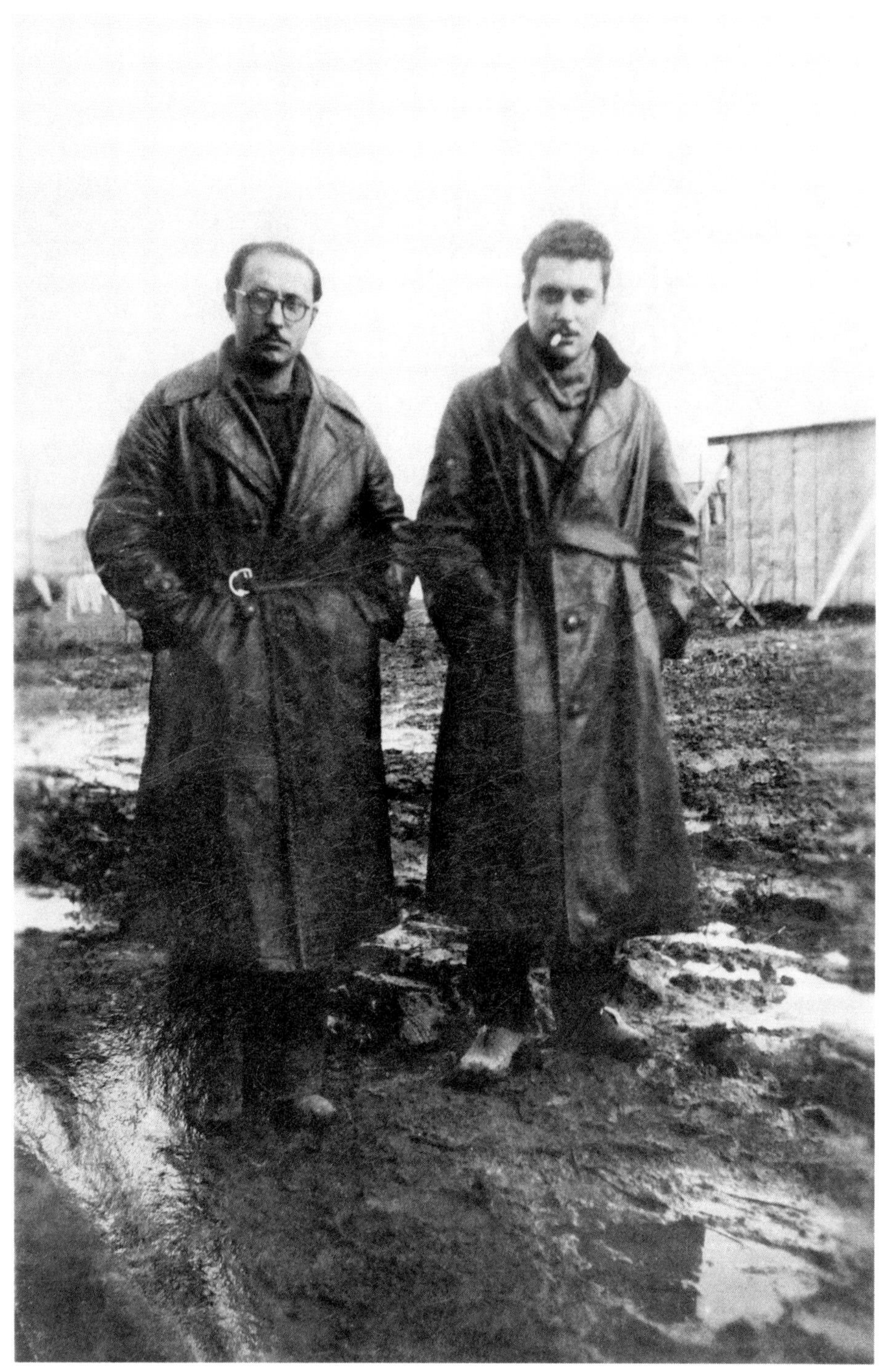

Francesc Tosquelles and Jaume Sauret at the Septfonds camp, 1939

Psychiatry Everywhere

The outbreak of the Spanish Civil War, in the summer of 1936, marked the beginning of a long trajectory of experimental practices—beyond the walls of any hospital, off the map and without dedicated spaces—with which Tosquelles redefined the collective imaginary of psychiatry. The actions of those years extended into new territories in the wake of what Emili Mira called "extensive psychiatry." Rooted in pragmatism, for Tosquelles the extensive dimension of psychiatric practice involved precise, possible action tied to people's various social activities. These actions were not restricted to the curing of patients and to the therapeutic staff, but rather focused on people and their human condition. This expanded psychiatric practice was carried out from limitations and contingencies, and distanced itself from the utopic and revolutionary ideas on how to eradicate mental illness: either by destroying psychiatric hospitals and their walls, or by integrating patients into the so-called normality of civil life. It was a practice geared toward sector psychiatry, which was deployed in situ as a radical critique of psychiatry as a self-enclosed discipline, with a specific objective and outlines. Disseminating psychiatry everywhere implied expanding psychiatric practice itself, dispersing its clinical competencies and blurring the rigid border separating madness from normality, insociability from society, and illness from health. Thanks to this expansion, sector psychiatry approximated social work and forms of implication and experimental pedagogy.

> Thus psychotechnics, child therapeutics, and the scenarios of the legal system constitute pragmatic spaces of what Mira defined as "extensive psychiatry." Destroying the psychiatric hospitals doesn't reduce madness to nothingness and shifting it onto community sites contributes in fact to ignorance about it.
>
> [...] Most often, the activities of sector psychiatry miss their objectives for the fact that the psychiatrists continue to concentrate solely on what they call "the treatment of mental illnesses."
>
> In order for sector psychiatry to have an operative impact—including upon the so-called mental illnesses—we (the caregiving personnel) must take part in numerous precise social activities which reach every person as such; more exactly, we must involve ourselves in the vagaries of extensive psychiatry.
>
> It's not at all a matter of going out to do "psychiatry" wherever there are human beings; rather, the psychiatrists themselves have to foreground their own human dimension in their work, at the risk of a certain scattering.[1]
>
> François Tosquelles, *L'Enseignement de la folie* [The lessons of madness], 1992

This diffuse, scattered psychiatry was carried out during wartime. In that political context, Tosquelles leads a child and adolescent psychotherapy center in two farmhouses on the road to Salou, which had been requisitioned by Josep Hortoneda, head of medicine and social aid for the Reus Anti-Fascist Committee. Since the nationalization of hospitals and schools both lay and religious, the pedagogy was coeducational and modern, and that therapeutic experience was aided by such figures as the teacher Joan Ganigué and Jesús Montaner, an athlete who led playful psychomotor activities with the children, in a continuation of Tosquelles's work at La Gota de Llet and with therapeutic mothering.[2] One of those farmhouses, Mas de Macià Vilà, which was later called Mas del Quer and Mas d'en Boule, requisitioned by the Republican

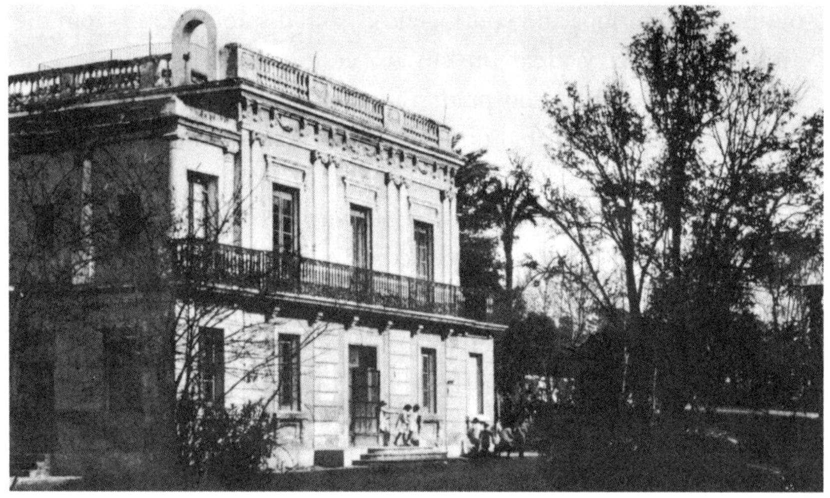

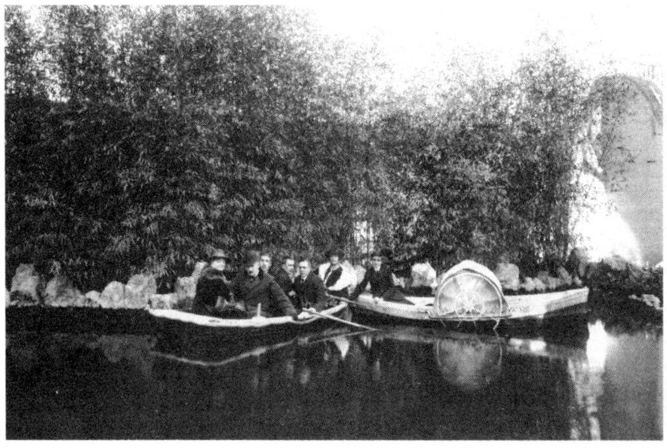

Above, the Mas del Quer, built in 1851 on the road to Salou

Left, the pond of Mas del Quer, circa 1920

Generalitat in 1936, was demolished in 1968, but over the years had retained traces of its successive uses: clinic, child and adolescent therapeutic center, family home and luxurious upper-class residence, women's school, farm, orchard with fruit trees, warehouse and offices of the family business.

After General Franco's coup d'etat against the Republic in July 1936, the working classes in Catalonia developed forms of collective economy based in expropriation, socialization, and self-management. They requisitioned and occupied privately owned and ecclesiastical buildings, farmhouses and estates belonging to large landowners, workshops and factories, more than ten thousand businesses that were the basis of the Catalan economy. That included the socialization of wood and other raw materials; unions and cooperatives worked to organize production around the humanization of work. And that was possible thanks to the creation of new schools, reading rooms, libraries, gyms and pools for the working classes, while transforming working spaces and the capacities and competencies of all in a moment of crisis for social order and hierarchies. The Republican forces—which included libertarian and anti-fascist groups and the political parties and unions (POUM, FAI, CNT, UGT, PCC, PSUC)—carried out the collectivizations, and organized the anti-fascist militias who went to fight on the front. From Reus, volunteers from the POUM and the ERC (Esquerra Republicana de Catalunya, or the Republican Left of Catalonia) youth groups, including Francesc Tosquelles, went to the Aragon front to work in the various spaces that had been requisitioned and collectivized.

On August 5, 1936, the Generalitat of Catalonia confiscated the Institut Pere Mata. More accurately, this was perpetrated by the Central Committee of Anti-Fascist Militias of Barcelona, which was the true organ of power in those moments. On August 13, the Workers' Control Committee was created at the Society of Various Professions and took over the institution. The former members of the administrative council were outside of the city and, in some cases, of the country. However, the takeover did not cause any radical changes to the life of the institution. Many of the nuns remained in their usual jobs and Sister Ana Fernández Rojas became the head of the field hospital that was established in one of the wings. As the months passed and the war front drew closer, the Institut, then the military-base hospital of the Ebro army, was moved in October 1938 to the Montesquiu castle in the Osona region. In 1939, the facilities were turned into a Francoist "Campo de Concentración de Prisioneros y Presentados."[3]

Josep M. Roig, Joan Navais, Frederic Samarra, and Montserrat Duch, "Entre dues dictadures: 1923–1975," in Pere Anguera's *Història General de Reus*

MINUTES OF THE WORKERS' CONTROL COMMITTEE

Dr. Tosquelles enters: [...] He formulates the following questions: "Is the Institut Pere Mata a militarized organization, beholden to the discipline of the War Health Committee? Or is it an organization of social aid? If that is not the case, is the Institut Pere Mata an industry taken over by worker control? [...] How has it been or how should it be structured?" He also says that a coordinated action of new organization must be undertaken.[4]

Book of minutes of the l'Institut Pere Mata Workers' Control Committee, minutes of the October 24, 1936, meeting

Working with the War

Tosquelles took part in the psychiatric services organized by the Catalan militiamen on the Aragon front. Working beside traumatologists, surgeons, dentists, nurses, and practitioners associated with the Clínic hospital in Barcelona, he was an active member of the Sariñena sanitarium as a general practitioner and surgeon's assistant, and he made caring for the medical community the focus of his practice. He cured more doctors than patients. His contact with the medical corps' experience of the anguish and violence of war, along with those of the patients, allowed him to expand his experience of working with the collective. The men and women who volunteered with the POUM, including a number of doctors, comprised the first column that arrived to Sariñena, where they created a collective community and opened a hospital at the stately home of the Penén-Paraled family, which had been requisitioned. Testimonies of the period describe the hospital as one of the best organized on the Aragon front, located in a space transformed by new uses and new practices, as in the Mas d'en Boule.[5] Tosquelles described his time in Sariñena in relationship with other in situ therapeutic experiences, such as in Benabarre and Bujaraloz, recalling attempts to adapt the task of sector psychiatry to the situation of the war.

There Tosquelles deployed a psychiatry that worked with the war and from the war, and that didn't separate wartime psychiatry from peacetime psychiatry. This radical continuity is seen throughout Tosquelles's practice; he understood the war as a place of reencounter between the catastrophic experiences of humanity and madness, where the end of the world in the society "of normal people" coexists with the psychic suffering of those who are excluded from that society. In the experience of the end of the world inflicted by war, Tosquelles simultaneously recognizes the human character of madness and the drama of

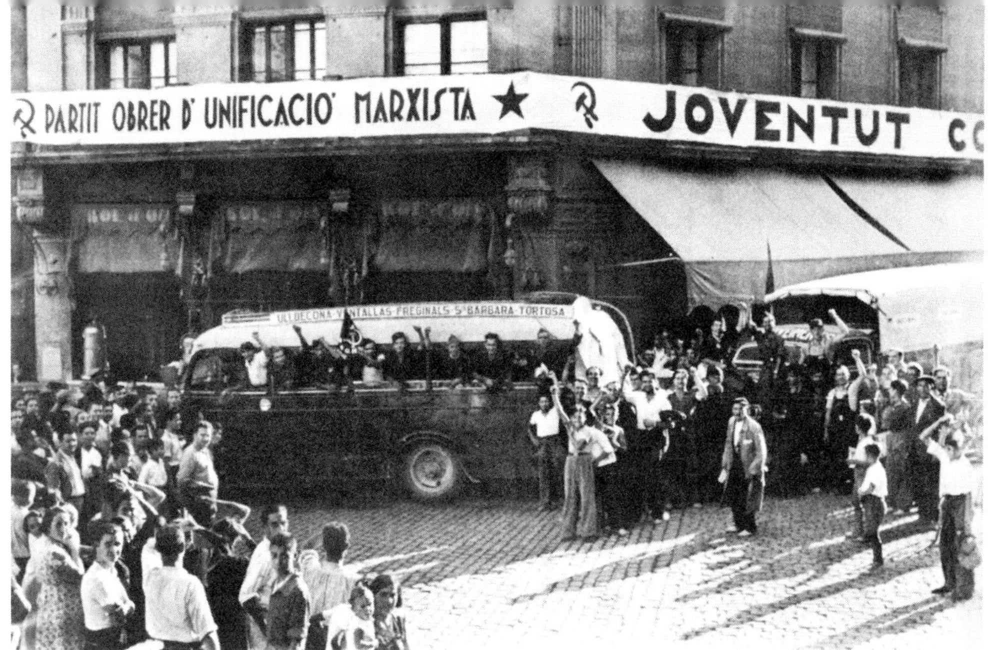

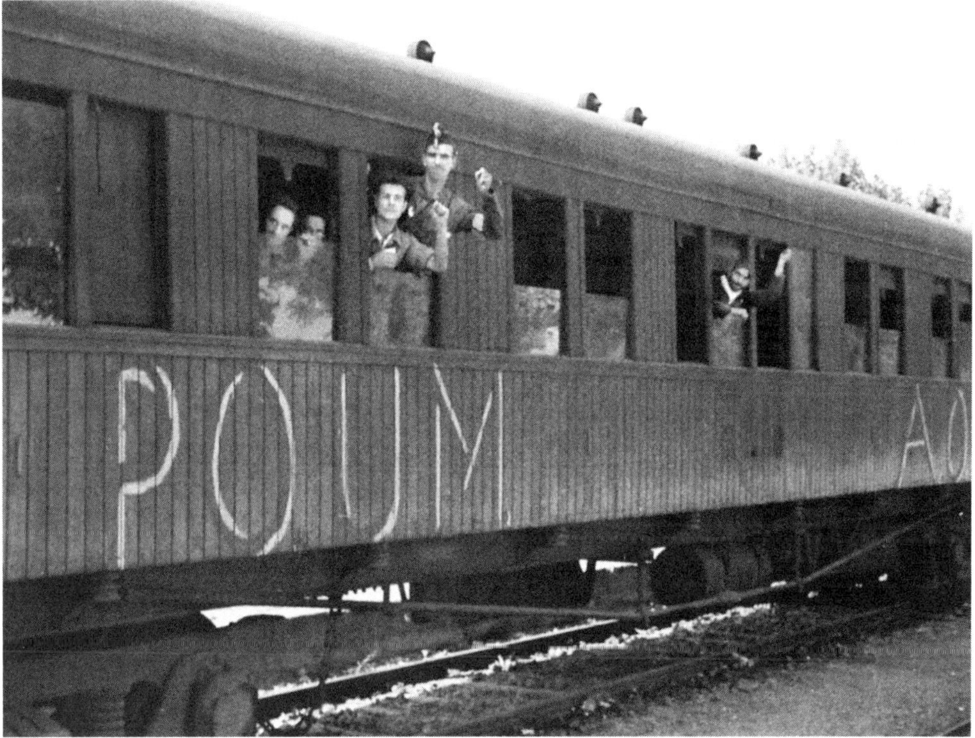

Top, militiamen of the POUM and the JCI (Iberian Communist Youth) leaving for the Aragon front on August 18, 1936. They are in front of party headquarters, located at the Casa Vilanova in the Plaça General Prim of Reus, which had been expropriated.

Bottom, the train of POUM militiamen on its way through Grañén, in Aragon, on September 14, 1936

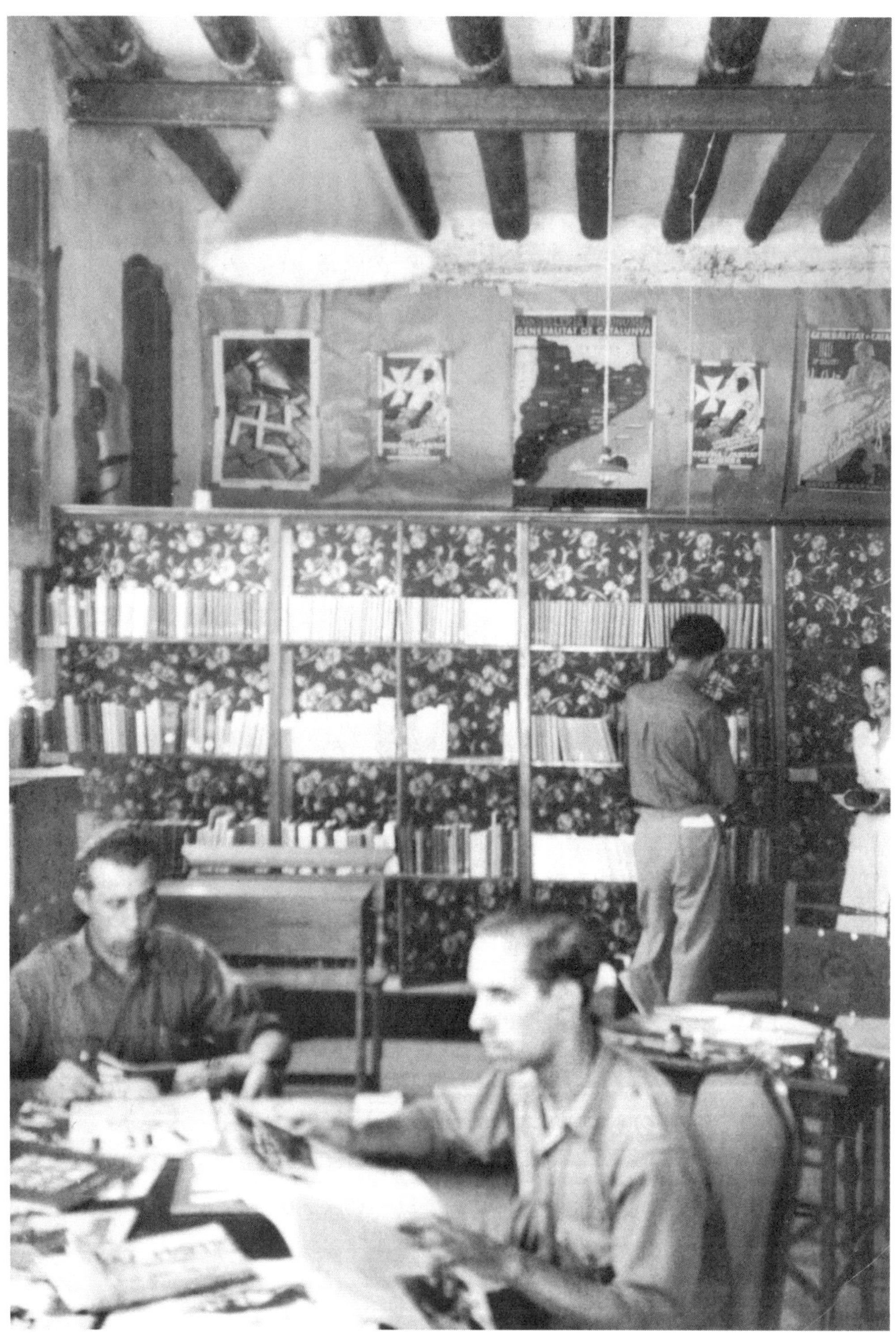

Library Services to the Front, Sariñena substation, on August 13, 1937

delirium in illnesses such as schizophrenia. For him, the experience of war, of the disappearance of a world and the end of his own times, is a political experience that links each individual's spiritual suffering with the possibility of becoming a person. Not knowing how to live through wars deprives us of our humanity.

Over the course of the 1940s, when he was already at the Saint-Alban hospital, Tosquelles elaborated lived experiences both from the Spanish Civil War and the Second World War in France in a study that became his doctoral thesis, defended in Paris in 1948. With the title *Essai sur le sens du vécu en psychopathologie: Le témoignage de Gérard de Nerval* (Essay on the meaning of lived experience in psychopathology: The testimony of Gérard de Nerval), he gathers the words of the patients and poets who narrate wars, bombings, earthquakes, cataclysms, commotions, and suicides. They are voices that speak of long nights that last days, in which Tosquelles listens to the lack of future the war forces them to live through. But he also listens to their desire to remake the world: the desire to give birth to the world, to make it be born again. To speak loudly and have a child, said one patient woman, adding: "I gave birth to myself, there's nothing more absurd … but it's true … I think about it all day long; otherwise, nothing would work, food wouldn't work, people, ice, winter."

In 1944, we recorded the following conversation (thanks to Dr. Chaurand). […]

—*What are your future projects?*
—*The future, very promising, for those who are sensible. We'll soon have earthquakes. It will be dark, day and night, casting the world into perdition. As with Noah's ark, those who see the light will take their leave. The end of the world, the world can't go on living. […] There'll be no more housing, all that will be rubble … People will live outdoors … They'll eat a piece of whatever will get them through the day … No more roads, they will be cut off by the bombs …* […]

What is one to do? The patient finds themselves facing a task that they can't visualize. *One has to save the world.* Françoise announces two methods: "speak loud, loud" (recreate the world via the Word) and "have a child." […]

"I made stories out of all that. I believed I was pregnant. The streetlights got me excited in a terrible way. The sparks from the tramways, it seemed to me that they were ultraviolet rays. Their intermittent glow with the passing of trains appeared to confirm what I was saying as if there was a correspondence. I lived the end of the world. I believed there was war. […]

PATIENT—*I'm broken, I'm not undone, not broken, I'm like you; I've often thought that I am dead but now I am here.*
DOCTOR—*How did it happen to you, your death?*
PATIENT—*It happened all of a sudden, we all disappeared.*
DOCTOR—*And now what do you do?*
PATIENT—*One is always waiting.*
DOCTOR—*For what?*
PATIENT—*I don't know.*
DOCTOR—*Who are you?*
PATIENT—*I don't know.*
DOCTOR—*Who are you?*
PATIENT—*The creator, the maker, the creator.*
DOCTOR—*What have you created?*
PATIENT—*Everything, the whole world.*
DOCTOR—*Including yourself?*
PATIENT—*Yes, me too. I gave birth to myself, there's nothing more absurd … but it's true … I think about it all day long; otherwise, nothing would work, food wouldn't work, people, ice, winter …*[6]

François Tosquelles, *Le Vécu de la fin du monde dans la folie: Le témoignage de Gérard de Nerval* (1948), 1986

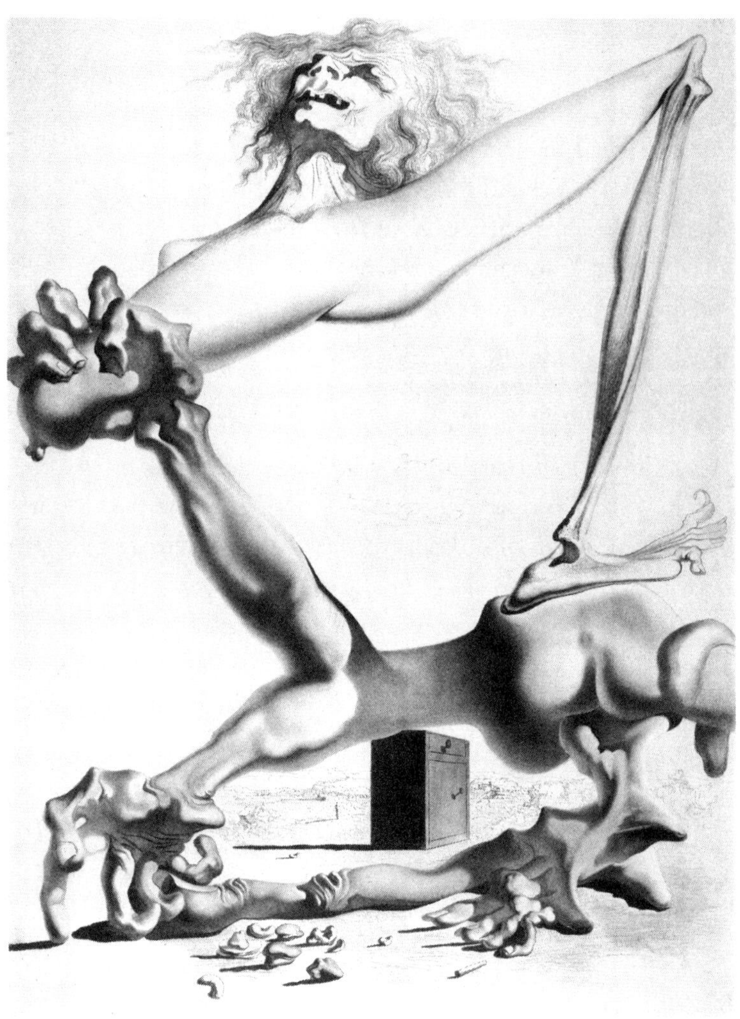

Salvador Dalí, study for *Premonición de la Guerra Civil* (*Premonition of Civil War*), 1935

Around 1936, with the outbreak of the Spanish Civil War, artistic representations of the end of the world proliferated. Tosquelles distinguished the Catalan surrealism of Salvador Dalí, with its situated landscapes, from the Aragonese surrealism of Luis Buñuel or the French surrealism of André Breton. Gérard Vuillamy, who was also linked with French surrealism, made, in collaboration with Paul Éluard, a series of portraits of Saint-Alban nurses during his stay at the hospital; in the novel *The Aesthetics of Resistance*, Peter Weiss, a writer and filmmaker, narrated the experience of sexologist Max Hodann in homes requisitioned and turned into hospitals or convalescent homes by the International Brigades during the Civil War.

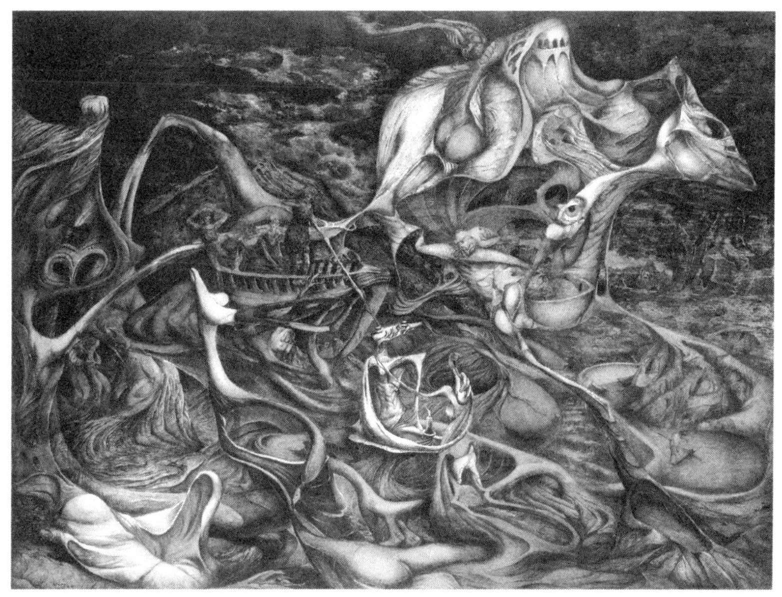

Gérard Vulliamy, *Le Cheval de Troie*, 1936–1937

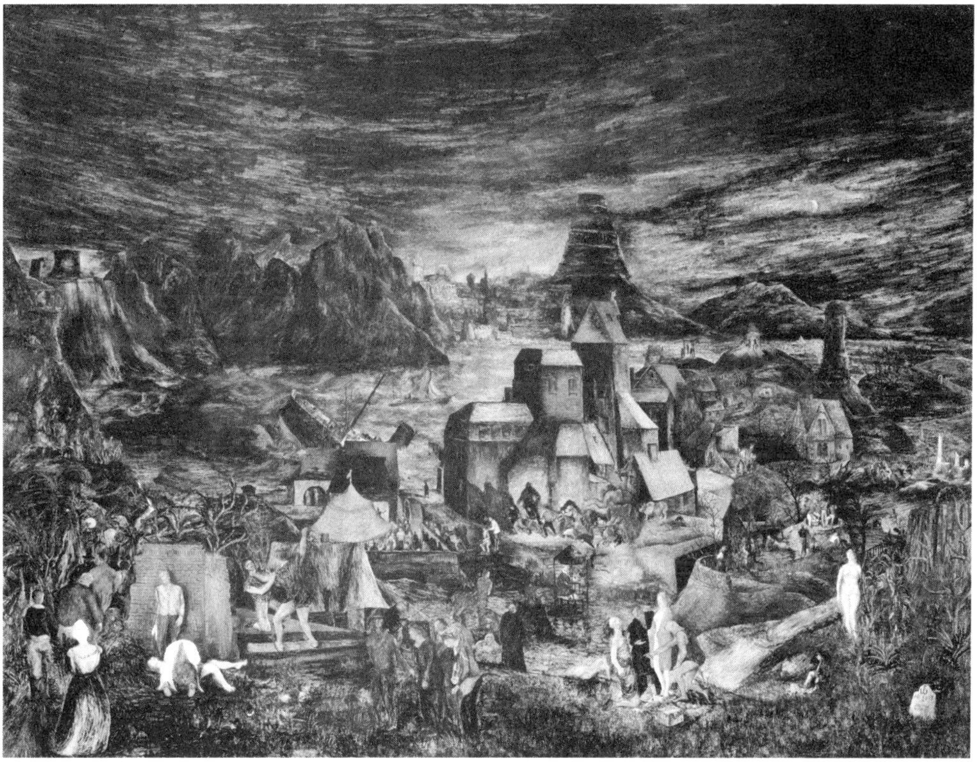

Peter Weiss, *Das Grosse Welttheater*, 1937

Literary language is at the heart of Tosquelles's reflection on the end of the world and he uses it to speak of delirium, war, and the human future. As Baudelaire expressed: "Le monde va finir. La seule raison pour laquelle il pourrait durer, c'est qu'il existe" (The world is ending. The only reason it might endure is that it exists). Or Gérard de Nerval, who—in the Passy clinic, in collaboration with Dr. Émile Blanche, to whom he addressed the brief prose texts that documented the doctor's listening to his illness—wrote of Aurélia's descent into hell, three months before he committed suicide in 1855: "C'est moi maintenant qui dois mourir et mourir sans espoir! [...] Le soir, lorsque l'heure fatale semblait s'approcher ..." (It is I who must now die and die without hope. [...] At dusk, as the fatal hour drew near ...). Or Ferrater, through the damage inflicted on him by the Civil War, his distress, and his suicide. And also Artaud: "Une lumière de fin du monde remplit peu à peu ma pensée" (A light of the end of the world gradually fills my thoughts).

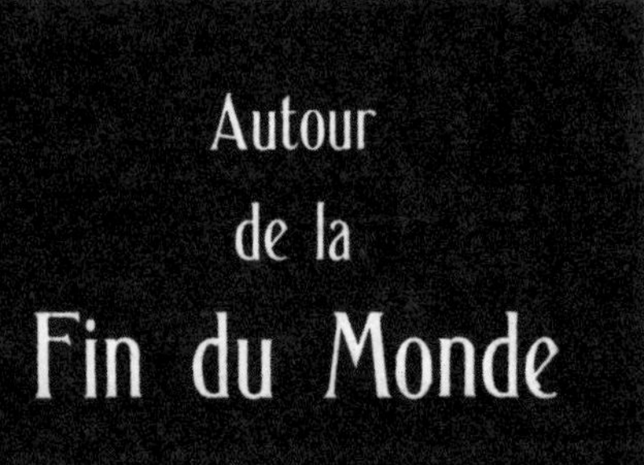

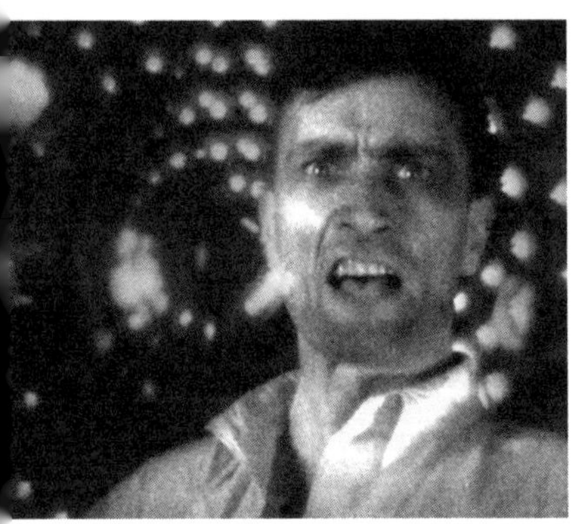

"Why lie, why try to place on a literary plane something that is the very cry of life itself, why give a fictional appearance to what is made of the ineradicable substance of the soul, which is like the plaint of reality?" (Artaud, *Correspondence with Jacques Rivière*, May 25, 1924). That poet who, as you know, was already suffering from schizophrenia in this period noted the difference between his life experience and that of other poets "afflicted by the weakness of the whole age, such as Tristan Tzara, André Breton, Pierre Reverdy. But in their case the soul is not physiologically damaged, it is not damaged substantially, but at all the points where it joins something else, it is not damaged *outside of thought*," "In me, this lack of connection to the object which characterizes all of literature is a lack of connection to life. As for myself, I can truly say that I am not in this world, and this is not merely an attitude of the mind." A few years later we were present for a visit which Voronica paid him at the psychiatric hospital of Rodez, where Ferdière surrounded him with the best care and in this way protected Artaud's lived poetry. Administrative and uncomprehending in equal measure, Voronica tried to remind Artaud of what the world of letters had lost with him. "You're France's greatest poet. Write. Don't abandon poetry." To which Artaud exclaimed with visible contempt, "Everything I do is poetry!" His poetic work would continue in the same vein that had always produced it, in his constantly endangered existence; the extravagant call (his inarticulate cries) that he now addressed to the demonic powers was in fact the same "cry of life" by which "literary" poetry had tried in vain to save him.[7]

François Tosquelles, *Le Vécu de la fin du monde dans la folie: Le témoignage de Gérard de Nerval* (1948), 1986

The title of Tosquelles's thesis echoes the film by Abel Gance, *La fin du monde*, and the 1930 film by Eugène Deslaw, *Autour de la fin du monde*, in which Artaud appears alongside Abel Gance, Sylvia Grenade, and Gina Manès.

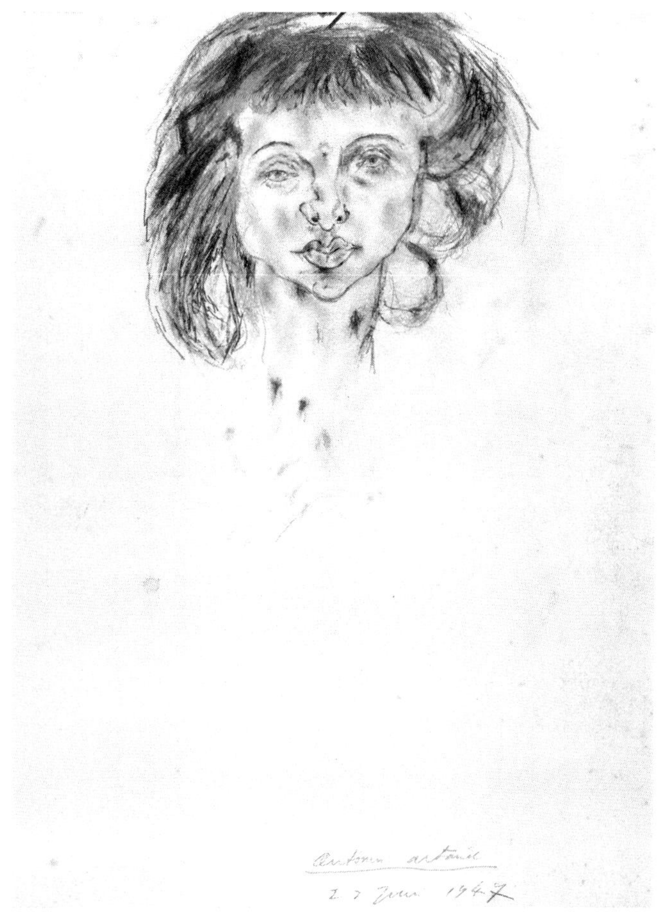

Antonin Artaud, *Portrait de Lili Dubuffet*, 1947. This drawing was a gift from Jean Dubuffet to Francesc Tosquelles, who had visited Artaud in the psychiatric hospital of Rodez during the last years of his life.

Therapeutic Experiences, Amateur Practices

War was the paradise where Tosquelles lived the therapeutic experience at Almodóvar del Campo, alongside Drs. Sauret, Peña, and Marín. In May 1938, he was named head of psychiatric services of the Extremaduran Army and director of the Almodóvar clinic in the province of Ciudad Real, located at the foot of the Sierra Morena surrounded by green and yellow plains. It was Emili Mira, Josep Solanes, and Tosquelles who made possible the creation of this community in Almodóvar after having defended the organization of local clinics for each army and frontline support services at each campaign-base hospital, unlike other centralizing proposals within the organization of the Republican army.

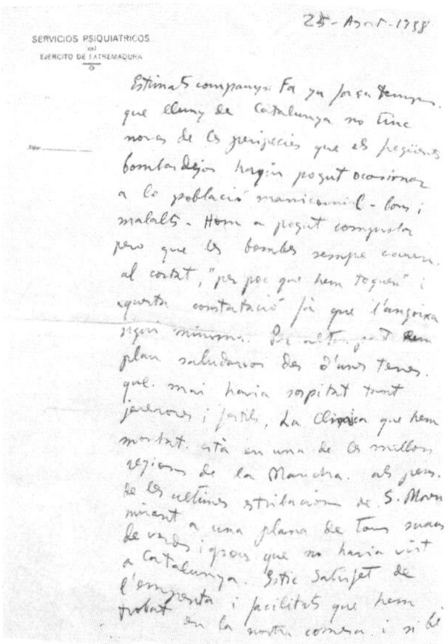

25-Agost-1938

SERVICIOS PSIQUIATRICOS
del
EJERCITO DE EXTREMADURA

Estimats companys: Fa ja força temps
que lluny de Catalunya no tinc
noves de les peripecies que els freqüents
bombardejos hagin pogut ocasionar
a la població manicomial - bons i
malalts. Hom a pogut comprovar
pero que les bombes sempre cauen
al costat, "per poc que hem toquen" i
aquesta constatació fa que l'angoixa
sigui minima. Per altra part [illegible]
plau saludar-vos des d'unes terres
que mai havia sospitat tant
generoses i fertils. La clínica que hem
muntat està en una de les millors
regions de la Mancha. als peus
de les ultimes [illegible] de S. Morena
mirant a una plana de tons suaus
de verds i grocs que no havia vist
a Catalunya. Estic satisfet de
l'empenta i facilitats que hem
trobat en la nostra comesa i si be

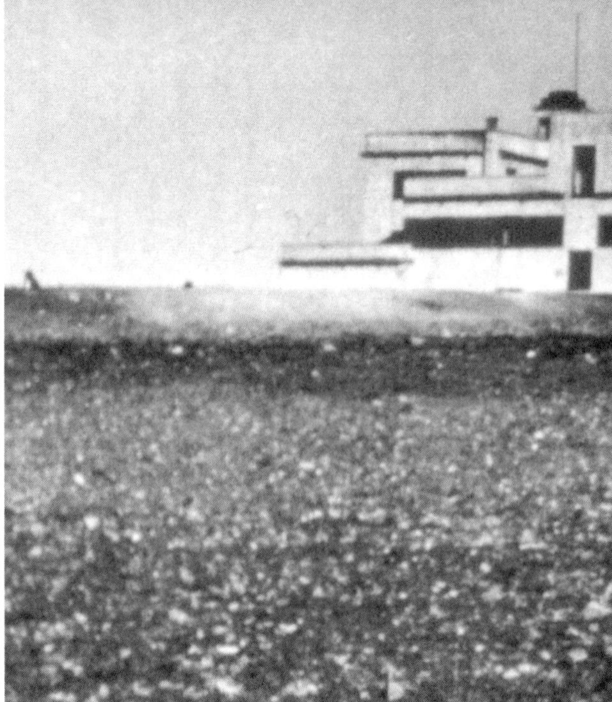

Psychiatric services of the Extremaduran Army, August 25, 1938

Dear comrades,

For some time now, being far from Catalonia, I've had no news of the effects—good or ill—the frequent bombings may have had on the asylum population. It's been proven, however, that the bombs always fall nearby, "almost hitting me," and that determination makes my anguish minimal. On the other hand, I'm pleased to be writing to you from lands I'd never suspected were so generous and fertile. The clinic we've set up is in one of the best regions of La Mancha, at the foot of the estivations [*sic*] of the Sierra Morena, facing a plain with two soothing tones of green and yellow I've never seen in Catalonia. I am satisfied with the effort and ease we've found in our task, although one is obliged to work quite a lot, despite the heat. We can also say that the war is some sort of paradise for us. Among the colleagues they've assigned to me is our friend Sauret, who has taken command of the psychoneurotic clinic and is working as a pure psychotherapist. The others, I don't believe you know them, since they are from the central regions; Peña, from Sant Andreu, is in the epilepsy clinic, where he works quite a lot. (In these two months more than two thousand people have come in for epilepsy testing.) A guy named Marín from Madrid, who works with real crazies, etc. We also have some neurology things, quite interesting, Babinski-reflex paralysis and other hysterias, etc. All in all, to be immodest, I believe we have one of the finest clinics in the army. We are also working on the professional selection of the future "high officials" and for automatic weapons, machine guns, etc. The enthusiasm of all our colleagues perhaps compensates the lack of a top-quality "showgirl" in our organization.

And you? Are Massot and Hoïc still at the asylum or are they soldiers? And Boné? And your families? Is Don Josep still sick?

I send my greetings to all.

Francesc Tosquelles[8]

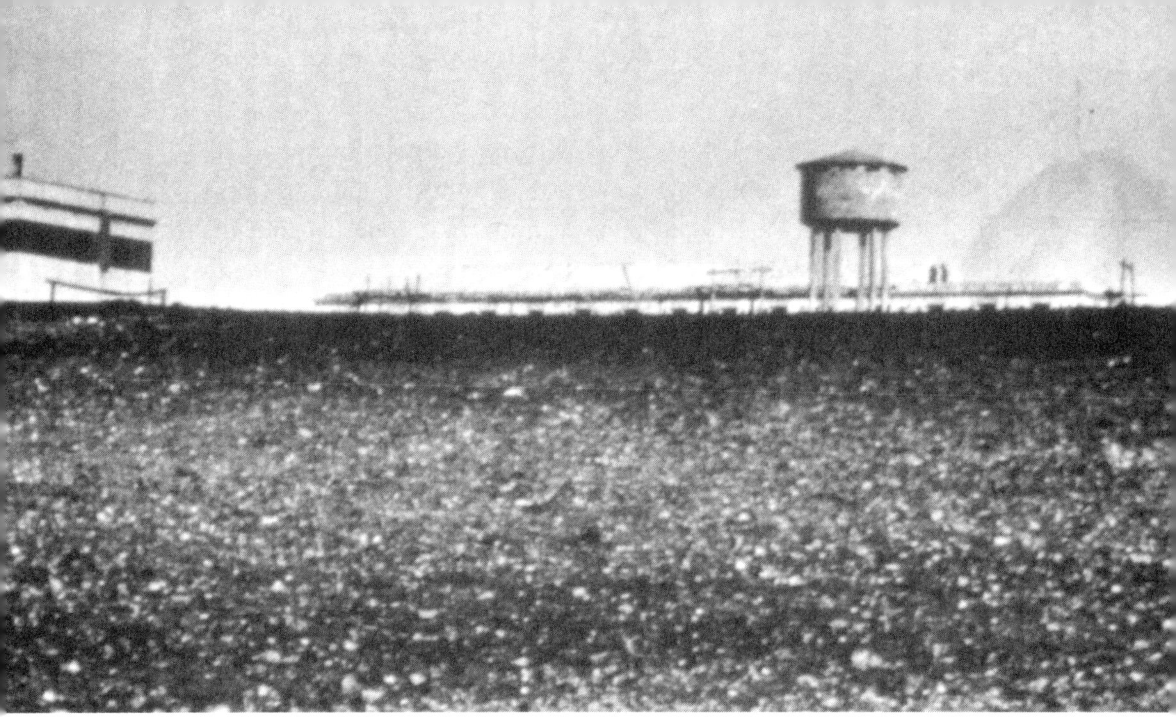

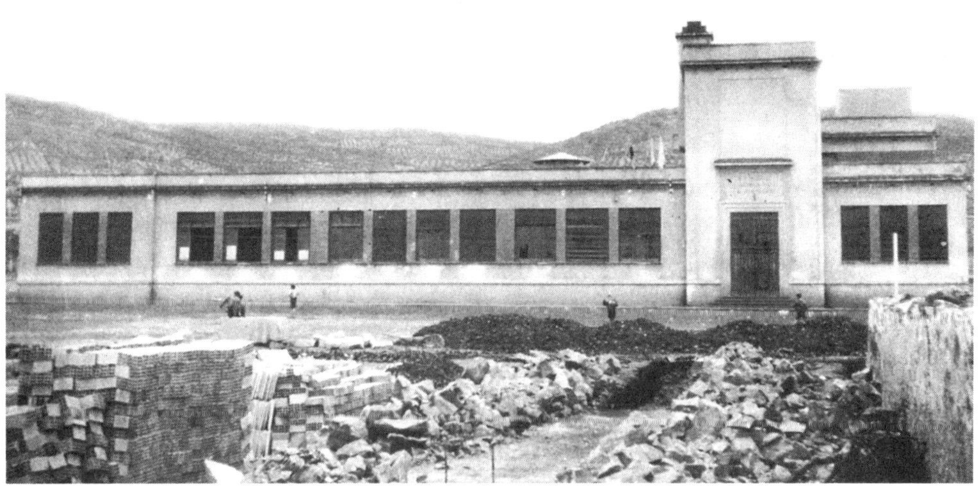

Top, the building that was turned into a field hospital and psychiatric hospital in Almodóvar del Campo, and where Tosquelles worked during the Civil War.
Bottom, the front façade of the overseers' building of that same complex. The images are from November 1954.

The ambulances traveled to the combat zone to practice psychiatry in situ, in order to avoid separating the treatment of war trauma from the place where it occurred. For Tosquelles it was important to not separate the curing of the war ill from the war itself. Because the war ill, once removed from the front, became the chronically ill. There was also a hospital in the rear guard that had three clinics with different medical specialties and a farm where the ill could work. However, Tosquelles's big battle in Almodóvar was rejecting the classic figure of the psychiatrist limited to caring for patients. He was involved in the organization of the life of the General Staff and took part in the professional selection of civilian soldiers within the army's organigram. Participating in the selection of people based on their capabilities, as Tosquelles would also do at the refugee camp and at the Saint-Alban hospital, involved intervening and modifying the naturalized forms of social, political, and military hierarchy. The mere act of

> I have to admit that I only saw myself as someone wanting to apply psychotechnics to radically human pursuits, in the field of psychiatry and education. I launched myself into a futile battle against windmills, where politics and more or less religious structural ideologies play the main roles. [...]
>
> At a certain moment, I was named chief of psychiatric services of the Extremaduran Army, and right away I approached my activities from the perspective of a true extensive psychiatry and not at all from that of medically directing a particular psychiatric clinic, as the chief of staff of the Army of the Central and Meridional Regions of Spain pretended to understand it. I refused from the start to be regarded as a classical psychiatrist reduced to treating mental patients. I demanded, before the group of generals and their aides, my indispensable participation in the activities of the army General S,taff to which I had been appointed, and this in the capacity, I told them, of a "permanent technical adviser" for everything relating to the mental health of the armies and the people they were sworn to defend. After a few hesitations, the thing was granted. So I found myself, among numerous other activities, charged with setting up the professional selection of the soldiers assigned to handle tanks and machine guns.
>
> [...] I was almost immediately listened to concerning the selection of soldiers who had to operate tanks and fire machine guns. But in my very detailed, foundational report, I proposed in passing that there be a selection process for lower-ranking commanders (sergeants and corporals). There was a certain conscious irony in this: I knew very well that the Communist Party, above all, wouldn't accept this project, since the latticework of its little "command posts" constituted the real scaffolding of its own political power there. So that was that, I wasn't given any response. [...]
>
> What would it have been like if I had proposed the selection of psychiatrists, or for that matter judges ... the selection of the selectors ...[9]
>
> François Tosquelles, *L'Enseignement de la folie*, 1992

proposing, as he did in the Extremaduran Army, that a selection be made for positions of responsibility, and for the selection panel itself that chooses the selectors, shook up the natural order of the military and psychiatric hospital, introducing approaches that were radically linked to exploring forms of equality and amateurism.

This community informally arose before Thomas Main, in 1946, and Maxwell Jones, in 1952, coined the term "therapeutic community" to give a name to the cohabitation between the medical staff and the patients within new common spaces that didn't previously exist. Therapeutic communities explored ways of organizing life around assembly methods and horizontal decision-making. In the case of Tosquelles, it was primarily informality and amateurism that led his work with the local community of Almodóvar, in which there were a painter and a priest, lawyers and farmers, some prostitutes who worked as nurses while the bordello was closed, and other people from the civil society unfamiliar with mental illness. The localness of that experience and the open community trace a geography that sought to redraw what was inside in relationship to what was outside. They drew a landscape of life in wartime in which psychiatric hospitals seemed to belong more to the civilian population than to a military order.

Tosquelles's work with the local community found its most singular expression in the collaborations with the prostitutes of Almodóvar del Campo. At a time when sex workers were forced to stop working because the brothels were closed, Tosquelles helped to maintain their jobs by transforming them, within the spaces they already occupied. For a while the bordello was annexed in service to the hospital. As such, in the former brothel space, the prostitutes were paid to receive soldiers transferred there by the hospital. They ceased to use the bordellos to have sexual relations and, while they continued working, they were able to have a different relationship to sex. They exchanged one job for the other within the same space. Periodically, these women would write up reports discussing the soldiers' sexuality as part of the therapeutic procedure. And that should be understood within the framework of Tosquelles's objective of creating community. In the 1980s, Tosquelles referred to these women retrospectively as "sexual assistants," a term that today would be linked to contemporary reflections on disabled people's right to sexuality and to the remuneration of sex work.

For certain doctors, going out and "doing community" allows them simply to no longer see patients, to run from madness. Similarly, certain anti-psychiatrists have said about hospital patients "but they're not crazy," so as not to commit themselves to that long and uncertain adventure of the therapeutic process.

I could treat this principle of exclusion in terms of two variants: the schizophrenic and the prostitute, without saying, of course, that the crazy person is a prostitute or vice versa, but they are both destined to be excluded.

The mad one is kept in the hospital and the prostitute in the street or the brothel: forms of inclusion the better to exclude. From time out of mind, there has been this attempt to suppress by means of the asylum and the brothel. Often, wanting to get the prostitutes out of the brothels is a Catholic position, in good faith of course, which consists in making prostitutes of future nuns who will work for nothing or for less money.

I myself take another position. At Almodóvar del Campo, there were two brothels: the first reserved for rich farmers, the second, less luxurious—let's say, one for the captain and the other for the soldier. I was against their shutdown. I went there, accompanied by a doctor from the region. I needed a homegrown doctor to lead the negotiation. I was successful in preventing the closure of those houses of prostitution by offering three choices to the girls. The first proposal was: "You can get the hell out, your future is none of my business." The second suggested that the prostitutes continue their trade, on one condition: they would receive soldiers whom I would refer—at a modest price, I would make up the rest—and they would give me a technical report on the sexual relations the soldier might imagine. All this had the therapeutic aim of learning about the fantasy element. They wouldn't spy, they would do a task which they knew to be of interest for curing the type of patient in question, as any nurse would. A dozen girls chose the third option: they became nurses in the external services as what I would call "sexual assistants." They had this quality: the need to accommodate the desire of the other, which it is better to exploit for scientific purposes than simply for money. None of them went so far as to have sex with a patient, they had the possibility of sublimating the business of sex and talking about it. In reality, the nurses or people in charge don't talk about the patients but about themselves.

It was necessary, therefore, to create a therapeutic community so the staff could meet and talk about the patients. In speaking of them, these girls would end up talking about themselves. And thanks to this activity, they were able not to correct themselves morally but to modify their psychosexual structure. In this manner, I was able to transform a number of prostitutes into nurses.[10]

François Tosquelles, interview with Bernard Favre, 1983–1985

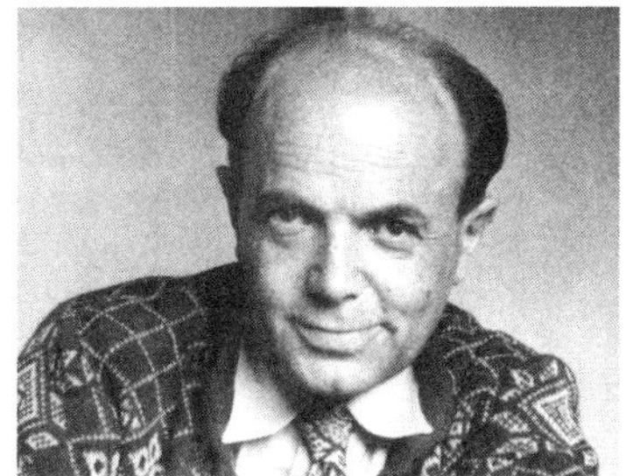
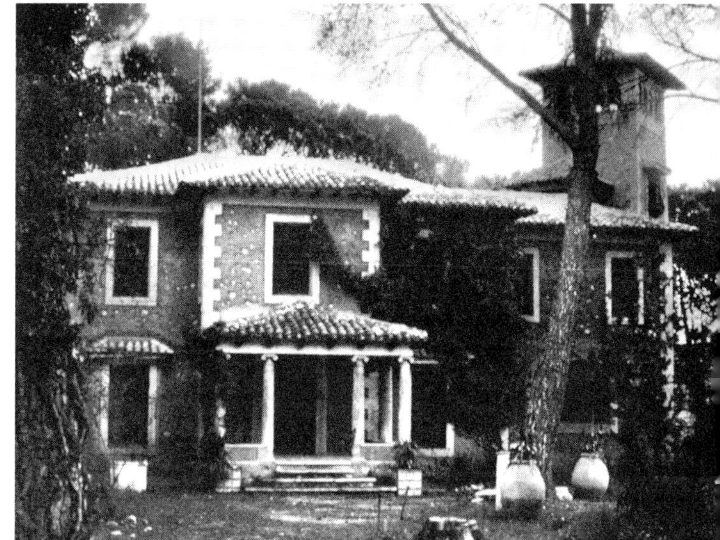

Javier Montejo, in his research into "therapeutic communities" during the Civil War, has restored, along with Tosquelles's experience in Almodóvar, the work of sexologist Max Hodann, director of a sanatorium for soldiers of the International Brigades, popularly known as the Cueva de la Potita hospital, in Albacete. Hodann was the author of *Geschlecht und Liebe in biologischer und gesellschaftlicher Beziehung* (Sex and love in biological and social relationship), published in Spain in 1936, a book that became the first sexology manual for the working class. Hodann did not publish any writing on his day-to-day work at Cueva de la Potita, but Peter Weiss, in his novel *The Aesthetics of Resistance*, rewrites the experience based on a notebook of Hodann's.[11]

It is necessary to teach that onanism is harmless. But that is not enough. Educating for the comprehension of a new morality, the struggle against constant bad conscience in sexual conduct, is a task that, from the perspective of strengthening our capacity for nervous endurance, must be added to the political work with troops. We should also consider gathering, from our health centers and our political commissariats, the questions from our comrades in relation to the sexual environment, and either respond to them in our magazines and newspapers, or use them as a starting point for discussions.[12]

Max Hodann, "Consideraciones sobre el problema sexual en el Ejército" [Considerations on the sexual problem in the army], 1937

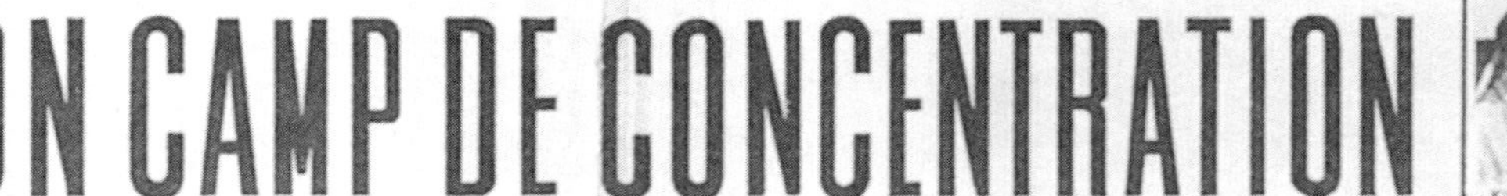

LE MEILLEUR REPORTER D'EUROPE AVAIT PHOTOGRAPHIÉ

SON CAMP DE CONCENTRATION

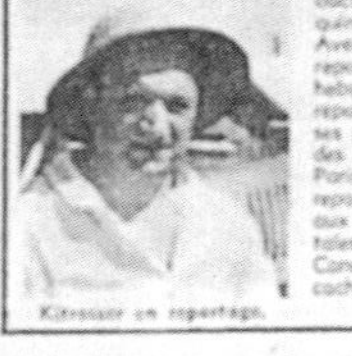

Kitrosser en reportage.

Kitrosser est un habitué de toutes les s[…] daction des magazines européens éd[…] quinze ans, où on l'appelle familièrement Avec Salomon à Londres, c'est le spé[…] reportage indiscret qui a fait la grande hebdomadaires d'avant-guerre. Des d[…] reportages ont fait sa notoriété et quelq[…] ses photos sont célèbres : Lord Halifax des spaghettis au wagon-restaurant d[…] Paris-Londres, l'exécution de Weidm[…] reportage provoqua un décret ministériel aux photographes d'assister aux exécut[…] tales et la réunion du Conseil d'Admin[…] Canal de Suez où Kitrosser réussit à p[…] cachant son appareil sous son gilet.

LE gouvernement de Vichy faisait interner, en 1941, au Camp de Septfonds, quelques centaines d'hommes qu'il estimait préférable, pour sa politique, de voir cesser toute activité journalistique, littéraire ou artistique. Kitrosser fut du nombre. Il ne tarda pas à voir, dans l'existence de ses compagnons, l'étonnant documentaire humain qu'il pouvait réaliser et à se procurer un appareil d'amateur. Il lui fallut plusieurs semaines pour terminer son travail et dut employer, pour le mener à bien, toutes les ruses que pratiquent les prisonniers pour obtenir par l'habileté tout ce qu'on leur interdit par la force. Les photos que nous publions ont failli ne jamais voir le jour. 90 % des compagnons de captivité de Kitrosser ont été déportés en Allemagne. Ils ont perdu dans ce transfert les quelques objets qu'on leur laissait encore ; et combien redeviendront un jour des hommes libres ? « Kitro » réussit à s'évader, vécut longtemps caché, changeant cent fois de domicile, gardant toujours sur lui les quelques rouleaux de pellicule, souvenirs de la plus dure aventure de sa vie.

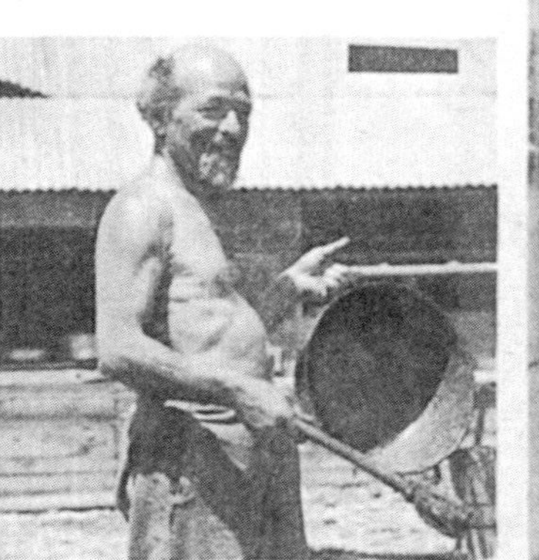

Grünfeld, directeur de l'Institut Freud, à Vienne, dans l'ancienne Autriche, a fondé au camp une université populaire clandestine.

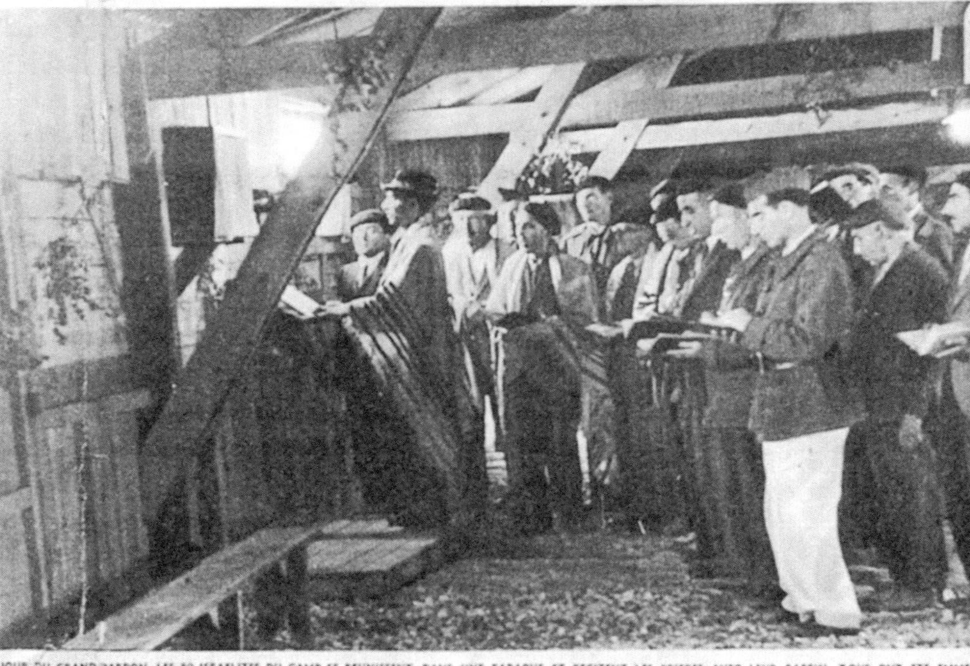

LE JOUR DU GRAND PARDON, LES 80 ISRAELITES DU CAMP SE REUNISSENT DANS UNE BARAQUE ET RECITENT LES PRIERES AVEC LEUR RABBIN. TOUS ONT ETE EMMENES […]

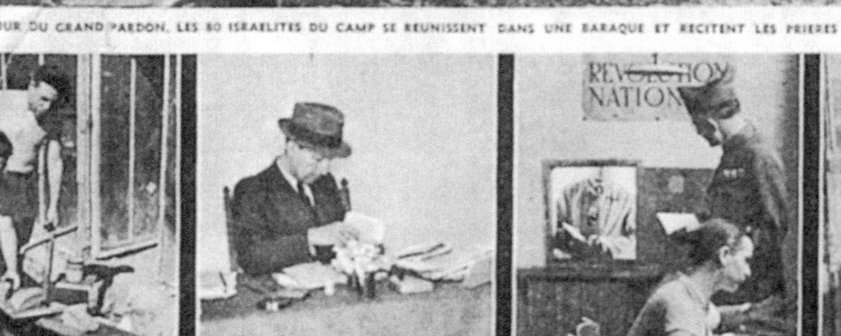

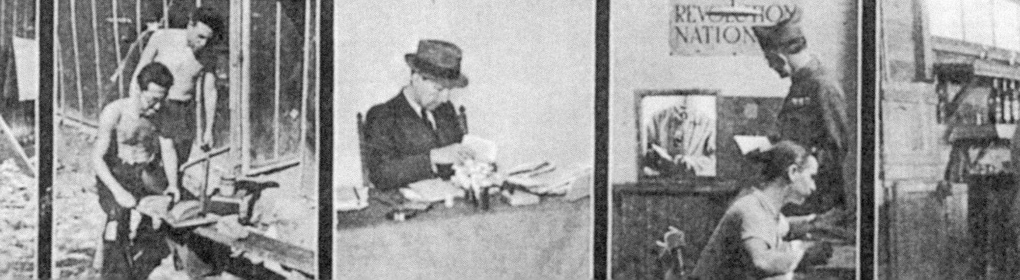

A Unit in the Concentration Camp

If more traces of the psychiatric unit that Tosquelles organized in the Septfonds camp had survived, perhaps we would know why, when he arrived there in September 1939, seeing the camp reminded him of entering a psychiatric hospital. Why did it look to him like the yard of a psychiatric hospital, so poorly organized that he requested authorization to transform it? Why did he ask for barracks at one extreme end of the camp, almost outside of it? To treat the war traumas of the Spanish Republicans—with a high suicide rate—or to help some escape from the camp? And why, one morning, did he enter a concentration camp and decide to stay there and work? For a whole year, between March 1939 and March 1940, Septfonds was a camp for Spanish militiamen. Despite being known as a camp for intellectuals and artists, there were metalworkers, farmers, mechanics, electricians, bakers, students, miners, doctors, teachers and stevedores, civilians and military, some of whom would be deported to Mauthausen, marked with the blue

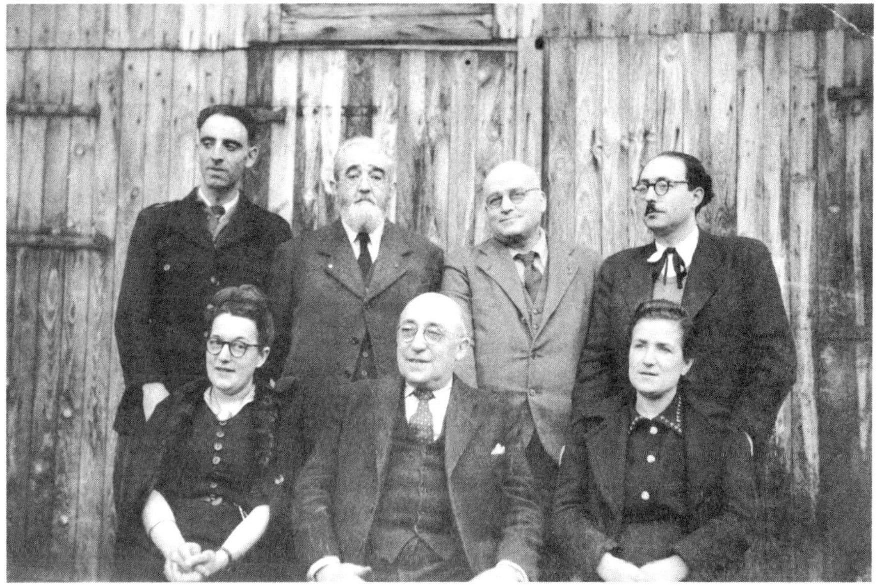

Above, Francesc Tosquelles at the Septfonds camp, 1939 and 1940, in one of the few photographs that remain. *At left*, a photo-essay on the camp made by Isaac Kitrosser, published in *Nuit et Jour* in January 1944.

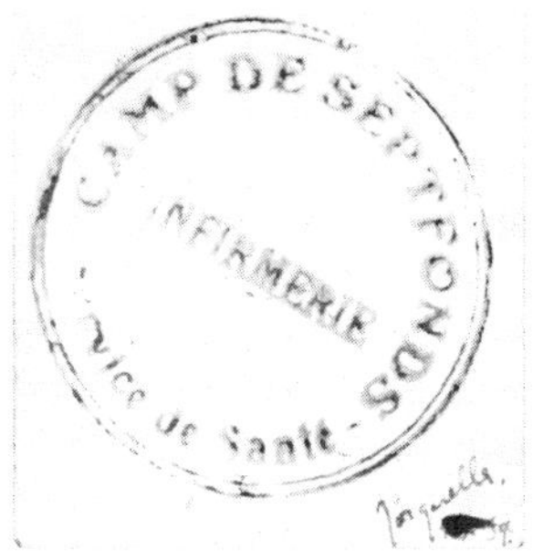

triangle of the stateless. Unlike other French camps, which began to be studied in the '90s, Septfonds was long a place whose narrative was forgotten in time. Compared to other camps such as Bram, Agde, Gurs, Saint-Cyprien, or Argelès-sur-Mer—in which nearly half a million refugees were interned—Septfonds was a small camp, a *camp d'accueil* (reception camp) that "only" ever housed sixteen thousand Republicans. After the forced internment of Austrian prisoners and Polish and Czech Jews, the camp and its administrative archives were destroyed in 1945.

But Tosquelles retained his memories of the experiences in the work clinic at the camp, and he evoked them in the 1980s in a dialogue with psychiatrists, psychologists, researchers, and social workers, a reflection on the condition of freedom: "The Freedom School." This dialogue unfolded as a long group meditation on the divergences between the institutional psychotherapy that he had experienced fully in France and the approach of Franco Basaglia and Italian anti-psychiatry, which, instead of institutional transformation of the hospitals, proposed eliminating the hospital as a space of internment. Tosquelles expresses profound disagreement with the Italian experience of negating the institution. His institutional psychotherapy, through extensive psychiatry situated beyond the walls, aspired to transmute spaces based on the conviction that institutional transformation was constantly in process. For him there were no spaces, no places, no landscapes that were not immersed in processes of institutionalization. From this commitment to material change, the Italian dream of a society without hospitals, prisons, schools, or walls could only be seen as an immaterial utopia.

Tosquelles was given this metaphor of the "school of freedom" by a patient who had lived the experience of the Saint-Alban hospital. It was an expression that, somehow, confirmed his suspicions regarding *freedom in normal times*. Freedom wasn't found outside of the asylums, but rather it could only be learned in those spaces that required much work of institutional transformation. Those places were the only ones where small schools of freedom could appear. Perhaps that is why, when Tosquelles spoke of his memories of life at Septfonds, he compared that French experience of reclusion in the refugee camp with his critique of the Italian anti-psychiatry without walls. The psychiatric unit at Septfonds where, for a three-month period, Tosquelles and Jaume Sauret treated some fifteen men suffering from the traumas of the Civil War and exile—while others with mental illness were transferred to the Montalban hospital and neighboring centers

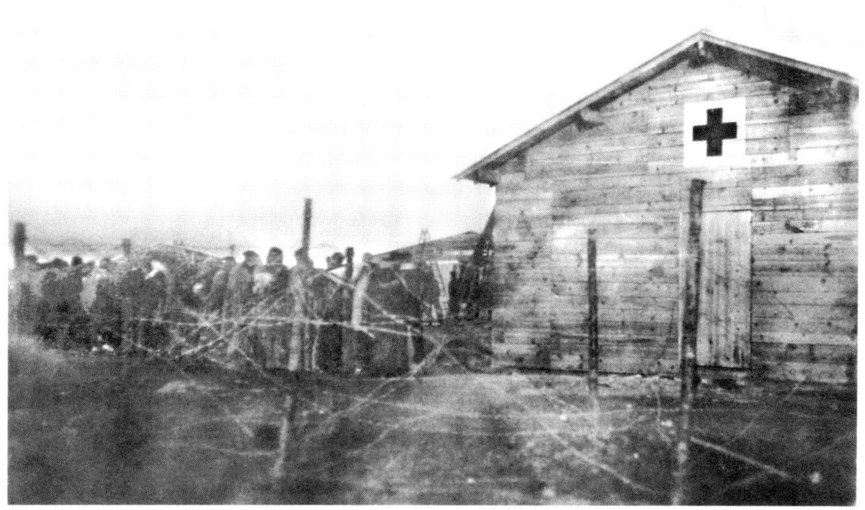

Above, the infirmary at the Septfonds camp, between February 1939 and June 1940. *Below*, *Groupe d' hommes à la toilette*, by José Roa, Judes camp (Septfonds), 1939.

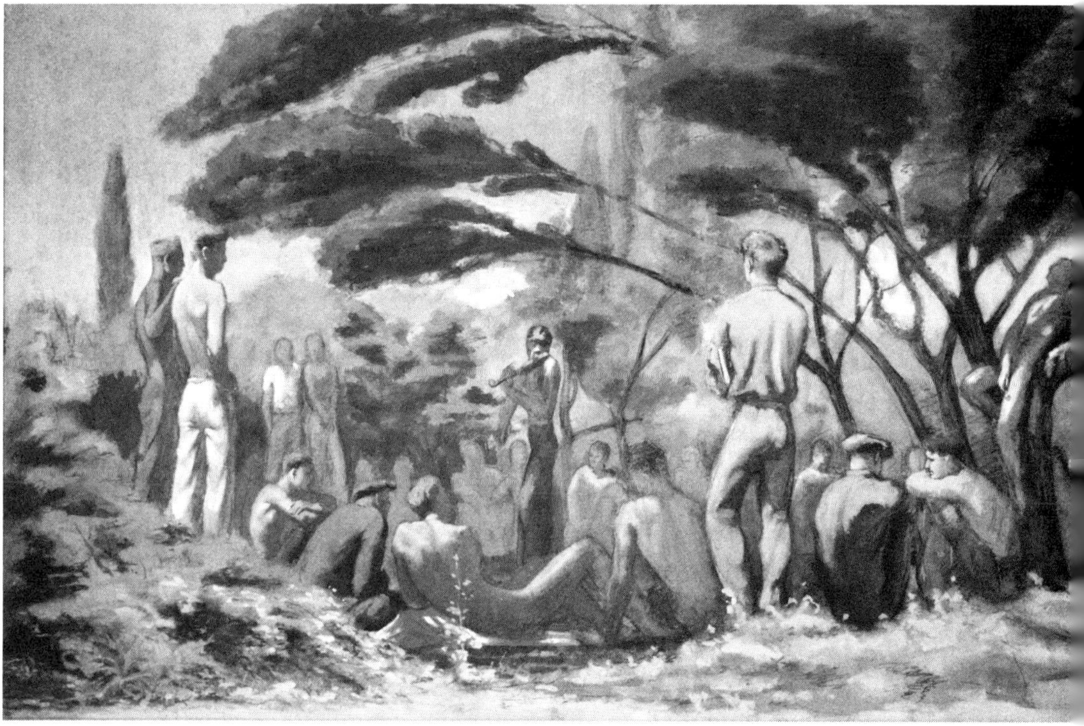

in the Lot region—is an experience that survives not through testimonies and photographs, but thanks to the humanizing artistic production carried out within the camp. Among the paintings made by the numerous artists who passed through the camp, along with postcards of the Judes camp and the important photographic documentation by Isaac Kitrosser, the transformative experience that took place at the camp seems to survive in a painting by José Roa: a gathering of men stretched out on the ground, talking and listening to music, the sun at their backs, the trees very green.[13]

The photographer Francesc Boix left that same French camp in September 1939; while we have photographs of his time at Mauthausen, no photographs survive of his stay at Septfonds. The Mauthausen images were published in the Communist press after the war and used in the Nuremberg trials to denounce the suicides, executions, and forced labor in the Nazi camps. What remains of Tosquelles's time at Septfonds are photographs with Sauret, their feet muddy, and group portraits in front of the barracks that mysteriously include women (the camp was only for men), as well as some administrative documents regarding his next destination, the Saint-Alban hospital, where he was invited by Dr. Paul Balvet.

Dr. Balvet, then the director at Saint-Alban, requested authorization from the prefect, via the psychiatrists Àngels Vives and André Chaurand,

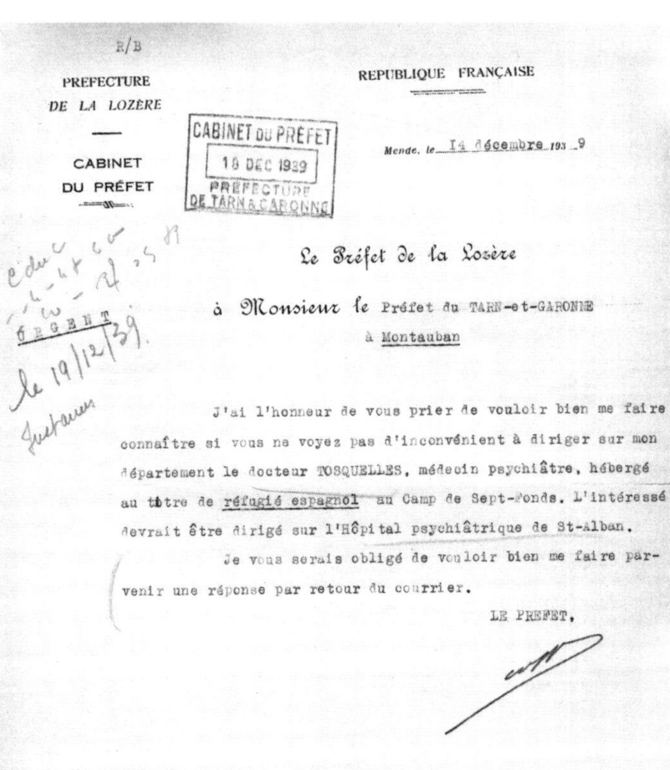

R/B

PREFECTURE
DE LA LOZÈRE

CABINET
DU PRÉFET

REPUBLIQUE FRANÇAISE

CABINET DU PRÉFET
18 DEC 1939
PRÉFECTURE
DE TARN & GARONNE

Mende, le 14 décembre 1939

URGENT
le 19/12/39

Le Préfet de la Lozère

à Monsieur le Préfet du TARN-et-GARONNE
à Montauban

J'ai l'honneur de vous prier de vouloir bien me faire connaître si vous ne voyez pas d'inconvénient à diriger sur mon département le docteur TOSQUELLES, médecin psychiâtre, hébergé au titre de réfugié espagnol au Camp de Sept-Fonds. L'intéressé devrait être dirigé sur l'Hôpital psychiâtrique de St-Alban.

Je vous serais obligé de vouloir bien me faire parvenir une réponse par retour du courrier.

LE PREFET,

Letter from the prefect of Lòzere requesting Tosquelles be released from the Septfonds camp in order to join the medical staff of Saint-Alban, dated December 14, 1939

Registry of departures from the Septfonds camp on January 22, 1940, which indicates Tosquelles's destination as Dr. Paul Balvet's home at the Saint-Alban hospital

-DEPART DE LA JOURNEEDU 22 JANVIER -

TREPAT SAMARRA Buenaventura- à Septfonds (T.et G.) Chez Mr. Andre Deramond.
MARTI ALEU Jose-à Septfonds(T.etG.) Chez Mr. Joseph Prior.
SOLANA PRIOR Ramon-à Carlat (Cantal) Chez Mr. Joseph Prior.
ALVAREZ SANCHEZ Grabiel - à Caussade (T.et G.) Chez Mr. Lugwig René Horloger.
BELLBER VALLS Joaquin - àLa Moulasse prés Saint Girons à 16 Ste. Job
PORTA VILANOVA Jaime - à la Moulasse " " " " " "
HERNANDEZ HERNANDEZ Jose - à Saint Etienne(Loire) Chez Mr. Abel Gaillard.
ESPINETA BALLESTER Pelmiro - à Montauban (T.et G.)à la Societé Pyrencene.
PLAZA GARRIDO Teodoro - à Albi (Tarn) à la STE. Pyréenne.
FERNANDEZ ALMANZA Leopoldo - à Albi (Tarn) " " "
FERIA DEL POZO Manuel - " " " " " "
GUALLAR GUALLAR Francisco - " " " " " "
ALBA CASO Grabiel à Mazerés (Arceje) Chez Mr. Valat Fernand coiffer
TOSQUELLAS LLAURADOR Franccoso- à Sant. Alban-Sur-Lomagnole(Lozere) Chez le Dr. Balset.
ALCARAZ ARACIL Jose - à Vincelies(Tarn) à L'Eutreprou Brenguer et Toudeut.
(56) METALLURGISTES - à Tarbes (H. Pyr.) à la Maison Hispano 1' Suiza.
(29) OUVRIERS DEVERS à Auch (Gers) à la disposition de l'Offic e departamental de la main d'oeuvre.
(50) METALLURGISTES à Fermyni (Loire) aux forges et Acieriesde Fermyni.

REFUDIES ESPAGNOLS INVALIDES DIRIGES SUR ALBAFEUILLE&LAGARDE&(T;tG

GALINDO RIBAS Agustin
ROMERO GOMEZ Francisco
CORTES ALVAREZ Leopoldo
RUZ PEREZ Francisco
ALVAREZ GARCIA Paulino
EGEA GARCIA Jose
GARCIA BOUEZ Laureano
LOSADA OLMO Antonio

for Tosquelles to leave the camp and join his medical team in January 1940. Tosquelles's passport that allowed him to travel from Septfonds to Saint-Alban was the 1934 French publication of clinical research he had done with Antoni Subirana, which had been widely read by French psychiatrists. That was how his psychiatric experience at the refugee camp, which for many was a way to escape reclusion and death, became the pathway to the place where he would spend more than twenty years practicing new forms of institutional psychotherapy: patient clubs, ergotherapy cooperatives, and cultural production through theater, cinema, writing, and debates over paid work.

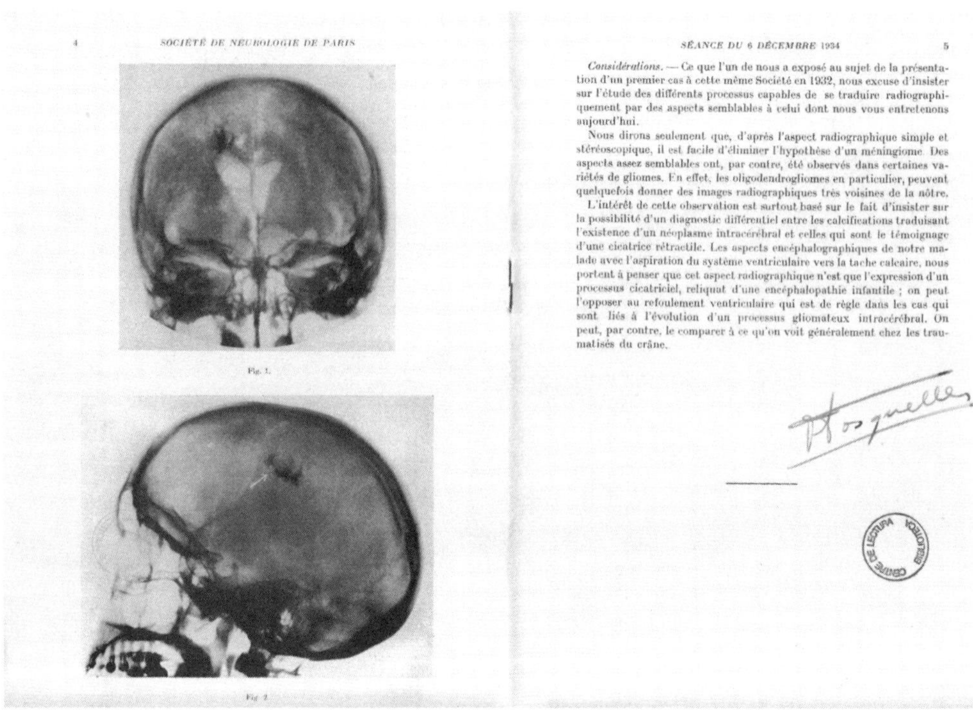

4 SOCIÉTÉ DE NEUROLOGIE DE PARIS

Fig. 1.

Fig. 2

SÉANCE DU 6 DÉCEMBRE 1934 5

Considérations. — Ce que l'un de nous a exposé au sujet de la présentation d'un premier cas à cette même Société en 1932, nous excuse d'insister sur l'étude des différents processus capables de se traduire radiographiquement par des aspects semblables à celui dont nous vous entretenons aujourd'hui.

Nous dirons seulement que, d'après l'aspect radiographique simple et stéréoscopique, il est facile d'éliminer l'hypothèse d'un méningiome. Des aspects assez semblables ont, par contre, été observés dans certaines variétés de gliomes. En effet, les oligodendrogliomes en particulier, peuvent quelquefois donner des images radiographiques très voisines de la nôtre.

L'intérêt de cette observation est surtout basé sur le fait d'insister sur la possibilité d'un diagnostic différentiel entre les calcifications traduisant l'existence d'un néoplasme intracérébral et celles qui sont le témoignage d'une cicatrice rétractile. Les aspects encéphalographiques de notre malade avec l'aspiration du système ventriculaire vers la tache calcaire, nous portent à penser que cet aspect radiographique n'est que l'expression d'un processus cicatriciel, reliquat d'une encéphalopathie infantile ; on peut l'opposer au refoulement ventriculaire qui est de règle dans les cas qui sont liés à l'évolution d'un processus gliomateux intracérébral. On peut, par contre, le comparer à ce qu'on voit généralement chez les traumatisés du crâne.

Final pages of the article by Tosquelles and Subirana published in the *Revue neurologique*, no. 6, December 1934

At the special session of the Société de neurologie de Paris, in 1932, one of us presented a case of intracranial calcification in an epileptic.

An analysis of observations recorded in the literature showed us the difficulty of classifying this case of "Hirsteine" de Schüller in one of the familiar forms.

As we noted on that occasion, intracranial calcifications can be divided into two large groups: the neoplastic group and the nonneoplastic group. Without a doubt, the case in question belonged to the second group, and we had compared it to a similar case described by Sullivan as involving in all probability an early-stage brain stone.

It seems to us that the case we're presenting today resembles the one we presented in 1932.

But in this patient the radiologically verifiable alterations can be attributed to a scar resulting from an ailment appearing at the age of four, which left her, in the clinical aftermath, with a cerebral infantile hemiplegia and epileleptic seizures. [...]

Considerations—What one of us laid out in our presentation of a first case to this same society in 1932 should excuse us from insisting on the study of the different processes amenable to radiography through aspects similar to the one we are discussing with you today.

We will only say that, according to the simple radiographic and stereoscopic view, it's easy to eliminate the hypothesis of a meningioma. Rather similar aspects, however, have been observed in certain varieties of glioma. Indeed, oligodendrogliomas in particular can sometimes give radiographic images very close to ours.

The interest of this observation is due especially to an insistence on the possibility of a diagnostic differential between calcifications showing the existence of an intracerebral neoplasm and those attesting to a retractile scar. The encephalographic aspects of our patient, with aspiration of the ventricular system toward the calcareous spot, suggest to us that this radiographic aspect is just the expression of scar formation, the remainder of an infantile encephalopathy. This can be contrasted with the ventricular backflow that is typical in cases linked to the evolution of an intracerebral gliomatous process. One can compare it, however, with what one generally sees in patients with cranial trauma.[14]

François Tosquelles and Antoni Subirana, "Un nouveau cas de calcification intracérébrale visible radiologiquement chez un hémiplégique de l'enfance avec crises épileptiques jacksoniennes: Aspects Encéphalographiques" [A new case of intracranial calcification, radiologically visible in a childhood hemiplegic with Jacksonian epileptic seizures: encephalographic aspects], session of the Société de neurologie, Paris, December 6, 1934

INSTITUT PERE MATA 3739

FULL CLÍNIC

d

lloc de naixement:
residència:
darrer lloc d'estada: "
data del naixement: 26 anys
estat civil: soltera professió:
Nom del pare: (d.)
naturalesa:
Nom de la mare: (V.)
naturalesa:
Nom del consort:
naturalesa:
Nom dels fills:

Entrades

Número	Data	Sol.licitant	Classe	Pessetes
11.571	I 16 de maig 1934	Instància pròpia	Ajt. de Reus, 1-28-2	85
	II 1 setembre 1936	Generalitat		95
S.A.860	III 13-Sepbre. 1945	Reingreso	Dip. Tarrag. 236 M.	240
	IV			
	V			
	VI			
	VII			
	VIII			

Sortides

Número	Data	Sol.licitant	Concepte
	I 31 agost 1936		Passa a 95.
685	II 11 Setembre 1938		Trasllat St. Andreu
2006V	III 28 Septiembre 1940		Defunción
	IV		
	V		
	VI		
	VII		
	VIII		

Dades diverses

Medical history of the patient whose case was the basis of Tosquelles and Subirana's research at the Institut Pere Mata

THE SPANISH CIVIL WAR

[...] From being a tradition throughout the West, and especially given the staggering number of victims of fascism, anti-Semitism has become an indicative factor, often a unique one, unfortunately, in many other deadly exclusions of the *other* defined as radically strange and dangerous. In truth, most often it's a matter of exclusions that are sly but just as deadly. The murderous *elimination* of psychotics in the same period stands as evidence.

In the last analysis, fascist anti-Semitism constitutes a criminal social practice that, analogously with a certain number of sacrifices or ritual and public murders, stems from a magical hope: that is, it involves a real wager, a real challenge, indeed a magical address to the gods—who are imagined to be playing with our future, without too many considerations for our shortcomings and our sufferings. The manifestations of apocalyptic despair that result in anti-Semitic phobia barely conceal what, in everyone's psychic reality, constitute phobic impulses that are among the most primary and radical, automatically set off by any hint of the presence of madness in others, seen as strange and malevolent.

Ignorance of the fear of the other then moves to the fore, in all the possible social scenarios. [...]

It's in this way, too, that the activation of the multitudes, the masses put in motion in the course of civil wars—such as ours, starting on July 19, 1936—poses an ethical problematic, in relation to which each combatant has to define themselves concretely.

Apart from the geographic distributions that intervened in the allegiances of a large number of combatants, each adult was called upon in fact to take part or not, according to their ethical perspectives, which did not always match up with the ideological formulations—often more partial and split than one might think.

This became apparent in the activity of all those who joined up, with a lucid spontaneity, during those first days of the war, especially in the victorious street battles—which the Catalan and worker militias mounted in opposition to the massive insurrection of the whole Spanish army. The case of Madrid, where the fascist army was also defeated, despite the lesser clout of the proletariat in that region, is to be explained in terms of political perpectives and a distributive structure very different from the relative weight of the social forces present.

I can't deal here with all the cleavages at play in that civil war—indeed with all the tendencies and other divisions manifested beyond the battleground in the whole world—that is, in other nations and among different states. [...]

Interview conducted in French by Françoise Picard, "François Tosquelles et la guerre d'Espagne" [François Tosquelles and the Spanish Civil War], *Vie sociale et traitements*, no. 172 (August–September 1987), pp. 35–38.

It was to underscore this problem of identity that I accentuated what constituted a pressing concern of the Spanish military insurrection: as on other occasions, the aim was to erase the culture, language, and history of Catalonia—which is to say, its identity. People often tend, perhaps you yourself, to minimize this aspect of the war. In the face of this misunderstanding, I can't help but recall a whole succession of historical events that essentially concern the engagement of Castile's authoritarian and inquisitorial feudalism, with the aim of controlling the entire Iberian Peninsula, and in fact the whole New World—as opposed to the Mediterranean, industrialist, and democratic outlook of Catalonia. One says Spain, thus hiding the fact that it's only Castile's actions that one has in mind. It's true that choosing the Bourbons as kings of Spain led to the persistent ignorance in France concerning these old and still-current problems; and I leave out of consideration the collaboration of the French in the long siege of Barcelona from 1714 to 1717.

That said, not all the latent and manifest tensions of the Civil War in question are reducible to the Castile–Catalonia antagonism.

There's never a single *cause*, either in the relatively dramatic historical events, or in any of the symptoms that emerge, or indeed that are provoked by certain *maladies*.

The very evolution of psychopathological crises—of the Spanish Civil War itself—always derives from a complex array of current factors inflecting the movement and the pressures of the older factors in play. For example, at the start of the war, no one could fail to recognize the characteristic scenario of the class struggle, brought into focus at that moment. Further, in 1936 the class struggle as the most concrete aspect of history's universal dynamic was omnipresent.

However, in May 1937, the proletariat, as the leading element, the protagonist of the class struggle, had already lost its specific role in our war. The Generalitat de Catalunya itself had lost all its real power in the conduct of the war and in the political life of Catalonia, when the central authority, more or less armed and inspired by the Spanish Communist Party, violently imposed itself in Barcelona on the powerful, originally anarchist, workers' movement, and on the organization that was very firmly implanted in the Catalan proletariat, the Workers' Party of Marxist Unification, the POUM [Partido obrero de unificación Marxista]—often labeled then as Trotskyist—in the well-known style of the Stalinist period. Little by little, everything became the fault of certain states and their politicians: Germany, Italy, and indeed Russia.

This was the Spanish war, not a localized civil war, but something with a universal dimension, aiming for the seizure of power by the proletariat. The International Brigades, present mainly on the Madrid front, it should be said, were withdrawn from combat and dissolved in December 1938, in the middle of the Battle of the Ebro, at the southern gates of Catalonia. The proletariat being disappeared from the historical movement in this way, everything was ready for the great war of the states—which as concerns France, commenced in September 1939. You know what ensued.

I could describe here the psychiatric activities and services implemented with the Catalan militias on the Aragon front, involving a quite useful change in the very form of psychiatric work, when at the beginning of 1938 the People's Army of the Spanish Republic ended up accepting—grudgingly on the part of the Russian agents—the need to organize psychiatric services appropriate to the wartime situation.

It was mainly the pressure from Professor Mira that accomplished this change of perspective that we very much hoped for in Aragon. So I was named chief of psychiatric services. I implemented the work of our core teams and mobile interventions in a vast space that encompassed Castile, in fact, bordering on Toledo, Extremadura, and the north of Andalusia. This lasted till April 1, 1939. I was able to successfully liquidate the affair and then miraculously escape with my life. After many twists and turns, by the 1st of September I was already in France.

So I participated, as a person in charge, in the two periods, and the different forms of psychiatric activities centered on phenomena that were directly or indirectly modulated by the war. The interest of this seems relatively secondary to me, although I concluded from these activities that one can and must always do the best psychiatry possible everywhere, while attending to concrete social situations, where one finds oneself with patients, and one knows more or less how they are relating psychically with their affinity or coexistence groups.

THE MEANING OF THE POUM'S SLOGANS

Political observers who do not have class-conscious, or more precisely Marxist, training have pointed out, almost to the point of obsession, the disparity of criteria revealed in the lack of correspondence between the main slogans of the POUM [Partido obrero de unificación Marxista, or the Workers' Party of Marxist Unification] and those of most of the organizations that are in the anti-fascist struggle alongside us.

The special interest of an organization—not ours—has made these differences take on an extraordinary importance with the objective of offering the "public" an unqualified interpretation that is ineffective with the working class, according to which we belong to or maintain concomitances with the fifth column or General Franco himself. The workers have memory and common sense and naturally have paid no heed to that gratuitous statement nor have they been able to believe that "Poumism" is an organization of "systemically oppositionist tendencies or innate interlopers." Common sense and memory have made them understand how facts of individual characterology become diluted in organizations, like ours, that are governed by a true internal democracy.

The workers are very familiar with our most prominent members and know that our history leaves no room for doubt about the firmness of our revolutionary ideal. The workers have been capable of seeing, in the example of the leaders of our youth ranks, the greatest guarantee of anti-fascism. Barcelona's Plaça Universitat, El Molino, near Huesca, the Sigüenza Cathedral, and recently Pozuelo are the eternally flaming tombs of our comrades who in life were members of the Central Committee of the heroic Joventuts Comunistes Ibèriques of the POUM.

SO WHAT IS THE MEANING OF THE POUM'S "OPPOSITIONAL" SLOGANS?

* * *

The main slogan of a Marxist party should be attested fundamentally by the historical interpretation based on the class struggle, which cannot be comprehended in a static fashion—in the present—but through its evolution. On the other hand, the slogans must be converted, through action, into an effective weapon, to the service of one of the classes in the struggle: the proletariat.

OPPRESSOR AND OPPRESSED, STOOD IN CONSTANT OPPOSITION TO ONE ANOTHER, CARRIED ON AN UNINTERRUPTED, NOW HIDDEN, NOW OPEN FIGHT, A FIGHT THAT EACH TIME ENDED, EITHER IN A REVOLUTIONARY RECONSTITUTION OF SOCIETY AT LARGE, OR IN THE COMMON RUIN OF THE CONTENDING CLASSES. (*Communist Manifesto*)

The triumph of the proletariat is not fated or historically inevitable; it depends on their "knowing how to defeat" the bourgeoisie. The Party is the brain, the general of this battle; the slogans of the Party are weapons indispensable to the victory.

* * *

Francesc Tosquelles, "Sentit de les consignes del POUM," *La Torxa: Portantveu del POUM i de les JCI de Reus*, no. 4 (January 30, 1937), p. 3.

On July 19, the "Spanish" army rose up in arms against the "Republican legality."

On July 19, the organized proletariat defeated the rebel army on the streets of the main capitals.

Since July 19, the struggle continues on the combat fronts.

But the world did not begin on July 19; July 19 had a calendar of years ahead of it, whose pages were linked not only by continuity but also by historical causality. It will be possible to comprehend July 19 if we find that causal link.

An unknown hero has spent two months obsessed with the memory of July 19, enraptured by the proletariat's heroic feat, "divinely" singing the epic deed; but our hero did not comprehend July 19.

July 19 is not an overlapping of days; July 19 is a consequence.

* * *

Spain did not achieve its bourgeois revolution in the eighteenth century, nor in the nineteenth century.

The secret of success is proper timing.

Spain became a semicolony of the British and the French; its economy is fundamentally agrarian, and its nascent industry grows stunted and parasitic on the hunch-backed torso of a feudal agrarian state. The export of farmed products means the import of manufactured goods; the continuation of the agrarian feudal state means foreign competition against national industry within the domestic market.

The development of the industrial bourgeoisie means the violent rupture of the economic bases of the agrarian feudal state, it means the realization of the bourgeois revolution.

The repatriation of the "colonial" army following nationalist insurrection in the Americas and the war of liberation against the French created a hypertrophic army.

The presence of the organized proletariat castrates the aggressive possibilities of the "revolutionary" bourgeoisie. The bourgeoisie moves callously from revolutionary to treacherous through hesitation and indecision.

Every attempt at bourgeois revolution in Spain has been thwarted by these two failings.

* * *

The world economy is constantly changing; all of a sudden the foreign agricultural markets are crashing; the agrarian crisis provokes a political change; the landowners and exporters become Republicans. The Republic will be a new instance of bourgeois revolution headed up by the bourgeoisie itself with the collaboration of their natural enemies: the farmers.

Consequence: failure.

The secret of success is proper timing.

Our former friend Miravitlles studied the budgets of the Republic.

POLITICS ARE CONCENTRATED ECONOMICS. (Lenin)

One can easily deduce that while the words have changed, the social alignment was the same as during the monarchy; the cold eloquence of numbers showed the bourgeoisie's inability to take the democratic revolution to its final consequences.

WINNING THE WAR ON THE FRONT REQUIRES
A WELL-ORGANIZED REAR GUARD.

FARMERS: LET'S STRUCTURE THE RURAL REVOLUTION
ON A SOLID FOUNDATION.

FARM WORKERS WANT ACTIONS AND NOT WORDS!

WE DEMAND CLEAR, CONCRETE, AND PRECISE POSITIONS
AND ROBUST ACTION ON RURAL MATTERS.

WHAT IS THE GOVERNMENT WAITING FOR
TO RESOLVE THE SOCIAL PROBLEM OF THE LAND?

FARMERS!!

BY STRENGTHENING AGRICULTURAL UNIONS
AND CREATING COOPERATIVES
YOU WILL GET RID OF THE INTERMEDIARIES.

THE UNITY OF ALL FARM WORKERS
IS YOUR GREATEST GUARANTEE.

A SINGLE OBLIGATORY UNION
IS THE BEST PATH TO THIS UNITY.

ALL FARM WORKERS UNIONIZED.
A SINGLE AGRICULTURAL UNION IN EACH TOWN.

THE COLLECTIVIZATION OF THE LAND
IS THE BEST GUARANTEE OF REVOLUTION.

COLLECTIVIZING THE LAND DOES NOT MEAN
WORKING IT COLLECTIVELY.

COLLECTIVIZING THE LAND MEANS GIVING IT
TO THOSE WHO WORK IT AND WHILE THEY WORK IT,
BE IT INDIVIDUALLY OR COLLECTIVELY.

Characteristics of the Republic:
STUNTED CAPITALISM AND GENDARME STATE.

* * *

Does the failure of the democratic revolution mean that the socialist revolution is far off?

The democratic revolution is not over.

Speaking of socialist revolution is either a subjectivist and voluntaristic error, or a Blanquist adventure.

That is how the Marxists in disagreement with us would speak if they wanted to criticize us calmly, the way we criticize them. That was how the Menshevik Kamenef spoke when criticizing Lenin.

The democratic revolution "is over" in the sense of the power takeover by the bourgeoisie. The Azaña biennium ended with the transfer of power to those like Gil-Robles and Lerroux, and the reconquest of November ended with the military insurrection.

The working class opposed those like Gil, the Red October.

The working class opposed the soldiers, their revolution.

The success of an action is evaluated once it is over. The economic structure of the monarchy has only been objectively broken by the proletariat up in arms.

The proletariat created the factory committees, the district committees, the farmers' committees. That wasn't a situation of dual power equivalent to 1917 Russia's!

The bourgeois democratic revolution must be completed and taken to its final consequences. Who should carry out this task? The petit bourgeois organizations that have already failed or the new workers' organizations that arose from the struggle?

THE LEADERS OF THE PETITE BOURGEOISIE "MUST" TEACH THE PEOPLE TO TRUST THE BOURGEOISIE. THE PROLETARIANS MUST TEACH THE PEOPLE TO DISTRUST THE BOURGEOISIE. (Lenin)

Are the farmers' committees not petit bourgeois organizations?

Are we to reject the farmers leading the revolution?

Do we want, or have we ever said we would implant, socialism by miracle—on the spot—or by decree?

We know that the capacity and revolutionary energy of the peasant farmer must be utilized to liquidate feudalism and for the proletariat revolution; but we will not let this revolution be led by the incapable petite bourgeoisie because they would waste the revolutionary energy, among other reasons. Stalin himself published a pamphlet, "The Theory and Practice of Leninism," in which he demonstrates the insufficiency of discussing whether in a particular, isolated country the objective conditions for a workers' revolution exist.

THE EXISTENCE WITHIN THIS SYSTEM OF SOME COUNTRIES WHICH ARE NOT SUFFICIENTLY DEVELOPED FROM THE INDUSTRIAL POINT OF VIEW CANNOT BE AN INSURMOUNTABLE OBSTACLE TO THE REVOLUTION *FROM THE MOMENT* WHEN THE SYSTEM AS A WHOLE IS ALREADY RIPE FOR THE REVOLUTION. (Stalin)

It is this very Leninist position according to which the capitalist front does not break in the place of greatest evolution but rather in the weakest place, precisely the place where there are more economic contradictions, more revolutions to wage, the bourgeois and the workers' revolution.

But to be clear, what breaks is the capitalism, the revolution that emerges is proletarian. In 1905, Lenin, thinking of the possibility of collaborating on a government of revolutionary coalition with the petit bourgeois (*Two Tactics*), presents the democratic revolution and the socialist revolution as two rungs of one single revolution.

THE BOURGEOIS DEMOCRATIC REVOLUTION MUST BE USED AS THE IMMEDIATE PRELUDE TO THE PROLETARIAN REVOLUTION. (Stalin, previously cited pamphlet)

As such, from an obviously Marxist perspective, it seems [clear] that:

The era of the democratic revolutions has ended.

Those who did not do it in time cannot carry it out with the same conditions as the pure democratic revolutions.

Only the proletariat allied with the peasant farmers can realize the democratic revolution and transform it into a socialist one and this transformation is fundamentally necessary.

Spain especially has demonstrated the inability of the bourgeoisie to bring about their revolution.

The fact of not having brought about democratic revolution was not an obstacle for strategizing the socialist revolution but rather more likely an advantage.

The revolutions in our era (of world capitalist crisis) are partial aspects, partial ruptures with the international capitalist chain …

* * *

July 19 was possible because the democratic revolution was failing and the workers had not decided to rectify it and take charge of leading the revolution.

July 19 did not only mean an obstacle to the progress of the revolution. Fascism—the political form of monopolistic capitalism—is the counterrevolution in the face of a failed revolution.

Spain, which does not have an efficient fascist party, had a hypertrophied army. Maurín pointed out this possibility in his books, in the meetings, and in Parliament. His last speech is an accusation of Republican ineptitude. "WHAT ARE YOU WAITING FOR TO START REPRESSING FASCISM?" he said days before, in Parliament itself.

The decision by the proletariat to crush the rebel army denotes a rectification; the proletariat moves to lead the revolution in order to quickly exhaust the democratic phase and thus join the socialist phase.

The slogans of the POUM do not lose sight of this interpretation; they all derive from this conviction, consolidated by the materialist dialectic and by the experience of class struggle and international revolutions.

Each slogan aims to enable this concrete objective: socialism.

PSYCHOTHERAPY AND POETIC FUNCTION: A READING OF "IN MEMORIAM" BY GABRIEL FERRATER

My response to the "indiscreet and pertinent" questions of my psychiatric colleagues at the Institut Pere Mata about the period before and during the war in Reus, about me, and about Oliva and Sol.

As always in therapeutic dialogue, the therapist's life events manifest in his commitment to his professional work.

Since nearly all of my colleagues at the Institut Pere Mata are from Aragon and settled in Reus after the Civil War, they never met Sol or Oliva, meaning that their reading of "In Memoriam" was when their questions arose about the events that took place in Reus in the early days of the war.

As such, I had to satisfy that curiosity, not because of its curiousness, but because any time we listen to a patient speaking—as a reader or as a psychotherapist—this brings with it connotations extracted from our own lives. Therefore, my analysis of the poetic function of language—with which Biel [Gabriel Ferrater] weaves the fabric of "In Memoriam"—could not leave out my own position as witness and actor in those moments of the war. As for Sol, there isn't much I can say about her that isn't easily surmised. As for Biel himself, or his family, also paradoxically, there is no need for me to go on at length. I can almost say that I never met them, and what I've been told is little. The only time I met Biel was at the Universitat d'Estiu in Prades, France. I found him to be a man who understood the complex problems of linguistics. I admired the precision with which he expressed himself and I told him that in our psychiatric profession linguistic issues were also highly important, and that I myself was from Reus. That was a mistake on my part. Biel "slipped" away from me and I never saw him again. I don't know if he was in a rush or if he was still afraid.

As for Oliva, as I told my colleagues at the Institut Pere Mata, I did indeed have dealings with him. Initially in a tavern, one evening and nearly in the dark—or at least now I remember it filled with cobwebs, smoke, and unpleasant smells. It was in 1930 maybe, or 1931, during the crisis that set Stalin and his people against the small core group that had struggled mightily during the first dictatorship to clandestinely form the Federació Comunista Catalano-Balear, a debate group I was part of as a student in Barcelona. My colleagues in the Bloc Obrer i Camperol, which emerged from that political crisis, asked me—since I was heading to Reus on vacation—to bring some texts and information to some militants there: Oliva, Hortoneda, and some others I can't recall as clearly. In Barcelona they believed that the militants in Reus, with the legitimate illusions that gave rise to the Russian Revolution, might follow the instructions decided by the agents of the "party," which according to Stalin had to come from

---

Francesc Tosquelles, *Funció poètica i psicoteràpia: Una lectura de "In memoriam" de Gabriel Ferrater.* Reus: Institut Pere Mata and Centre de Lectura de Reus, 1985; new revised edition, Barcelona: Arcàdia, 2022. We reproduce here the third part of the book as well as Gabriel Ferrater's poem "In Memoriam," which appeared as an appendix in the original edition of *Funció poètica i psicoteràpia*.

Moscow or Madrid, and had to go against the Republicans, against the socialists, and against the anarchists, as much or more as against the monarchists and the right wing. It was necessary, they said, to defend a single tactic that could be summed up as "all power to the Soviets." Someone joked that in any case, in Catalonia, that would have to be translated to "all power to the debate groups," because there wasn't a single Soviet in all the towns on the Iberian Peninsula. Very well. So, there in the dark, and to tell the truth somewhat reluctantly, I met up with Oliva and Hortoneda in a tavern, close to Sol's cathouse. Oliva listened to me with his eyes gleaming from more than just alcohol: they showed that he was not a man whose "vigilance" would be numbed by stories and falsehoods of people from the "party." He said that in Reus there was, it's true, many people who went to the movies and had a vicarious ball watching the cops-and-robbers heroes, like people inspired by Moscow or something similar—I didn't know he was speaking from personal experience, as an attendant and witness at the Sala Reus. But I do remember that he said many people went to the movies, stomped their feet, shouted, shrieked, and ate peanuts, impatiently awaiting the sequels. "They are hoping that someone else, those people on the silver screen, will pull their nuts out of the fire." I remember that he suggested I tell Quim (Joaquín Maurín) that here in Reus, in any case, if things went very badly, that the people of the BOC [Bloc Obrer i Camperol, or the Workers and Peasants' Group] would keep their own quacks to themselves. "The Reus group will not be a trolley for Stalin's Russia nor for the branch offices of Hitler's bragging idiots." We didn't talk about any women, not about Sol or about his wife, not even the film stars who sold the American dream to our young folk.

I didn't see Oliva again until a few days before Franco's coup, when it was clear that he, like myself and so many others, was afraid of the consequences it would have for all of our lives, and for Catalonia. We'd been chastened by the negligence, of varying degrees of good faith, by so many Republicans who trusted in the power of conviction, reason, and good sense.

I went to see him expressly to tell him that President Companys himself, who had come on Sunday to the Institut Pere Mata to see his son and speak with us, had told me that the most naive and eccentric of the men in the Madrid government—the innocent and hopeful Casares Quiroga—had just banned him from giving any weapons to the Aliança Obrera; but since our president was no fool, he would do it immediately, as the situation was so serious and urgent. So I told Oliva that we needed to see how we could connect the system of defense and counterattack with the people in the FAI and, to the extent that it was possible, control the anarchist's enthusiasm for violence. I saw him again on the 14th of July, with Jordi Arquer, who coincidentally was staying at my home for a few days, when the dealings with the anarchists in Reus became ambiguous.

Surely it eluded Biel's discernment that Oliva was smarter than he looked, although indeed often stubborn and with highly unusual ideas, but it wasn't the war that gave him his sense of "responsibility" and his brand of loyalty. Between being an attendant and ticket taker at the Sala Reus theater, and leading the committee in Reus, there was a continuity that Biel—due to the very effects of the social class where he was risking his life—couldn't see. But that's of no consequence. In regard to the poetic

n.b. Gabriel Ferrater's phonetical use of the "eu" sound is like scatting—*Reus*, *Bordeus*—in "In Memoriam" and in his later poems.

function woven in "In Memoriam," we have already mentioned the phonetic group *eu* found in both Re*us* and Bord*eus* (Bordeaux), the two landmarks or places where Biel and Oliva find themselves—or each other—dead or alive along the path of "In Memoriam." With phonetics and with his father's wine business, it is the same path that is traced and retraced; a path that is *s(eu)*—"his"—destiny. It would do Biel little good to be ironic about the people of Reus, condemned to trade with hens, or to consider them with the same *menyspr(eu)*—"disdain"—as he did Oliva. The poem will make the path, that of his own footsteps. It opens, as I said to my colleagues at the Institut Pere Mata, the *space-time* of a poem and *closes* with its 351 verses, lined up straight, one after the other. We look at how, after evoking the events in Reus, Biel's poetic work opens with other poetic constructions that he himself would say are pure "fables." The "hortus conclusus" alluded to in the "Second Fable," for example, is not merely a reference to Vilagut's cooking and the "blonde girl" but also to the "high gates" of poetry. He himself says it: "inside, the cool promises" that "spoke of a distant and long past / (he'd settle so much in a matter of years / of attentive affection), of parties and of rites / according to the calendar, and of a future / of imminent dehiscence." Nothing is finished in a single poem, or a single psychotherapeutic session, even though each time is a "whole," often in "imminent dehiscence."

Continuation of the account of some aspects of my life in Reus in 1936.

I also recalled, when speaking to my colleagues at the Institut, that I hardly ever saw Oliva again after that. During the first months of the war, I had more dealings with Hortoneda, another comrade in the POUM, who was in charge of Health care in the Reus committee. It is to Hortoneda to whom I owe or we owe the requisition of two farmhouses for the summer camps on the Salou road, now part of the Fortuny district. It was there where we were able to establish the bases of the children's psychotherapy, which had always been precarious. With the teacher Ganigué and with Jesús Montaner, an athlete who organized the psychomotor games for the children, we began operations that added to what Frias had already begun at La Gota de Llet and, in a truly dismal and hopeless way, at the Casa de la Caritat. Oliva was uninterested in the children's difficulties in life. I don't see why he should've been interested. He wasn't the only one who turned a blind eye and sought to flee his own childhood and the childhoods of others. Biel himself began his poem at fourteen years old, when he had clearly already spent many years struggling to be and become himself.

Oliva made fun of me, saying that there wasn't much to be done with those kids who still pissed and shit their pants. My projects were, to Oliva, nothing more than "an intellectual game." Often—from what can be seen in that world—I think that unfortunately one could say he was right. Even most psychiatrists manifest a true phobia of childhood. Perhaps in order to be able to make a clean break in their own lives between childhood and adult life, they've ended up organizing a "new specialization" between them. There are specialists in child psychiatry! Thus one could believe that manifestations of insanity in grown-ups arise spontaneously, or one could seek out some germ or elephant in the social park that is to blame.

Oliva again reproached me for my "intellectual game" when I spoke at the Fortuny "meeting" in the early days of the war. He told me that intellectuals—speaking of me and others—were of no use in politics. I agree, but nevertheless I thought that what I said at the Fortuny needed to be said, even if it was useless.

I spoke again from atop a truck in the Plaça Prim, with Mas, from Estat Català, and my friend Solé i Barberà, who had joined the PSUC [Unified Socialist Party of Catalonia]. That was of no use either. The objective was to inspire interest in the young and not so young, who were walking down the streets of Monterols and Padró, in creating shelters against the imminent bombings. When the bombs fell, I was no longer in Reus because I was practicing psychiatry on the Aragon front. And it is true—perhaps—that there are as many bombing victims or even more with the shelters than without them. It doesn't matter, what upset me was the lack of sensibility among many people to the dangers of being or becoming authentic men. I too believed that people needed to, looking toward the future, take responsibility. I was too young and had too little experience in the practice of *psychoanalysis with normal people* to realize that the indifference or lack of sensibility was an often-useful defense against unbearable fear and anguish.

I kept notes from my speech at the Fortuny and I can repeat them now, because they have a clear importance for what we are dealing with here.

Even without wars, politics and its effects leave marks on our destinies. The songs of love and war are always coupling and uncoupling our lives, even before birth. The ambiguities, phobias, and outbursts that coincide with, accompany, and impede the lives of each person with others always play the same song, for parties and funerals, particularly when one sheds their skin, as Biel says, at fourteen—and sometimes later as well. It is during the very shedding process that events come and go that, even when not as apparently tragic as the events that began in July 1936, move the political actions of us all—both those who join in the dance willingly and those for whom the music plays even if they are deaf to it.

Biel only makes a few allusions to his own—more or less discreet and more or less spectacular—"political-reactive" ambiguities. As in so many other things and occasions, he will treat them with irony and perhaps with hints of shame or repulsion. But everything has its importance and, in particular, that provides the always-present indicators that words lead to the realm of poetic elaborations and to the realms of each person's private and public lives.

What I said at the Fortuny in a short speech was this:

"Now, as everyone realizes, we are moving with history from one surprise to the next. Just as children do every day of their lives and they manage to keep on going. Like children, we must look at the things that are happening with our eyes wide open. We must inquire into uncertainty. We must learn to live with uncertainty.

"Since I know a little bit about the history of rogues, I can now say that the people of Reus should not believe that this civil war and revolution is an epidemic or a more or less tragic bit of nonsense dreamed up by people who are scatterbrained, woolgathering, or killjoys.

"*Here and in the world*"—I said—"an empty space has opened up that can never be covered with weak philosophies or lessons learned, not in Catalonia, not in Spain, and not around the world.

Death as a surprise and the enigmas of the deaths of our beloveds.

Considerations around certain lethal aspects of the political activities that often underscore a paranoid logic; the Marxist analysis of the processes of alienation, the need for Freudo-Marxist elaborations and the difficulty of living a concrete experience in the social camps. The difficulty of the indispensable elaboration of the death drive.

"The events we are witnessing break with the apparent continuity of each of our everyday lives. Each of us is breaking up. This break, at least for Mediterranean and European people, will be deeper than the one produced by the French Revolution and the Russian Revolution. It is not a matter of simple events we can find shelter from anywhere, because it is a matter of the concrete life of men themselves. The people of the POUM who have spoken to you have thought this over deeply and weighed the consequences. I don't know if what I am saying will be of any use to you. However, I believe that we must take the measure of the cut or the void installed in the story of each of us and in the history of humanity, so we can make the necessary leap correctly, all together and each of us on our own.

"This is not the time to lose our heads. Now is time to really think, with the difficult but essential serenity, in order to act with prudence and bravery. And if death comes or threatens us, may it be for us all a greater birth, as Maragall said. What the current historical events whisper in each of our ears is that no one lives or dies alone. Each and every one of us must take responsibility. Whether the revolution becomes a fruitful one or a simple and tragically violent comedy depends only on you, on each and every one of us together."

At the Fortuny—very few people, not even Oliva, could understand what I was saying—I think I wasn't far off. In other words, I knew that our war was not an isolated domestic event, or a simple game, or a clash of ideologies.

The logic of "ideas" is often managed by "ideologues" of all stripes, as if they were detached from the real fabric of political, social, and economic events.

Often people believe with passionate naivety that all social complexity is a mere consequence of the omnipotent personal ideas and opinions of each person. In that sense one can speak of a *paranoid logic* of political practices—which does not mean that politicians are always paranoid; they can become paranoid as easily or more so than others do in the limited and reduced ambit of their family and friends.

What is perhaps not known—*or avoided*—is that this paranoid logic has direct, often hidden, roots that absorb nourishment from each person's psychosexual problems, and give the expectation and spectacles of death a place of pride that is—as they often say—honorable. And it is here where the cause lies. There are many people—almost always "obsessives"—who would say that they are *condemned* to live until the death they sense and smell all around them finally comes. Beyond death, all they do is navel gaze.

Biel in "In Memoriam" also talks to us about the dead. What accounting of the events of that period—in prose or as the object of a poetic re-elaboration—could fail to mention it?

There was no need to go to the movies, or read adventure or detective novels, or even continue playing cops and robbers, as many of us used to do, for death to become a spectacle in our reach. There was no need to be obsessive or perverse to constantly, day and night, in public and in private, see our own imagined death, elusive, depicted or portrayed on the screen of the deaths of others.

In war, and particularly in civil wars, oft-imagined private death that gives way to the fear of losing our beloveds becomes a palpable and radically irreversible reality. Simple separation, the loss of one of our family members or friends, the feeling of being abandoned by those we love, these all inevitably mark everyday activities with angst over a death that seems possible, but which is luckily only temporary. Now, with the war, separations and deaths inexorably become definitive events.

In times of war, it is not even necessary that the death we encounter, often by surprise, is that of someone we know. Perhaps thanks to the surprise, but even more so due to the difficulties of identifying the corpse, this is precisely when we more often think, in a lucid and concrete way, about one of the aspects I will now discuss of the linked things that are almost always hidden or forgotten when dealing directly with the presence or imminence of death of those we know and love.

What I will say about this is not derived solely from my personal experience. It also—and primarily—comes from what is almost always said little by little in long psychoanalytical dialogues, when during the analyst's silence, the speaker progressively and openly evokes his personal experience with death. In the face of death, people—young and old, quickly or gradually—come to evoke or ruminate "new evidence" even more surprising than death itself. They realize that not even the thick fog of emotions or war can ever erase the disappointment or disillusionment evidenced by another's death: nothing more and nothing less than *realizing that, in fact, they didn't really know the person they'd been living with for so many years*. Something more or less hidden left with them. It becomes clear that having witnessed concrete actions and remembering words spoken by someone is not enough to even know what they thought; and much less to know their dreams, how they elaborated their desires, always somewhat thwarted or unrealized. Our beloved dead take their dreams with them, and if we still love them, we ask that they leave us a legacy.

Someone who, in the course of their analysis, explained their casual presence at the burial of a stranger then told me, significantly although his tone was joking: "Who knows who that dead man really was, who knows what he dreamed of!;" "You've never analyzed a dead man!;" "So you don't know what they dream of, either!;" "I do, because I stayed by my father's deathbed for some hours ... I fell asleep and dreamed; but it wasn't my dream, it was his, I'm convinced of that. Our parents pull out all the stops to make us the heirs to their dreams."

Which is why, for example, an analyst, Maud Mannoni, says that what is most important to the children she treats—mentally impaired or psychotics—is not what their parents have done or said to them but what their parents keep quiet. She refers primarily to what sometimes is still called—in melodramatic style—"a family secret." The children then come with their clinical symptoms to do something—suffering or making others suffer—that is always directly—and in significance—related to what their parents have concealed from them. That is often true, even though it does not explain the full fabric nor all the symptoms nor, to put it one way, the illness.

The case is, as everyone knows, that children often put much effort into realizing the dreams of their ancestors and also that other times they do the exact opposite—which also maintains the same dream very vividly in the minds of the offspring rather than erasing it.

Despite the objective twists and turns of life, and despite the breaks in history we create, it is there that the continuity and the very source of what can be called "a culture" lies. When observing a family, one often sees that even the resumption of the communication of unconscious desire and dreams can skip a generation or two. The chain of generations is as important and sometimes more so than the breaks. There are also those chains of the dead that represent us, for example, in a totemic tree such as the classic African baobab—a sort of cemetery sometimes real or reserved for special occasions, like a celebration or a party for the tribe's dead. Certain oak trees serve the same symbolic function, and we could even say that the bell tower in Reus is a stone tree, which sometimes invites the churchgoing living to eat traditional "bread and nuts" in the old graveyard—the one they call the Slaughterhouse—to repeat totemic meals in an attempt to recover the dreams of past generations and make them our own.

However, setting aside all lyricism, we find in certain (so-called) pathological forms of life patients who suffer and complain that an inner force or "voice" leads their life, and they cannot think on their own or do anything of their own volition. In classical psychiatry we call that "deliriums of possession." In fact, like in certain archaic cultures, it was said that the spirit of a dead person—sometimes of a demon—had taken control over the victim. And this is not a question of magic, or even of unfortunate loyalties and identifications. One is closer to the truth when one evokes "male-*dictions*" that strive to "re-*state*" what one never knows about the persistent dreams of certain of the tribe's dead ancestors. A kind of return, where one realizes that the dead and other disappeared things still form part of our lives. Sometimes we also find some patients and even some people who pass as sane—and who are—who tell us that they live with a dead person inside them, weighing on them, dragging on them, and creating a void within that is very hard to bear.

Keeping in mind all these contingencies of human suffering, I insist on the fact that it is when faced with the death of a loved one when we most realize how little we knew about them and obviously about what drove them, about their unconscious desires, or about their dreams. With their death, the "truth" of our loved one slips away from us. The possible regrets, which often grip a member of the family, are nothing more than another way to express or hide this real problem.

In any case, it is clear that the anecdotes evoked by Biel in "In Memoriam" cannot be considered a testimony of a series of politically significant acts. The very deaths evoked in relation with this catastrophe do not lead us to consider any aspect of the economic and political crisis, nor any of the expectations inherent in national and international history. I do not believe Biel portrays any of the dead as standard-bearers of a political battle for the future. The conflicts between men, in the poem he writes, move in an egocentric and homegrown perspective. Every dead man evoked, however, is weighed down by his own nature as a singular man and, in fact, then becomes an element of Biel's own process of personalization.

As such, I will now explain the interest that sociological considerations and analyses hold, particularly for us, in the evaluation and practice of our profession ... But it is also time to define the limitations and even the incapacity of leading us there where the uniquely personal disruptions lie, although somehow the disruptions themselves always lead us, with varying lucidity, to take part in the field of political events or to flee from it.

Sociological analyses can be reduced to descriptions of a collective scene as dramatic or comic, in which committed people co-determine their behaviors for concrete decisions, or for the opinions each member of the group forms of the others, or even for what we try to extract as constants and variables in the sociological analyses; the limitation of what sociological technique can establish always becomes an opaque obstacle, in terms of the subject's process of self-creation. That developed this way, transparent in regard to the work of Marx where all the signifiers of sex and death are left out of the circle of interests, whose dynamics and historical and commonplace distributions he tries to analyze. Even the "objects" he studies are analyzed more as values of change than values of use, even though values of use naturally involve movements of desire and the body. Admitting that still today the great directions or lines of development of the "tensions" and "exits" of the society Marx describes remain valid, they still do not offer us a path into our work if we do not also take into account, in a "radical" way, what Freud, through psychotherapeutic practice, has been uncovering about man. And even if we consider that Marx's sociological work, like all scientific works, is determined and limited by his time period, in fact it continues to be used by many sociologists and critics of history and by people of varied and often opposing political orientations. They often don't say they use it, but they do. And when they don't, their works as sociologists or historians are so foolish they almost make one laugh or cry.

Very well. What is now important for us is taking the social alienation that Marx tried to define in its forms and mechanisms and adding to it what each concrete man of flesh and blood, living or dead, has been uncovering—also with scientific and *rational* methods—precisely through the research projects regarding what is termed "mental alienation." People in general, and often in unison with the proclamations of the most outstanding spokespersons of each culture, utterly reject any consideration of what can be discovered or concealed by the facts of alienation. Mad ones are the always the first to pay the piper. In fact, death and madness still are two forms of taboo that hardly anyone dares to face. It is not a simple fear, but rather a true phobia and persistently prohibited. It is only acceptable to joke about them ... or to circle around them anonymously with philosophical elaborations, and sometimes with literary works that almost always entail a quick change of subject. I believe that Biel knew that.

As such, it is "logical" that it's been very difficult to take steps to smooth the path and create links and bridges beyond these two taboos in question, in order to piece together a theory that is practicable for the "subject" in relation, always, with the other, with language, with society. Without accentuating, with madness, the problems of sex and death. In any case, all the seeds of Freudo-Marxism that have been put forth for that have failed to find the necessary fields of experience for a scientific elaboration. Often, the Freudo-Marxist writings do not transcend simple statements of good intentions, describing utopian or polemical perspectives that approach and sometimes turn out to be truly "delusional" products. We would almost have to say that, lacking any concrete field of experience, many times they get lost along the paths of ideologies, of philosophical and aesthetic productions. It is well known that, when avoiding a rational and experimental approach to any scientific object, many "model" productions, in one way or another, have often circled and circled around the same axis or same void, like horses on a carousel or donkeys on a waterwheel. We will never get past the stories told around the fire if we lack a field of experience—a laboratory.

Without experimental repetition, none of the hypotheses of science amount to anything. And this is not the moment to retract what I could say about the experiences of what is termed institutional psychotherapy, as has been happening in France. Despite the concrete character of those experiences that many of my colleagues have been developing with me or in other places, I have always been aware of their failings as well as the impossibility of achieving "concrete exportations" of them within the psychiatric market. In any case, I have never accepted reducing their action to the task of a traveling salesman or a propagandist.

Here we must consider both what Biel tells us and the propaganda that a certain Freudianism, or even a certain Freudo-Marxism, has made of the problem of sex. Easily evoked, more delivered than released to everyday pedagogy—to exultant propaganda and to public acts—it is easy to take it too far, spontaneously. This makes it seem as if the elaboration of sexual problems can happen without stumbling blocks or reservations. In any case it is true that now people can talk about it naturally, without shame or remorse. Let us suppose that thus, via the miracle of the spoken word and pedagogy, sexual repression had magically disappeared along with its conscious and unconscious effects. I don't believe it has, but that's not what concerns us here. What becomes very clear, however, is that nothing of the kind has happened—in fact, more the opposite—with the death drive. We have already mentioned here that many people of good faith—and furthermore, professional scientists—have almost always made light of the concept of drive, relegating it to a pure manifestation of animal instinct. But what happened with Freud's death drive is much worse. When—with clinical experience, and by that I mean concrete psychoanalysis—he tried to endow the death drive with a rational statute, everyone—and most psychoanalysts as well—shouted that the question was scandalous and delusionally absurd. Once again they forgot that, as happens with all the specific drives of human destiny, the death drive also comes and goes, settles down and tirelessly repeats its charms, solely along the path of language. On the other hand, death, the one most people refer to, remains on the imaginary plane or on the plane of biology. Never, or almost never, is *symbolic death* dealt with, nor its links that, like all symbolic structures, are established in the field of social life.

The repetition.

Biel himself, despite his poetic work that is so measured and calculated, has been crushed by the "rock of suffering." I think that, thus, he was able to make his own death drive and perhaps all the deaths evoked in "In Memoriam" simply a "passage" to the biological act, even though surely he sees it as a lucid, even rationalized, act. Obviously, I can't know, but I see that as fundamentally a result of the insufficiency of his unconscious work to elaborate the death drive as such. Biel's death can only be "anticipated" and "experienced" as a "repetitive fate" in a visual manner and, in fact, finally released from the destiny of all the sexual drives or—to put it politely—of the eventualities and dimensions of love.

Verbal evocations of death are always among the most fruitful moments in all psychotherapeutic processes.

Thus now I will appeal to some personal references regarding the paths of children's worries, since dialogues between the father and sons—in any event—deal with the "mysterious" problems of imaginary death and symbolic death. I will talk about myself, because we've also said that in every act of psychotherapy the analyst's personal problems come into play, so no patient can get further in his work than his analyst has gotten with his own. That does not mean that the patient merely imitates the analyst. Quite the contrary, the analyst's previous work in terms of his own singularity guarantees the freedom of the reconstruction that is being analyzed.

So although this is about my father and me, and about the dead, I will leave aside the various possibilities that follow and repeat the oedipal legend, as it is not what interests me here. Although it's generally forgotten, King Laius appears as having abandoned his son to death, or at least as having failed to recognize him as the heir to the throne. Others prefer to think that it is the boy himself, Oedipus, who kills his father without recognizing him when they meet at the crossroads of Thebes. As we know, legends are a verbal mechanism that can be entered in various ways. Between a father and his son there is always a spoken and unspoken dialogue in which death is a problem. However, in the case of the Oedipus legend, we see that often people prefer to treat it as a sexual problem of incest: indeed, it is well known that erections and laughter are easily brought on and cast off.

So now I will explain how a dialogue on death emerged between me and my father.

It was at the end of the "European" war of 1914–1918. On November 11 we hung up a sheet on the balcony of our home, sewn with red letters that said "Long live peace." For me, the war was images on trading cards, and I knew that people got killed there, people who weren't Moors or Jews but people who were defending their land, their nations. I considered the Catalan volunteers heroes, and in my mental theater there was a jumble of ambulances and hospitals. A few months later, many boys—and girls?—from our town cheerfully paraded around, not wearing berrettinos but dressed as soldiers of each country. Like on the trading cards, but I was also expecting to see the dead, and I saw none. My unsatisfied curiosity led me to ask my father what they'd done with the dead. "In the present circumstance," he responded, "there is really only one, and it will be the straw dummy of the Carnival King." However, it seemed to me that they burned that Carnival King as if it were alive. Back at home, very angrily I told my father: "You tricked me, you said millions had died." His response: "Yes ... but no one knows them ... they are the anonymous dead."

That was how I learned that, in the Great War, what affected people, both the passionate and the indifferent, was the *leap death took toward general anonymity* as evidenced by the ridiculous monuments to the unknown soldier. The deaths of the Jews and the atomic bomb in the last war are events that connote the same *impersonal and anonymous death*.

I repeat that social and even mental alienation are related to the *ubiquitous anonymity based on the anonymity of death*. Perhaps that has happened at other moments in history. I wasn't there. But I often think how in many pre-Christian religions the problem of death was more of a personal elaboration. Of death or of immortality, one could say, like in those stories of successive reincarnations in different forms of animals or objects. There is an enormous difference between *reincarnations* into some other body and *resurrection*.

When Christ disappeared from the tomb—they say—he left a story or a text with some angels, with memories of past events. So the angels carried the story to the women who were waiting to celebrate the great burial. Absent body, in the same place as the disappeared body, through the spoken or written word of the angels becomes the place of all possible rebirth. Perhaps it is not a coincidence that Biel has an angel's name, and that his word still reaches us here and now when his body has become completely absent.

Since the story—or legend—of Christ, it would make sense—at least in our culture—that everyone would be permanently resurrected *by the very spoken and retransmitted word.* This is precisely the objective of the word's poetic function, which is not a quality exclusive to professional poets and should not be confused with memory. An unspoken memory does nothing or, at most, is a nuisance and an obstacle.

There is no other mystery to *resurrection* than the work with words, day in and day out. There is no other incarnation than our children—yet the relationships between parents and children are only structured through verbal exchanges. Facts matter, but they matter, as far as the subject is concerned, only when they become a literary construction: fables and fabulation are only one particular case that matters to those who listen and discuss them, because *up until now, indirectly,* the texts always made metaphoric or metonymic reference, obliquely, to a personal, authentically lived story. The facts themselves—note what Biel tells us in passing—"In the moment it didn't affect me much." Yet despite that, he doesn't manifest in his poem the lack of interest of a heart insensitive to the tragedies recounted: he bears witness only to a structural fact inherent in the poetic function of language. And it is precisely that which makes psychotherapy possible as a human activity *radically projected in the place where the subject lies*—which is not, I will repeat, *his consciousness.*

Obviously, psychotherapy is an activity we provide through technique. What happens in session is no mystery or magical effect. It is what is always in reach of everyone, even though everything depends fundamentally on the other to whom the messages are addressed, "patim-patam," as the song goes. Madness and sanity are notions that, on this level of interhuman relations and their effects, are completely irrelevant.

* * *

At the beginning or end of a book to which many people have contributed their efforts, one must thank them.

I hope that all the readers of my work realize how indebted I am—and over many years—to numerous patients, now more or less anonymous, and to their *caregivers.*

This began at the Institut Pere Mata with a certain intention that had striven to be lucid since I was eight or nine years old, even though it really took root in 1929, and especially after 1933, when I began to practice medicine there.

Of all my colleagues—teachers and friends—the first one I met (without forgetting the debt I owe to Dr. E. Mira i López for all he taught me and encouraged me to do), and in my very home, was Dr. Emili Briansó. Being a precocious child, I learned much about his anxieties and hopes from the long conversations and friendship he had with my godfather, Dr. Francesc Llauradó.

I also knew that in the technical journal published at the Institut Pere Mata he'd written that he foresaw that psychoanalysis would bring radical changes in how patients were treated. Surely that was the first time a Catalan doctor paid any attention to Freud. That was in 1911.

Starting in Reus and later in France, over many years, as much as possible I've continued persevering in that effort.

The humanization of hospitals and treatments—inside asylums and out—is not enough to provide care. Good will and enthusiasm buffer the disappointments. Concrete health care policy, locally and generally, results from a technique elaborated with effort over years. If it is not conducted this way, it won't last and everything will be lost in polemical debates that are merely a hindrance.

It has almost been seventeen years since I resumed regular contact with the people who work at the Institut. It goes without saying that without them I never would have even dreamed of writing this book. I don't want to name anyone in particular, because everyone there has contributed, directly or indirectly.

I feel that in any case putting down in writing these many uncommon ideas and concepts, which are often confusing and not in keeping with what many professionals teach or what circulates in cultured environments, will be useful for everyone.

It may be that bearing witness to the radically human character of the difficulties that stall and surprise patients—provoking a whole series of exclusions from the social groups they live in—is an indispensable hygienic task prior to all caretaking and prevention of madness.

People who are of sane spirit—or believe themselves to be—are not radically different from patients. They also use similar psychic mechanisms and social situations to continue on as best they can. What very often happens is that the sane are even more afraid of these stories than others are. Which is why, often, they don't want to hear them.

As I express my gratitude for all my colleagues at the Institut and those who've had the patience to read me, I want to make a special mention of Mr. Macaya i Gausset. He has been, from the beginning, in charge of the annual secretarial tasks for the Jornades d'interès psiquiàtric that have been organized annually in Reus over the last fifteen years around Easter week. I am also indebted to him for the wearying job of typing up my text numerous times, and I wish to acknowledge his willingness, his efforts, and his loyalty.

IN MEMORIAM
Gabriel Ferrater

When the war first broke out, I was
fourteen and two months old. In the moment
it didn't affect me much. My head was fully
turned by something else, which I still now
consider more important. I discovered
Les Fleurs du Mal, which meant
poetry, certainly, but there is
something else, I don't know what to call it
and it is what matters. Revolt? No.
That was what I called it then. Lying in
a hazel tree; at the heart of a rose
with soft and very green leaves, like
the skins of a flayed caterpillar, there,
in the world's crotch, I thickened in
happy revolt and, while the country
cracked with revolt and counter-
revolt, perhaps not happy, but
more in revolt than I. Moral
life? Sort of, but more ambiguous.
Perhaps the better term is *selfishness*,
and it's best to remember that at fourteen
we have to shift from the first person:
the plural is too tight around us, and the exercise
of the singular stylite, the nausea of
the one atop himself,
seems like a good plan for the future.
Then come the years, and luckily
they also go, and we grow weary of
the hand caressing the stubborn brow
of the lamb inside, and we adopt
the plural, perhaps out of modesty,
and renounce the singular, leave it behind
while thanking and rewarding it. Enough.
But when vacation ended, I saw that
someone had given my world
a new face. Blood and fire.
They didn't seem horrible, but they were
the same old blood and fire as ever. They burned
down my Catholic school, and Guiu,
who was the sergeant who made us do military-style

gymnastics, and whom we all hated
(back to the plural, because life is
one step forward, two steps back), Guiu
had been shot dead, and they told us
that it had been hard to do, because he wore
chain mail under his disguise of little
old farmer lady, carrying a basket with
three grenades hidden beneath the eggs.
They killed him in the corner of Hercules
Square, right by the high school,
which is where we went between classes,
and I don't remember that the square seemed
somehow marked, or that we
searched for a bullet in the plane tree,
or any other sign. As for the blood, needless
to say the wind carried it off the very
same day. It made the dust
a bit heavier, that's all.
The scorched walls of the primary school,
I don't know if I remember them or imagine them.
We didn't go inside. We shed
our skin, and had no interest in
the tattered old skin. We could smell the fear
that was the aroma of that autumn,
but it smelled good. It was a grown-up
fear. We were emerging from childhood fear
and were lucky that the world made it
so easy for us. The more afraid
they felt, the freer we were.
It was the same old process, and we
obscurely understood that with us the
wheel was spinning faster. We were happy.
Together, and always, and very much so.
They made us join the union, and the union
gave us vivid and varied pleasures.
Inside a requisitioned flat, which for us
was a flat taken from the enemy
(our enemy, not the official one),
behind poker smoke, we brought in
books and furniture, we traded
in pistols and bullets, we gave
the Roman salute (our side was
more likeable, but the others
had more evil prestige), we
wanted to bring girls into dark corners

but failed, and we burned our nervous
energy going up and out on the balcony.
We discovered whores and stealing.
Stealing wasn't that new. As for the whorehouses,
we'd soon have been old enough,
but we got a few extra months. The first
bombing we spent in the shelter beneath
Sol's cathouse, and we were all afraid
we'd be caught there. Although very
diminished, our parents still held the power.
Isidre was the first of us
to get the clap, and his father
chose the best wrong moment to
buy him the bicycle he'd been asking for.
Every day one of us had to
ask to borrow it, to give him an excuse
not to ride it. Bicycles
fill my memories of those days.
They were what we stole most. We had
set up a whole workshop to repaint them
and recompose them: the frame of one with the
wheels of another, and the inner tubes of yet another.
I don't know how, one afternoon when
we'd all slipped out of the house
halfway through lunch to ride to
Tamarit castle, when it was time
to leave, I had no bicycle. I wanted
to rent one but I found the shop
where they knew me closed. Didn't seem
fair and I refused to give up. I banged and
kicked the door, and it opened.
No one was there. I grabbed
the bike, and left a note.
The trip was agonizing. A relentless
wind forced us to duck. And on the
way back it was in our faces.
Standing on the pedals, as if climbing
a steep slope, I stood firm
and trembling but made no progress.
And we lost each other.
Agustí and I stretched out for a long while
in the shelter of the ditch
near the fields they razed to make
a military airfield. By night and
half walking, we finished the route.

In the first few houses, we found
an open bakery. We pounced
on it, and we were kids, much littler
kids than we actually were, and we dropped
to the floor and lying on the cool mosaic
we ate bread fresh from the oven, sticking
our whole faces into it,
crazy with the pleasure of
being pure fatigue and hunger and weight.
Anything could happen, and I wasn't
surprised by the sudden racket, the
shouts and the footsteps,
nor the greasy rifle barrels they pointed
vertically toward the floor,
nor that someone lifted me up, and pushed
me into a van, nor that my father was
waiting for me in a strange place and
arguing with a lot of men, and my
friends' fathers were there too, and mine
seemed to be imposing himself little by
little and he took me home. The next
day I found out the shop
had been collectivized. Furious,
the committee had chased us
all afternoon, to charge me for the bike
the former owner might have considered
rented, but they didn't. For a few days
our fathers were important to us.
We stole other stuff. For a while we
were obsessed with briefs.
Whole gang would go into a store,
look around, rummage, not buy anything,
and stuff our shirts and sweaters with
briefs. I don't know why we did it. I can't
explain how we didn't get caught either.
I guess that in those days they
were always dizzy, and all
stunned, and perhaps also perverse,
and their reflexes of order had been
damaged. They didn't care, or it excited
them to be robbed. All we knew were
those sidelong watery glances of the
shop owners, like a woman defeated
by her rapist. I remember one day
we chose again Subietes's shop,

as we often did, never coming out
empty-handed. The owner himself
would help us; he laid the boxes
out on the counter, he opened them, and then
took them far from our hands, and
counted them out loud. We didn't
insist, and he counted them again.
When we were outside, full of pride,
I pulled out the briefs I'd swiped
before he'd started counting. And Albert
had a pair, too. Everyone was sleeping
and everything buzzed in their ears.
Mr. Subietes was murdered
too. When I remember him now,
I see black and white clothes, with
someone inside them who seemed
quite old. Maybe he wasn't. As for
the black, I don't think he was in mourning:
he was a believer and in those days they
wore black to Mass, as did
elegant old men, and some regular
old Republicans. Old Subietes
went to prison for being Catholic.
He was unlucky. When he was in jail,
one day there was a big panic. They
were in Salou. The Italians. They'd
landed. The committee in Reus
requisitioned three or four buses,
got in with all their prisoners and
took them to the ditch. It was quick:
it was over as fast as that false
alarm. Ton is one of the drivers
who, requisitioned with his bus,
had to witness it. Distressed,
he watched the prisoners leave
the bus, passing right by his seat. He knew
almost all of them. Mr. Subietes
saw Ton's distress
and felt sorry for him. As he passed,
pausing for a moment, he put a
hand on his shoulder, and said: "You see,
Tonet, it is what it is." A grim
consolation. The president of the committee
in charge of the executions that day,
I knew him too. He was named Oliva.

It's Oliva I want to talk about now.
Before, he worked as a doorman at
the movie theater we went to on Sundays
to sully our hands with love. I haven't seen
him since. The only image I have of him
is dressed in leather, carrying a Luger
with a blond wood butt,
longer than his thigh, more of
an insignia than a weapon. The spirit
of symbolism blooms in times of war.
Both Oliva and his wife
were ritualists. They requisitioned
a house from the rich, to live in
themselves; she soon decided
every wealthy home needed a
cactus. In succulent plants the woman
had learned to see the supplement of
the life of the rich: a shadow of
the soul, slight beneath the immense
sun of possession. Then she possessed
and laughed, and they all laughed, and
bought a life of things, finally
material, emptied of hope.
It was just a moment, two or three months.
The proles went on laughing,
but not taken by surprise, laughing
like always. Hope returned
and they bought in secret, mostly
the rich. We took the turn,
and the way back, bit by bit,
was closed to us by the familiar margins.
Oliva and the rest of the committee, I
often saw them waiting at some
café table, or walking quickly down
the street, to sit and wait.
One night there was an orchestral concert.
My father took me and I
trembled with impatience. The music
parfois nous prend comme une mer, and I
was taken then swept away by a sea
of a time about to be lost, that one could see
losing itself and reneging, excited was I
by the idea of giving myself over to another,
more personal, flow, or at least flowing
unaccompanied, even by my father. I heard

Beethoven and Ravel, and I can't
say where they led me to, if they even did carry me off.
When the concert ended, they played anthems:
the "Himno de Riego," the "Internationale,"
"Els Segadors," and the "Warszawianka," which
was the FAI's anthem. People
clapped most for "Els Segadors." Oliva
didn't like that and poured out
of his proscenium seat, screaming. We tried
to clap ourselves deaf. He looked at
the laughing faces, and shouted
mute, like a flame, and we laughed and clapped,
flowing as water. My father and I were
buddies then, as we would be often later,
and didn't want to go straight home
and we sat to have a coffee together.
We talked about politics, and I think
I thought that there was no need for any
revolt (I don't mean of the political order)
and that our fathers could be part of our gang.
At night, in a café, one can have a father.
Oliva came in, and I now know that
he had had three or four too many drinks.
We were sitting by the door, and he saw
us right away. Gripping his big rifle butt
that must have been helping him remain standing,
he looked at my father and said: "You were
the one responsible." (Those days were
filled with people responsible. Everyone
was responsible for something, and they couldn't
keep track of what, and were always searching
to see if there wasn't someone else, someone
more responsible.) My father was able
to distract him easily, and Oliva
put down his gun. When my father
told the story later, the dialogue went on
much longer. I couldn't understand
why he wanted to disperse such concise
virtue. Now I can clearly see it for what it was:
dispersing a fog his voice didn't
reveal, but which showed through in
his eyes. I was fascinated,
and didn't call it by its name, the name
it had when it clouded my eyes.
As it did briefly, three days later, when

I found myself face-to-face with Oliva
in the hallway at Sol's. As boys
in a cathouse, we sensed
vaguely that it was our rightful
realm, and that the interlopers
were them, even with their pistols.
Then came a time of many paths, and
someone was shuffling a deck of cards
that were places and us people. My
mother met Oliva, six or seven years
later, when we were not expecting it.
One evening in Bordeaux, when she
was alone at home, she opened the door to him.
He had climbed our stairs
because he knew that people from his
town lived there. He asked for help.
He said he'd been working in an *usina*,
a German one, in Royan I think.
Bombing had destroyed the factory
and the attached encampment.
Oliva wasn't there, by chance, but
he'd lost everything, his clothes
and his money, everything, except his life,
which had become foreign to him, and he was
no longer the one responsible for it: the Germans
took charge of his new destiny.
Perhaps my mother was the last
woman who ever spoke to Oliva
who knew anything about him. She gave him
a few pieces of clothing, which he might
not ever have worn. Two days
later, another English bombing
caught up to him.
Since I'm not an Oranian
from Saint-Germain, I don't believe
fear is any great subject for literature
or philosophizing. I do know that many
men have felt fear, and we should talk
about them, too. Oliva felt fear, and he
inspired fear in many people, not so much
in my father and me, Ton somewhat more, and
in others as much as he felt, or even more.[1]

THE FREEDOM SCHOOL (I)

MAX AUVRAY—I work at Bourg-en-Bresse, but before that for six years I was at the psychiatric hospital of Le Puy-en-Velay, very close to Saint-Alban. We went there several times and still talk a lot about those places. In that period, I was part of the Auvergne team of the Centers of Training in the Methods of Active Education (CEMÉA).

FRANÇOIS TOSQUELLES—And you worked at Sainte-Marie-de-l'Assomption?

MAX AUVRAY—Yes, it was difficult.

FRANÇOIS TOSQUELLES—But the life is difficult because you have to perform in places occupied by the enemy brothers, so to speak. This story is a very curious one. This morning we talked about Albi and about the psychiatric hospitals that don't trace back to those created by the French Revolution, after the law of 1838, and which remained in private hands: the community of Saint-Jean-de-Dieu for the men and Sainte-Marie-de-l'Assomption for the women. But we didn't talk about Le Puy, although it was via Le Puy that I arrived at Saint-Alban.

It's a strange story ... of war and psychiatry. And then, there's a woman, there's always a woman. In my case, a French one, a native of Le Puy, who, in 1912 or 1913, had married a psychiatrist from Barcelona named [Àngels] Vives. Immediately after the fall of Barcelona to Franco, Vives left for France with his wife, and just upon arriving in Le Puy, he decides to visit the hospital of Sainte-Marie-de-l'Assomption. In the course of this visit, he reencounters an old acquaintance, André Chaurand, a psychiatrist who would later work with me at Saint-Alban, and who at that moment was having a lot of trouble. Practically banned by the proprietary sisters of the hospital who thought he was a communist spy and regarded him as a clandestine syndicalist. It was the Vichy epoch.

They shared talk about the Spanish Civil War and the refugees ... Chaurand had a certain Catalan culture: he had an interest in the languages of Occitania—of Provence and Catalonia. He was also interested in Catalan psychiatry and had busied

---

In October 1987, over the course of three days, a group of psychiatrists, psychologists, researchers, and senior officials from Normandy, Lyon, Geneva, and Trieste gathered with François Tosquelles in his home, in Granges-sur-Lot, to talk about the transformative experiences that had been carried out in French, Italian, and British hospitals in their various situated ways: institutional psychotherapy, anti-psychiatry, and therapeutic communities. The recording of this extensive conversation lasts twelve hours. A longer excerpt appears in the next part.

Excerpt from the dialogue between Max Auvray, Maurizio Costantino, Alain Dupont, Jacques Ferrages, Errol Franko, Giovanna Gallio, Max Lafont, and Marie-Noëlle Piednoir with François Tosquelles. "L'École de la liberté," in Giovanna Gallio and Maurizio Costantino, *Per la salute mentale, pratiche, ricerche, culture dell' innovazione*, 1987, pp. 73–100.

himself with the refugees; so Vives tells him that a Catalan psychiatrist (Chaurand didn't know me) is in France, in a concentration camp. Words that, at the time, fell into a void. However, a few days later Chaurand went to Saint-Alban to see his friend Balvet, who was its director, plus other colleagues. They took their seats at the table and proceeded to eat like lords entertaining peers: "The children are growing up nicely" and things of that sort (psychiatric dignitaries, in short). While they were eating, Balvet told him that he had gone to visit the prefect, who had suggested that he take into Saint-Alban some workers from the concentration camp of Septfonds: Spaniards, bargain rate, for the little jobs to be done at the hospital. Balvet, who was right-wing at the time, had replied that for his part, he didn't want any "reds," and he had added: "If there happened to be a psychiatrist, it's worth considering ..." To which the prefect replied, "But monsieur, you're quite right: at the camp there are only criminals, so no psychiatrists!"

It was then that Chaurand, still eating, told Balvet that the prefect had got it wrong, because at Septfonds there was an excellent psychiatrist! But since Balvet was Catholic (Chaurand was, too, but the other man was more so, and inclined toward mysticism) ... Later, while being driven in the prefect's car, Chaurand said to him, "Monsieur Prefect, you misled me! There's an excellent psychiatrist in the Septfonds camp ..." Chaurand wasn't lying in stating that I was a formidable guy, that I had published I don't know what, and done this thing and that thing ... He actually made up everything because Balvet was going solely on the idea that since I was Catalan, I must be okay! That's how I came to receive a telegram from the prefect saying, "Would you accept a position at Saint-Alban?" I looked at the map and I didn't find any Saint-Alban, so I said yes. I really like going someplace where I don't know where I'm going.

MAX LAFONT—At the Septfonds internment camp, you were a prisoner or there to help the detainees suffering from psychic disturbances?

FRANÇOIS TOSQUELLES—Even that story is a little paradoxical. On my arrival in France, I stayed hidden in the mountains for several days, in a refuge managed by some women called Hospice de France. Those courageous women tended to my feet, they gave me bread to eat. After a week of this life of ease, I descended into the town of Bagnères-de-Luchon and, by chance, I met a guy ... a policeman ... We ate together; he was in counterespionage, he wanted information.

I didn't find anything troubling in that, it was the beginning of the war, the first days of September ... I told him what I knew, which seemed to be my duty as an anti-fascist ... Franco's army had stationed itself in the port of Barcelona and I had chanced to hear certain officers say that Franco and Hitler would be arriving in Paris in a week. I had arrived in France with a satchel, inside of which were all the reports of actions during the Spanish war: the actions of selection for the machine gunners, for the tank crews, and even of our "extensive psychiatry"—so to speak. Because I had dealt with mental health in the Spanish army, and not just mental patients. I thought all that might interest the French army and I told this man that I intended to enlist. He replied that the best thing for me to do was to enlist in the Foreign Legion, but I said that I wasn't, didn't feel that I was, a foreigner. If they wanted to lose the war they could do that, but as for me, I was disposed to work like a good Frenchman, which in fact I was (because all Catalans are French), during the anti-fascist war.

So then he gave me two messages: the first was permission to remain free, in Toulouse, and the second was rather a piece of false information: it's that there existed at Septfonds a concentration camp where there were only intellectuals ...

So, as we had no more money, a friend (Dr. Sauret) and I, with no one forcing us to, made a tour around the outside of the camp early one morrning, convinced there were only intellectuals inside. We had arrived in the cold and fog, and we toured the perimeter, because we didn't dare enter at six or seven, with the agents not yet on the job.

Viewed from the exterior, the grounds resembled a psychiatric hospital. One could see shadowy figures coming out of the buildings, arguing over a cigarette butt, or such talk ... They were running about. In sum, it resembled the courtyard of a psychiatric hospital. The commandant of the camp, who was named Vigouroux, soon became my kin. As he said himself, he belonged to the family of that Vigouroux who was a collaborator of Charcot's. The one who had done hypnosis, and built electric cars.

Starting from this name business, we had a conversation with him and learned that he was worried: there had been many suicides in the camp and when someone from the Cahors psychiatric hospital was brought in, it was the end, because they were locked up for life, abandoned. They don't do miracles at Cahors! That's how the idea of trying to do something at the Septfonds camp was born.

I requested a building on the edge of the camp, outside the barbed wire, or rather, with one foot in, one foot out. The thing worked and I was given carte blanche. In this wooden building, the most pathetic of all, we opened a little psychiatry service, choosing as aides, from among the camp folk, a painter, a guitarist, etc. None of them knew anything about psychiatry, but they were people who knew art. And I should say, there was a psychiatric nurse—a single one—and he was more than sufficient. This little service looked after the patients with success, and moreover it is true, too, that I made use of it to bring in people by one door and see them out by the other, the door that opened to the outside. Because it is easier to escape from a concentration camp by passing through a psychiatry service than by going directly.

A psychiatry service is not just a way station. As a Saint-Alban patient once said, when he was at a film club a dozen kilometers from the hospital. He spoke up while we were talking about escapees from the camp, saying he actually lived at the psychiatric hospital and the hospital was a school of freedom. That is what was lacking in Basaglia: the realization that a hospital worthy of the name is a freedom school. It's necessary to be a "school of freedom"—freedom that isn't possible in present-day social life.

GIOVANNA GALLO—There you've touched on a real problem.

FRANÇOIS TOSQUELLES—That's the difference between Basaglia and me: my desire was for the psychiatric hospital to be a school of freedom above all. I didn't say: "Close the building!" Because, after that, it's not the school of freedom in our actual social life, it's just the school of administrative alienation.

GIOVANNA GALLO—Please excuse me, you dwell on this point and I feel provoked … I need to say certain things …

FRANÇOIS TOSQUELLES—I interrupted the story precisely to provoke.

GIOVANNA GALLO—Fine then. Perhaps you haven't had the chance to visit Gorizia and aren't aware of the content of the experience that's described in the transcriptions of the patients' assemblies. We've recently rewatched a film (*The Gardens of Abel* by Sergio Zavoli) that takes footage from the Gorizia hospital: it was in 1967, I believe. Basaglia had worked, with his team, for ten years in that psychiatric hospital and had created a situation which, I believe, completely corresponds to what you call a "school of freedom." In the film and in the minutes of the meetings, what one sees clearly is how the patients speak and move around. It's a long road of internal transformation, from the inside toward the outside. However, around 1968, the question was raised in terms of more radical choices: "Freedom, the school of freedom, to do what? To remain in the enclosure of a hospital, without any rights, etc.?" First of all, there was a crisis for an administration that did not have a real open-door policy. And then, there was an incident where a patient, out for Saturday and Sunday, killed someone.

FRANÇOIS TOSQUELLES—We said this morning that outside, they, the prefect and the peace police, don't want any disturbances … and let no one accuse them of letting a madman roam free! There are so many murders, committed by crazies and by those who are not crazy, at least officially. If someone kills, one always finds reasons why: jealousy, a family trouble, or they had an irrepressible urge … etc. But someone is not considered dangerous if they are not crazy, because they are not in a state of permanent criminality! To cite Lombroso, the mad person is regarded as one of the variants of the born criminal who will always, perforce, end up in social catastrophes: they will not only be a source of scandal, of disorder, but also of murder, once on the outside. Therefore, you should always expect certain administrative defensive reactions in the interest of peace, the honor of the country or of the administration, reactions against the mad. Even the family, which doesn't want to be overtly faulted in its internal equilibrium, will demand that its rights be recognized. Initially, they will say that the individual in question is a little strange, an artist, badly brought up … But as soon as the discussion turns to the equilibrium of the whole family, internment is the solution. Case closed, let's not mention it again!

GIOVANNA GALLO—So, you think that there's always the need for a protected space?

FRANÇOIS TOSQUELLES—No, not that! I mean, yes, "protected from the outside"! Fear of madness is a natural state of the human race. Human groups exclude madness in their very formation, and that's why the status of therapeutic action in a community is a utopia, which must be handled with kid gloves, you understand. If you don't maneuver carefully, you don't prepare the release, the exit. I'm not against release from the hospital … I started by telling you about a movie theater, which was twenty kilometers from the hospital, and the patients would go there and mix with the "civilians."

III

MATERIAL LIFE: A PSYCHIATRIC REVOLUTION

SAINT-ALBAN 1940–1962

I have never gone in search of something radically new. I've never imagined myself to be an inventor by trade. I've never thought of constructing and promoting anything whatever that might be patented. I am partial rather to plagiarisms, or if you like, to the theft of ideas that I glean here and there and that seem to constitute little pebbles that can be used in my therapeutic task. In fact, paradoxically, it's in my work as a psychotherapist that I've most frequently been able to glean. But also in all the events of my concrete life.

FRANÇOIS TOSQUELLES

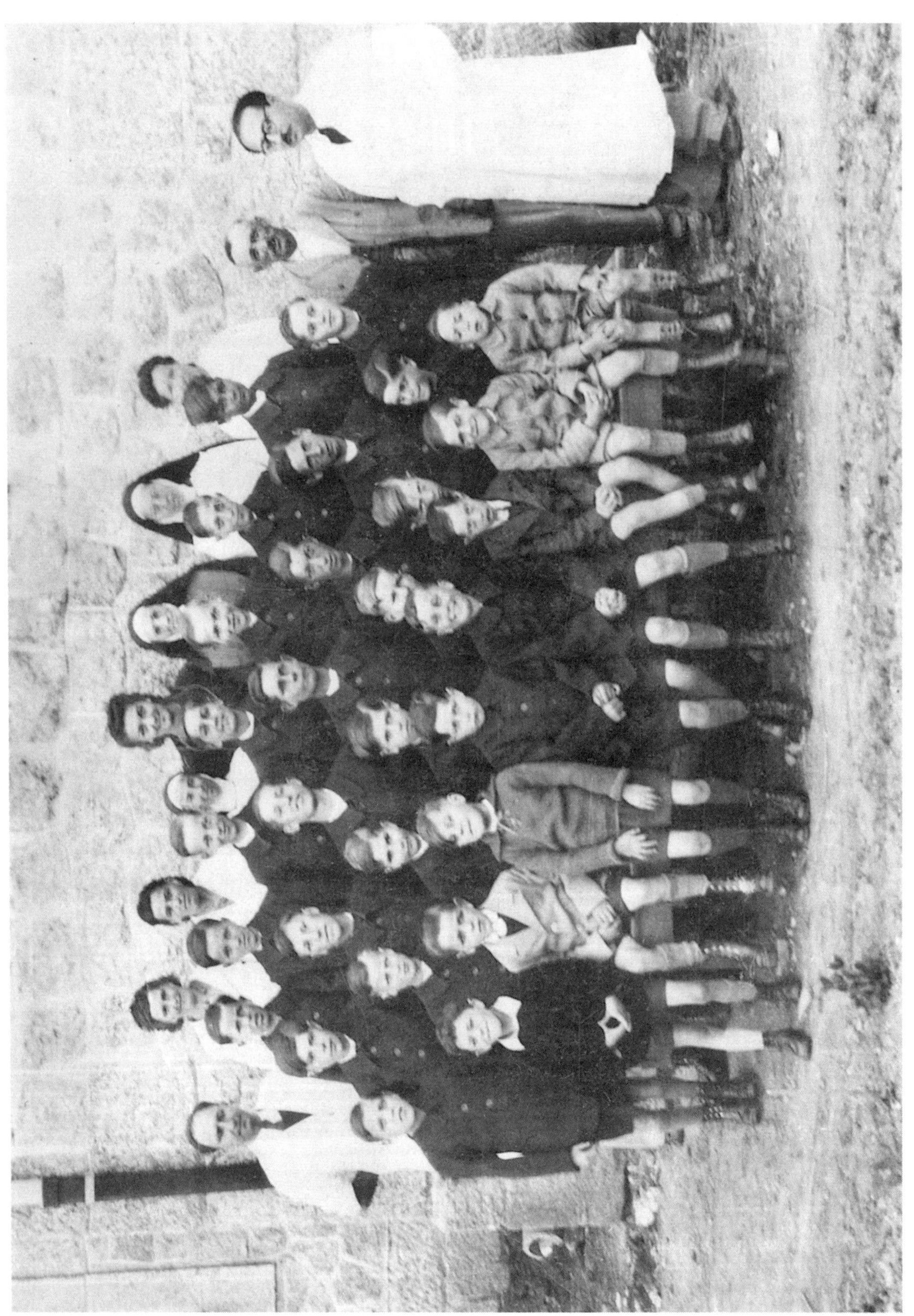

Francesc Tosquelles at the Institut Théophile Roussel's program for adolescents, in Le Villaret, 1942

Transformations: Dealing with Circumstances

Material life was the context of a revolution that was made by pushing limits: hunger, cold, exile, deportations, escapes, isolation, the impoverished countryside of Lozère in Nazi-occupied France. Working with the limits of material life meant authorizing life as a space of transformation. Without an instruction manual but with experimental pragmatism: without programmatic utopias but with untread paths where one had to relearn how to walk. Similarly, Tosquelles left Septfonds with a map where he searched for Saint-Alban-sur-Limagnole: he couldn't locate it but decided to go there anyway, without knowing where he was headed. Three years after he arrived, the psychiatrist Lucien Bonnafé, in a 1943 letter, described Saint-Alban as a prodigiously backward and isolated place, a harsh region, with a hospital that was literally in ruins and absurd architecture that dated from the start of the century. There were still solitary cells for patients. The only well-organized facilities were the infirmary, the farmhouse, and the medico-pedagogical institute, thanks to a team of doctors formed by the psychiatrist André Chaurand and Tosquelles's speculative pragmatism. During the years of the occupation they organized a structure of weekly meetings to discuss the patient cases with a community of doctors, a working group they called Société du Gévaudan. Thus they created a whole series of activities, some of which took place in the library, or the common room, or outside: film projections, a wall newspaper, gardening, crafts with wool and raffia fiber, singing sessions, mushroom-hunting excursions, and reflections on the responsibility of madness.

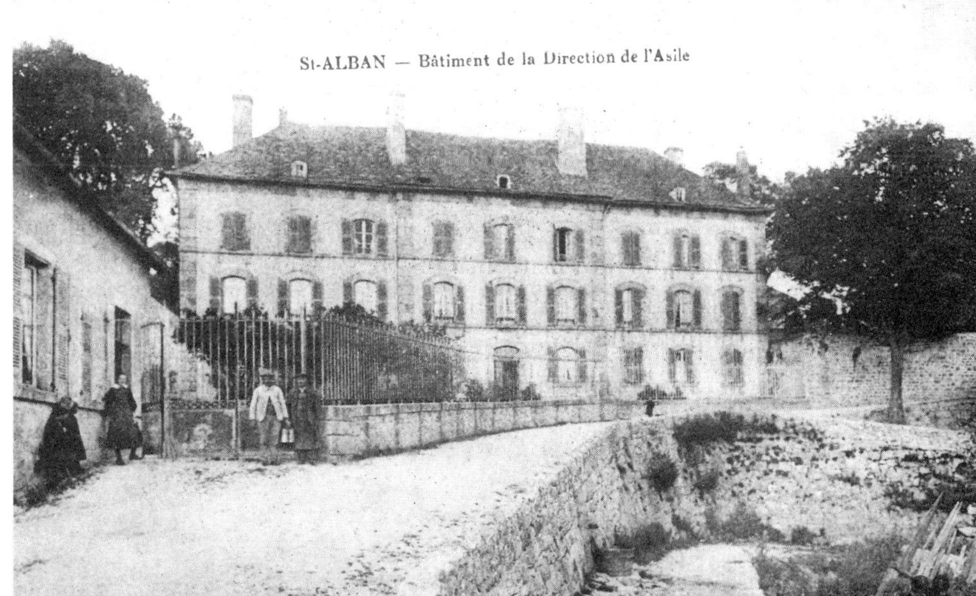

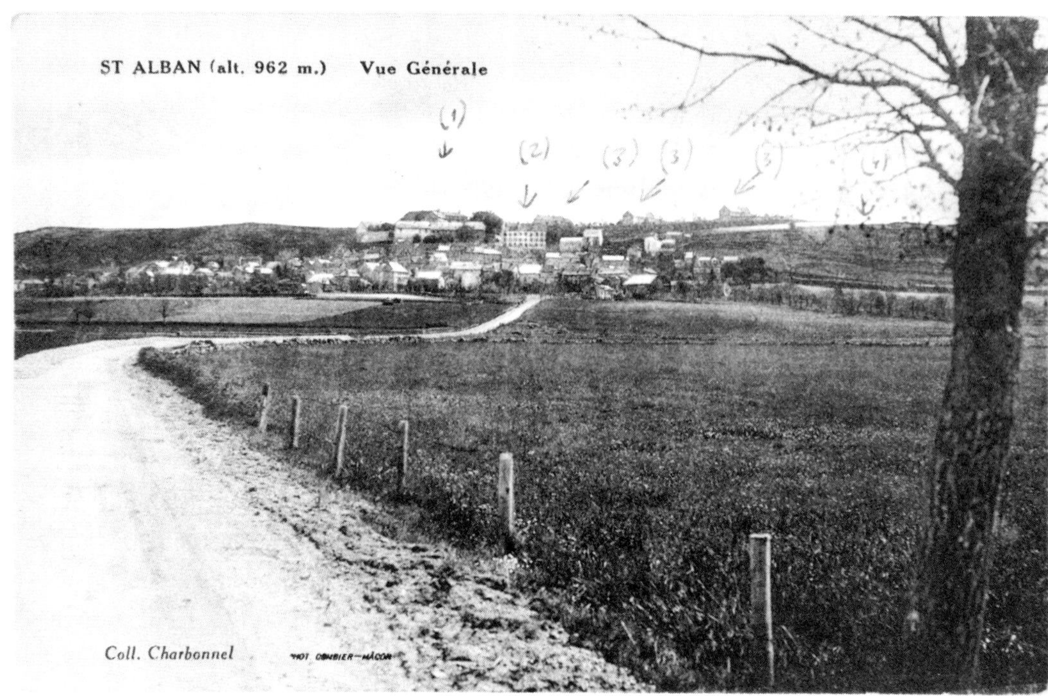

Postcard Tosquelles sent to his wife, Elena Álvarez, in December 1940, before she arrived in Saint-Alban: "(1) These buildings are those that hide the castle and that shelter the women's service of the hospital. In the lower part of one of them I have a small men's service. These are the evacuees from Alsace. (2) This building houses the administration, the head office, the library; it's where I live at present. (3) These are the wards for men—that is, my service. (4) On the other side is our little house."

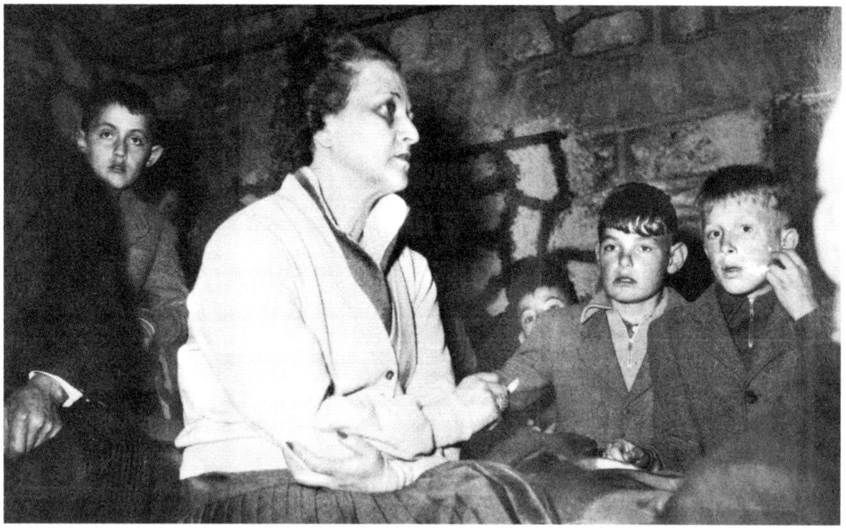

Elena working on theatrical activities with autistic children in Le Villaret, a former agricultural colony that the hospital acquired in the late 19th century

CARTE POSTALE

(1) Estos edificios son los que esconden el castillo, y son destinados al servicio de mujeres del hospital, en la parte baja de uno de ellos tengo un pequeño servicio de hombres, son los evacuados de Alsacia.

(2) Este pavellon, es la administracion, direccion, biblioteca etc. es donde vivo actualmente.

(3) Son los pavellones de hombres, o sea mi servicio

(4) En la otra vertiente esta nuestra pequeña casita.

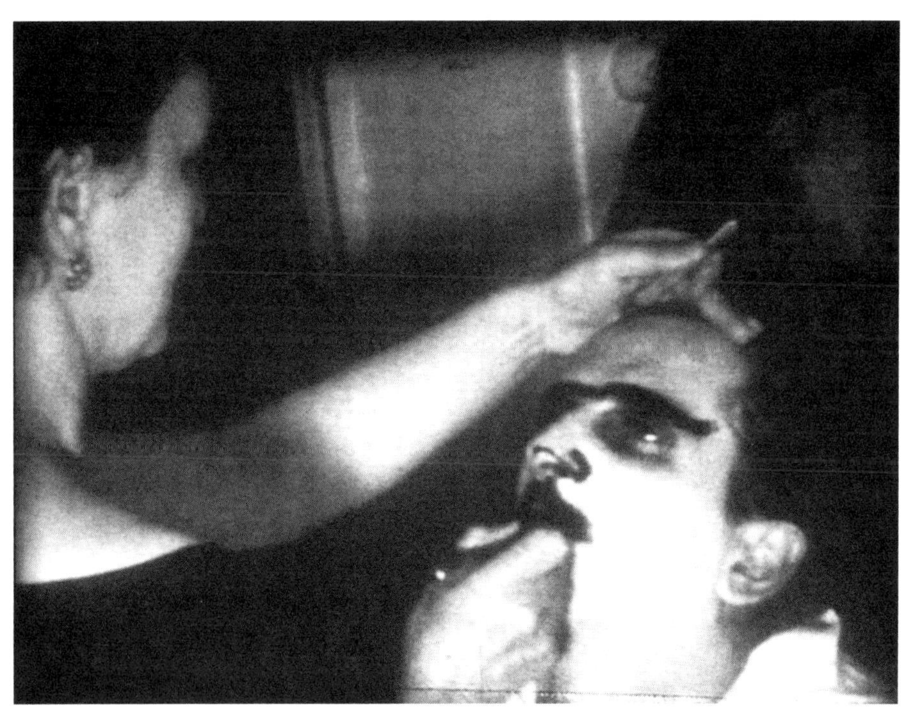

Elena during one of the theater nights at the hospital. (Still from *Film Tosquelles*, 1958.)

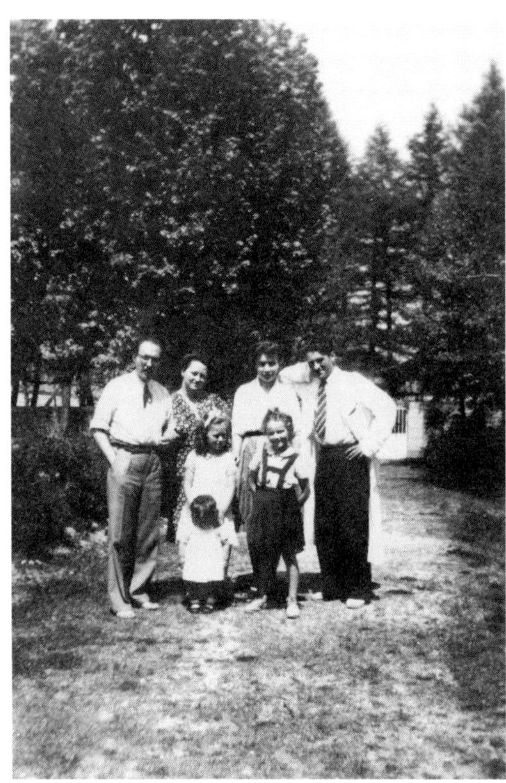

Francesc and Elena Tosquelles,
Lucien and Jeanne Bonnafé,
and their children, 1943 or 1944

In addition to Chaurand and me, the medical service consists of two residents (a post presently vacant for a short time) and a priceless treasure, Tosquelles, a Catalan refugee here—Balvet's doing—a quite exceptional guy, with truly excellent ideas, a worker like no other who has participated tenaciously in the reorganization of the hospital under Balvet. It's hard to say what is most remarkable about him, whether intellectually or pragmatically. Needless to say, it's a treasure for me to see him lavishly spend his insatiable activity in the service. [...] Evenings, personal work, personal correspondence, meetings of the Société du Gévaudan (entire medical personnel), I'll send you some of our minutes. This teamwork is functioning admirably. Tosquelles is in fact the secretary of the society and my secretary types up the minutes. The Gévaudan sits in session every Wednesday, sometimes Gévaudan business, sometimes literature related, etc. Moreover, once a month, meeting of the Gévaudan at the Villaret Medical-Pedagogical Institute in a childhood session. [...] Ergotherapy is the axial preoccupation of the service. Therapy via work is only the structure, the essence being the deep cultivation in every patient of non-alienated capacities: social competence, responsibility, dignity. That goes from the carding of wool or the sorting of colored pearls to theatrical performance, by way of horticulture, gymnastics, singing, etc. The achievements in this domain are contingent on fully exploiting the concept of a village asylum. I can't set out the material framework here but the spirit will show through. The vital center of this humanizing activity is the common room, library, game room, entertainment room, hangout space, etc. [...] I've left out an important detail: in the common room you'll find the monthly wall-posted newspaper resulting from the joint effort of everyone, from the director to the patients.[1]

Letter from Lucien Bonnafé to Paul Bernard, 1943

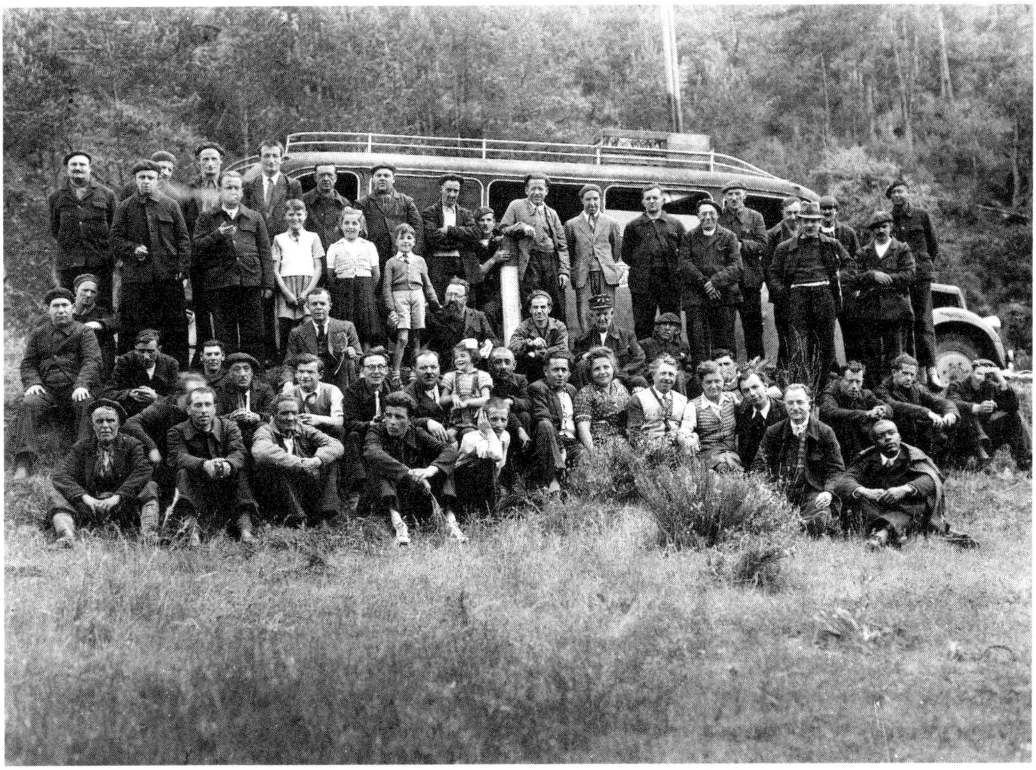

Patients from the Saint-Alban hospital during an excursion to Garabit, Cantal, on Whitmonday 1952; in the second row, sitting on the ground, wearing a military cap, is Auguste Forestier.

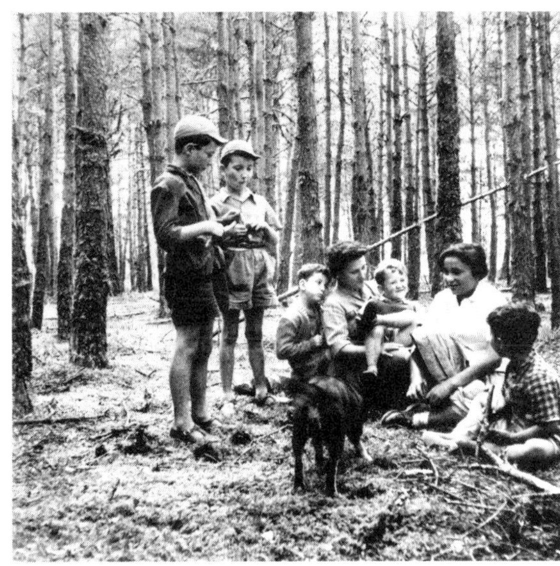

A field trip to the forests of Franquet, in Saint-Alban

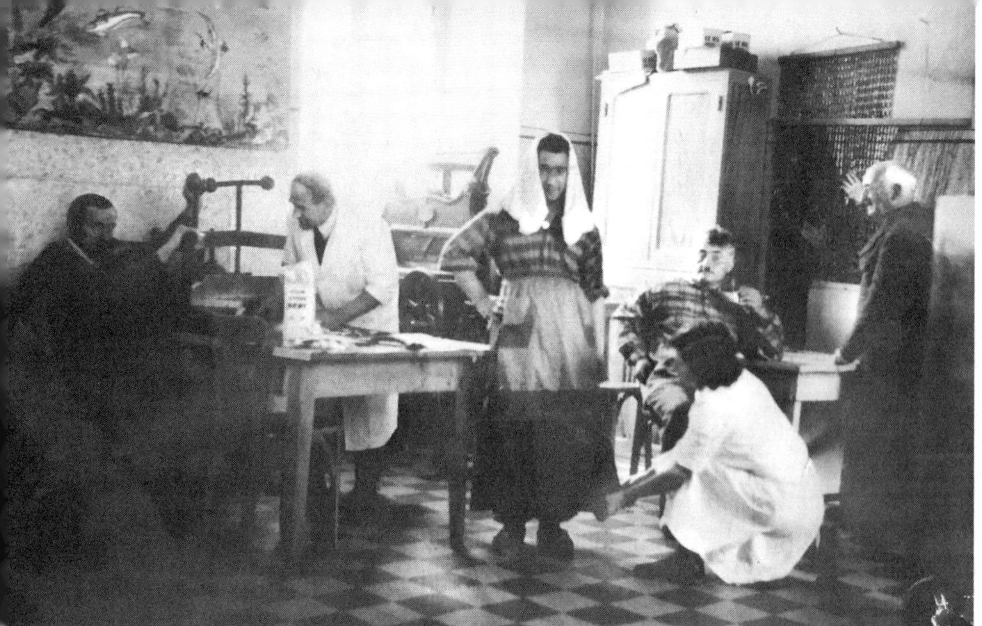

Above, everyday scene inside Saint-Alban. *At right*, a wall newspaper from the military clinic in Manresa, no. 3, 1937.

Wall newspapers were used as a tool during the Spanish Civil War, both on the front and in the rear guard. Halfway between a poster and a magazine, between a bulletin board to write on and share thoughts, ideas, and concerns and a collective collage of photographs and news cut from hard-to-get newspapers, which allowed information to circulate. Military units, hospitals, children's camps, unions, and international organizations used this tool for public and participative communication that made possible a different reading experience, because it blurred the line between writer and reader. Everyone could read and write on it. The wall newspaper held an important position in the Saint-Alban common room, continuing those forms of communication used during wartime and in spaces historically condemned to reclusion, enforced passivity, and a lack of social bonds, such as psychiatric hospitals.[2]

> In 1947, at Saint-Alban, a common room was created and a newspaper that hung on the wall was published. Those pages became an ideological position; that was when a struggle between nurses would appear, or between parties and unions. The time came when I had to make a decision and I fired the two Christian Democrats.[3]
>
> Francesc Tosquelles, "El Club (June 26, 1986)"

HOSPITAL MILITAR CLINICA Nº 3

PERIODICO MURAL

(editado por los enfermos y heridos de este hospital)

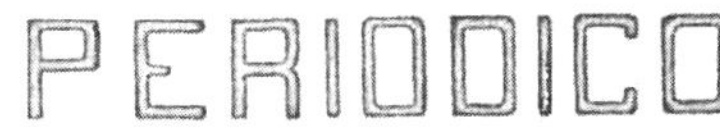

La disciplina es la base de la victoria

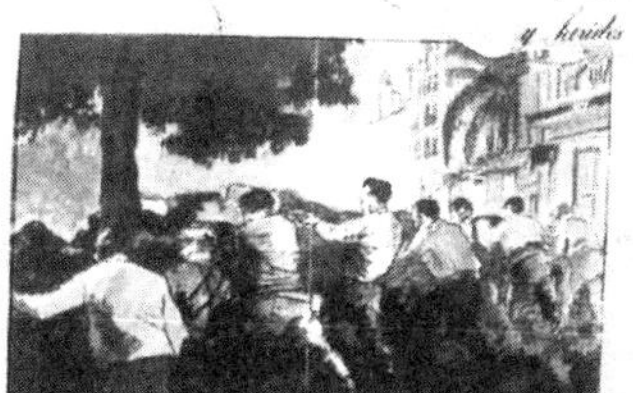

Una vida...

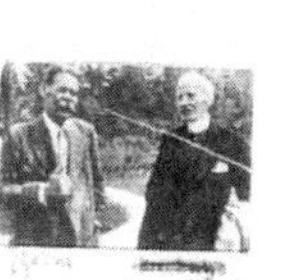

Gorki ... Romain Rolland

Curiosidades

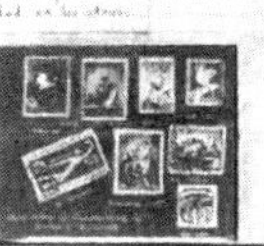

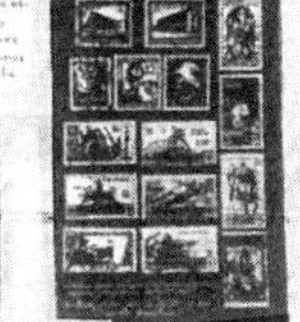

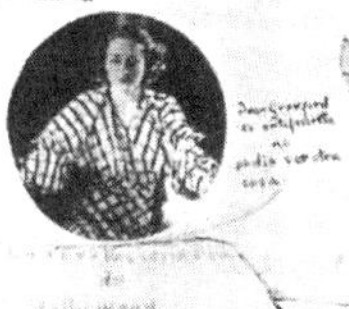

Hay que descubrir a los emboscados

Comentarios

Abnegación de las enfermeras de la República

... ¡Compañeros, ayudad tan humanitaria obra!

¡Viva la República!

¡Viva la Cruz Roja!

Eugenio Lombera

Guerra

Pontoneros

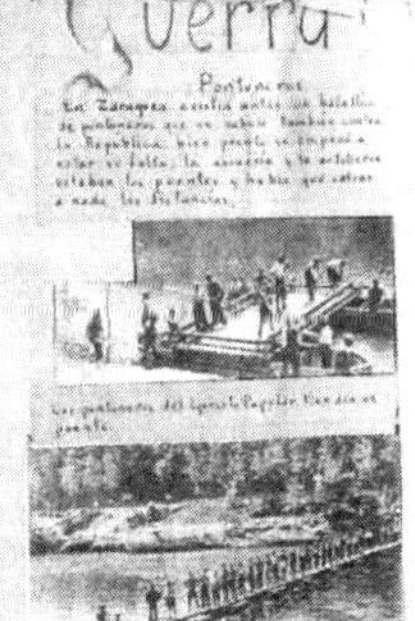

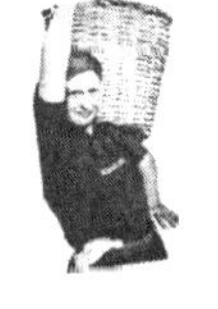

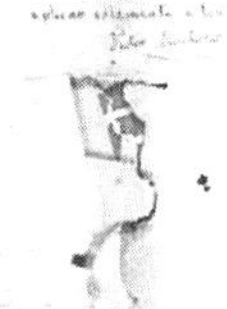

A los campesinos

Pedro Gimeno Fleta

El deber del hospitalizado es el de ayudar a descubrir y aplastar al agente provocador

Cultura Popular
"COMPAÑERAS"
ACUDID
A LA EXPOSICION DE
PERIODICOS MURALES

LE CHEMIN

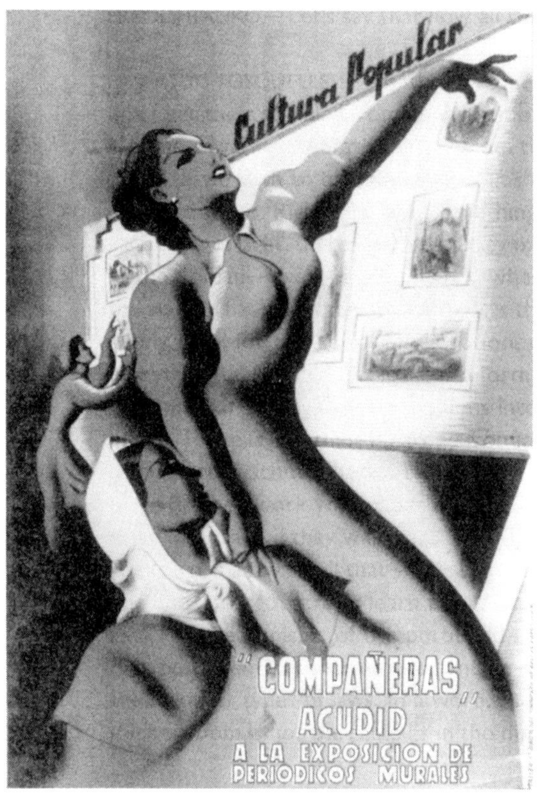

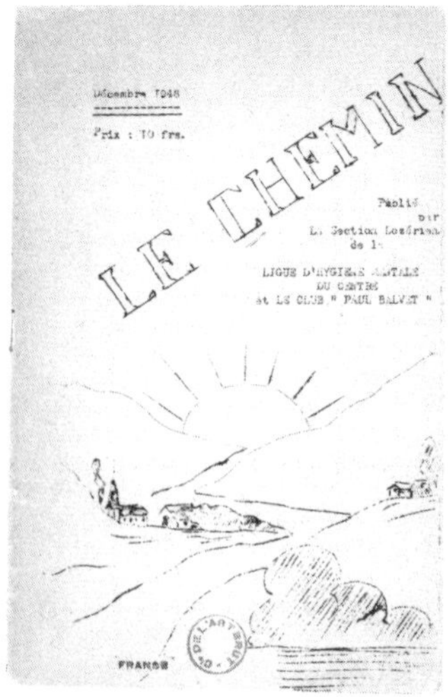

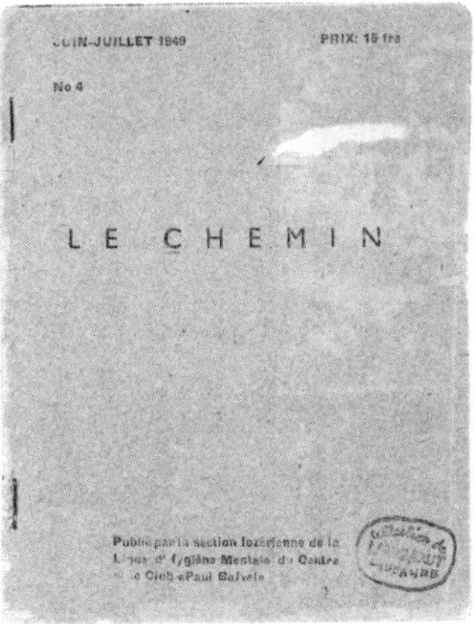

Above, invitation to the exhibition of wall newspapers, *Cultura Popular*, Madrid, 1937. *Right*, 1948 and 1949 issues of *Le Chemin*, a magazine created at the Saint-Alban hospital to facilitate communication with the outside world.

The work of the collective wall newspaper led the way to other writing practices, such as *Le Chemin*, a magazine first published in 1948 that was distributed outside of the hospital, and *Trait d'union: Journal intérieur*, a magazine published from 1950 to 1981, produced on a Freinet press by the patients, doctors, and nurses, for internal distribution only. Understood as a therapeutic tool and a new instrument of collective life, *Trait d'union* reported on local current events, featured poems, reports, and editorials, announced the film program, and described the objects made by patients in the workshops. The reading and selection of texts by doctors, patients, nuns, and nurses was carried out in an editorial assembly. It was heir to several publications created in psychiatric environments, such as those published in the early nineteenth century in England and the United States, and in Catalonia, *La Razón de la Sin Razón*, from the Sant Boi asylum, in the mid-1800s. *Trait d'union* was contemporaneous with *L'Écho des bruyères*, from the Fleury-les-Aubrais hospital (begun in 1947), *Le Tremplin*, from Ville-Évrard (begun in 1948), and *Le Bon-sens*, from Bonneval (begun in 1950).

It was in the pages of *Trait d'union* where Tosquelles wrote about his desire to reorganize the hospital yard without having a clear idea of how it should be, and also where he wrote about his primary concern: the patients' fear of isolation. "Helping each of them discover the existence of the others. Learning to comprehend and respond to their calls," he wrote in the October 31, 1952, issue. In the December issues, Frantz Fanon elaborated the political distinction between abandonment and repose: abandonment is neither rest nor leisure, but the refusal to go on, the rejection of life when plagued by the pressure of anxiety. And in an article in March 1953, in reference to the psychiatric hospital, Fanon defended the urgency of being able to maintain the time sequence—yesterday, today, and tomorrow—to avoid lives being lost in the past, lives with no present, and all those who live in fear of the future.[4]

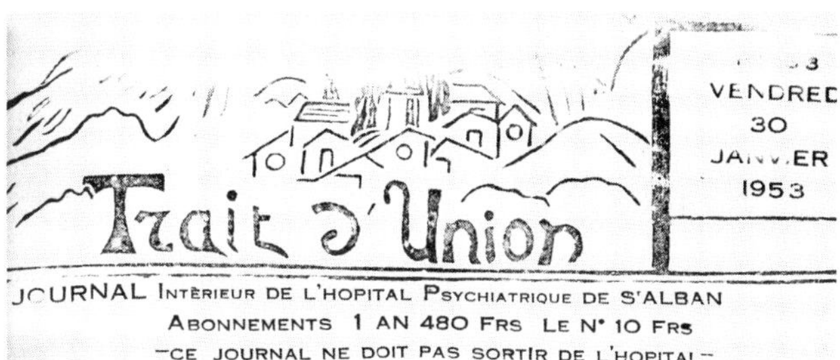

Trait d'Union

VENDREDI 30 JANVIER 1953

JOURNAL INTÈRIEUR DE L'HOPITAL PSYCHIATRIQUE DE S'ALBAN

ABONNEMENTS 1 AN 480 FRS LE N° 10 FRS

—CE JOURNAL NE DOIT PAS SORTIR DE L'HOPITAL—

L'HOMME FACE AUX CHOSES

Dans le monde, il y a des objets, des arbres, des champs, des voitures, des avions; dans le monde il y a des choses. L'homme qui regarde ces objets, ces choses peut rester indifférent. Il peut aussi les désirer. Vouloir ou désirer une voiture, c'est vouloir n'avoir plus le désir d'une voiture. Désirer quelque chose c'est ne plus vouloir désirer. On répond habituellement que le désir voit plus loin que la chose désirée. La chose désirée est toujours une limite.

Il se produit un changement de plan lorsque à la place d'une chose on met un homme. Tout homme appartient à une institution, s'incarne dans un cadre. C'est un militaire, il est officier ou deuxième classe. C'est un maçon, ou un entrepreneur, ou un paysan. Il est marié ou célibataire; il a des enfants ou il n'en a pas, aime la lecture ou le cinéma, ou les dominos. Quand on rencontre un homme, il y a presque toujours une certaine timidité. Un nouveau paysan arrive dans une ferme: les autres d'abord le regardent de loin, puis ils s'approchent de lui: on lui dit bonjour... A midi, l'acte social de manger et de boire déliera les langues, si l'on peut dire. Mais au début, on s'est respecté on s'est mesuré du regard.

Dès qu'on rencontre un homme nouveau on parle, on ne peut que parler. C'est le langage qui rompt le silence et les silences. Alors on peut communiquer ou communier. Le prochain au sens chrétien est toujours un complice. Un complice qui peut trahir comme tout complice. Se fâcher avec quelqu'un c'est constater qu'on n'a rien de commun. Communier, c'est communier en face de quelque chose.

Il y a à la base de toute communication une intention, mais il faut que cette intention soit sincère. Pour découvrir et vouloir cette sincérité, il faut distinguer le monde et la somme des objets qui se trouvent sur terre.

En face des objets, nous agissons différemment qu'en face d'autres hommes.

Nous mangeons pour manger, nous respirons pour respirer. En faisant cela nous vivons. Et nous mangeons ou respirons sincèrement. Vivre est une sincérité. Il ne faut pas dire que manger ou boire ou fumer, ce n'est pas vivre. Il ne faut pas mépriser ce qu'on appelle le quotidien. Il ne faut pas être à la recherche de l'inhabituel.

C'est à partir du commun que pourront surgir les inventions créatrices. Mais je continuerai un autre jour.

Samedi matin à la réunion du journal on a discuté un peu du sommeil. Et le Docteur Tosquelles nous rappelait que beaucoup de malades réclament des cachets pour dormir. Cette difficulté à trouver le sommeil s'appelle l'insomnie.

Qu'est ce que l'insomnie?

L'insomnie est une manière de vivre qui veut se croire valable. On veille quand il y a raison de veiller. Le quotidien est celui qui peut suspendre sa veille. Sa sincérité est telle qu'il possède la liberté de se suspendre. L'insomnique n'a pas cette liberté de sommeil, de détente, d'assoupissement. L'insomnique ne veille pas; c'est la nuit qui veille. Ça veille.

Dr Fanon

Article by Frantz Fanon published in *Trait d'union* on January 30, 1953

In the context of the vast restriction imposed by the Vichy regime under the Nazi occupation, the "Club Paul-Balvet" was created in 1942 to promote self-management among the patients for the organization of parties, dances, courses, and theater, and in which the practice of writing and the printing press took on various forms. In Louis Gauzy's recollection of the patient cooperatives, the film screenings that took place in the common room followed dynamics more closely linked to free association and learning to speak up within the group than to the typical dynamics of a film club. Sister Marie Saint-Jules wrote about the experience of some of the women who went to the towns near Saint-Alban to sell the crafts they had made in the ergotherapy workshops. She explained that such outings allowed them to experience various situations: facing the disappointment of failing to sell anything by the end of the day; the sadness and joy of seeing families and little children; making decisions about the collective money and organizing the cooperative till.[5] In the late 1950s, Hervé Bazin, author of such novels as *La Tête contre les murs* and the essay *La Fin des asiles*, recorded Tosquelles's voice for *France-Soir*, explaining the experience of demolishing one of the hospital's wings with the patients themselves, as well as the complicity they shared with the mother superior of the nuns of the order of Saint-Régis.

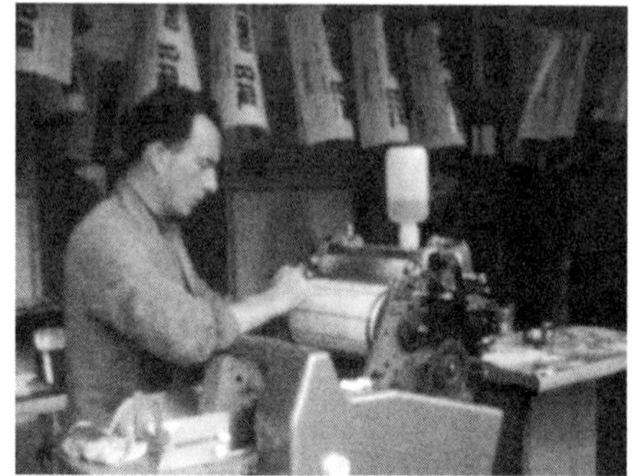

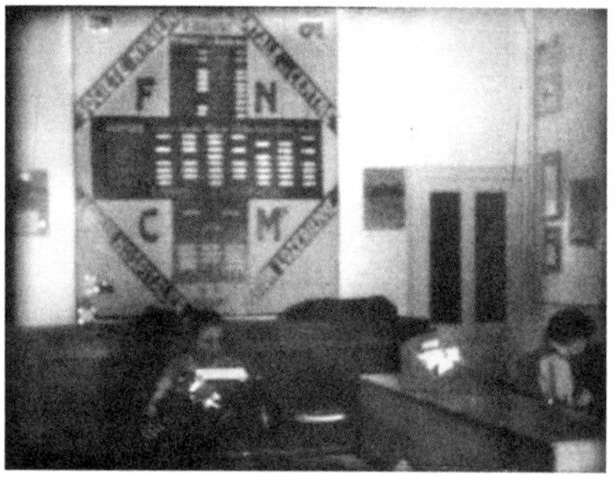

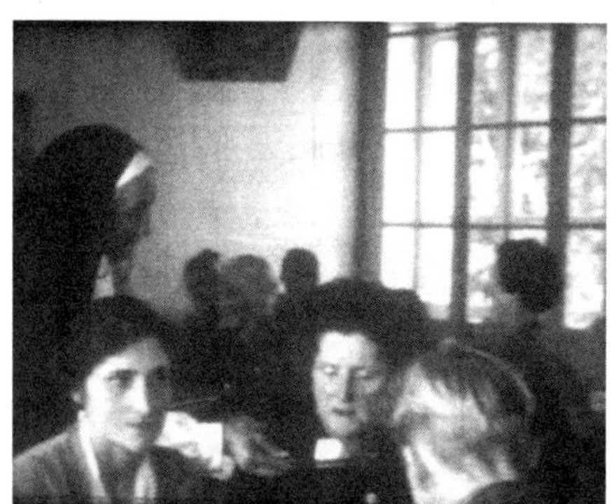

Stills from the film *Société lozérienne d'hygiène mentale*, by Tosquelles, 1958, that show the printing press, some offices, and the dining room in Saint-Alban

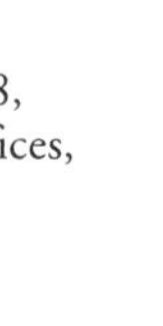

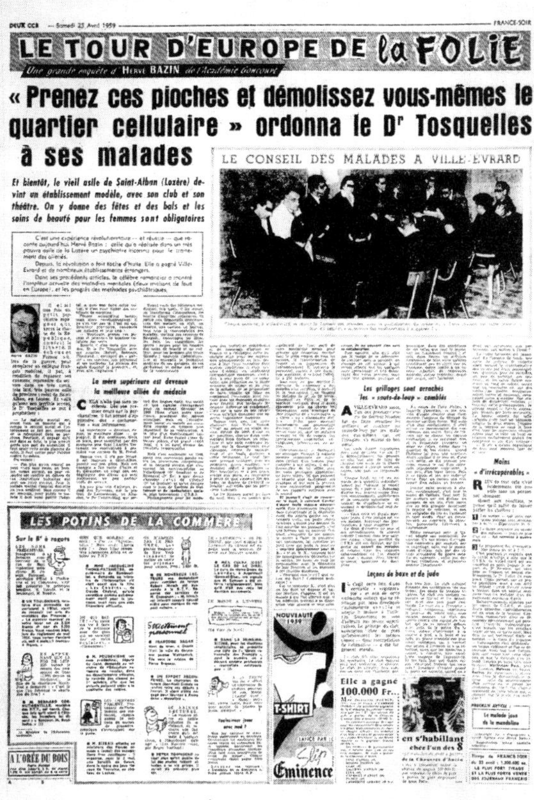

DEUX CCB — Samedi 25 Avril 1959 — FRANCE-SOIR

LE TOUR D'EUROPE DE la FOLIE

Une grande enquête d' HERVÉ BAZIN *de l'Académie Goncourt*

« Prenez ces pioches et démolissez vous-mêmes le quartier cellulaire » ordonna le Dr Tosquelles à ses malades

Et bientôt, le vieil asile de Saint-Alban (Lozère) devint un établissement modèle, avec son club et son théâtre. On y donne des fêtes et des bals et les soins de beauté pour les femmes sont obligatoires

C'est une expérience révolutionnaire — et réussie — que raconte aujourd'hui Hervé Bazin : celle qu'a réalisée dans un très pauvre asile de la Lozère un psychiatre inconnu pour le traitement des aliénés.

Depuis, la révolution a fait tache d'huile. Elle a gagné Ville-Evrard et de nombreux établissements étrangers.

Dans ses précédents articles, le célèbre romancier a montré l'ampleur actuelle des maladies mentales (deux millions de fous en Europe), et les progrès des méthodes psychiatriques.

LE CONSEIL DES MALADES A VILLE-EVRARD

La mère supérieure est devenue la meilleure alliée du médecin

Les grillages sont arrachés les « sauts-de-loup » comblés

Leçons de boxe et de judo

LES POTINS DE LA COMMÈRE

THE EUROPEAN TOUR OF MADNESS

Once upon a time there was a little Spanish psychiatrist who, after the fall of the Republic, chose liberty. He made his way to France where, the war being on, he was to replace a mobilized French colleague. And so, after retaking the required exams, he managed to resume service, this time in a very old, very ugly, very poor provincial asylum: that of Saint-Alban, in Lozère. Thereupon, with his terrible accent, Dr. Tosquelles commenced to prophesy:

—The mental patient is, above all, a person who has broken the social contract and internment becomes their accomplice by getting them back in touch with their psychosis. Yet, however engaged they are in their madness, even the most afflicted retain a share of sociability. One has to take hold of this one lifeline. One has to bet on the insane against themselves.

Or further:

—Just as an animal can't live without kidneys, a man, even a normal one, can't resolve his conflicts outside these human institutions that are his social kidneys. For the patients, the hospital must be an artificial kidney. But since it is bad, in order to heal the patient, we must also heal the hospital. What good is it to practice our trade, if it boils down to signing maintenance certificates?

Remarks that are commonplace today, but revolutionary then. He didn't stop there. It was he, the provisional director, who assembled his patients and shouted:

—Messieurs, do something for me! Take these pickaxes and knock the cell quarters to the ground!

Soon only dust and dirt remained. And Dr. Tosquelles, with his associates (Balvet, Bonnafé, Chaurand …), undertook to "heal" his services, his staff, and his methods. The isolation of agitated patients disappeared … and with it the "agitation."

Making good use of mediocre buildings, as they were, he opened them up, transformed their atmosphere, filled them with collective activities, instigated an internal democracy, created workshops, a club, a theater, a cafeteria, a newspaper, all of them staffed by the patients; started meetings of delegates, encouraged parties, dances, excursions, sports; insisted on beauty care and a hairdresser for the women, decent clothing for the men; shook up the administration, saw to the medical instruction of his male and female staff and even the nuns of the community.

All this didn't proceed without incident. Already with his first course in psychoanalysis, he was accused of teaching "smutty business" to the nurses.

The mother superior—later his best ally—voiced a complaint. He was obliged to continue, Bible in hand, the allegedly spicy explanations of Freud by sanctifying them with examples from the Old Testament.

Since then, he has not budged. He is still at Saint-Alban, perched on his rock. But his example has resonated and from Gévaudan, twenty years worth of students have rippled out to become medical directors just about everywhere. [...][6]

Hervé Bazin, "Le tour d'Europe de la folie" [The European tour of madness], *France-Soir*, Saturday, April 25, 1959

In France, the space of freedom that the hospital was gradually occupying had a situated genealogy. On June 10, 1838, a new law endorsed by the psychiatrists Étienne Esquirol and Guillaume Ferrus, protégés of Philippe Pinel, marked the beginning of a change in the relationships between psychiatric hospitals and the *départements* and regions. From then on, every French *département* had to have its own public hospital with a psychiatrist in open communication with the political and administrative structures of the region. As Michel Foucault has written, that initial moment of sectorization created a shift from the justice system to the medical system, as the psychiatric hospitals directly inherited the power to treat madness, which gradually moved away from its association with social disorder, criminality, and, as a result, prison. It is replaced by "mental illness," treated by the medical system through new structures of reclusion. Three years before that law was passed, in 1835, Pierre Rivière, confessed murderer of his mother, sister, and brother, had originally been sentenced to death but this was commuted to life imprisonment after the court recognized his murders as an act of madness, and this change in interpretation occurred thanks to the efforts of psychiatrists such as the aforementioned Étienne Esquirol. Robert Castel, who in the 1970s collaborated with Michel Foucault at the Collège de France in the working group dealing with the publication of Pierre Rivière's confession, points out that this new modern frontier between mental illness and criminality is the turning point upon which, in the nineteenth century, the new medical power and the grand figure of the alienist doctor were constructed.[7]

But the 1838 law, which according to Foucault marked the beginning of psychiatric autonomy and power in the nineteenth century, was also the start of a prehistory of sectorization in the territory and of the psychiatrist as civil servant. Where Foucault situates the new psychiatric power and new forms of government, Tosquelles glimpses a new world of possibilities: different material relationships between hospitals and regions, families and prefects. For Tosquelles, the 1838 law protected the ill from the abuses of the administration and of the familiar institution; it allowed for pushing the limits of administrative powers, and for doing institutional work in a network, embodying the figure of the psychiatrist based on new forms of possible freedom and developing a local economy. Understanding the figure of the psychiatrist as a true public civil servant allowed Tosquelles to link his medical practice with other forms of commitment.

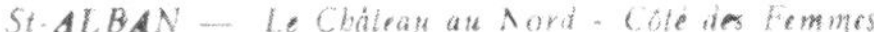

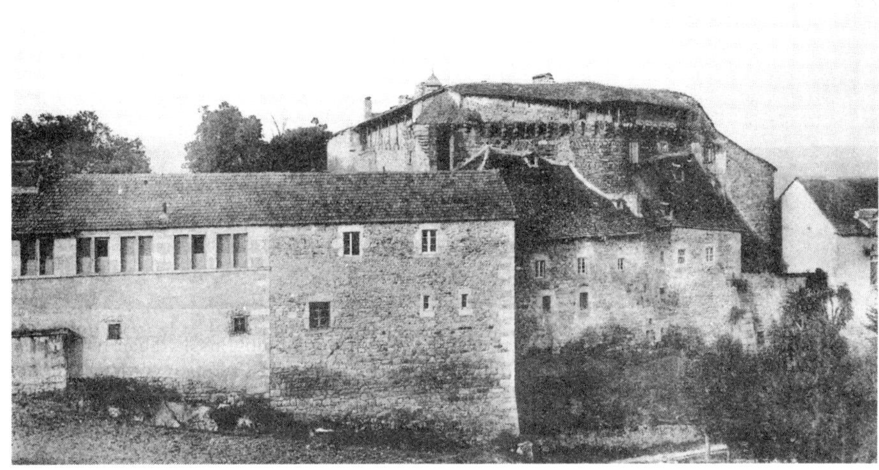

In his writings, Francesc Tosquelles situates the earliest experiences of anti-psychiatry at Saint-Alban in the 19th century, in conceptual continuity with the sectorization project of the 1838 law. The hospital had originally been a religious foundation, with a church and a feudal castle. In 1821 Hilarion Tissot, a medical student and a monk of the order of Saint-Jean-de-Dieu, bought the castle on his pilgrimage to Santiago de Compostela. With the help of the townspeople and the nuns of the congregation of Saint-Régis, Tissot turned the castle into a hospital and, as he saw more and more patients, it became the main hospital center in the region of Lozère. Mireille Gauzy wrote that Tissot was a strange, atypical monk, some sort of madman who created spaces and a discourse of healing the insane that involved great freedom, but that he soon came into conflict with the prevailing social and political order. The asylum became property of the *département* of Lozère in 1823 and for a long time it took in men and women imprisoned in the capital, Mende, holding up to six hundred inmates.

MINISTÈRE
DE L'INTÉRIEUR

DIRECTION GÉNÉRALE
POLICE DE LA
~~SURETÉ~~ NATIONALE

[RÉ]GION de MONTPELLIER
INTENDANCE de POLICE
RENSEIGNEMENTS GÉNÉRAUX
[Co]mmissariat de MENDE

N° 929

RI/YC

ÉTAT FRANÇAIS
~~RÉPUBLIQUE FRANÇAISE~~

MENDE, le 8 Avril 1943

Le Commissaire de Police
des Renseignements Généraux, RISPOLI,

à Monsieur le PREFET de la LOZERE
- Cabinet -

OBJET: Situation politique de la commune de St ALBAN.

J'ai l'honneur de vous rendre compte que mis en possession récemment de certains renseignements pouvant laisser supposer qu'une sourde agitation antinationale se manifestait dans la commune de St ALBAN, notamment à l'Hôpital Psychiatrique, et était susceptible de prendre la forme d'une reconstitution clandestine de cellule communiste, j'ai procédé sur place à une enquête, et vous communique ci-après les renseignements qui ont été recueillis sur les personnes mises en cause, les nommés CAYZAC, PIC Jean, BERTUIT, BRUNEL Jean, BRUNEL Augustin, BONNET, BOULET Jean, GASC père et fils, FAVIER et TOSCALES.

A première vue, il ressort de l'enquête qu'il n'y a pas à l'heure actuelle à St ALBAN de cellule communiste organisée, étant donné qu'aucune manifestation clandestine de propagande par tracts, papillons, inscriptions murales, n'a eu lieu à ce jour.

Il n'en existe pas moins un certain nombre d'individus dont le loyalisme à l'égard du Gouvernement et du régime est des plus douteux, qui ne cachent pas leurs sympathies pour les puissances anglo-saxonnes et qui attendent avec impatience, non pas l'instauration du communisme peut-être, mais le retour de la République et d'un Gouvernement "Front Populaire".

A report by General Intelligence signed by Police Commissioner Rispoli at Mende and addressed to the prefect of Lozère, April 8, 1943. The Vichy police surveilled Tosquelles and other members of the medical staff of Saint-Alban. The report contains the only written trace of the monthly allocation sent to Tosquelles for a few years by the Mexican government due to his status as a Spanish exile and in solidarity with the Republic.

TOSQUELLAS-LLAURADO Francisco, was born at Reus (Spain). He is married to ALVAREZ FERNANDEZ Hélène and has two children aged 7 and 1. All three live with him.

A psychiatric doctor in Spain, he was mobilized into the Spanish Republican Army during the Civil War as a doctor-lieutenant, then a doctor-captain. In September 1939, the subject took refuge in FRANCE and was interned in the Septfonds camp (Tarn-et-Garonne).

In January 1943, at the request of the medical director of the asylum, who was short of doctors in the wake of the hostilities, TOSQUELLAS was authorized to come to the Saint-Alban psychiatric hospital as a nurse.

Subsequently, he was made an assistant to the doctor in charge.

Housed and fed by the administration, he was to receive no salary.

From the professional standpoint, he gives every satisfaction.

For a long time, the subject benefited from a monthly allowance from the Consulate of Mexico in France, as an immigrant approved by the government of that country.

A cultivated individual, speaking our language correctly, TOSQUELLAS rarely leaves the commune or even the hospital.

He only frequents the mayor of the commune, Monsieur Buffière, the departmental councillor, who holds him in high esteem and portrays him as an anti-Francoist Spanish Republican.

The director of the hospital has nothing but praise for this Spanish immigrant whom he considers extremely competent and to whom he attributes no political activity.

He didn't hesitate to say that the day when the police decide for whatever reason to obtain the dismissal of this man, he would do everything in his power to oppose it.

The attitude of this new director is, furthermore, rather abnormal and has caused him to specify that the subversive political doings of his subordinates are not his concern and that he would be reluctant to communicate to the police whatever information might come his way by chance.

As concerns TOSQUELLAS, one cannot reasonably impute to him any definite misconduct.

It is quite possible that, happy to have secured his situation in FRANCE, he is content to exercise his profession scrupulously and he manifests toward our regime, which he cannot affirm, an attitude of complete neutrality.

And yet, his presence at Saint-Alban, where there existed a communist cell before the war, seems undesirable to many persons, especially those belonging to the legionary and militia circles.

They stress the intelligence of TOSQUELLAS and his education, and assert that for three years he has found it easy to attract the sympathies of the personnel and to engage discreetly in a skillful propaganda dangerous to the country.

In our national milieu, it's difficult to accept that this Republican Spaniard has kept his position while severe sanctions have caused many Israelite French doctors to lose theirs.

An equitable resolution of this affair seems difficult, consequently.

It's advisable, however, to bear in mind that TOSQUELLAS obtained his appointment to the Saint-Alban hospital only at a time when numerous doctors were being mobilized and to mitigate the shortfall of key personnel in that establishment.

If the competent authorities decide that this situation has not changed since 1940 and that the number of doctors is still too small, we think that TOSQUELLAS could be retained in his employ.

In the contrary case, there is no reason to keep in place a Spaniard unsupportive of our regime and to whom the common law should therefore be applied.[8]

Report signed by the police commissioner of Mende, addressed to the prefect of Lozère, April 8, 1943; drawn from the archives of Tarn-et-Garonne

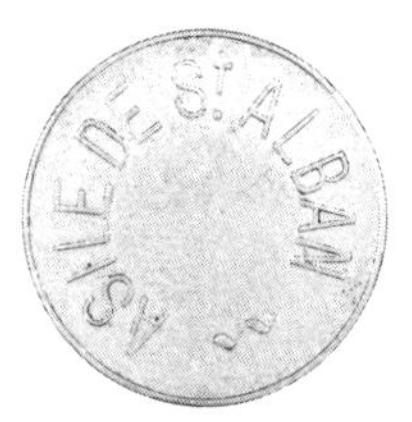
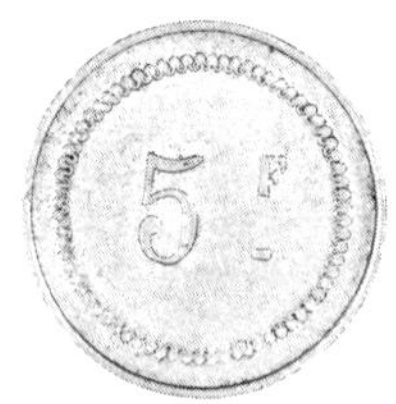

Coin that Dr. Agnès Masson put into circulation within the hospital in 1934; the patients could exchange them for food and items at the hospital store. After Paul Balvet's arrival, the coins disappeared.

Faith in the transformation of the ways of embodying medical authority was one of the legacies Tosquelles inherited from the psychiatrist Agnès Masson, director of Saint-Alban from 1933 to 1936, a period in which geopsychiatry was promoted. Despite being one of the first female psychiatrists in France and having directed institutions, Masson is as unknown as her doctoral thesis published in 1935, *Le travestissement: Essai de psycho-pathologie sexuelle*. Today we can only read it in contrast with her radical project of humanizing life at Saint-Alban, since it deals with transvestism through the lens of the prejudices of the era: stigmatization, biological pathology, and the need for institutional reclusion.

Agnès Masson could as easily be seen driving around Lòzere in a van to gather up escaped patients as managing with the administration the installation of the first measures to humanize collective life at Saint-Alban: electricity and heating; bathtubs and toilets to halt a typhus epidemic; two infirmaries; a laundry and a system of coins that served as currency within the hospital … She also introduced silent films and a library. When Dr. Paul Balvet arrived in 1936, he created the common room, the canteen, the sports club, a kitchen council, and the Théophile Roussel pavilion in the agricultural colony of Le Villaret, outside of the hospital grounds, where Tosquelles would work with children and was photographed in 1942. A few years later, when talking about his experiences there and in Reus, Tosquelles said that in every revolution one had to recover their own childhood.

Over the following pages, a report on the 1935 renovations carried out in the Saint-Alban hospital to improve the quality of life of the inpatients, in which Agnès Masson speaks of natural light and tile flooring, of mirrors and courtyards with flowers

DÉPARTEMENT DE LA LOZÈRE

Asile Public d'Aliénés de Saint-Alban

RAPPORT

MÉDICAL et ADMINISTRATIF

PRÉSENTÉ

par Mme le Docteur MASSON

DIRECTEUR-MÉDECIN

Exercice 1935

MENDE. — IMPRIMERIE IGNON

1936

ASILE DE SAINT-ALBAN

MODERNISATION
1933 - 1936

Tous ces travaux, sauf les grosses installations de chauffage central et une grande partie de l'installation électrique, ont été faits par l'Etablissement (plans, devis, surveillance)

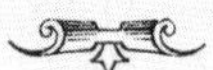

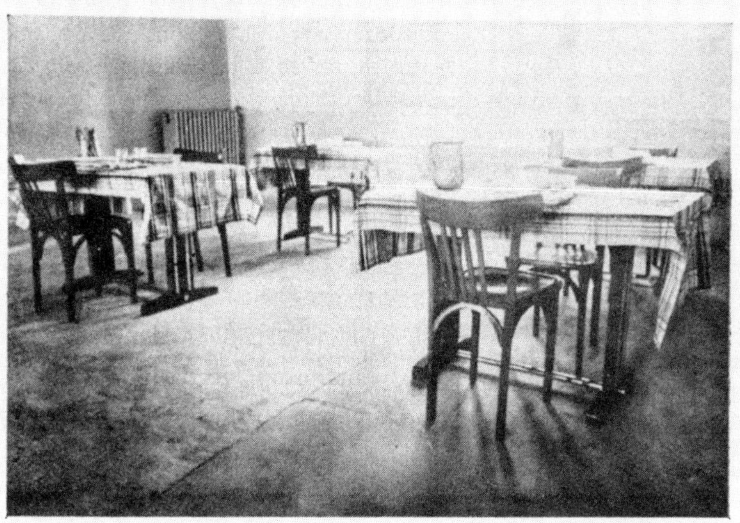

PAVILLON DE LA TERRASSE : REFECTOIRE

Réfectoire comprenant 8 tables à 2 places, type restaurant.
Un autre réfectoire identique vient d'être installé au Pavillon Pinel (service des hommes).

PLANS

Les plans et projets suivants ont été approuvés par le Conseil général :

1° Les plans et le projet d'agrandissement du service des enfants anormaux du Villaret. comprenant : 3 pavillons de 20 enfants, 1 infirmerie grabataires, 1 infirmerie maladies incidentes, 1 pavillon de service médical (dentisterie, etc...), 1 pavillon de classes avec salle de fêtes. Ces pavillons s'inspirent des principes suivants: 2 dortoirs de 10 lits par pavillon, lavabo individuel dans la salle de lavabos annexée au dortoir, plus les lavabos de service (réfectoire, salle de jour, etc...) ; salle des lavabos située sur le parcours entre l'escalier et le dortoir et, au rez-de-chaussée, entre la salle de jour et le réfectoire ; escalier de secours extérieur pour les pavillons à étage ; boxes dans l'infirmerie des maladies incidentes. Ce projet est actuellement soumis à l'approbation du Ministère.

2° Le projet concernant les nouveaux pavillons des services généraux et des nouveaux services des femmes, destinés à remplacer les anciens, a déjà été approuvé par le Conseil général dans ses grandes lignes et est actuellement à l'étude ; les pavillons du service des femmes s'inspireront des mêmes principes que les pavillons du service d'enfants. La buanderie en construction s'intègre dans ce plan d'ensemble.

3° L'adduction d'une nouvelle source d'eau, déjà approuvée par le Conseil général, est à l'étude, ainsi que le réseau d'égouts.

Tous ces travaux, pour lesquels l'approbation du Conseil général a déjà été obtenue, seront exécutés par tranches, en utilisant les disponibilités budgétaires présentes et futures.

4° Le Conseil général est appelé à se prononcer, dans sa session de Novembre 1936, sur le projet de la construction d'un laboratoire, constituée par un petit pavillon indépendant comprenant : 2 salles de laboratoire, 1 chambre noire, 1 petit magasin, 1 bibliothèque-cabinet médical, 1 vestibule et les annexes habituelles.

Photographies Vve Langlois,
à Marvejols.

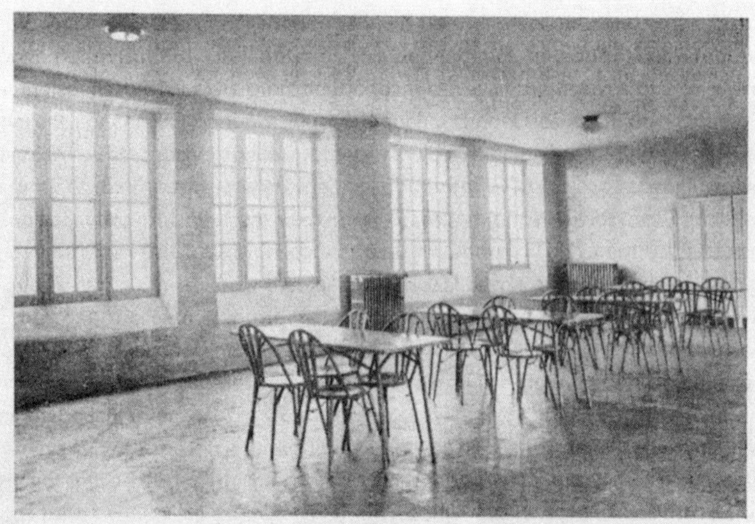

PAVILLON DE LA TERRASSE : SALLE DE JOUR

Fenêtres comme celles des dortoirs. Tables et chaises métalliques. T. S. F. Salle pour quinze malades.

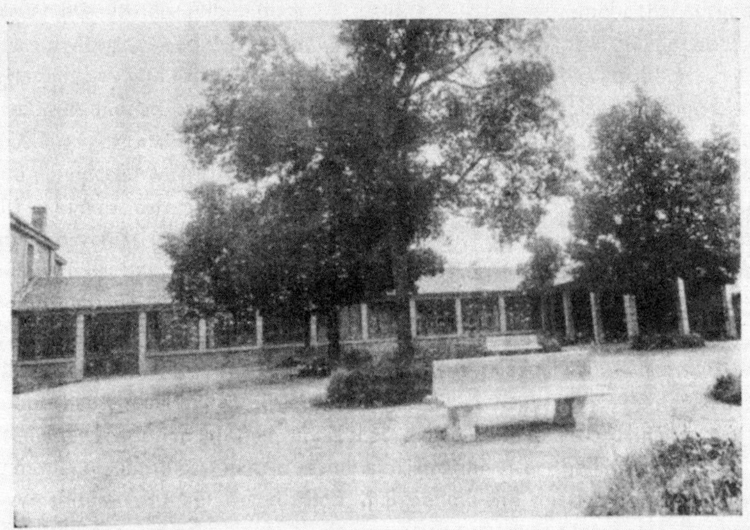

SERVICE DES HOMMES : PAVILLON BAILLARGER

Nouvelle aile appuyée au mur de la cour. Préau en bout. Bancs doubles en ciment (modèle de l'Asile de Naugeat, à Limoges, d'après un plan dû à l'obligeance de M. Dupas, directeur de l'Asile). Quarante-huit places pour trente malades. Des bancs analogues sont en voie de construction dans les autres cours des trois services.

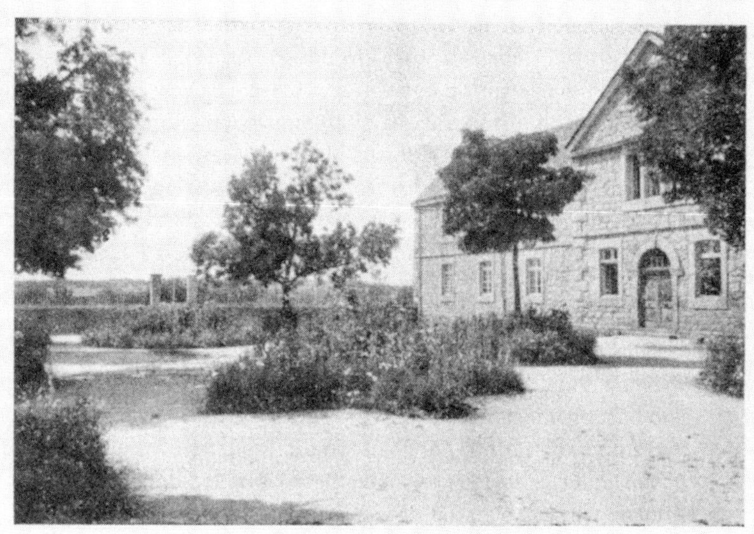

UNE COUR FLEURIE : PAVILLON ESQUIROL

Toutes les cours du service des hommes, y compris la cour des agités, ont des plates-bandes fleuries, que les malades respectent et entretiennent. A gauche, ample vue sur les collines environnantes (la presque totalité des cours de l'Asile a la même vue).

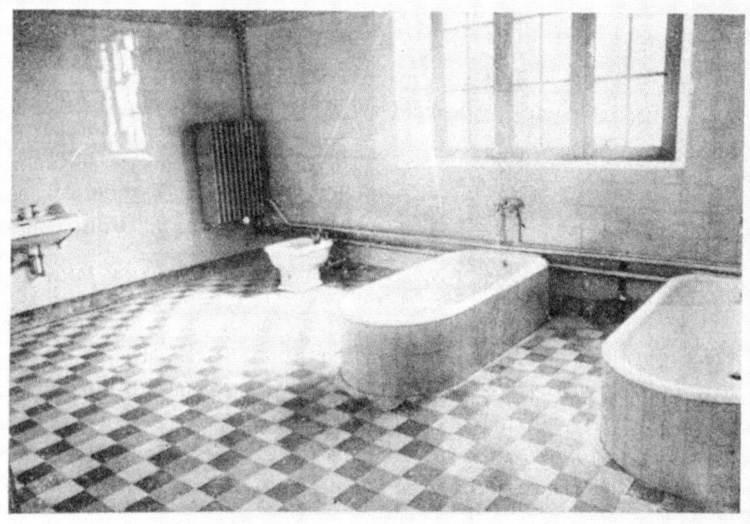

PAVILLON BAILLARGER (aile nouvelle) : SALLE DE BAINS

Toutes les sections du service des hommes vont recevoir (dans des locaux plus petits existants) le même aménagement. Le carrelage, au lieu d'être arrêté à deux mètres comme ici, montera jusqu'au plafond.

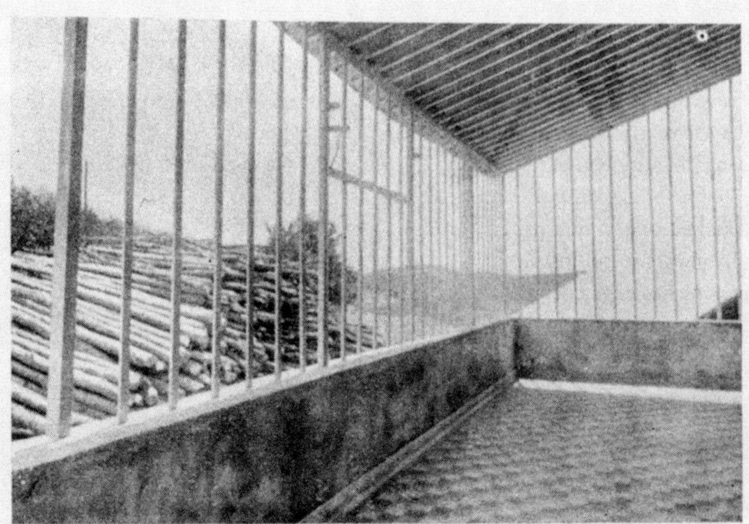

PAVILLON DE LA TERRASSE : VERANDA

Construction nouvelle en appentis, ouvrant sur le réfectoire. Elle a, dans son troisième côté (non visible), une porte et un escalier métalliques (de **secours** *en cas d'incendie). Deux châssis ouvrants à crémones ordinaires (un est visible dans la photo) et un pivotant horizontalement à ressorts (id.). Dimensions :* **6 × 3,50.**

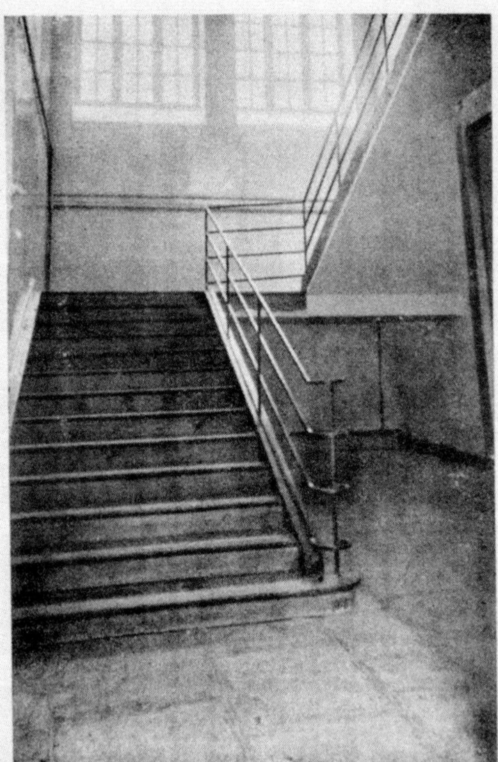

PAVILLON DE LA TERRASSE :

ESCALIER

Création nouvelle à l'intérieur d'un bâtiment réadapté : largeur de la cage d'escalier, 4 m. 50 ; largeur de l'escalier : 1 m. 80 ; marches de 0 m. 35 × 0 m. 145.

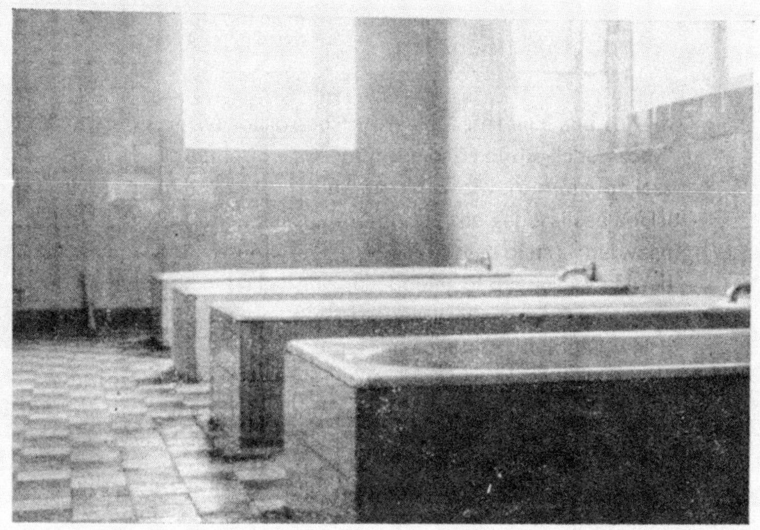

SERVICE DES HOMMES : PAVILLON ESQUIROL

Ancienne salle de bains modernisée. 5 baignoires carrées légèrement enfoncées dans le sol, revêtement faïence. On voit dans le fond, à gauche, une installation non encore terminée (lavabo). Robinetterie des baignoires enclavée.

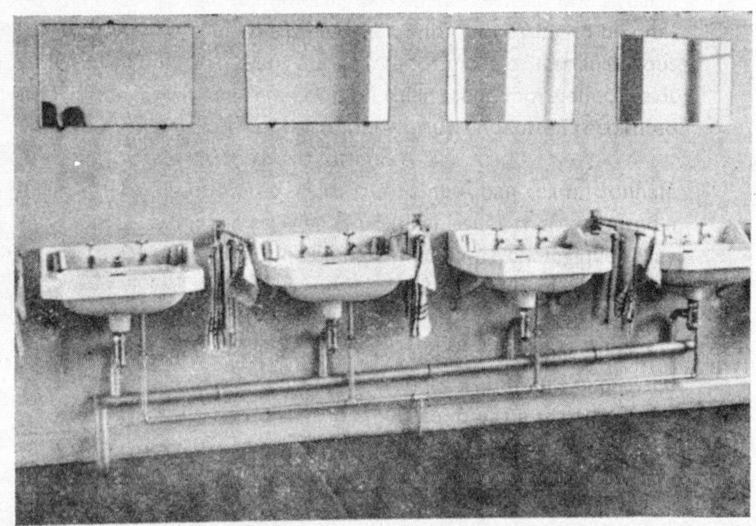

PAVILLON DE LA TERRASSE : LAVABOS

Dans les dortoirs du Pavillon de la Terrasse, il y a deux lavabos pour trois malades (six et quatre pour les deux dortoirs). Dans les pavillons en projet (enfants, femmes), il est prévu dans les dortoirs un lavabo par malade (lavabo individuel), sans compter les autres lavabos prévus dans chaque pièce (réfectoires, salles de jour, etc...). Les lavabos mis à la disposition des malades sont en grès émaillé (danger minime en cas de bris). Au Pavillon de la Terrasse (femmes tranquilles), chaque malade dispose d'un porte-serviettes à trois branches, avec deux serviettes et gant éponge. Les robinets (eau froide et chaude) sont commandés librement par les malades. La même disposition est prévue pour l'installation sanitaire de tous les quartiers actuellement en cours.

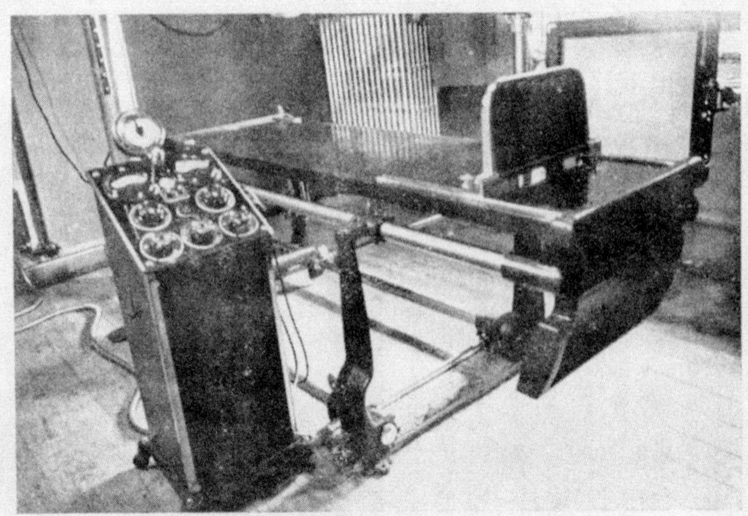

SALLE DE RADIOLOGIE

La salle de radiologie est peinte en bleu foncé.
L'appareil est un « Orienta-Sécurix » de la Compagnie Générale de Radiologie.

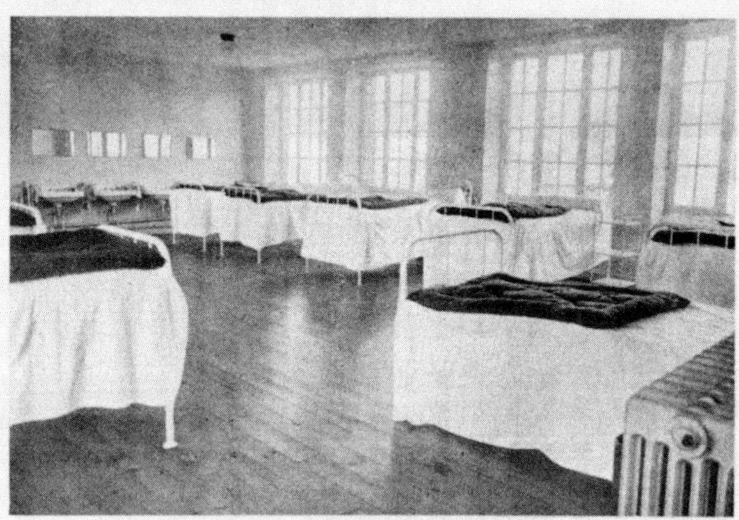

PAVILLON DE LA TERRASSE : UN DORTOIR

Ce pavillon n'a été affecté au service des femmes qu'en 1934. Il contient deux dortoirs (9 + 6 lits), une grande salle de jour, un réfectoire, une salle de bain, une véranda, deux salles d'infirmerie, la salle de radiologie et le laboratoire photographique annexe. Les châssis des fenêtres se composent de trois parties, dont la partie centrale, pivotante et munie de crémones ordinaires, peut être ouverte librement par les malades. Comme dans tous les pavillons, l'installation électrique comporte des diffuseurs (4 dans ce dortoir).

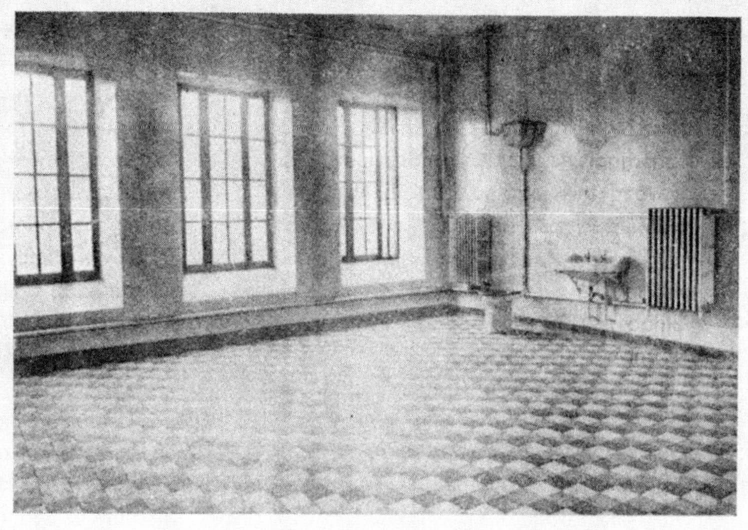

PAVILLON DE LA TERRASSE : INFIRMERIE (2 salles)

Locaux adaptés, fenêtres repercées. Les châssis des fenêtres se composent de trois parties ; les deux parties latérales, plus petites, sont pivotantes (comme il s'agit d'une infirmerie, les châssis pivotants dégagent une ouverture moins grande que ceux du dortoir précédent). Les deux infirmeries contiennent 6 + 2 lits. La baignoire est une baignoire de forme courante, à une tête, légèrement enfoncée dans le sol et carreiée avec des carreaux de faïence coupés à la forme.

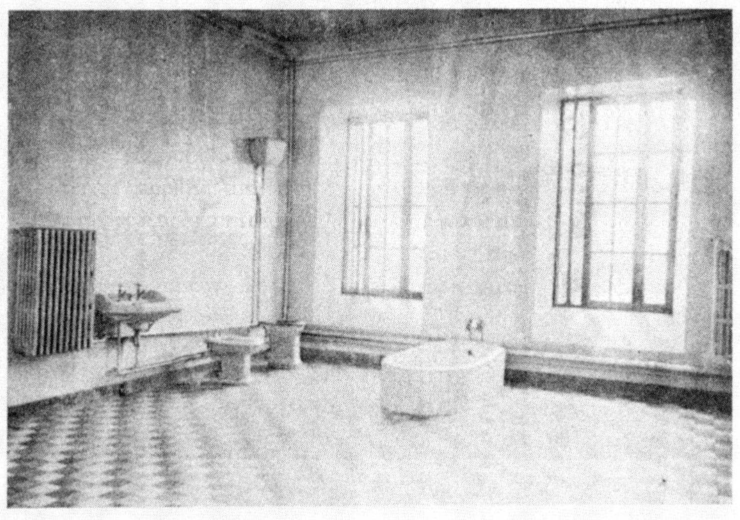

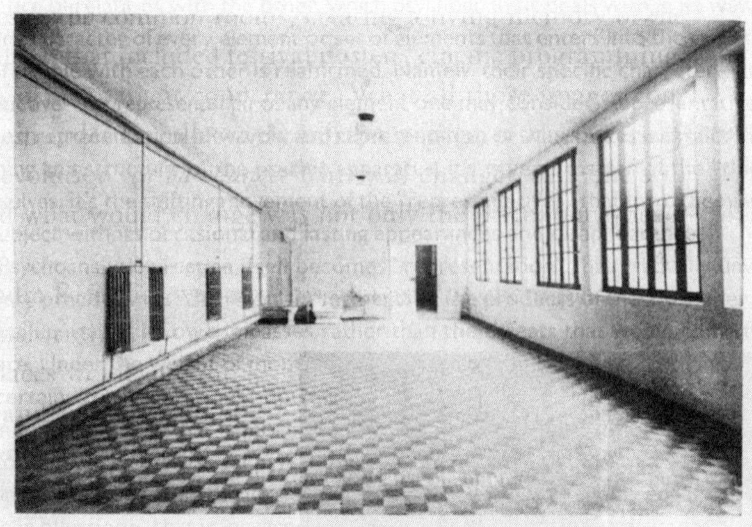

PAVILLON BAILLARGER (aile nouvelle) :
INFIRMERIE

Une seule rangée de lits. Fenêtres avec deux châssis à la disposition des malades.

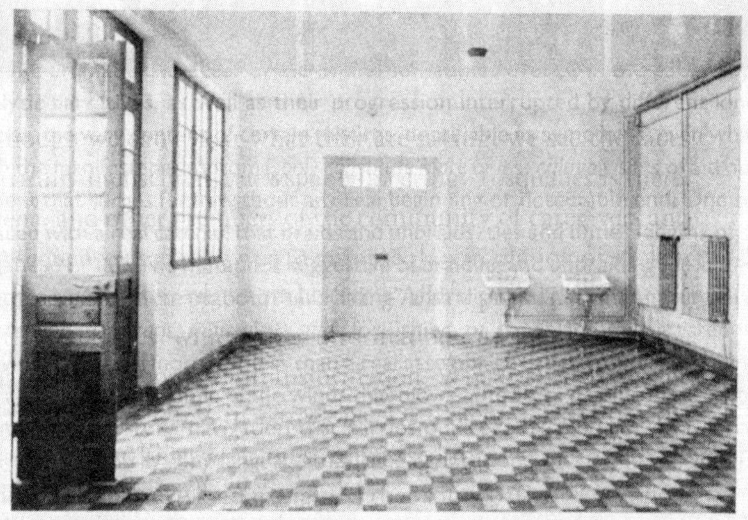

PAVILLON BAILLARGER (aile nouvelle) :
REFECTOIRE

Deux lavabos, comme dans tous les réfectoires (deux à six suivant le nombre des malades dans les installations en cours). Le carrelage va être étendu progressivement à tous les locaux de l'asile au rez-de-chaussée (plus de 300 mètres carrés posés en 1935, d'autres en projet).

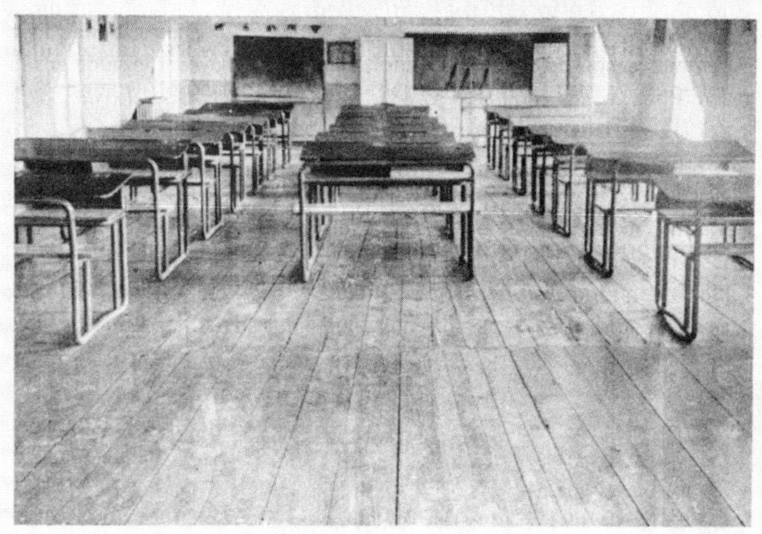

PAVILLON TH.-ROUSSEL, AU VILLARET
(à 2 kilomètres de l'Asile)

Salle de classe (local adapté). Ameublement en tube et bois. Cette classe doit être supprimée lors de l'agrandissement du service, un des nouveaux pavillons devant contenir les classes et les locaux annexes.

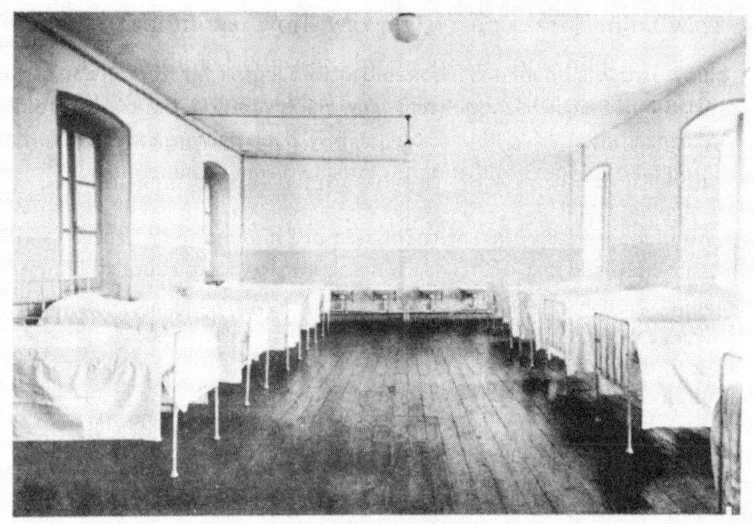

PAVILLON TH.-ROUSSEL : UN DORTOIR

Dans le fond, six lavabos et même disposition dans l'autre dortoir. Des lavabos sont en train d'être installés dans tous les dortoirs du service des hommes dans les limites de la place disponible (en général six lavabos par dortoir). Des glaces sont également envisagées comme au Pavilon de la Terrasse (sauf dans la section des agités). Quelques lavabos vont être installés, à titre provisoire, dans les vieux bâtiments des femmes qui doivent être démolis.

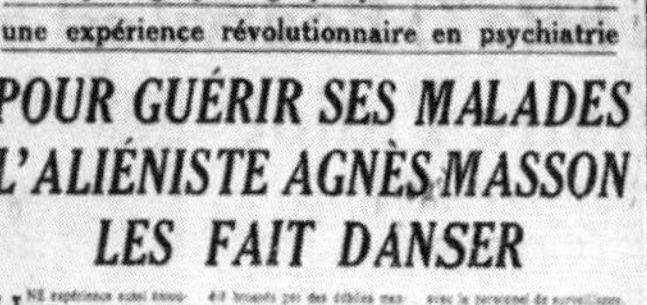

Un reportage photographique sensationnel sur une expérience révolutionnaire en psychiatrie

POUR GUÉRIR SES MALADES L'ALIÉNISTE AGNÈS MASSON LES FAIT DANSER

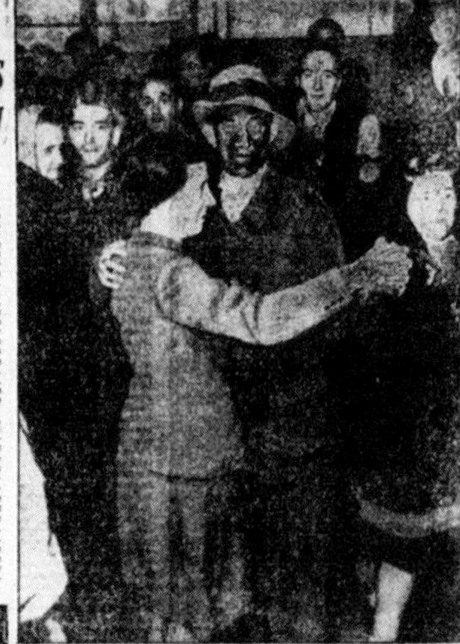

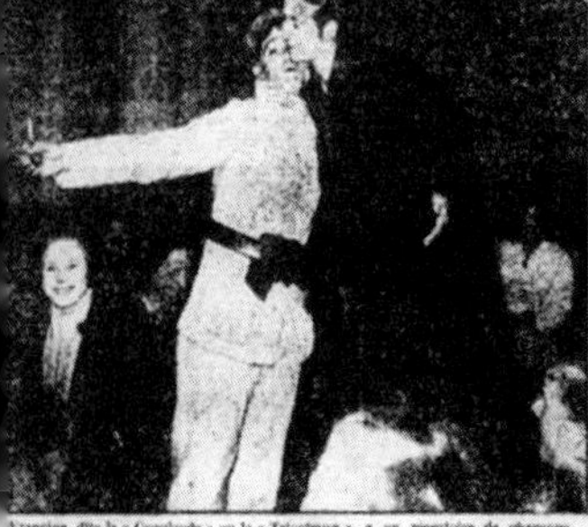

Mi-Carême : ils s'amusent follement

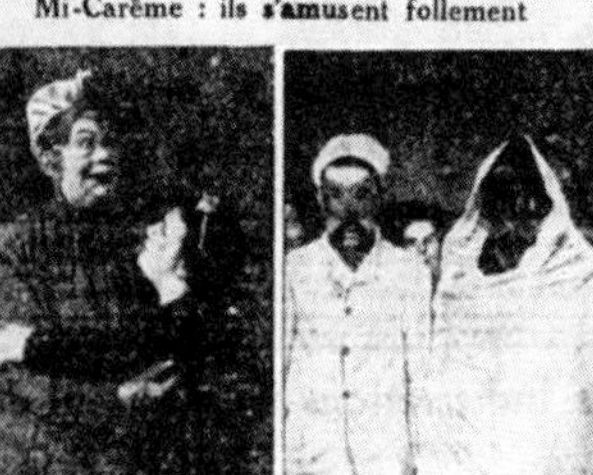

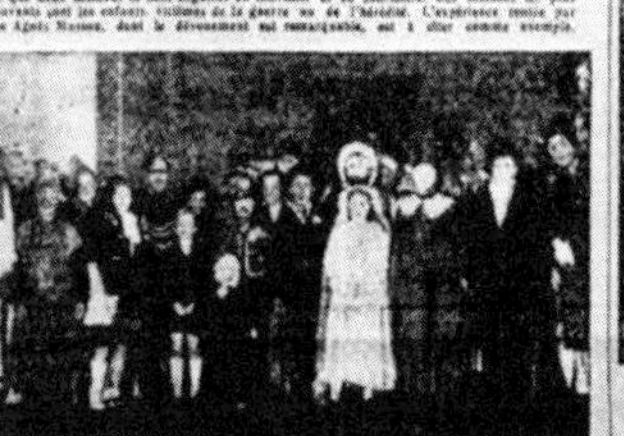

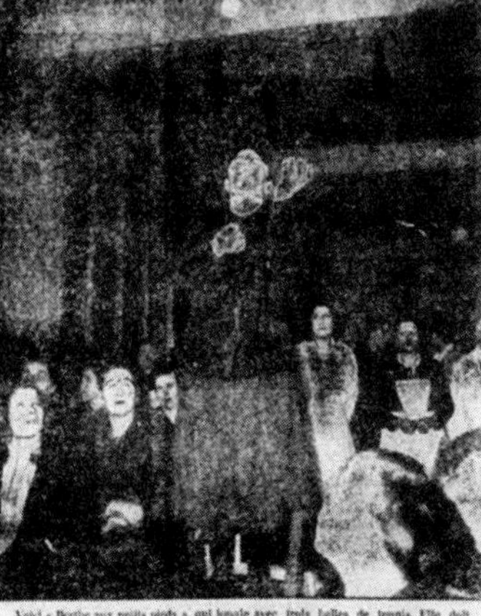

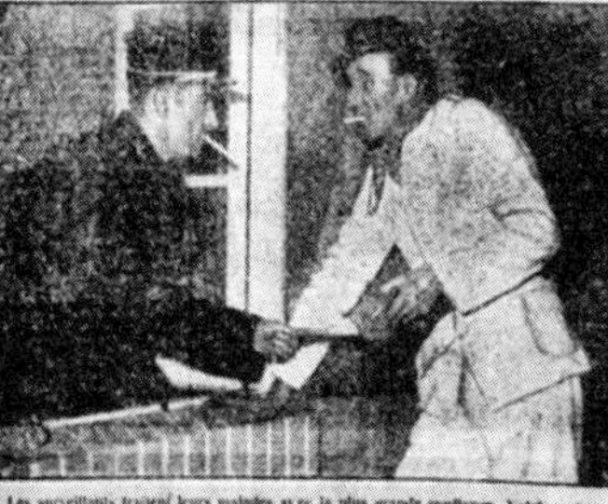

Captions to photographs (*from top to bottom, and right to left*):

"The director of the Châlons asylum, Madame Agnès Masson, dances with one of her patients, who asks to be called God. Agnès Masson has literature and medical degrees and is a chief physician of asylums, a laureate of the Academy of Medicine, and a socialist militant in her free time."

"Francine, aka 'the Loudmouth,' or 'the *Tricoteuse*' ['the Knitter,' a figure from the French Revolution], has a varied repertoire of songs. Her favorite number is 'C'est mon petit chéri d'amour' [That's my little sweetheart], whose refrain the audience repeats in chorus. Francine feels a real passion for the director."

"Here is 'Berthe of the Little Feet,' who juggles three tennis balls. She owes her internment to a shock suffered in 1914 when a German shell exploded close to her. Many children currently in treatment have undergone a comparable shock."

"Here is a group of costumed patients assembled on the stage of the entertainment hall. Note that two patients are got up as a male and a female nurse. [...]"

"The monitors treat their patients with a great deal of trust. Here is a nurse (in white fatigues) who's about to play a role in the skit of a patient outfitted as a common soldier, one who will give him an order. The patients have requested hundreds of our photos."

Agnès Masson and her contribution to the French history of community psychiatry are little known. Italian by birth, she defended her medical thesis in 1929 at the University of Lyon, under the name of Agnès Chiarli. After Saint-Alban, she practiced at Naugeat-Limoges, in Haute Vienne, before being named medical director at the psychiatric hospital of Chalôns-sur-Marne in 1944. She was also a Socialist municipal councillor from 1945 to 1947, as well as secretary of the Group of Elected Socialist Women—Municipal and Cantonal.

TO HEAL HER PATIENTS, THE PSYCHIATRIST AGNÈS MASSON HAS THEM DANCE

An experiment as moving as it is fascinating is being attempted by Madame Agnès Masson, directress of the psychiatric hospital of Châlons-sur-Marne.

Madame Agnès Masson is France's youngest psychiatrist entrusted with running an asylum. Nicknamed "Chérie" [Darling] by her residents, she has revolutionized the methods of treatment of the insane. She applies to her patients a cure from which the straitjacket and the cell are banned. She replaces those "remedies" from another time with dancing, theater, and cinema.

Her appointment dates back to the month of December 1944. Naturally the administration was shocked to learn that Agnès Masson had set her crazies to dancing. They considered recalling her, but "Chérie" had already been adopted by her patients. She kept her post.

Her idea is simple: she offers her residents a situation of semi-liberty that eases their readjustment to normal life. She doesn't want them to be absorbed in contemplating the gray walls of their cells. Of the three hundred women she cares for, more than half knit sweaters for themselves or their families. The men do odd jobs. Theater sets, tending to the surrealistic, have been painted by mental incompetents still subject to periodic crises.

The monitoring staff wholeheatedly support the efforts of the directress. An exceptional climate of trust was able to be created. Patients and monitors collaborate amicably. The collaboration becomes very close for the preparation of entertainments. The theater plays are performed by "mixed" troupes, where the staff have crazies as partners. On stage it becomes impossible to tell them apart.

The star of the galas at the Châlons asylum is named Arsène. He declares himself "prince of all the Europes, all the Arabies," and "duke of La Tourne-Tournefeuille." He is both a good painter and a good actor. Our reporters have photographed him and his fellow stars: the juggler "Berthe of the Little Feet" and the chanteuse Francine, "the Loudmouth."

The dances at the Châlons asylum are very much favored by the police of the prefecture, who go to them with their families. There is one per month. For Mardi Gras and Mid-Lent, the patients are disguised. To be sure, only the "inoffensive" are authorized to attend. One frequently sees them dancing with the surveillance staff.

Dr. Masson's methods have produced astonishing results. The number of patients has clearly declined. A very short stay is generally enough to restore the patients to their mental equilibrium. This is especially true for the adults. For the old people and the children, the degrees of progress are slower to come, the cures more infrequent. But some of them make so much progress that they can be allowed to go shopping in the town. They never try to use that semi-liberty to strike out on their own. The asylum is their home. They are pleased to go back there.

Madame Masson is not entirely satisfied, of course: she wants to turn her establishment into a model of its kind. She needs 15 million francs to redo the decor of the place. For her patients' benefit, she's gotten rid of the gray uniforms that recalled those of convicts. She employs a housekeeper who takes herself for the wife of Hitler, a cook who, more modestly, is only the führer's fiancée, and a bookkeeper who claims to be the duchess of Hohenzollern. (The prestige of Germany appears to be substantial in the Châlons asylum.)[9]

"Pour guérir ses malades, l'aliéniste Agnès Masson les fait danser" [To heal her patients, the psychiatrist Agnès Masson has them dance], unsigned article, *Samedi-soir*, March 22, 1947

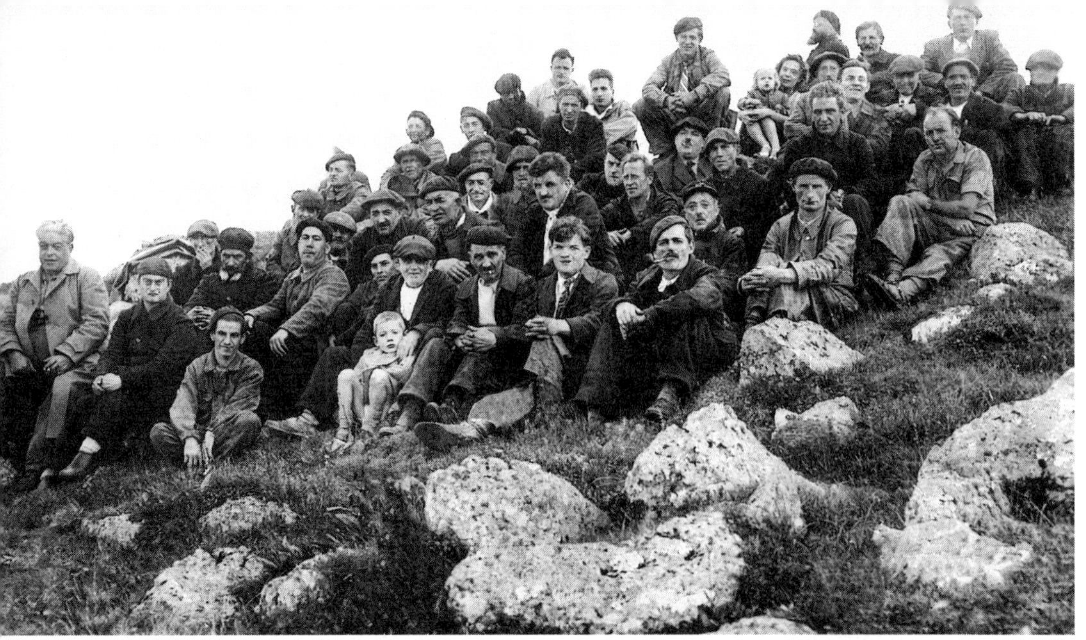

Hiking trip for male inpatients at Saint-Alban, circa 1950–1955. Seated in the second row, second from the right, is Auguste Forestier.

Resistances

With Paul Balvet, Francesc Tosquelles shared ways of maintaining life under the Nazi occupation that became blurred into the local history of the Resistance during the Second World War. After the liberation of France, Lucien Bonnafé, who had worked at Saint-Alban, and Georges Daumézon, who along with Philippe Koechlin had given the name "institutional psychotherapy" to the practices they'd developed at the hospital, were charged with carrying out the census of how many patients had died in French psychiatric hospitals. They estimated that, between 1940 and 1944, the "soft extermination" had allowed forty thousand of the patients to starve to death, a tragedy that was collectively silenced until the 1980s. Until then there was no talk of the indifference shown toward the patients who had been excluded from circuits of family and collective solidarity; it was not said that, despite occupied France not having an official eugenics program—as there was in the Nazi hospitals and elimination programs in Germany—in French hospitals like Le Vinatier, with large tracts of farmland and great profits under Vichy, they had let two thousand mental patients die; it was not said, as the editor and writer François Maspero wrote in his novel *Les abeilles et la guêpe*, "I lived a hundred meters from the soft extermination and I had no idea."[10] The lack of official recognition for these deaths is at the heart of the great books by Max Lafont and Isabelle von

Bueltzingsloewen, with an explicit commitment to reverting this oblivion with accounts of fascist acts during the war. Within this history there were also humanizing experiences, such as the battle for material life in Saint-Alban, where there were no deaths and the patients and the farmers shared work in the fields and the carding of wool to be able to barter their products for meat, wine, potatoes, and butter. Other informal economies made life livable at the hospital through more imperceptible knowledge and practices that don't form part of the larger story of Saint-Alban, like those carried out by Germaine Balvet. She was a psychiatrist, like her husband Paul Balvet, but she did not hold any official post at the hospital. Knowledgeable about the properties of herbs and medicinal plants, she would organize gardening tasks with the patients and trips into the forest to collect mushrooms, within a larger open understanding of the landscape and of the actions that comprised an institution.

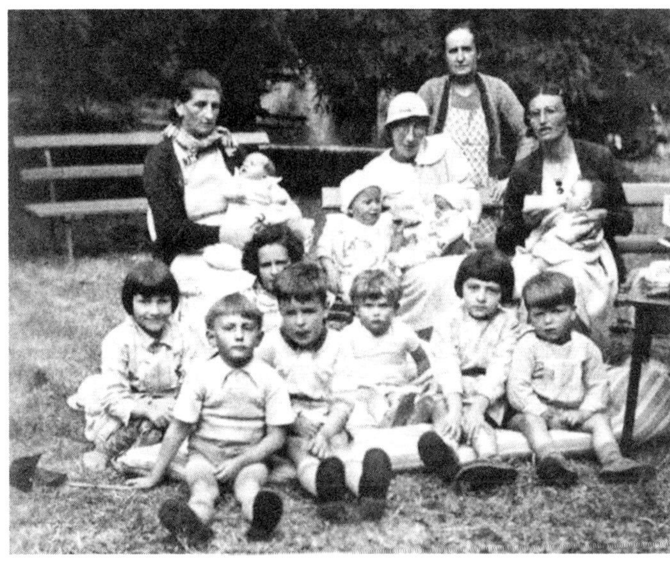

Germaine Balvet (*on the right*) with other wives and children of the doctors and staff who lived at the hospital

Germaine Balvet, a psychiatrist, did not officially occupy any post at Saint-Alban. Yet she did involve herself in various activities there that would inject more humanity into the services. In particular, she helped to form "caregivers and patients" teams that would go out to gather mushrooms and wild fruits. Her botanical knowledge was precious, and the nutritional value of these harvests helped to prevent any of the residents from dying of hunger despite the governmental restrictions. She was an ecologist before the ecologists started to draw attention to themselves. At her home, for example, one would eat nettle soup. She wasn't a sophisticated lady; she was simple, a great walker, a lover of nature and plants. Olivier [Balvet] said that this might be partly due to her grandfather's having been a herbalist. I remember the hospital's gardens being very carefully maintained in the time of Mrs. Balvet. Shaded by three majestic firs, as many chestnuts, a few acacias, beeches, and yews, the raked paths wound through the bordering box trees. Lilacs, rhododendrons, peonies, forget-me-nots, marigolds, rose mallows, sweet alyssums, lilies, fritillaries, and roses imparted colors and fragrances to this enchanting garden. A hospital patient, Father Alexandre, an old man with a white beard, looking like a Russian pope, was the gardener. He had a privileged status that he owed no doubt to his passion for gardening, which agreed with that of Mrs. Balvet.[11]

Marie Rose Ou-Rabah, *À l'ombre des poiriers: Hélène et François Tosquelles* [In the shade of the pear trees: Hélène and François Tosquelles], 2014

In the face of the occupation, numerous Jews, members of the Resistance, and other political dissidents found refuge at Saint-Alban thanks to the engagement of the doctors and the nuns in the Resistance. Lucien Bonnafé welcomed into his home the poet Paul Éluard and the philosopher, doctor, and science historian Georges Canguilhem. As the film critic Georges Sadoul—who took refuge at Saint-Alban during the Resistance—recalls, Éluard had a relationship with the clandestine press of René Amarger, leader of the Mouvements Unis de la Résistance (MUR) in Saint-Flour, and Canguilhem had a link to the bookstore in Toulouse run by Venetian anti-fascist Silvio Trentin. Despite not being at Saint-Alban at the same time, they both participated in the meetings of the working group of the Société du Gévaudan. In those meetings, Canguilhem led an experience of clinical observation with Tosquelles. In the report on the case of

The asylum rose up in the lofty solitudes haunted by the Beast of the Gévaudan. To me Saint-Alban looked like a castle stronghold out of a thriller novel … Paul and Nusch lived there in a white room that was well heated. Éluard was happy like I've seldom seen him. He had just met a printer from Saint-Flour with whom he had exchanged many signs of appreciation and had gotten the artisan, without too much difficulty, but without strong guarantees of security, to agree to secretly print some booklets from the Bibliotéque Française. Maupassant, Hugo, Aragon (Arnaud de Saint-Roman), Charles Cros, Verlaine, and Jean du Haut (Paul Éluard). My friend Éluard then read me his *Sept Poèmes d'amour en guerre*. He also read me Verlaine, with warmth and passion. Verlaine, once held in contempt by the surrealists, where now he found one of the fonts of his "natural flow." Lastly, he read me certain poems whose titles he had taken from Goya, *"Enterrar y Callar," "L'Aube dissout les monstres."* He recited this last poem, whose title paraphrased the saying of the painter, "The sleep of reason gives birth to monsters."[12]

Georges Sadoul, "Portraits du poète à plusieurs âges de sa vie" [Portraits of the poet at several ages of his life], *Europe*, vol. 1, 1953

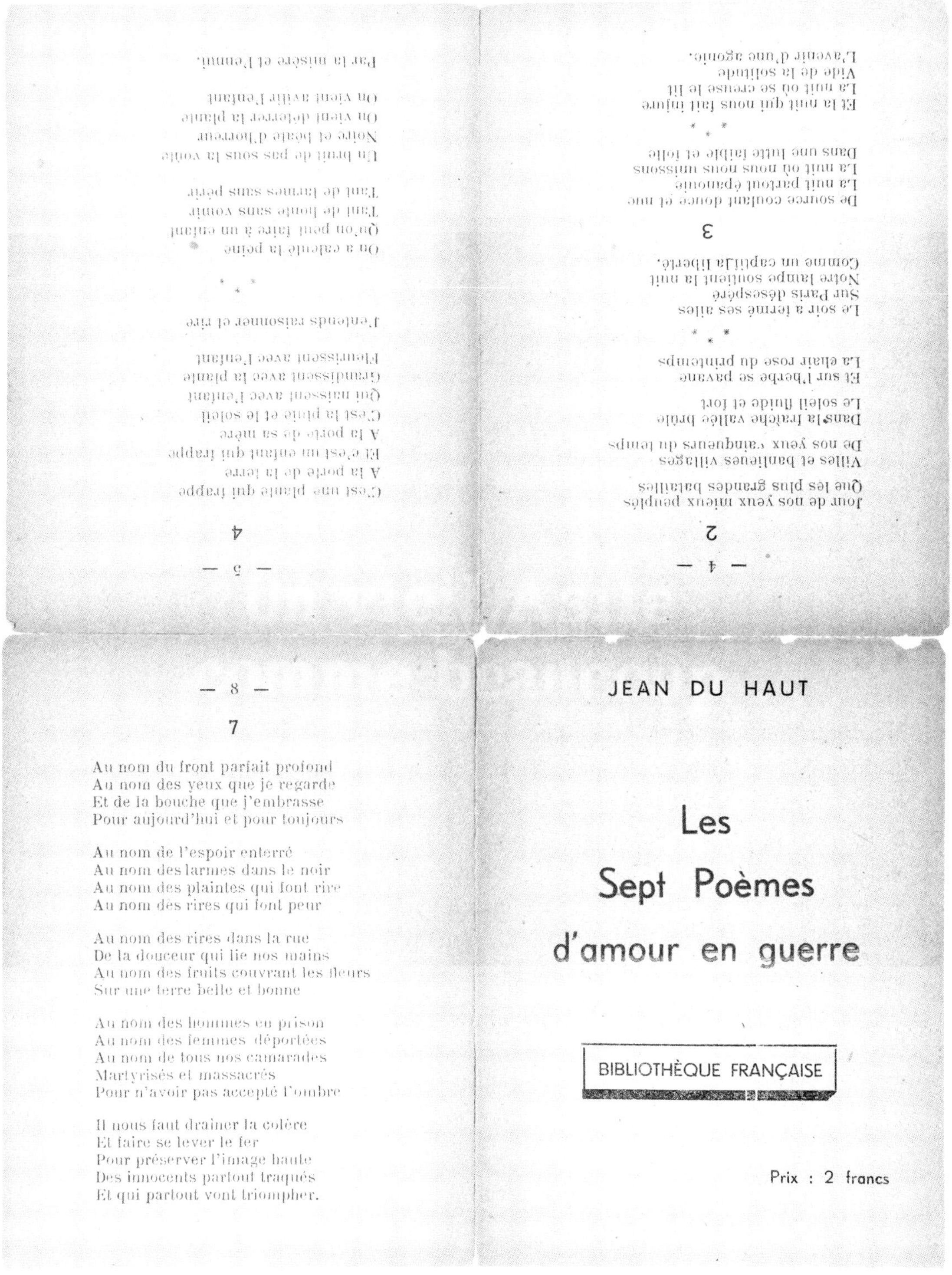

JEAN DU HAUT

Les Sept Poèmes d'amour en guerre

BIBLIOTHÈQUE FRANÇAISE

Prix : 2 francs

— 4 —

2

Jour de nos yeux mieux peuplés
Que les plus grandes batailles

Villes et banlieues villages
De nos yeux vainqueurs du temps

Dans la fraîche vallée brûle
Le soleil fluide et fort

Et sur l'herbe se pavane
La chair rose du printemps

* * *

Le soir a fermé ses ailes
Sur Paris désespéré
Notre lampe soutient la nuit
Comme un captif la liberté.

3

De source coulant douce et nue
La nuit partout épanouie
La nuit où nous nous unissons
Dans une lutte faible et folle

* * *

Et la nuit qui nous fait injure
La nuit où se creuse le lit
Vide de la solitude
L'avenir d'une agonie.

— 5 —

4

C'est une plante qui frappe
A la porte de la terre
Et c'est un enfant qui frappe
A la porte de sa mère
C'est la pluie et le soleil
Qui naissent avec l'enfant
Grandissent avec la plante
Fleurissent avec l'enfant

J'entends raisonner et rire

* * *

On a calculé la peine
Qu'on peut faire à un enfant
Tant de honte sans vomir
Tant de larmes sans périr

Un bruit de pas sous la voûte
Noire et béate d'horreur
On vient déterrer la plante
On vient avilir l'enfant

Par la misère et l'ennui.

— 8 —

7

Au nom du front parfait profond
Au nom des yeux que je regarde
Et de la bouche que j'embrasse
Pour aujourd'hui et pour toujours

Au nom de l'espoir enterré
Au nom des larmes dans le noir
Au nom des plaintes qui font rire
Au nom des rires qui font peur

Au nom des rires dans la rue
De la douceur qui lie nos mains
Au nom des fruits couvrant les fleurs
Sur une terre belle et bonne

Au nom des hommes en prison
Au nom des femmes déportées
Au nom de tous nos camarades
Martyrisés et massacrés
Pour n'avoir pas accepté l'ombre

Il nous faut drainer la colère
Et faire se lever le fer
Pour préserver l'image haute
Des innocents partout traqués
Et qui partout vont triompher.

Pages of the book by Jean du Haut (Paul Éluard) clandestinely printed in Saint-Flour in 1943

MC, an inpatient, he himself noted the dates of his stay at the hospital: from June 23 to July 5, 1944. Éluard, who also evokes MC in his poems, was there from November of 1943 to February of the following year.

When Canguilhem arrived in Saint-Alban he had already defended his thesis, *Essai sur quelques problèmes concernant le normal et le pathologique*, in July 1943; it would be published in expanded form as a book more than twenty years later, in 1966, with the title *Le normal et le pathologique* (*The Normal and the Pathological*). In that thesis, Canguilhem elaborated the concept of pathology as a socially determined construct, with no objective scientific dimension, as well as the function of medicine in the establishment and restoration of the "normal," a question that Foucault would make the central focus of his writings. In the working notes Canguilhem wrote at Saint-Alban, particularly those from July 1, 1944, through MC's voice emerges this concern for the ill body in the hands of normative medicine and ways of taking responsibility for it: "What are the responsibilities of those who take care of me throughout the day? [...] Like a statue! She doesn't live in a statue. I am like a statue. They observe me all the time, make me live. Do you hear it, the device? [...] Look into my eyes, they are suffering. Can you possibly give me my true reflection, my true features? But do not lead me into error. What responsibility must one assume when we see a person constantly complaining and suffering. [...] Even though you tell

au Docteur Francesc Tosquelles
et à Madame Helena Tosquelles,
avec mes vives amitiés,

POÉSIE ET VÉRITÉ
1942

St Alban 1943

While my doctoral thesis in medicine, in 1943, mainly concerned problems of physiology, inquiring into the normal and the pathological led me also to consult authors like Karl Jaspers, Eugène Minkowski, and Henri Ey, as well. In the summer of 1944, as a doctor in the Maquis of Auvergne, I hid and treated wounded combatants, over several months, at the psychiatric hospital of Saint-Alban, in Lozère, and its environs.[13]

Georges Canguilhem's introduction to the collection *Penser la folie: essais sur Michel Foucault* [Thinking madness: Essays on Michel Foucault], 1991

I spent two months in the Maquis, at a place that has become the symbol of the Resistance in Auvergne, at Mont Mouchet, and I happened to pay a visit to the psychiatric hospital of Saint-Alban, where I found someone from the Toulouse days, namely Bonnafé, and a Spanish psychiatrist in exile from Francoist Spain, Tosquelles, who became famous. I could tell you about my formal questioning of a lady from the psychiatric hospital, under the supervision of Tosquelles.[14]

Georges Canguilhem, interview with François Bing and Jean-François Braunstein, 1995

me I am like this rather than like that, I won't believe it. Even if you give me my portrait, I will not be able to believe you."[15]

The voice of MC—which, according to Canguilhem, denounced the malaise of the medicalized body, the malaise of medicine—had already appeared some months earlier in verses by Éluard published in *Souvenirs de la maison des fous*. There at the hospital, Éluard conceived that book as a new way of registering faces and words through six poem-portraits of female inpatients, with illustrations by his son-in-law, the painter Gérard Vulliamy, the partner of his daughter Cécile. Louis Parrot has called those texts descriptive poems within the surrealist project of registering the words of all those who speak from a voice outside of the social order. While surrealism wanted to make madness a revolt against mundane appearances, conventions, hypocrisy, and quotidian life, the words of MC that appear in the poem do not say much of revolt. They do not express the opposition or lack of discipline in the female patient who looks into the eyes of medical responsibility. In Éluard's poem, the women of soot are savagely wretched beasts, buried, burned, and frozen in an earth without seeds and without roots, without bonds, without kinship, eternally alone; women who do not know how to be wives, who do not know how to be mothers, nor laborers, nor shop clerks nor dressmakers, much like Marguerite Sirvins, who appears there drawn with her embroidery needles. The revolt of these women is a revolt devoid of hope. Like them, their revolt lives only to age, to be buried. As if their lunacy, instead of speaking of the ailments of the common world, speaks only of their cloistering, their lack of world. The poems in *Souvenirs de la maison des fous* bequeath us this unease at the heart of the project of revolutionary madness: the lunacy of the women would not speak of society; it would speak only of them, in the third-person plural.

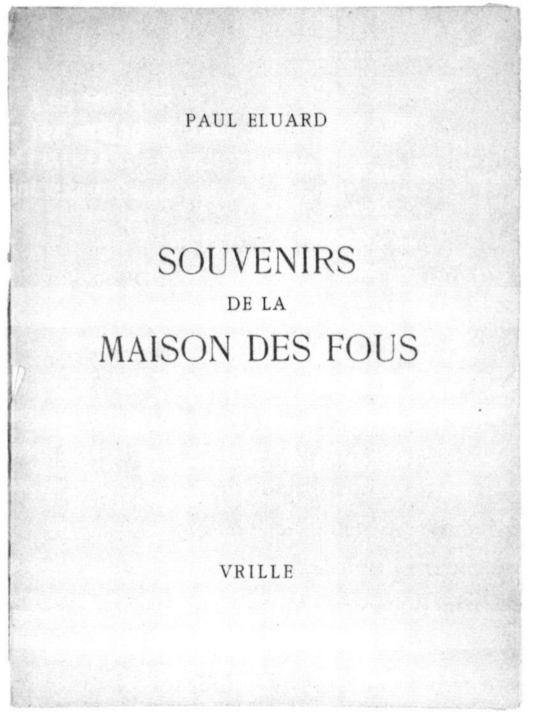
PAUL ELUARD

SOUVENIRS
DE LA
MAISON DES FOUS

VRILLE

Souvenirs de la maison des fous, created between 1943 and 1945, situates Éluard far from the essay where he had established, twenty years earlier, the programmatic relationships between surrealism and madness in dialogue with drawings of the patients.

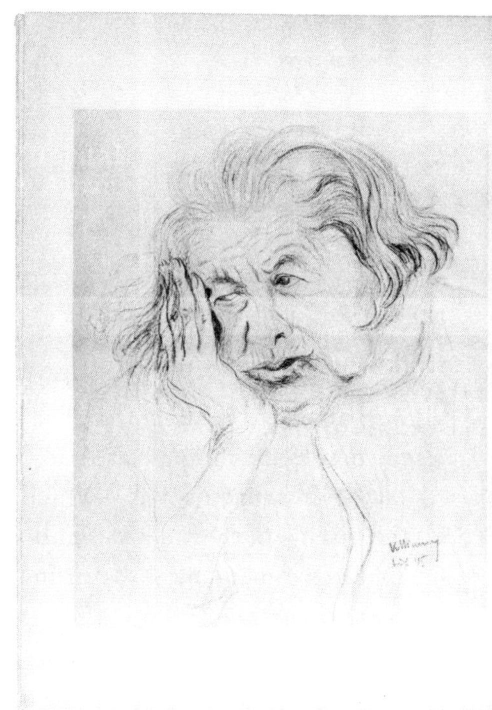

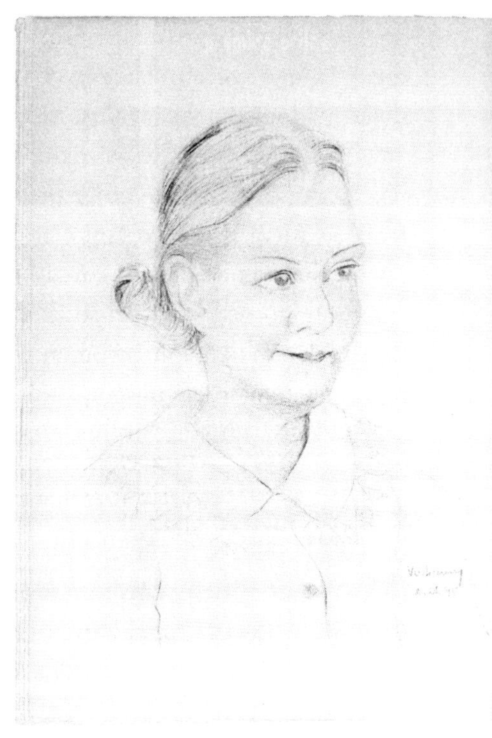

The crazies are locked inside ominous cells and our delicate hands inflict knowing tortures on them. Don't imagine, however, that they succumb. The land they have discovered is so attractive that nothing can draw their minds away from it. Maladies! Neuroses! Divine means of uncomprehended liberation. [...] Let's be clear, it is we who are locked up when they close the doors of the asylum: the prison is all around them, freedom is inside. Let us go to Sainte-Anne! Consider the cells of the Salpêtrière![16]

Paul Éluard, "Le génie sans miroir" [The mirrorless genie], *Les feuilles libres*, 1924 (with texts written by Pierre Drieu La Rochelle, Pierre Reverdy, Tristan Tzara, Erik Satie, Pablo Picasso, and "some crazies")

Fausses guenons et fausses araignées
Fausses taupes et fausses truies
Et parfois l'ombre d'une biche
Sauvagement bêtes et malheureuses
Timidement femmes illuminées

Ensevelies secouant leur linceul
Femmes de craie femmes de suie
Brûlées le jour d'un feu nocturne
Glacées la nuit par un monstre visible
Leur propre image éternellement seule

Chantant la mort sur les airs de la vie
La terre leur est familière
Terre sans graines sans racines
Sans la lumière agile du dehors
Sans les clefs d'or de l'espace interdit.

False monkeys and false spiders
False moles and false bitches
And sometimes the shadow of a doe
Savagely dumb and discontent
Timidly illuminated women

Interred shaking their shrouds
Chalk women soot women
Daily burned by a nocturnal fire
Frozen at night by a visible monster
Their own image eternally alone

Singing death to the tunes of life
The earth to them is familiar
Earth without seeds without roots
Without the nimble light of the outside
Without the golden keys to forbidden space.

Petite et belle elle peut vivre sans miroir
Petite et belle elle peut vivre sans espoir

Les longs charrois de nuit et l'aube à petit feu
Ont dégradé son corps ont dévasté son cœur

Vivre toujours peut-être et patient je regarde
Le jour pâle épouser sans plaisir ses yeux vagues.

Diminutive beauty she can live without a mirror
Diminutive beauty she can live without hope

Night's long cartages and the slow dawn
Have degraded her body have devastated her heart

Living forever perhaps and patient I watch
The pale day wed her pleasureless eyes.[17]

Paul Éluard, *Souvenirs de la maison des fous*
[Recollections of the madhouse], 1943–1945

Photographs by Jacques Matarasso taken at Saint-Alban during the winter of 1943–1944

Top, Paul and Nusch Éluard; *middle*, Paul and Nusch Éluard with Léo Matarasso; *bottom*, Éluard, *le dormeur du val*

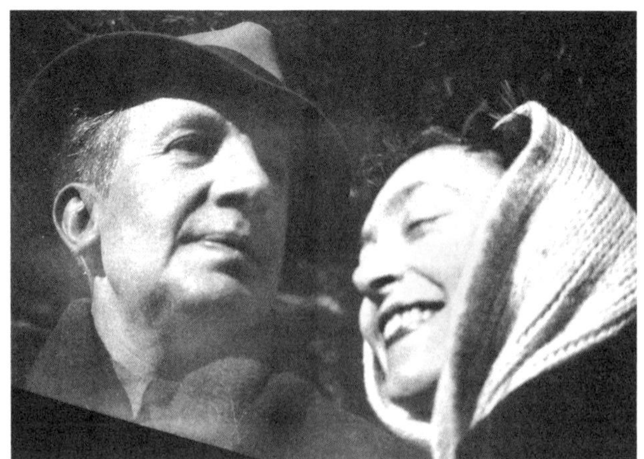

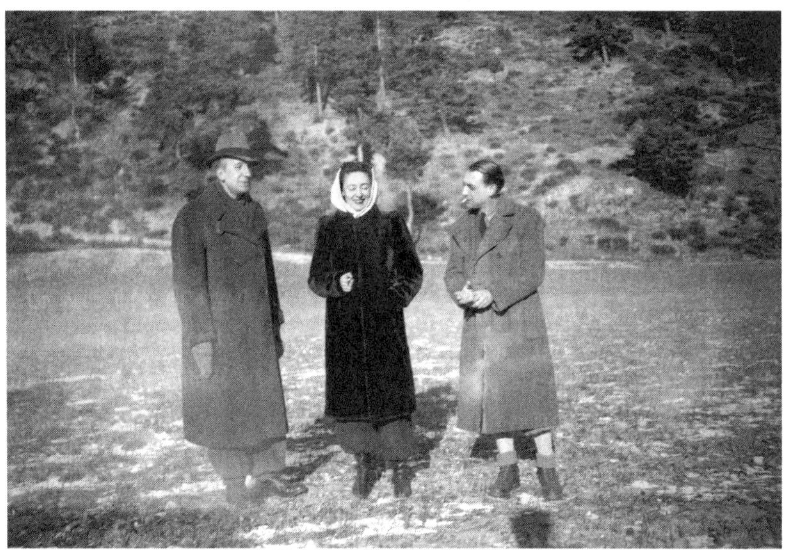

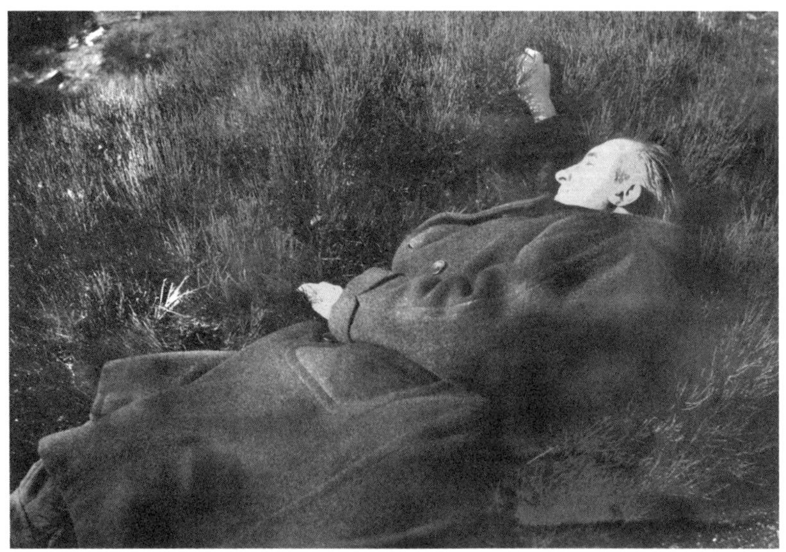

At right, writing by a hospital patient, which Lucien Bonnafé sent to Paul Éluard in 1943

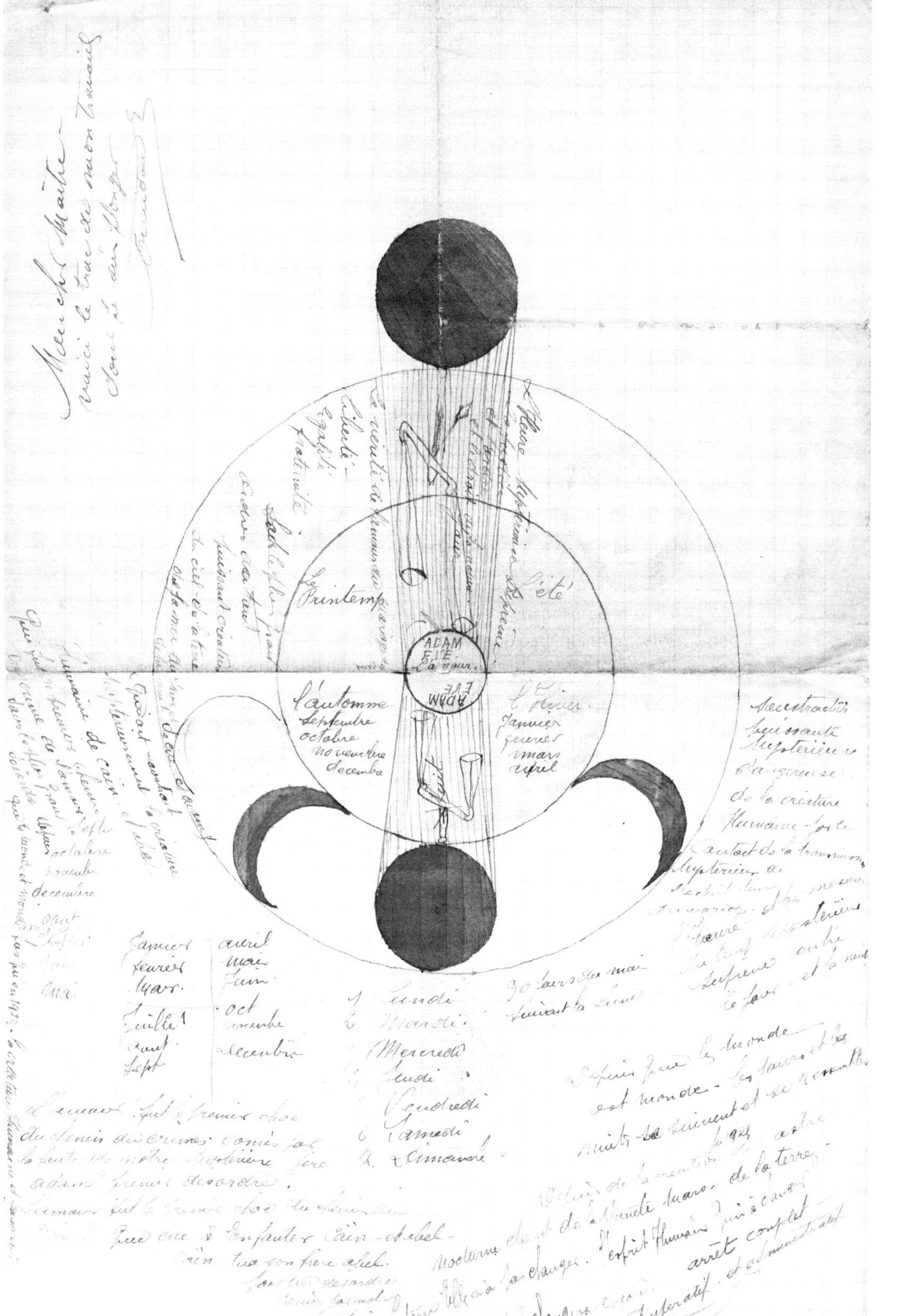

Merci cher Maître

ADAM
EVE
L'amour

ADAM
EVE

Le Printemp

L'été

l'automne
Septembre
octobre
novembre
decembre

l'Hiver
Janvier
fevrier
mars
avril

Liberté
égalité
fraternité

Mystérieuse
dangereuse
de la créature
Humaine par le
contact de la transmission
Mystérieux de

l'heure Mystérieuse
le temps entre
Suprême
le jour et la nuit

Janvier	avril
fevrier	mai
Mars.	Juin
Juillet	oct
aout	novembre
Sept	decembre

30 jours de mai
suivant la Lune

1 Lundi
2 Mardi
Mercredi
Jeudi
Vendredi
6 Samedi
7. Dimanche

Depuis que le monde
est monde - les jours et les
nuits se suivent et se ressemblent

Pour cela il a enfanté Caïn - Abel -
Caïn tua son frere abel.

l'esprit Humain
arrêt complet
Imperatif. et administratif

At Saint-Alban, Paul Éluard also wrote the collections *Les Sept Poèmes d'amour en guerre* and *Lingères légères*, in which, with an alternating use of "I," "you," and "us," he echoes the collective life of the hospital, not only the voices of women isolated by lunacy.[18] It will be his daughter Cécile Agay—pseudonym of Cécile Éluard—who makes public that dialogue that speaks of and with the female inpatients at Saint-Alban, in the newspaper *Les Étoiles*, organ of the national writers committee of the southern region. Her article features these institutionalized women who are entrusted with domestic tasks in the hospital: women with young gazes, and smooth, taut skin; women who can engage in conversation. They are some of the patients who care for and play with the children and who work with the doctors and hospital administrators through bonds we would now consider forms of "extended kinship."

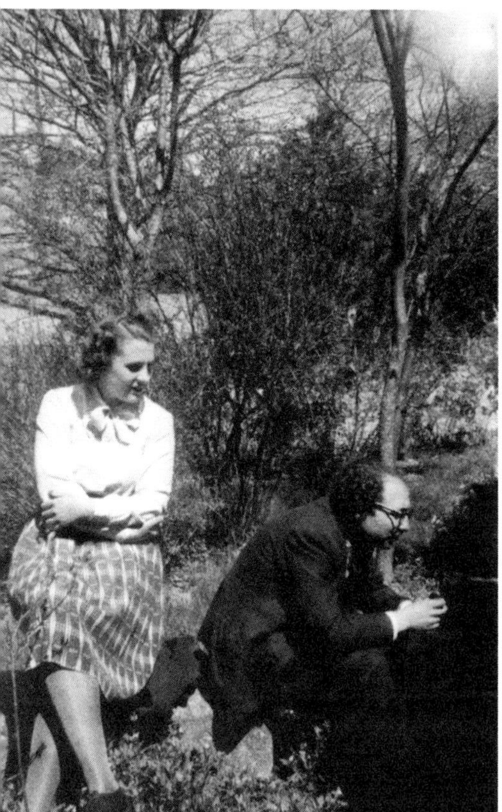

Left, Cécile Vulliamy and Tosquelles, at Saint-Alban, in the summer of 1945

Below, Cécile with one of the wooden houses made by Auguste Forestier, the same year

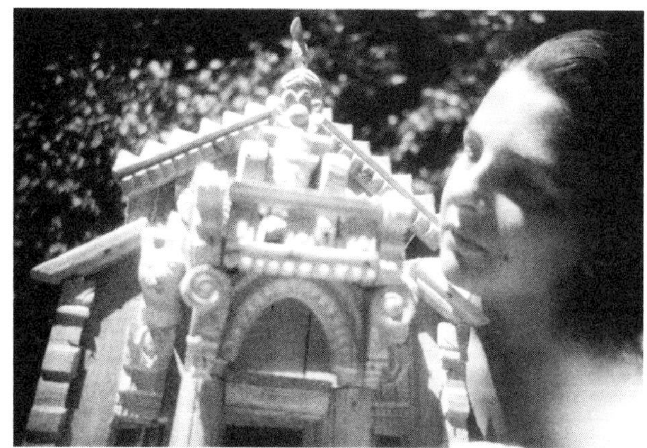

J'AI VISITÉ DES FEMMES
enfermées dans leur propre univers

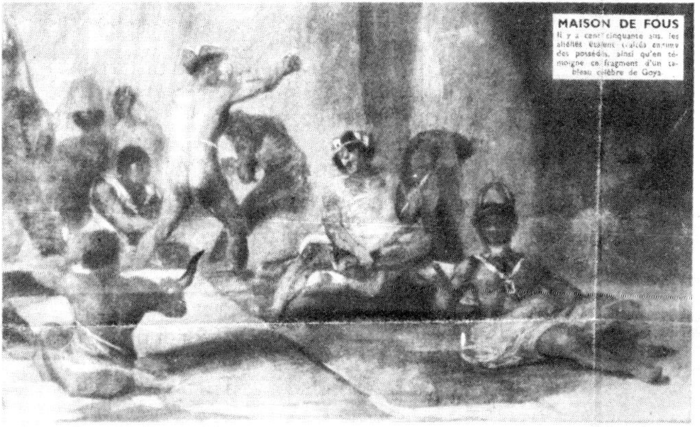

MAISON DE FOUS

Il y a cent cinquante ans, les aliénés étaient traités comme des possédés, ainsi qu'en témoigne ce fragment d'un tableau célèbre de Goya.

L'asile que notre collaboratrice Cécile Agay a visité pour nos lecteurs a servi de refuge pendant la clandestinité au poète Paul Eluard. La fréquentation des internées lui a inspiré quelques poèmes réunis dans un récent recueil intitulé Le lit la table *(Editions des Trois Collines, Genève). C'est pourquoi quelques-uns de ces poèmes servent d'épigraphe à ce reportage.*

L'HOPITAL psychiatrique est demeuré pour beaucoup de gens un lieu mystérieux ou effrayant. On n'en imagine guère la véritable atmosphère qui est celle d'un monde sans hypocrisie et sans mesquinerie. Les malades ont souvent des regards aussi purs que des enfants et paraissent en général plus jeunes qu'ils ne sont. Ils sont rarement méchants. Ce sont eux qui souffrent, persécutés par leurs obsessions.

Je reviens de visiter un de ces asiles, situé dans un site romantique et sauvage, en plein Gévaudan, tout au haut d'un rocher. Plus haut encore, il n'y a que le cimetière qui déroule ses croix de bois, toutes simples et toutes pareilles, sans un nom...

J'ai passé une matinée en compagnie des femmes — au quartier des agitées (elles sont séparées suivant le caractère de leur maladie).

6 h. du matin : Dans les dortoirs, quatre-vingts femmes se lèvent, celles du moins qui en sont capables. Cinq d'entre elles sont restées couchées, deux sont aveugles et gâteuses, deux sont malades, la cinquième porte la camisole de force. C'est la seule. Ce n'est pas une punition mais une protection, car sans cela elle se déchirerait le visage.

Une petite vieille gémit :

« Je suis malade, je veux boire du sirop le soir, j'ai mal à ma tête... » Elle secoue la tête avec un rythme obsédant.

Des infirmières et des religieuses aident les idiotes à s'habiller. Dans une grande salle, trois lavabos pour quatre-vingts personnes, c'est peu...

On se lave, sommairement en général, mais il faut se peigner et se laver même si l'envie vous en manque car l'infirmière veille. D'ailleurs il y a les coquettes : celles qui adorent les cocardes dans les cheveux, les rubans multicolores et mutins.

6 h. 45 : On déjeune d'un bol de bouillie de châtaignes dans une grande salle — de longues tables et des bancs.

Grand brouhaha. Beaucoup de malades parlent seules, agitent les mains et les bras avec des gestes mécaniques et arbitraires. Une Arabe tatouée, à la chevelure courte et frisée, se touche à chaque seconde l'oreille gauche. C'est une fonction aussi vitale pour elle que de respirer. D'ailleurs personne ne songe à l'en empêcher. Je suis très frappée d'une chose : chaque malade a son monde à elle, aucune correspondance entre elles, aucune conversation, aucun échange de regards, un mur invisible entoure chacune de ces proscrites.

LA MALADE PHILOSOPHE

Le visage pourri par des flots de tristesse
Comme un bois très précieux dans la forêt épaisse
Elle dormait aux rats la fin de sa vieillesse
Ses doigts leur égrenaient gâteries et caresses
Elle ne parlait, elle ne mangeait plus.

Je m'assieds à côté d'une femme à la peau lisse et fraîche comme une assiette et qui se pose sans arrêt des questions :

« Qu'est-ce que cette soupe ? Pourquoi n'est-elle pas sucrée ? »

Les autres l'injurient avec véhémence :

« Espèce de folle, tu es dans un hôpital, pas dans un salon... »

Mais elle, très digne, très droite, calme et les cheveux tirés, continue sans se troubler :

« Qui suis-je ? Entre moi et le Créateur, il y a une différence énorme, moi je m'ignore et l'ignore. Je suis nulle et dans l'impossibilité de vivre. Je suis le néant. Qu'est-ce que vivre ? C'est créer ce corps. Est-ce que je suis un peu plus que ce bout de bois ? (elle montre la table) avec un peu de vie — à 47 ans je pose la question... »

Je lui demande : « Pourquoi vouloir tout savoir ? » Elle me répond : « Mais c'est atroce, je veux savoir : pourquoi les fleurs se fanent, pourquoi il y a des colères. Qu'est-ce qui crée tous ces mannequins ? (elle montre les autres femmes). Qu'est-ce qu'il faut faire quand on se lève ? Comment expliquez-vous que vous puissiez créer quelque chose avec rien ? Un corps, c'est un être, un hêtre, c'est un arbre. Elle écarte les bras, tend l'oreille lorsque je lui parle. Elle souffre, dit-elle. Et cette angoisse paraît fort vraisemblable. Cette femme se pose les questions que se sont posées avant elle des philosophes comme Pascal, Platon ou Sartre.

Elle s'est enfin mise à manger — d'ailleurs avec appétit.

ELLE A SON LANGAGE A ELLE

Un peu plus loin, une femme brune, aux prunelles fixes dans de grands yeux noirs sourit comme une princesse lointaine. Elle m'apprend qu'elle doit partir le lendemain pour l'Algérie (c'est son pays — voici deux ans qu'elle s'apprête à partir.)

Elle me demande de l'aider à quitter l'hôpital, elle paraît très douce et m'est fort sympathique, mais que puis-je — elle n'est pas guérie. Elle invente un vocabulaire extraordinaire et son langage est souvent incohérent.

« On m'a promis à la « locologique » que je partirai — mon mari m'attend. »

« Que fait votre mari ? »

« Il est menuisier — c'est-à-dire « hydropidique » — moi, j'ai été malade, j'ai eu de la « popadixie », mais je veux travailler, raccommoder : je sais « initialer » même des nippes. »

Elle me confie mystérieurement que « l'autre jour, l'âme lui coulait par les oreilles... »

7 h. 15. Le déjeuner est terminé. Quelques malades balaient, font le ménage. Puis on les met au travail. Lorsqu'elles sont occupées, elles sont plus calmes, leur état s'améliore. Il y a beaucoup plus de guérisons depuis qu'on emploie le travail comme thérapeutique. Jadis, elles seraient restées à ne rien faire.

UNE MENINE DE VELASQUEZ

Dans la salle où l'on carde la laine, voici une étrange apparition : une naine pas plus haute qu'une enfant de dix ans et qui, malgré son âge, garde une expression enfantine. Vêtue d'une robe d'un magnifique rouge vermillon, elle est digne de figurer dans un tableau de Velasquez. C'est une arriérée, dont le niveau mental ne dépasse pas deux ans. Elle rit et pleure tout aussi facilement. Elle s'amuse d'un rien. Je lui donne un œillet, qu'elle respire avec ostentation, puis essaie de manger. Une vieille enfant ! Les jours de beau temps, on la conduit aux champs par la main, et elle arrache les légumes. Elle a une toute petite activité.

Ce sont les « idiots » qui ont l'aspect le plus frappant, dont la dégénérescence mentale s'accompagne souvent d'une déformation physique. On obtient en les éduquant, sinon une guérison complète (car il s'agit-là d'un état congénital), mais une amélioration considérable.

Une de ces petites filles de 50 ans (une naine elle aussi), est arrivée à l'asile, ne sachant ni marcher, ni manger seule, ni parler : un paquet informe et remuant, renfermant un être humain. Maintenant, elle marche, elle s'habille seule, mange proprement (sur une chaise plus haute que les autres), elle sait même mettre la table pour les autres. De cet être vagissant et lamentable, on a fait un être humain.

Une autre, grande et disgracieuse, se dit médecin. Son menton s'orne d'une petite barbe, sa tête est couronnée d'un cercle de métal. Elle se plaît au quartier. Cependant elle irait volontiers à Rome chercher des vêtements pour les religieuses. Elle s'imagine que ce doit être le pape qui leur donne...

De bonnes vieilles aux petits yeux vifs d'écureuil : ce sont les plus gaies (elles ont beaucoup dansé au quatorze juillet !) — des persécutées que les esprits martyrisent jour et nuit — une ancienne religieuse qui a fait vœu de se laisser mourir de faim : elle est maigre comme une déportée et il faut la nourrir à la seringue depuis un an. Toutes ces femmes sont enfermées dans leur propre univers où j'arrive difficilement à pénétrer, mais elles restent humaines : coquettes, gentilles, curieuses ou boudeuses. Elles s'habituent à moi. Deux ou trois seulement marmonnent des injures ou des malédictions, mais d'une façon impersonnelle.

Fausses guenons et fausses araignées
Fausses taupes et fausses truies
Et parfois l'ombre d'une biche
Sauvagement bêtes et malheureuses
Timidement femmes illuminées

Ensevelies, secouant leur linceul
Femmes de craie, femmes de suie
Brûlées le jour d'un feu nocturne
Glacées la nuit par un monstre visible
Leur propre image éternellement seule

Chantant la mort sur les airs de la vie
Leur terre leur est familière
Terre sans graines, sans racines
Sans la lumière agile du dehors
Sans les clés d'or de l'espace interdit.

Paul ELUARD.

J'AI DEUX MILLIONS

Une femme forte et rouge vient vers moi :

— Je vis depuis deux mille ans, me dit-elle. J'ai vécu au temps de Tut ank Amon et j'ai eu trois maris.

— C'est beaucoup ! lui dis-je.

— Mais non, c'est très peu en deux mille ans !

Elle m'explique ensuite la formation du monde : « Des vapeurs se sont élevées de la terre et se sont condensées, il en est sorti un cerveau ». Tut ank Amon la préoccupe beaucoup et tient dans son système une place de premier plan :

— Il n'était ni homme ni femme, il a d'abord été homme, puis femme...

11 h. 30. C'est le repas. Les malades se réunissent de nouveau dans la grande salle. Elles déjeunent d'une soupe de légumes, de haricots verts et d'un ragoût de mouton. Chacune a un morceau de pain et un verre de vin. (Le vin n'est pas rare dans ce pays.)

Je vais maintenant quitter le quartier.

Toutes les malades ne restent pas enfermées. Certaines d'entre elles (et pour les hommes, il en est de même), peuvent sortir dans le village, dans la campagne, en toute liberté. D'autres travaillent à l'extérieur, chez les médecins ou dans les fermes. On leur confie des enfants à garder. Elles les aiment beaucoup. Une agitée est devenue très calme depuis qu'elle s'occupe de l'enfant d'un médecin. On devait lui mettre auparavant la camisole de force. Maintenant, elle n'a plus de crises. C'est la transition qui la ramènera vers la vie normale et la guérison.

Cécile AGAY.

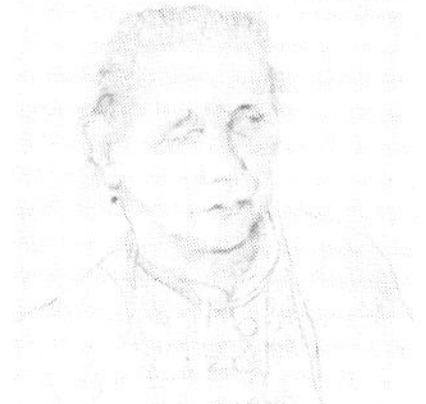

Dessin de VULLIAMY.

Femme, accablée, appliquée à vieillir
Et mes sœurs me devaient quinze millions de siècles
La cadette voyait plus clair à travers moi
Qu'à travers l'Algérie trapue un continent
Moulé pétri laqué par des chaleurs d'argent.

Article by Cécile Agay (Éluard) published in *Les Étoiles*, October 9, 1945, with a detail of the Goya painting *Casa de Locos* (1812–1819), a drawing by Gérard Vulliamy, and excerpts from poems by Paul Éluard

The asylum that our colleague Cécile Agay visited for our readers served as a refuge during the clandestine life of Paul Éluard. His time spent with the mental patients inspired him to write some poems assembled in a recent collection entitled Le Lit la table *[The bed the table] (Éditions des Trois Collines, Geneva). Some of these verses are offered as an epigraph to this reportage.*

For many people, the psychiatric hospital has remained a mysterious or scary place. One can't really imagine the atmosphere, which is that of a world without hypocrisy or pettiness. The patients often have gazes as pure as children's and for the most part look younger than they are. They are rarely mean-spirited. It is they who suffer, persecuted by their obsessions.

I have just visited one of these asylums, situated in a wild and romantic locale, in the middle of Gévaudan, atop a rocky hill. Higher still, there is only the cemetery that spreads forth its wooden crosses, simple and uniform, with no names inscribed …

I spent a morning in the company of the women—in the quarters of the agitated ones (they're separated according to the character of their illness).

Six o'clock in the morning. In the dormitories, eighty women are getting up, at least those who are able. Five of them have stayed in bed, two are sick, the fifth wears a straitjacket. She's the only one. It's not a punishment but a protection, for without it she would tear up her face.

A little old one whines: "I'm sick, I want to drink my syrup in the evening, my head hurts ..." She shakes her head with an obsessive rhythm.

Nurses and nuns help the idiots to get dressed. In a big hall, three washbasins for eighty persons, it's too few ...

One washes, perfunctorily in general, but one has to comb one's hair and wash oneself even if the desire is lacking because the nurse is watching. But there are also the style conscious, those who adore rosettes in their hair or whimsical rainbow ribbons.

Six forty-five. One breakfasts on a bowl of chestnut mush in a large hall—long tables and benches.

A big hubbub. Many of the patients talk to themselves, move their hands and arms about with mechanical, arbitrary gestures. A tattooed Arab woman, with short, frizzy hair, touches her left ear over and over. It's a function just as vital to her as breathing. Moreover, no one thinks of stopping her. I'm struck by one thing: every patient has their own world, nothing shared between them, no conversation, no exchange of glances, an invisible wall surrounds each one of these outcasts.

THE PHILOSOPHICAL PATIENT

Her face ruined by waves of sadness,
Like a very precious wood in the thick
forest
She gave the end of her old age to the rats.
Her fingers treated them to morsels
and caresses
She no longer spoke, no longer ate

I seat myself next to a woman with skin as smooth and cool as a plate, one who asks herself an endless round of questions:

"What is this soup? Why isn't it sweetened?"

The others scold her with vehemence:

"You crazy thing, you're in a hospital, not a salon ..."

But she, very dignified, calm and straightening her hair, continues as before:

"Who am I? Between me and the Creator, there is a huge difference. Me, I don't know myself and I don't know Him. I am hopeless and unable to live. I am nothingness. What is it to live? It's to create this body. Am I a little more than this piece of wood? [She indicates the table.] With a little life, at forty-seven I ask the question ..."

I ask her: "Why want to know everything?"

She replies: "But it's awful, I want to know: Why do the flowers wither, why are there angry fits? What creates these mannequins? [She indicates the other women.] What needs to be done when we get up? A body is a being [*un être*], a beech [*un hêtre*] is a tree."

She opens her arms and cocks her ear when I speak to her. She suffers, she says. And this anguish seems very credible. The woman asks herself questions that philosophers like Pascal, Plato, or Sartre asked themselves before her.

She finally sets to eating—with appetite, moreover.

SHE HAS HER OWN LANGUAGE

A bit later, a brown-skinned woman, with a fixed gaze in big dark eyes, smiles like a princess of old. She informs me that she must leave the next day for Algeria (she's from there—for two years now she's been getting ready to leave).

She asks me to help her depart the hospital. She seems very sweet and seems very likeable to me, but what can I do? She isn't cured. She invents an extraordinary vocabulary and her talk is often incoherent.

"They've promised me to the 'locologic' that I will be leaving—my husband is waiting for me."

"What does your husband do?"

"He's a woodworker—that is, a 'hydropodic'—me, I've been ill, I've had the 'popadixy,' but I want to work, to mend things: I know how to 'initial' even old clothes."

She tells me in mysterious confidence that "the other day, my soul leaked out through my ears ..."

Seven fifteen. The meal has ended. A few patients sweep and tidy up. Then they are accompanied to work. When they are occupied, they are calmer, their condition improves. There are many more cures now that work is used as therapy. Before, they would have had nothing to do.

A VELÁZQUEZ MENINA

In the room where wool is carded, a strange apparition: a dwarf no taller than a child of ten, who has kept a childish expression. Wearing a dress of a magnificent vermilion hue, she is worthy of appearing in a painting by Velázquez. She is learning disabled, with a mental level no higher than a two-year-old. She laughs as readily as she cries. She's amused by a trifle. I give her a carnation, which she sniffs with ostentation, then attempts to eat. She's an old toddler! When the weather is good, she's led by the hand to the fields, where she pulls out a few of the vegetables. Her activity has a very narrow range.

It's the "idiots" that are outwardly the most striking. Their mental degeneration is often accompanied by a physical deformation. By training them, one can obtain not a complete cure (for we're talking about a congenital condition), but a substantial improvement.

One of these fifty-year-old little girls (a dwarf as well) arrived at the asylum not knowing how to walk, eat unassisted, or talk: a shapeless and fidgety package, enclosing a human being. Now, she walks, gets dressed by herself, eats in a proper manner (on a higher chair than the others); she even knows how to set the table for the others. Out of this mewling and pathetic creature, they have made a human being.

Another woman, large and unsightly, calls herself a doctor. Her chin sports a beard, her head is crowned with a metal circle. She enjoys the place. Yet she would gladly go to Rome in search of vestments for the sisters, imagining that it has to be the pope that provides them …

Charming old ladies with lively squirrel eyes: these are the most cheerful (they danced a lot on the 14th of July)—persecuted women whom the spirits torment day and night—a former nun who made a vow to let herself die of hunger: she is as skinny as a deportee and has needed to be fed with a syringe for a year. All these women are closed up inside their own universe that I manage to penetrate only with difficulty, but they remain human: coquettish, sweet, curious, or sulky. They are getting used to me. Just two or three mumble insults or curses, but in an impersonal way.

I'M TWO THOUSAND YEARS OLD

A strong red-faced woman comes toward me:

"I've lived for two thousand years," she says. "I've lived in the time of Tutankhamen and I have had three husbands."

"That's a lot!' I say.

"No, it's not. It's very few in two thousand years!"

She then explains the forming of the world: "Vapors rose up from the earth and condensed. A brain grew out of it." Tutankhamen occupies her mind a great deal and holds a preeminent place in her system:

"He was neither man nor woman, he was first a man, then a woman …"

Eleven thirty. It's mealtime. The patients reassemble in the big hall. They lunch on a vegetable soup, green beans, and mutton stew. Each one has a slice of bread and a glass of wine. (There's no shortage of wine in this region.)

I'm now going to quit the women's ward.

Not all the female patients stay locked in. Some of them (and likewise for the men) can go into the village or the countryside in complete liberty. Others work on the outside, at the doctors' homes or on the farms. They are entrusted with children to watch over. These women love the children. An agitated patient has become calm since she's been taking care of a doctor's child. Before, she had to wear a straitjacket. Now, she has no more crises. This is the transition that will bring her back to normal life and healing.[19]

Cécile Agay [Éluard], "J'ai visité des femmes enfermées dans leur propre univers" [I visited women confined in their own universe], 1945

Another facet of this dialogue takes shape in *Parler seul*, the long poem that Tristan Tzara wrote in the summer of 1945, also at Saint-Alban, where he was in the company of his son, and Cécile Éluard, and Gérard Vulliamy. It was published in 1948 with illustrations by Joan Miró. Tzara composed it after the end of the war, having suffered the experience of the persecution of Jews under the Nazi occupation, during his first stay at a psychiatric hospital, after Éluard had told him about Saint-Alban. The poem—about which Michel Leiris said that the words spoke for themselves, with no punctuation or guide—was addressed not only to the female patients, the foreign, the deviant and the disoriented, but to women with much more familiar names, such as Cécile (Éluard?), Jeanne (Bonnafé?), Françoise, and Tamara (Leibowitz?), and suggested that they all formed part of one single world, far from the surrealist mysticism of female lunacy.[20] It was a world situated somewhere in Lozère, where a Catalan psychiatrist treated madness with common sense, as Tzara wrote to Michel Leiris.

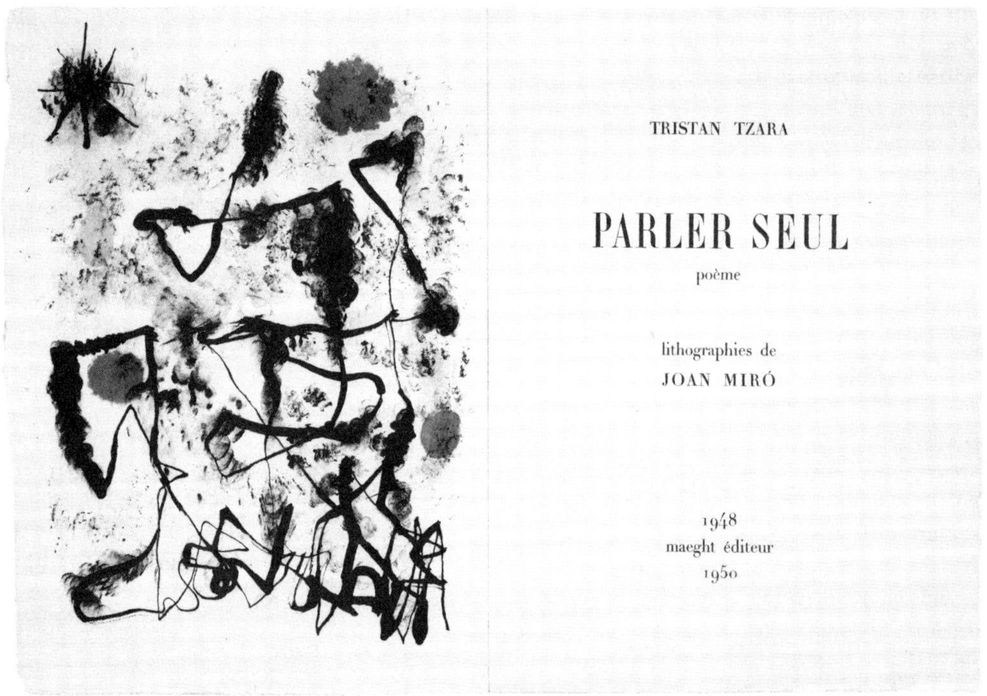

Tristan Tzara and Joan Miró, *Parler seul*, 1948–1950

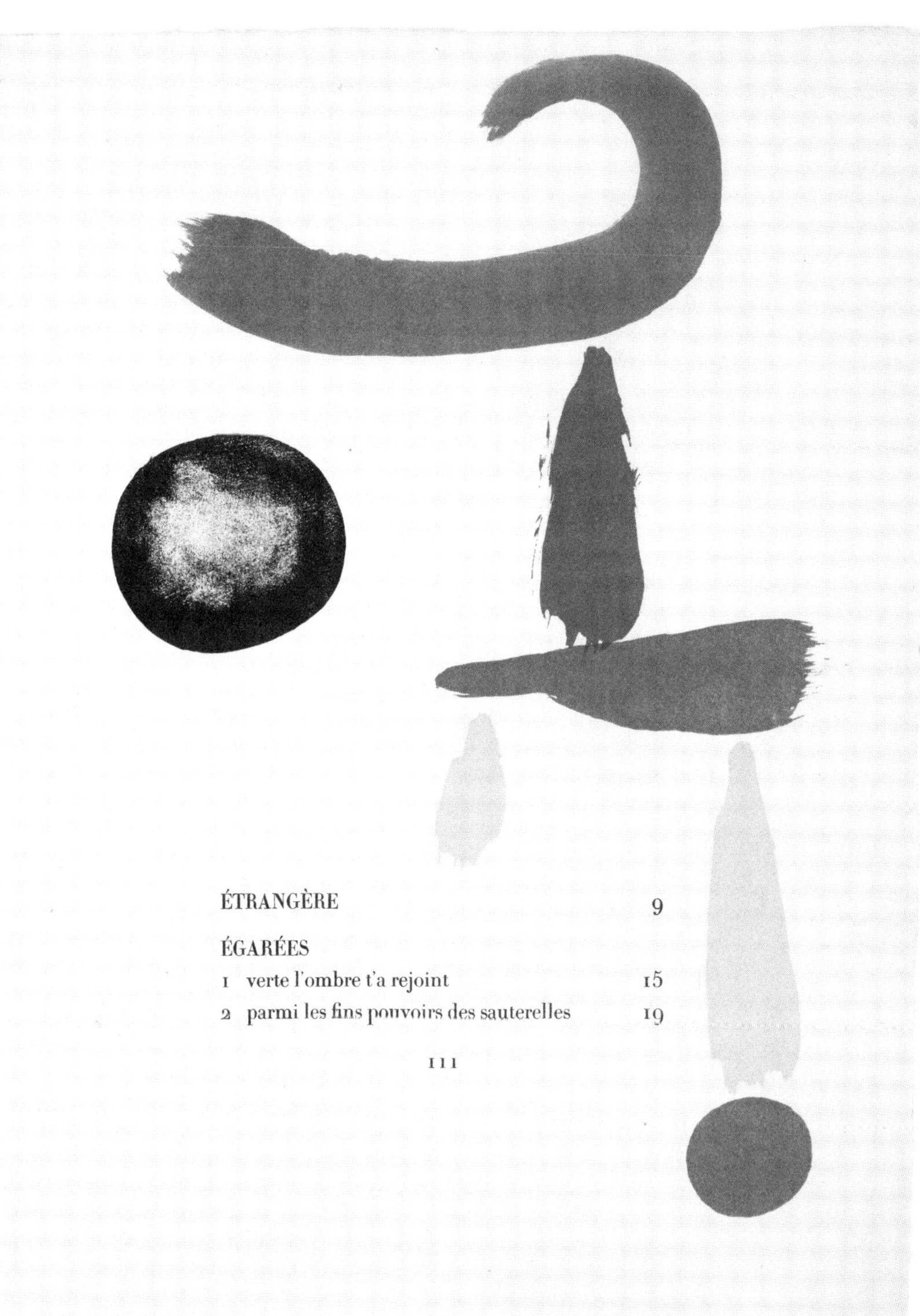

ÉTRANGÈRE 9
ÉGARÉES
1 verte l'ombre t'a rejoint 15
2 parmi les fins pouvoirs des sauterelles 19
111

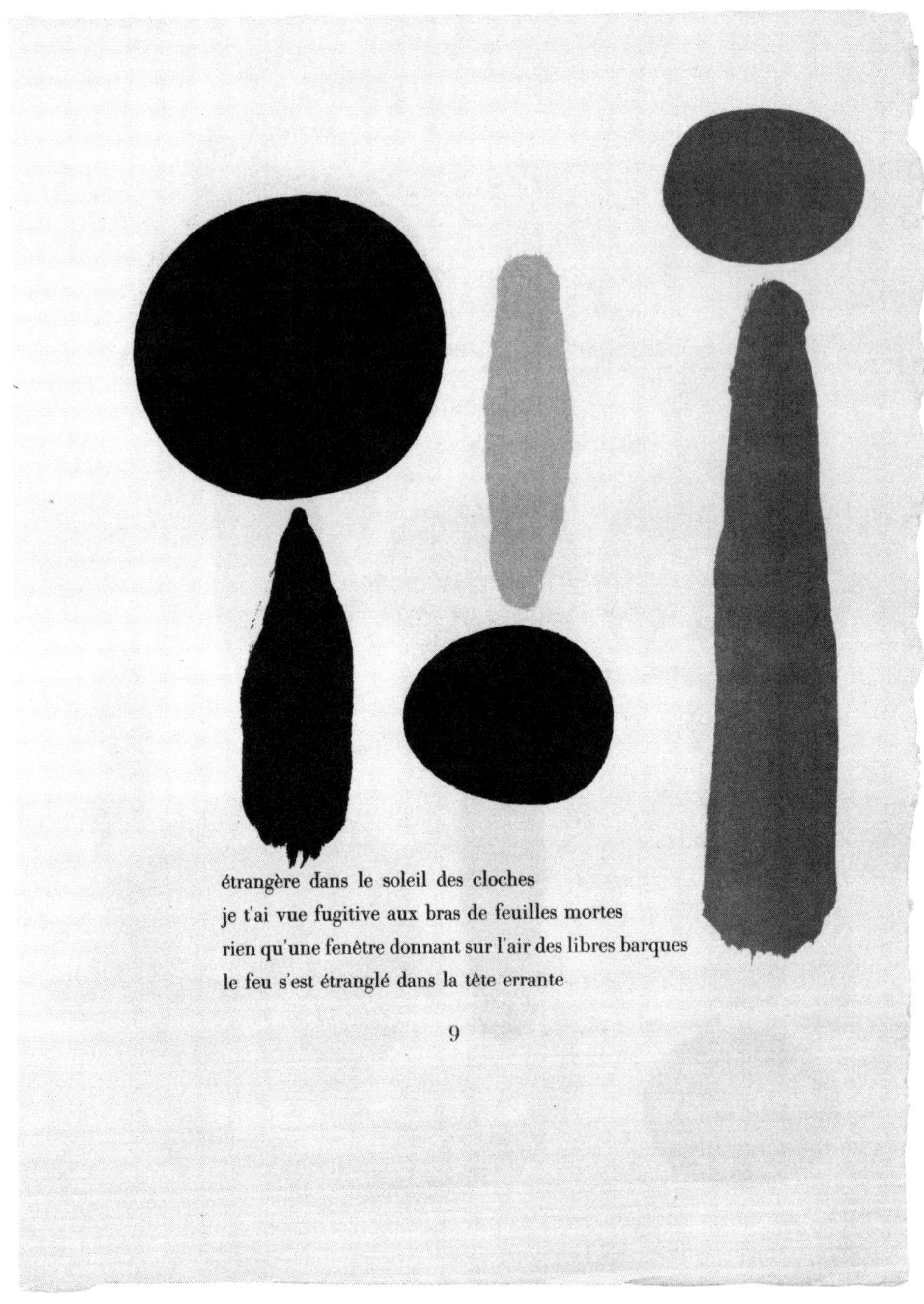

étrangère dans le soleil des cloches
je t'ai vue fugitive aux bras de feuilles mortes
rien qu'une fenêtre donnant sur l'air des libres barques
le feu s'est étranglé dans la tête errante

9

a stranger in the sunshine of bells
I saw you fugitive in the arms of dead leaves
nothing but a window open to the air of free boats
the flame lost its breath in the errant head

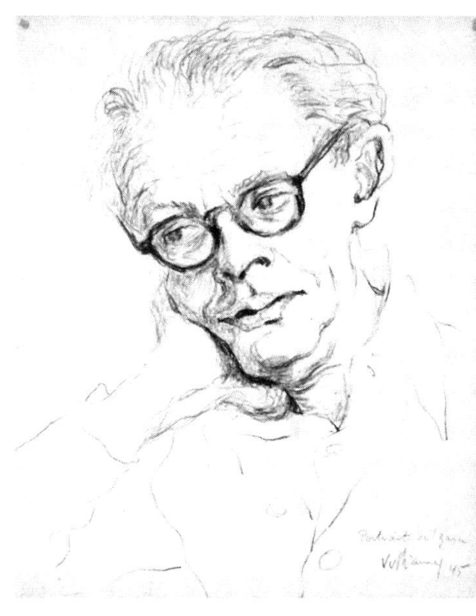

Gérard Vulliamy, *Portrait of Tristan Tzara*, Saint-Alban, 1945

I'm living here within the asylum compound, which is like a little town—it's totally relaxing—one learns extremely interesting things. It's a bit like traveling to a foreign country. And so much more engaging than what happens—generally—in civilian life. There is in particular a female patient who would interest Sartre—she's known as "the existentialist." She is very intelligent and both of us get caught up in her game that, obviously, could take one far. There is also a very interesting psychiatrist, a Catalan who would like to restore "madness" to its everyday common meaning—and who arrives at an impressive percentage of cures.[21]

Letter from Tristan Tzara to Michel Leiris, Saint-Alban, August 20, 1945

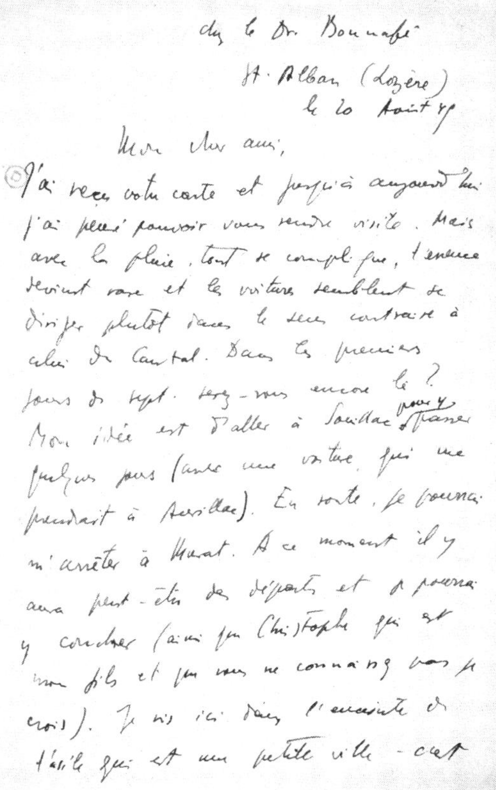

chez le Dr. Bonnafé
St. Alban (Lozère)
le 20 Août 45

Mon cher ami,

J'ai reçu votre carte et jusqu'à aujourd'hui j'ai pensé pouvoir vous rendre visite. Mais avec la pluie, tout se complique, l'essence devient rare et les voitures semblent se diriger plutôt dans le sens contraire à celui du Cantal. Dans les premiers jours de sept. serez-vous encore là? Mon idée est d'aller à Souillac pour y passer quelques jours (avec une voiture qui me prendrait à Aurillac). En route, je pourrai m'arrêter à Murat. A ce moment il y aura peut-être des départs et je pourrai y conduire (ainsi que Christophe qui est mon fils et que vous ne connaissez pas je crois). Je vis ici dans l'enceinte de l'asile qui est une petite ville – c'est

Ms. 44: 335

tout-à-fait reposant – on apprend des choses extrêmement intéressantes. C'est un peu comme un voyage à l'étranger. Et tellement plus sensible que ce qui se passe – en général – dans la vie civile. Il y a surtout une malade qui intéresserait Sartre – on l'appelle "l'existentialiste". Elle est très intelligente et souvent je me perds avec elle à son jeu qui, évidemment, pourrait mener fort loin. Il y a aussi un psychiatre très intéressant, catalan, qui voudrait rétablir "la folie" dans son sens commun journalier – et qui arrive à un pourcentage impressionnant de guérisons. — Et vous cher ami? Travaillez-vous? et Kahnweiler? Voulez-vous lui dire que les quelques heures passées en sa compagnie en juillet m'ont rempli d'un réel plaisir. – J'espère vous revoir bientôt et de toute manière en Octobre.

Très amicalement à vous

Ainsi qu'à Zette et à Kahnweiler TZARA

Art Brut and Situated Practices

In a letter dated February 17, 1949, Jean Dubuffet recalls that in 1945 he spent twenty-four hours at the hospital, where Tzara and his son had wooden objects made by Auguste Forestier, sculptures that had, through Éluard, reached the hands of Picasso and Dora Maar and also Gaston Ferdière, Artaud's doctor. At Saint-Alban, initially, both Dubuffet and his project of collecting art brut (which had begun at the end of the Second World War, when the artistic avant-garde began to be institutionalized) were received coolly. In July 1945, Dubuffet started a methodical search in France and Switzerland for what he called "art brut": works made by autodidacts with no artistic background. Thus was born an artistic practice that could be understood as a critique of culture, but also and above all grew out of the figure of the artist-patient as producer of a body of work that had not been touched or damaged by culture. It grew out of the myth of the "completely pure, raw, brute, expressive artistic operation," which is how Dubuffet described his programmatic book, in which he juxtaposed these "raw productions" against "cultural art" marked by mimesis and conventionalism.[22] Most of all, it grew out of a large program of preservation and museography, which allowed for the identification of these objects and practices carried out in hospital settings, and distanced them from their places of experience through a network of relationships between doctors and collectors.

Art brut was thus connected with a custom begun some years earlier by Hanz Prinzhorn, psychiatrist and art historian, who gathered drawings and books by the patients at the psychiatric hospital in Heidelberg between 1890 and 1920, and with the work of Marcel Réja, doctor, poet, art critic, and author of the book *L'Art chez les fous: Le dessin, la prose, la poésie*, published in 1907. Two years earlier, Auguste Marie had established the Musée de la Folie in the Villejuif asylum, where he was the head doctor.

From the correspondence between Jean Dubuffet and Jean Oury in 1948 and 1949, and the letters between Dubuffet, Tosquelles, and Dr. Roger Gentis (the director of Saint-Alban after Tosquelles left in 1962), one can surmise the resulting economic exchanges from the transfer of pieces from Saint-Alban and Dubuffet's Foyer de l'Art Brut. Beginning in 1948, and for several years, two boxes (68 × 55 × 72 cm and 110 × 60 × 40 cm) circulated, transporting objects between Lozère and Paris. On Dubuffet's request, Jean Oury was in charge of the shipments. Oury also wrote the first texts on the work of patients such as Auguste Forestier and negotiated with Francesc Tosquelles, who, although reticent at first, eventually accepted the patients' work being sent to the Art Brut Collection. In turn, Dubuffet sent Tosquelles a drawing by Artaud; the book by Dr. Walter Morgenthaler on Adolf Wölfli, *Ein Geisteskranker als Künstler* (*Madness & Art: The Life and Works of Adolf Wölfli*), which had been published in 1921; numerous volumes for the patients' and doctors' library; the complete works of Proust; some books by Artaud, including *Les nouvelles révélations de l'Être* (1937); and as Élie Faure's art-history volumes. He also sent colored pencils, paintbrushes, and ink as Christmas presents and ordered payments of 1,000, 2,000, and 5,000 francs to the Club Paul-Balvet for the purchase of a printing press and to make possible the production of the newspaper *Le Chemin*. A part of those funds was also given to patients including Auguste Forestier, Aimable Jayet, and Clément Fraisse. The latter received 50,000 francs instead of the car—and garage to keep it in—he had asked for in exchange for his work sculpting wood paneling.

Dubuffet also requested texts from the patients, which he compiled with Jean Paulhan; he even spoke with the townspeople of Saint-Alban who had bought objects from Forestier to see if they wanted to sell them to the Foyer de l'Art Brut. Later, in the 1960s, he suggested that the director of Saint-Alban, Roger Gentis, acquire Forestier's pieces from the nurses in exchange for amounts sometimes as high as 60,000 francs. From then on, this was a regular practice and Gentis continued sending to Paris works produced or found at the hospital over the course of years.

On the occasions of the exhibitions held at the Foyer de l'Art Brut or on-site at the Collection de l'Art Brut, Dubuffet asked himself about how to present these patients as artists, and with what public names ("For" or "Forest" instead of Auguste Forestier, or using the name of his hometown; "Mademoiselle Sir" instead of Marguerite Sirvins; "Arnal" instead of Benjamin Arneval). Dubuffet's correspondence also reveals his insistence with the medical community at Saint-Alban to obtain details, biographical fragments, and memories of the artist-patients' day-to-day life at the hospital. The project of the Art Brut Collection was built on this aporia: the objects made by inpatients at Saint-Alban, which were separated from the experience of the places where they were made, had to retain, once in Paris, living traces of their condition as objects created in contexts that had nothing to do with the art world. For Dubuffet, these works not only had to contain the world from which they'd been distanced but also, once they

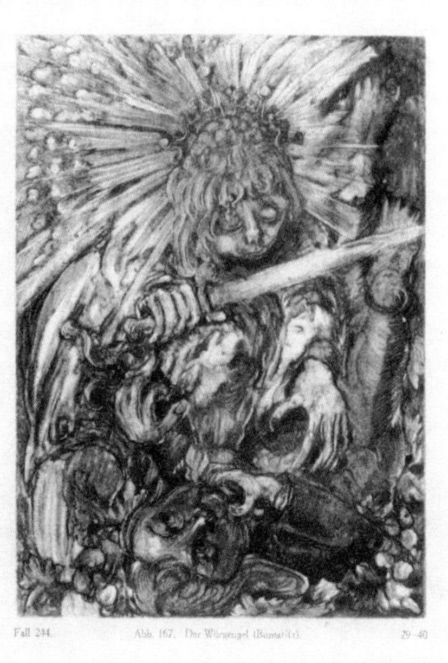

BILDNEREI DER GEISTESKRANKEN

EIN BEITRAG ZUR PSYCHOLOGIE UND PSYCHOPATHOLOGIE DER GESTALTUNG

VON

HANS PRINZHORN

DR. PHIL. ET MED. NERVENARZT IN HEIDELBERG

MIT 187 ZUM TEIL FARBIGEN ABBILDUNGEN IM TEXT UND AUF 20 TAFELN VORWIEGEND AUS DER BILDERSAMMLUNG DER PSYCHIATR. KLINIK HEIDELBERG

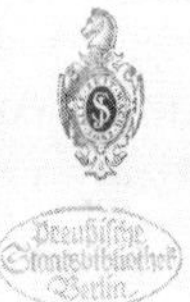

Preußische Staatsbibliothek Berlin

VERLAG VON JULIUS SPRINGER · BERLIN · 1922

Hans Prinzhorn, *Bildnerei der Geisteskranken*, 1922

AU
DOCTEUR DUBUISSON
SOUHAITS
DE BONNE ANNEE
POUR
1899
J. H. GIRARD

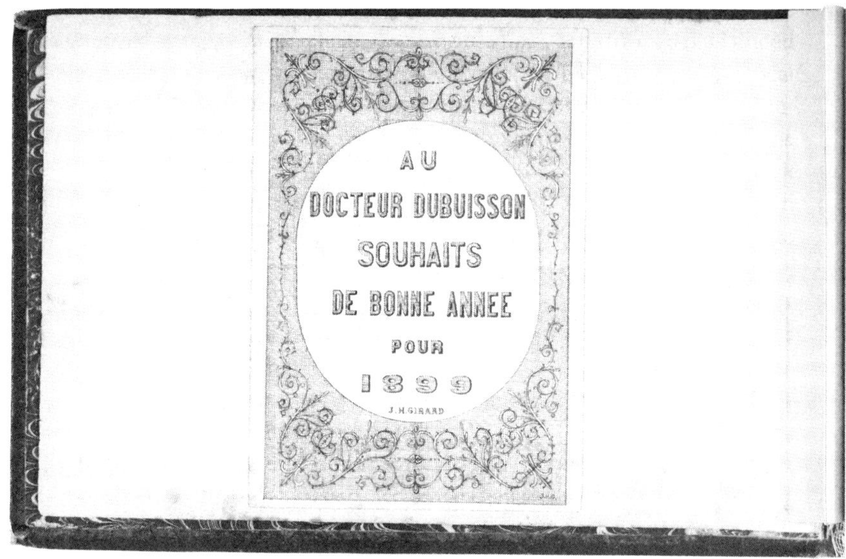

First page of the album of drawings that Dr. Maxime Dubuisson collected between 1899 and 1915

were exhibited as works in the collection, had to remain inaccessible to the larger public. So, for a long time, Dubuffet showed them in private homes or exhibition centers, in dark spaces with gray walls and amid many other objects. Initially, to ensure limited access, only four people could visit at a time. And he also decided to guide the visitors with his own commentary so that the objects echoed their lived context, of which they'd been stripped, and their intimate nature, which was no longer the case either once art brut found its audience. That lived context and intimate nature had disappeared in the very act of deciding to maintain them.[23]

Michel de Certeau, when writing about forms of popular art and everyday practices, pointed out that as soon as these artworks became objects of study and conservation they lost their disruptive power, which was eclipsed: they had made "art out of something dead." Through the process of idealization, which captured the forms of popular expression and praised the figure of the autodidact, any possible overflowing into other fields these practices could have was deactivated. For Certeau, practices like those that Dubuffet gathered under the name art brut only had strength when they had the capacity to "reorganize the setting where the discourse takes place."[24] This is the case, for example, of the wooden figures made by Auguste Forestier, who had been committed in 1914 for having derailed a train. His Beast of Gévaudan, horse-drawn carriages, and his military obsessions had managed to overflow the limits of the hospital because the nurses and nuns would buy his sculptures in exchange for tobacco, wine, and oil, and they would gift them to their friends and family, or to the townspeople on market days. The fact that Forestier's beasts and ghosts left the hospital and created an exchange value beyond the institution reorganized the meaning of what it was possible to do and how it was possible to live in a psychiatric hospital. As in the case of Clément Fraisse, who was locked in an isolation cell from 1929 to 1931 because he'd attempted to burn down his family home with the banknotes of his inheritance. Fraisse sculpted in relief on the wooden paneling of the walls, depicting his experience of isolation, a work that Tosquelles was able to partially save from destruction. And the case of Marguerite Sirvins, who embroidered collective scenes within the hospital and who in 1956, in *Trait d'union*, described her inner resistance: "Pay no heed to what is written about this person. I am innocent and I ask that this comedy end, I rebuke myself nothing and, by night, they write in my dossier, and I send you these words to quiet the rumors."[25]

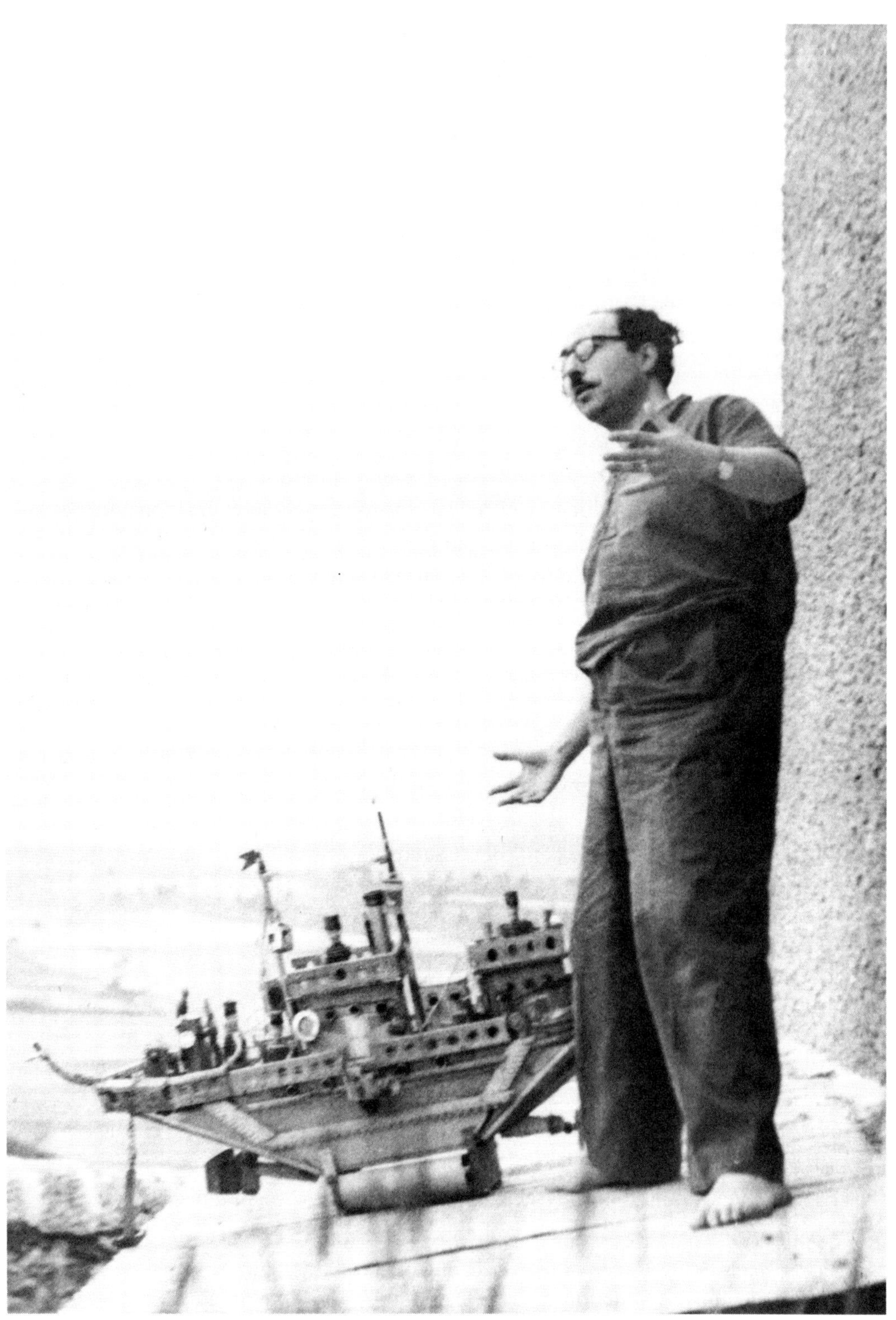

Tosquelles on the roof of the administrative building at Saint-Alban, with a boat constructed by Auguste Forestier

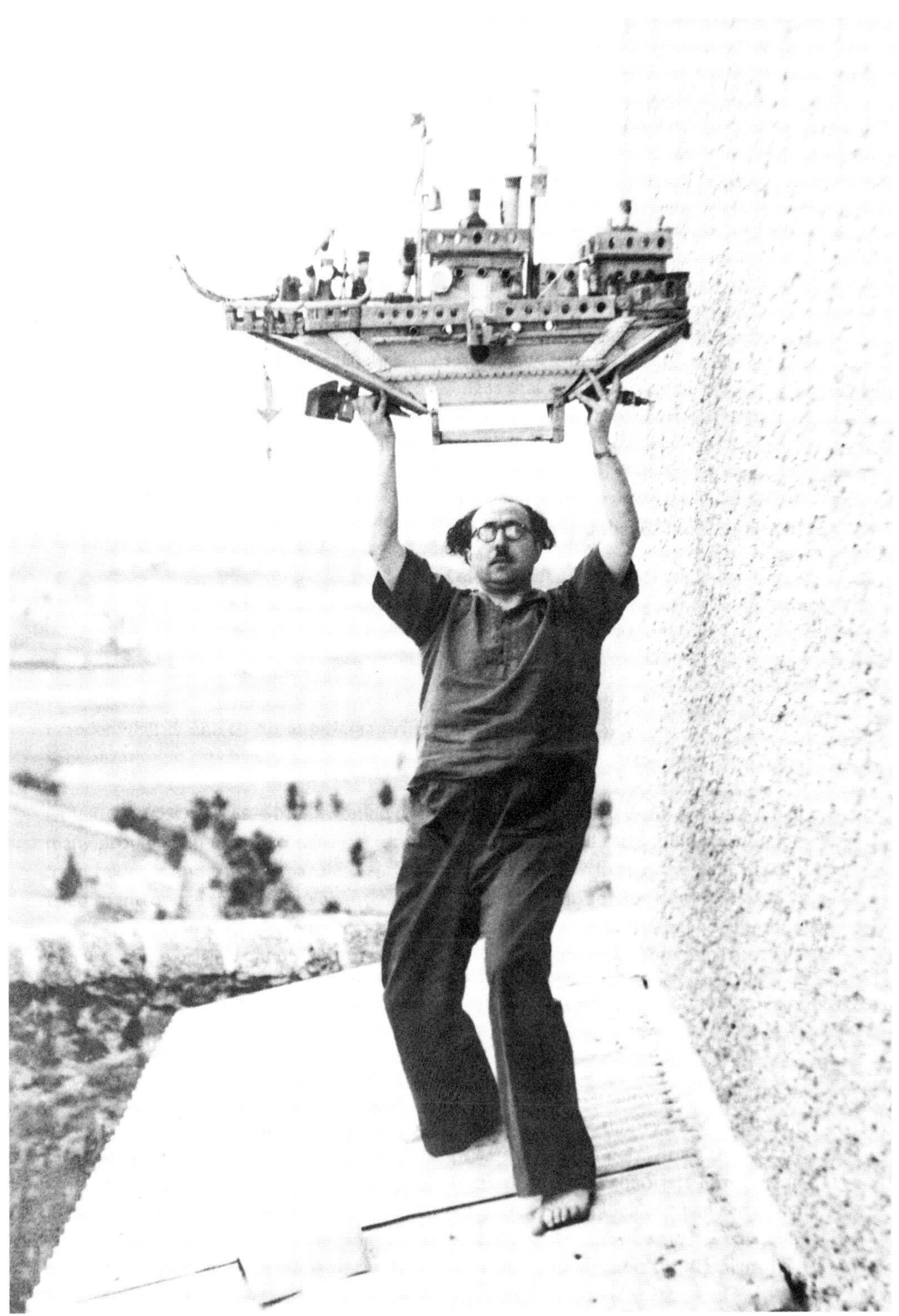

Separating the work made by the inpatients at Saint-Alban from the "living whole" of which they were part is one of the concerns raised by Jean Oury in his writings of the late 1940s that comprised the bulk of his doctoral thesis, defended in Paris in 1950 and published more than half a century later in 2005. Oury did not agree with the opposition of "brut" versus cultural practices—as he made clear years later, recollecting his meeting with Dubuffet—and he was also critical of the fetishization of the objects. His primary concern was how to carry out sincere ergotherapy in the production of the works without contributing to the suffering that certain patients felt when having to give them up. Oury was particularly attentive to the emotional bond established between the patient and their works and the pain produced by being separated from them, as well as the feeling of exploitation the patients might feel.

THE EXCHANGE FACTOR

In these artworks, there is a crucial factor: the exchange factor. It's a desire to exchange, existing on the plane of the cogito or the pre-cogito, but which appears essential.

In the case of F., this exchange is above all commercial in nature; he exchanges his sculptures for tobacco, money, or different objects.

With Jayet, it's primarily an affective exchange; for example, when I give him news of his wife, I note a real joy associated with a phenomenon of "safeguard of the affective ego" (Freud), which leads him to offer me all his notebooks.

With A., it's an affective exchange, but tinged more with automatisms.

With Mademoiselle S., the exchange is manifested mostly in the form of a childish gift (simple schizophrenia).

With Mademoiselle D., it's an amorous exchange of drawings or watercolors (erotomania).

THE EXCHANGE PROJECT

In all these cases, we can discern a certain aim during the construction of the work. There exists a project of exchange during the creation. Bringing it to light is a rather delicate matter, but one can register it by an indirect method instead. For example, A. started drawing for me only in September 1948. It took several tries for him to agree to it. He was afraid of mutilating himself. The pencil, he would say, "could cripple me." He made me a dozen sheets of drawings. At the beginning of October, I was obliged to leave the hospital for about a month. Immediately after my departure, all drawing ceased and it was impossible to persuade him anew. So what had happened? Was it merely a coincidence, with the processual development alone explaining this abrupt halt? [...]

My departure having erased this concrete project, the intentional arc went slack and the act of drawing sank into A.'s autistic world. It is quite obvious that A.'s drawing is not purely gratuitous; it is a mode of affective relation that ties him directly to me, a transitory emergent affectivity in an apocalyptic world. And it is this living substance that is the project of A.'s artistic act.[26]

Jean Oury, *Essai sur la conation esthétique* [Essay on aesthetic conation], 2005

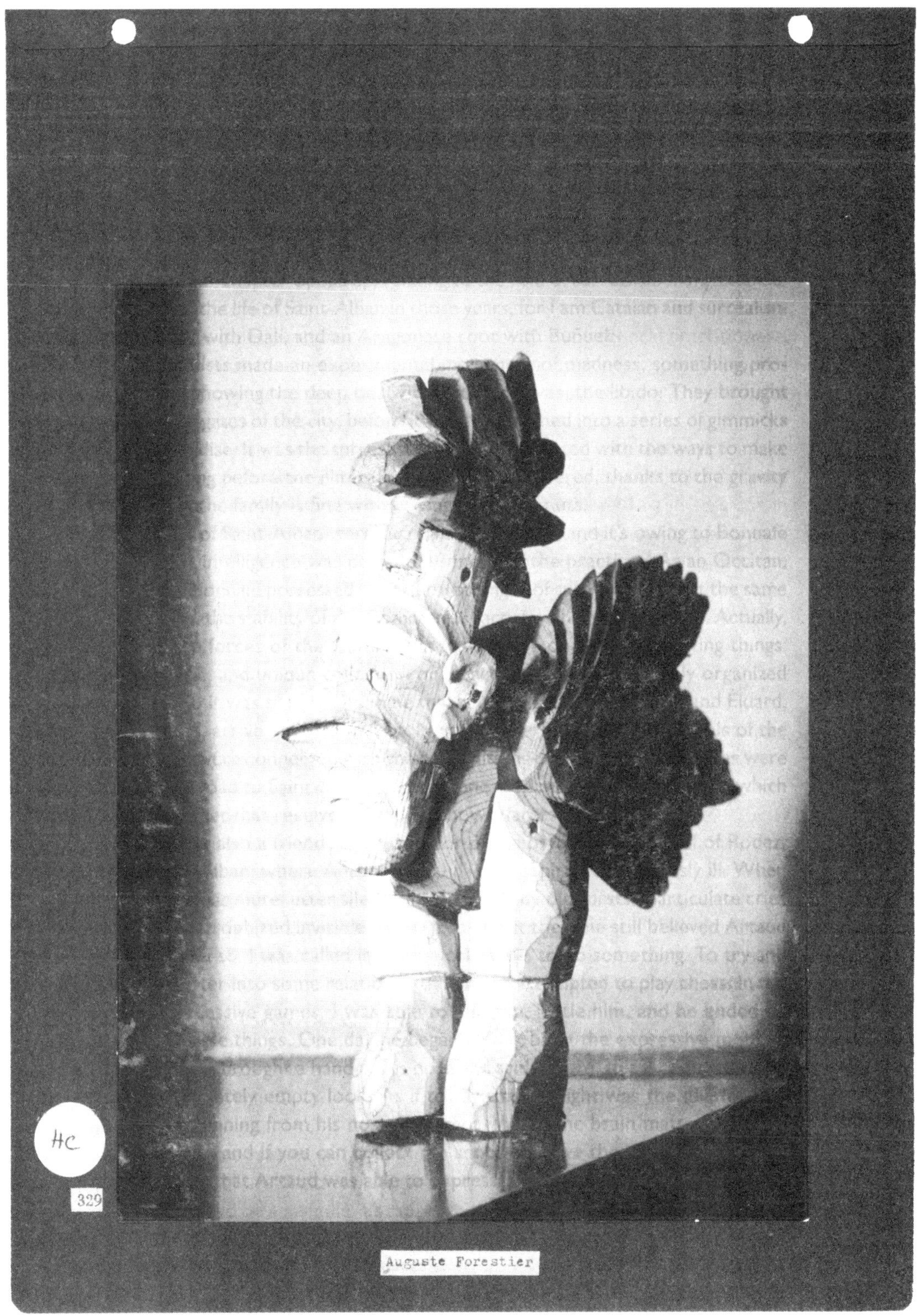

Page from one of the albums created by Jean Dubuffet, circa 1948, with a photograph of a rooster sculpted by Auguste Forestier

So it takes a certain delicacy to deal with F. Unfortunately, one can be tempted to exploit him, as much for selfish ends as for apparently philanthropic ends. One musn't forget that his work has value only because of its deep spontaneity, that his work is an integral part of his being, and that causing the disintegration of the one has an immediate repercussion on the other. This exploitation factor, whether on the objective or subjective plane, is a highly important phenomenon that should always be considered when one wants to undertake an honest ergotherapy. It must always be borne in mind that a simple exchange can be experienced by the patient as an act of exploitation.

In spite of that, F. is always pleased to show his pieces. This exhibitionist tendency is still very strong. Lately, one saw on the walls of the hospital courtyard the quarter-length figures of wooden soldiers. Many of the village children have little houses or oxcarts made by F. His productivity is impressive.[27]

Jean Oury, *Essai sur la conation esthétique*, 2005

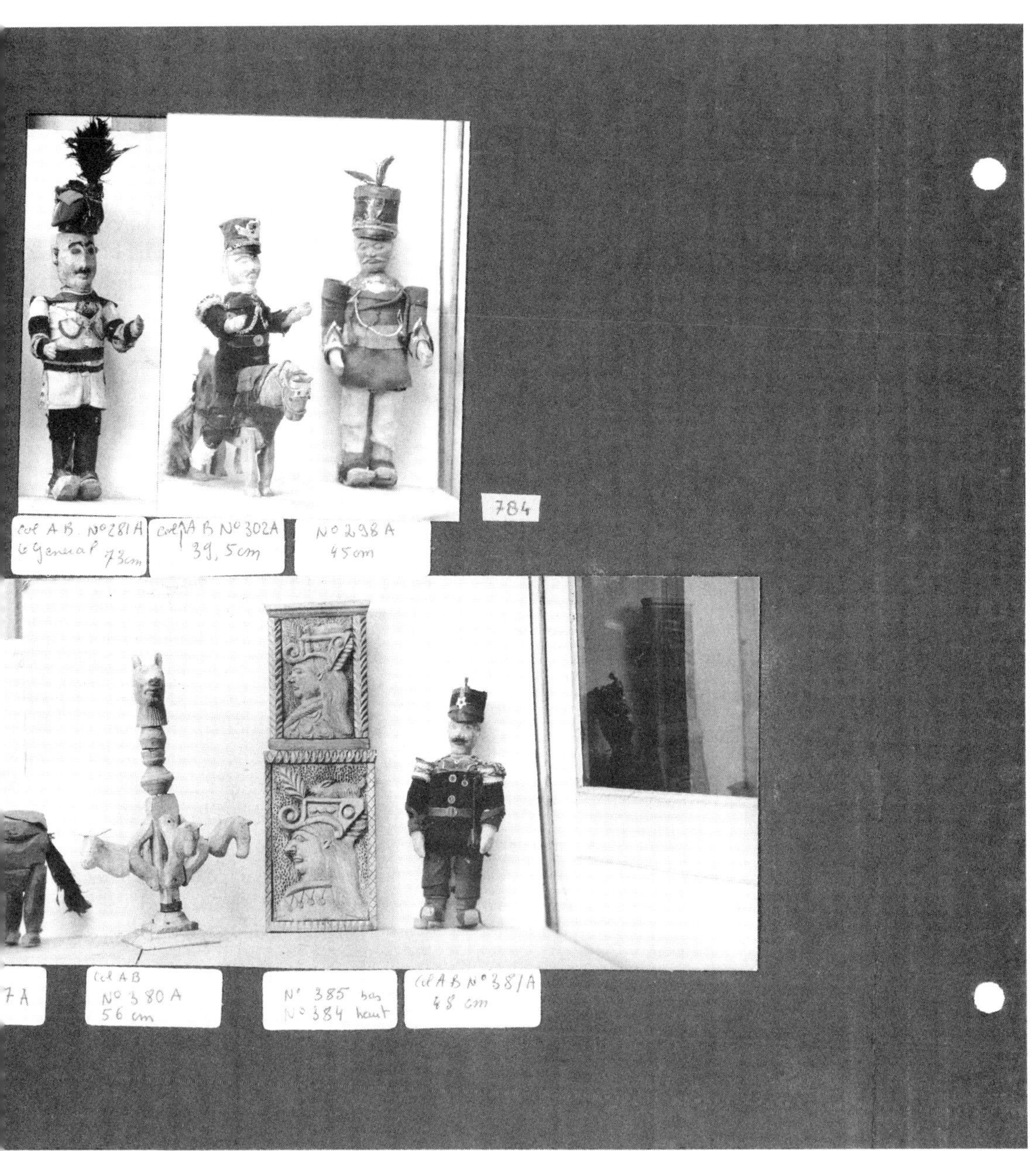

Page from an album created by Jean Dubuffet, with photographs of Auguste Forestier's sculptures, circa 1948

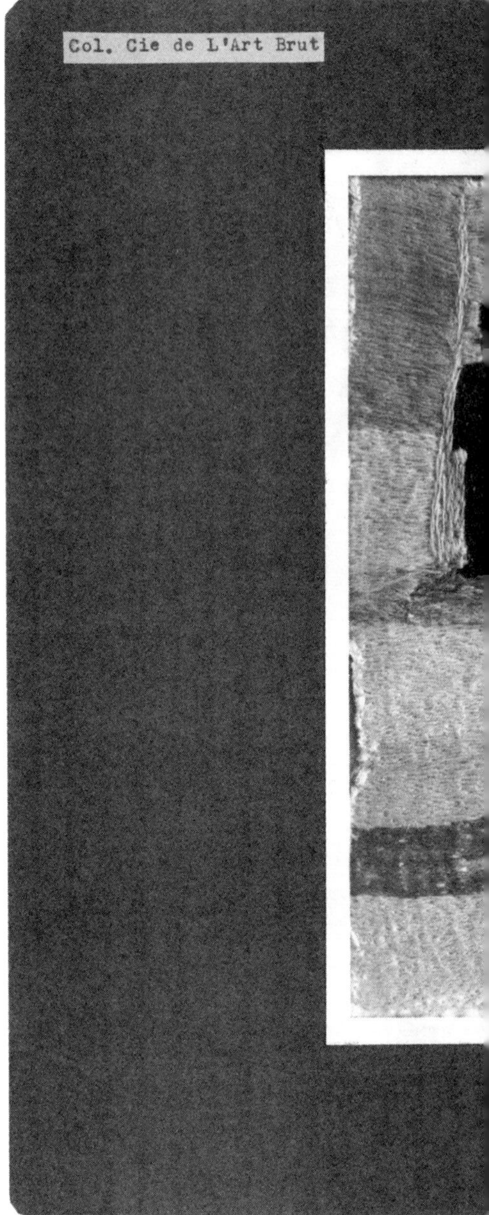

Still today we continue to celebrate art brut as an autodidactic practice produced in contexts of reclusion: psychiatric hospitals and prisons. It continues to be exhibited in museums on dark walls and with dim lighting to evoke its isolation and solitude. It is spoken of as a practice with no public, as anti-cultural or outside of the culture. It is an art of others. Of the poor, more than of the rich. Of women, more than of men. However, during the twentieth century, all those who historically had been considered outsiders and excluded from culture began to form part of it, thus demonstrating that "outside of the culture" doesn't actually exist. Paradoxically, this is what artist Jean Dubuffet's modern attitude affirmed when, in his search for anti-cultural objects, he reproduced one of the artistic gestures of the French avant-garde: like Marcel Duchamp with his readymades, Dubuffet shifted these objects from their uses and contexts to bring them into the world of culture.

Initially, Tosquelles resisted this decontextualization, which ripped the objects from the framework of the therapeutic practices in the hospital. Today, recontextualizing art brut means resituating the boat, the Beast of Gévaudan, and the wall paneling into the landscape of Saint-Alban. It means, above all, giving a name to this operation that speaks of cultural appropriation. These objects that formed part of a barter economy and small, informal exchanges were not stolen, but they were forced into a cultural economy of collecting. The cultural appropriation consists of having turned them into artworks that belong to a collection, erasing the contexts of domination and inequality in which they were produced. The ownership, therefore, does not precede the appropriation but derives from it. And this is why, today, art but is linked to the post-colonial world and to museums of primitive art, with their demands for reparation and restitution.[28]

Éric Fassin and Joana Masó, "Art brut i apropiació cultural" [Art brut and cultural appropriation], 2021

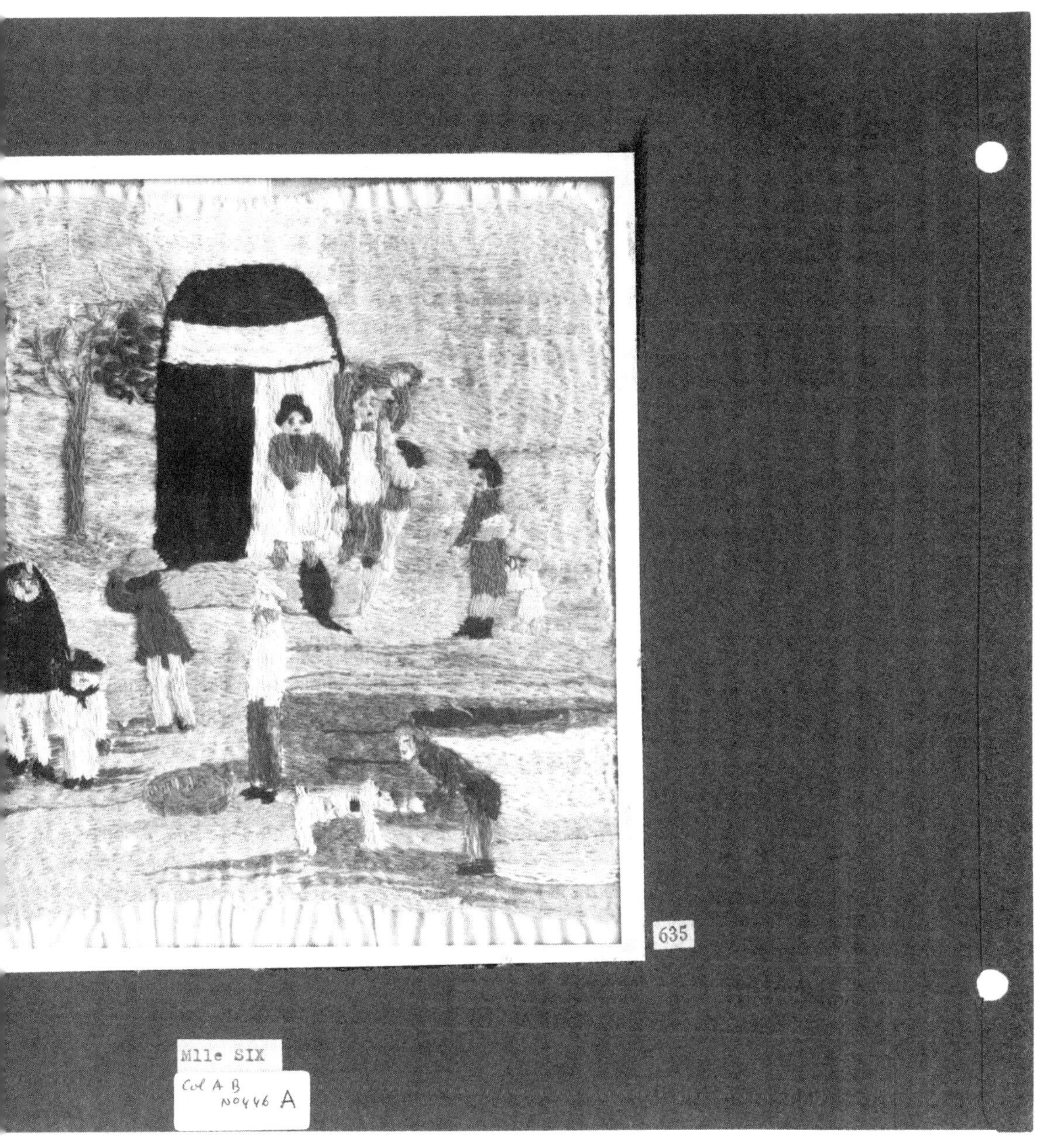

Page from the album created by Jean Dubuffet, with photographs of embroidery by Marguerite Sirvins, circa 1948

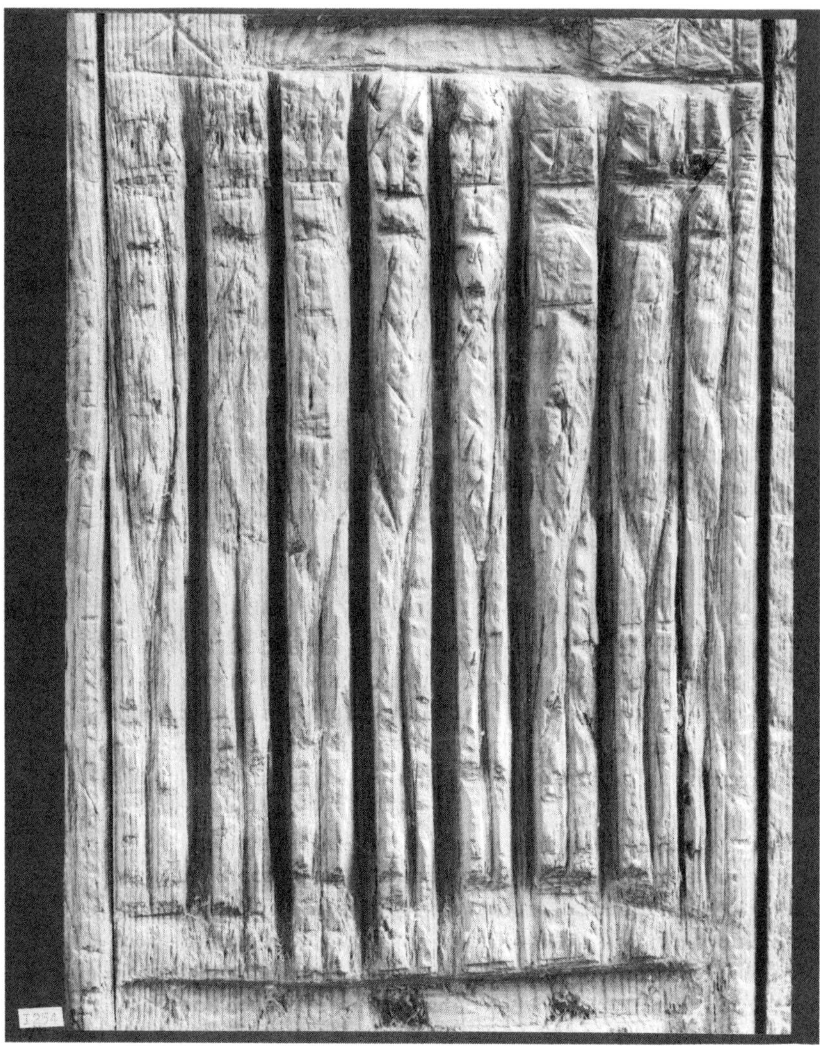

Photograph of a detail of the wooden hospital-wall panel that Clément Fraisse sculpted with a spoon, between 1930 and 1931. The image was published in the first volume of the series *Fascicules de l'art brut*, begun by Jean Dubuffet in 1964.

These fraught cultural experiences now seem far from what Dubuffet described in the 1940s as untainted artistic cultural practices, because the twentieth century has constantly brought contemporary art closer to experiential contexts, weaving bonds between culture and necessity. Perhaps this is why those bonds are nearer to experiences such as Artaud's, who spoke of a culture whose living strength would be identical to hunger, of a culture that would hold the power of hunger.

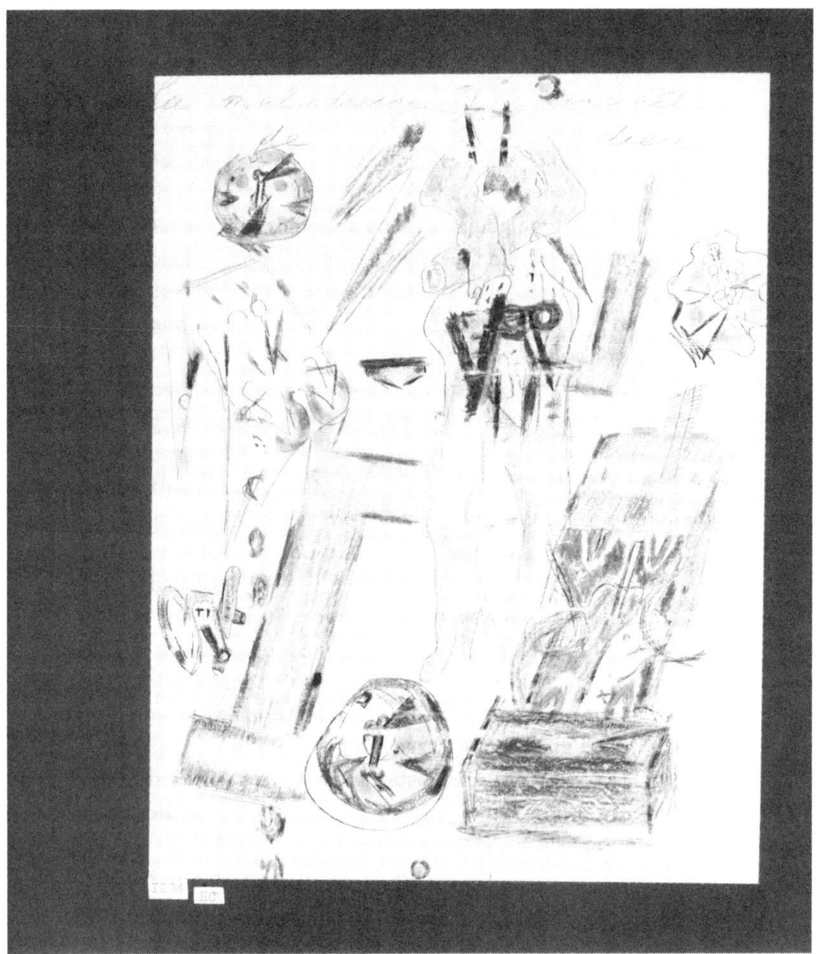

Page from an album created by Jean Dubuffet in 1963, with a reproduction of a drawing by Antonin Artaud, *La Maladresse sexuelle de Dieu* (The sexual clumsiness of God)

The most pressing thing, it seems to me, is not so much to defend a culture whose existence has never saved a human being from their concern with living better and with being hungry as it is to extract from what is called culture ideas whose life force is identical to that of hunger. Above all, we need to live and to believe in what makes us live. And what comes out from our mysterious inner being must not perpetually return to us in the form of a grossly digestive concern.

I mean to say that if it is important for us to eat without delay, it is more important not to squander our simple force of being hungry on the sole concern with eating right away.

If the sign of the times is confusion, I see at the root of this confusion a rupture between things, words, ideas, and signs that are its representation.[29]

Antonin Artaud, *Le Théatre et son double* [*The Theater and its Double*], 1938

The Movement of the Institution

In 1953, Gilles Deleuze presented a compilation of texts that invited reflection on the relationships of institutions, or institutional environments, with necessity. The collective reflection proposed by the book *Instincts et institutions* (Instincts and institutions) through fragments of Freud, Lévi-Strauss, Malinowski, Kant, Hume, and Balzac, among many other voices, inspired Ginette Michaud's book *La Borde … un pari nécessaire* on the idea of institutionality in psychotherapy, drawing on his own practice at the experimental clinic La Borde. Tosquelles wrote the prologue for that book, tracing the red thread that linked it to the institutional experience at Saint-Alban.

In his introduction to *Instincts et institutions*—which was published in a collection edited by Canguilhem—Deleuze discussed the institution as a system of possible means that could satisfy a tendency or a need. A system of possible means in opposition to the law. Against laws that limit concrete actions, the institution emerged as a positive model of possible action. Against the excess of laws that characterize tyrannies, the multiplication of institutions had a democratic root. From that starting point, Deleuze considered the theories and practices of the institution as radically inventive, capable of imagining original forms of satisfying the needs of the various institutional contexts. This confidence in inventiveness, which he associated with institutions, can only be experienced as a strength to the extent that every institutional process managed to deal with its own urgencies and needs. An institution had to be able to touch its own forms of hunger, sustenance, and protection.

> What is called an instinct and what is called an institution essentially designate processes of satisfaction. In the first instance, by naturally reacting to external stimuli, the organism *draws* from the exterior world the elements that satisfy its tendencies and its needs. For the different animals, these elements form specific worlds. Secondly, by instituting an original world between its tendencies and the exterior world, the subject *constructs* artificial means of satisfaction, which free the organism from nature while subjecting it to something else, and which transform the tendency itself by introducing it into a new environment. It's true that money frees one from hunger, provided one has some, and that marriage spares one from the search for a partner, while subjecting one to other tasks. This means that all individual experience presupposes, as an a priori, the prior existence of an environment in which the experience is *brought about*, a specific environment or institutional milieu. Instinct and institution are the two organized forms of a possible satisfaction. [...]
>
> The institution always presents itself as an organized system of means.

This is the difference, moreover, between the institution and the law: the latter is a limitation of actions, the former a positive model of action. Contrary to the theories of law that place the positive outside the social (natural rights) and the social in the negative (contractual limitation), the theory of the institution places the negative outside the social (needs), and presents society as being essentially positive, inventive (original means of satisfaction). Such a theory will give us, finally, political criteria: tyranny is a regime in which there are many laws and few institutions, democracy a regime in which there are many institutions, very few laws. [...]

Furthermore, if need only finds a very indirect, "oblique" satisfaction in the institution, it is not enough to say "the institution is useful," one must still ask: To *whom* is it useful? To all those who need? Or rather to a few (privileged class), or just to those who make the institution function (bureaucracy)?

Every institution imposes on our body, even in its involuntary structures, a series of models, and gives our intelligence a knowledge, a possibility of projection, of a project. We are led to the following conclusion: man has no instincts, he creates institutions. This being the case, instinct would signify the *urgencies* of the animal, and the institution would answer to the *exigencies* of man: the urgency of hunger becomes in man a demand to have some bread. Finally, the problem of instinct and the institution will be grasped most acutely not in animal "societies" but in the relations between the animal and man, when the exigencies of man are brought to bear on the animal by incorporating the animal into the institutions (totemism and domestication), and when the urgencies of the animal encounter man, either to flee him or attack him, or in the expectation of food and protection.[30]

Gilles Deleuze's introduction to *Instincts et institutions*, 1953

In Tosquelles's thinking, confidence in the transformative condition of institutions when they manage to link themselves with their own needs translated into the practice of movement. Tosquelles speaks of institutional work as work that elaborates situated strategies, that promotes events, exchanges, and concrete recognitions, quotidian actions that cannot be done without the movement of the whole community of patients and doctors, caregivers and nurses, including the immediate surroundings. This movement is never the result of a magical action or well-intentioned voluntarism on the part of the medical authorities. Institutional work only lives during this movement in process, which requires theoretical articulations of the way in which establishments—psychiatric, educational, political, familiar—live as anti-institutions, from multiple resistances that impede their true institutional implementation. This movement implies a heterogeneity that Tosquelles calls "institutional plurality." When reflecting on the relationship institutional psychotherapy has with its spaces, he builds on the reflection Ginette Michaud did for La Borde, because institutional psychotherapy is above all a practice of transformation of spaces through a system of mediations, or through a "technique of setting," as Jean Oury called it. For Tosquelles and Oury, a place emerges from the crossroads of a group of institutions. At La Borde, these places were called "workshops," like La Kalo—the workshop of "kalotherapy" (hairdressing and makeup)—and the henhouse, where they grew tobacco, and the calendar of daily meetings, the rotation of professional roles, the driving school, the workshop to create the newspaper, the club, and the reflection group on institutional work among the collectives of La Borde and Saint-Alban.

What is a club? Above all, it's place where one goes. It's not an association of individuals with a purpose in mind, and if this form of association is called a "club" in society, that's because it has to do with visits to a given locale by people who come there for the same thing as you.

A club can be a sports club, a games club, some other kind of club, or a nothing-at-all club—the latter being that club par excellence where one doesn't come with the aim of doing something definite, if it's not visiting others in a place where one is sure of encountering them.

It makes sense that in a psychiatric hospital designed to "resocialize" the patient, as it's commonly put, one would think of creating this privileged organization.

It's obvious that the club should be suited to those who will frequent it, and it seems just as obvious that they will be the ones to give it its shape, because it's true that interhuman relations are also situated in space and that no organization is possible for a group without there being spatial reference points, without a "spot" where it can be situated. The same necessity is found at the level of the group as that noted by Halbwachs at the level of society:

"Although a society is essentially made up of thoughts and tendencies, it cannot exist, its functions cannot be exercised, unless it installs and extends itself somewhere in space, unless it has its place there. It must be tied in its whole and its parts to a certain expanse, of a certain position, a certain size, a certain configuration of the material ground ..."

When a Trobriand woman wants to talk to others, she takes her jug and goes to the well.

When a Bororo man wants to talk to others, he goes to the men's house.

For the woman villager of a century ago, the washhouse.

For the present-day French, the café.

Every milieu has its privileged place where one exchanges conversations or money, a game of cards or a round of drinks.

One of the first acts of Dr. Oury, a psychiatrist of the nearby Institut Médico-Pédagogique [special needs school] as well as director of La Borde, was to look for a place with a table and chairs for the children, to sell small bars of soap or ballpoint pens, play cards or read illustrated magazines. By organizing "the club" he was only following Makarenko's example.

The experience of Dr. Frantz Fanon, at the psychiatric hospital of Blida, also deserves to be cited. On the theoretical principle which seems obvious, that the "club" concept should be different for every cultural milieu, he created at Blida a club of a particular kind. Since the patients he had were Muslims, he gave them the opportunity to meet in a Moorish café, being aware of its importance in Muslim social life. There, no tables or chairs, but mats placed on a sort of raised platform where Muslims settle themselves sometimes for hours to smoke kif and drink Moorish coffee or mint tea.[31]

Ginette Michaud, *La Borde ... un pari nécessaire: De la notion d'institution à la psychothérapie institutionnelle* [La Borde ... a necessary wager: From the notion of institution to institutional psychotherapy], 1977

On June 4 and 5, 1960, Francesc Tosquelles, Jean Oury, Roger Gentis, Horace Torrubia, Jean Ayme, Yves Racine, Jean Colmin, Maurice Paillot, and Hélène Chaigneau met in Saint-Alban for the first gathering of the Groupe de Travail de Psychothérapie et de Sociothérapie Institutionnelles (GTPSI). Over the years they were joined by Félix Guattari, Ginette Michaud, Claude Poncin, Henri Vermorel, Michel Baudry, Nicole Guillet, Robert Millon, Jean-Claude Polack, Gisela Pankow, and Jacques Schotte in various annual meetings of monographic debate around problems common to different French psychiatric institutions: the circulation of money within the hospital; multi-referential psychotherapy; the phantasm and the institution. Tosquelles always considered these problems through a political lens.

> It's the fact that Tosquelles, from the beginning no doubt, has positioned himself as a political militant. I mean ... it's not that he's full of political ideas. It's that his way of being, whatever the situation, is political. Perhaps it's hard to describe but ... maybe I'm judging this in comparison with myself ... and in that regard I think there is a certain affinity and antagonism with Tosquelles that has played a part in our relationship. But I myself, when I came to La Borde, I too came as a militant. I set about organizing the activities at La Borde, the meetings, the workshops, the schedules more or less as I organized groups of young people, cells of political groups in which ... within which I was involved, [...] I believe that Tosquelles acted that way right out of the gate, with the good sisters of Saint-Alban and with all the personnel, with all the protections he created, he acted with a kind of militant logic, which is more an existential logic than a matter of content.[32]
>
> Félix Guattari in the film by François Pain, *Félix Guattari sur un divan* [Félix Guattari on a couch], 1986

During the Second World War, in the Armentières psychiatric hospital (near Lille), another figure had carried out an action analogous to Saint-Alban's, without knowledge of the psychiatric revolution that was going on, simultaneously, in Lozère. Fernand Deligny, after a year of deployment as a noncommissioned officer and liaison officer, returned to the psychiatric hospital where he had previously spent several months as a specialized teacher. Until 1943, when he was suspended, Deligny held the de facto role as educator, in charge of a wing filled with "unteachable, profoundly retarded" children. In the context of an institution completely altered by the absence of medical staff (who were on the front) and exposed to the chaos of war, Deligny, apparently alone, beneath the bombs, took a good number of initiatives: suppression of punishments, work with the guards (unemployed textile workers, artisans, former prisoners), occupation of spaces outside of the typical circuits of hospital life (basements, stairwells), organization of excursions, games, sports activities, and workshops. There was no therapy, no theoretical elaboration, no medical team, no psychoanalysis or transferential constellation … Nonetheless, in action and improvisation, his intuitions were very similar to Tosquelles's: making use of the war, rethinking the role of the space and the movement in space, working with nonprofessionals, who are less limited by their knowledge and socially closer to the patients. And writing, since Deligny was a writer. Writing a report that gathers all those experiences, in the form of narrations and essays. Those principles founded the thinking and its practical application, over the course of the subsequent attempts: La Grande Cordée (1947–1962), an association sustained over the network of popular education (particularly the CEMÉA) and the network of informal fostering of autistic children, in Cévennes (1967–1996, the year he died). At the heart of this idea and practice, the project of creating the conditions of a living environment inspired in their—they being psychotic, autistic, or criminal children and teens—own ways of being, based, among other models, on ethology. As he showed in the cartography of his "lines of errancy," the areas in the Cévennes where the autistic children lived with their "nearby presences" (workers, farmers, students, unemployed people) were equivalent to the places Tosquelles spoke of: places themselves filled with micro-spaces (the shelter, the dining room table, the laundry, Jacques Lin's carpentry workshop, etc.) that provoked the emergence, like a spider with its web, of an environment or a "common body" produced by the sequence of everyday tasks collectively accomplished by speaking adults and children without language, and by their constant coexistence. Deligny was not a psychiatrist nor a psychoanalyst and his stay at the La Borde clinic, where Oury and Guattari had invited him to organize some workshops in 1965–1967, reaffirmed his decision to make, from the mutism of Janmari, the model of his network. But the network was also a "raft," an image that Jean Oury used to talk about La Borde: a precarious institution, a vessel for those shipwrecked from society, a light craft whose knots and tethers had to be constantly reworked. Oury had met Deligny during his Grande Cordée period, in the popular-education setting, and at Saint-Alban one of his earliest initiatives was cyclostyled excerpts of *Les Vagabonds efficaces*.

Deligny's search led him far from institutions, but his critique rested more on "the instituted" than on the institution and, like Tosquelles, he wanted to preserve the notion of psychiatric hospital with his corollary, the invention of an environment organized for the material and psychic survival of crazy children. An in-depth study of the relationships between institutional therapy and his attempt in the Cévennes remains pending.

For Deligny, cinema quickly became one of those places where something could happen, prompted by the camera-tool. The filming of *Le Moindre Geste* was the incarnation of the cinematic projects at La Grande Cordée, theorized by Deligny in his programmatic text "The Camera as Pedagogical Tool" (published in 1955), none of which ever succeeded. The film, with no script or director, was improvised by autodidacts (Josée Manenti did the camerawork) and describes the adventures and epic burlesque ravings of its protagonist, Yves G., a psychotic teenager taken in at La Grande Cordée, in a territory defined by his "lines of errancy" around a hole into which one of his fellow inmates had fallen. Later, cinema became, for Deligny and his network—as well as for Tosquelles, although from a different perspective—one of the tools for documenting these attempts and, beyond that, an opportunity to reflect on the image and its relationships to language.

> My first contact with Tosquelles occurred by chance. I was working and living at the time with Fernand Deligny, his companion Huguette Dumoulin, and their two daughters, my son, and the boys who lived with us, in the valley of Thoiras, so not very far from Saint-Alban.
>
> One day we received a visit from Fernand Oury, who was on his way to Saint-Alban, and a few days later, we saw a black half-track car roll up: it was Tosquelles. He disembarked. We lived in one of those Cévennes-type houses with an overhanging second floor, and down below a yard. Toquelles descended with his bearing, his look, of an International Brigades general. He was accompanied by four or five male nurses. They opened the big trunk of the vehicle and pulled out a wicker basket. And those strong lads commenced to transport the basket to us, fifty meters above them. They arrived at the terrace. I came down to greet them. Tosquelles introduced himself: "François Tosquelles."
>
> What I saw first of all was someone whose presence radiated a considerable warmth. His hands spoke very, very fast … but these are feminine impressions. I began with that. I found him utterly charming. He said to me, "I would like to see Deligny." "Well, that's easy." We climbed the stairs together to Deligny's office. They spoke to each other briefly, then Tosquelles said: "The nurses are down below, I would like for them to join us." So they all came in with the wicker basket, and inside it were enough victuals for all of us, including bread. He had planned on bringing the meal and on arriving at mealtime. It was noon. We installed ourselves together, the conversation went full tilt between Tosquelles and Deligny. What did they talk about? I don't really recall. I was captivated by the vivacity of this new person in our midst, this rapidity he had of flipping situations over, to make something playful out of them; and then I was amazed by a poetic dimension that was always opening up. It's hard to describe how he managed to make that happen. It was through a piling on of witticisms,

which finally scintillated, yielding a different meaning from the one that had obtained a few sentences before, in such a way as to please, to gain one's attention if possible. I would say in such a way that a transference took hold, and took hold very quickly! We were switched on, and after a certain moment, he was leading us, as if he had a conductor's baton and was willing everyone to speak, which we all did. If we were a little uptight at the beginning, there was very soon an explosion of spontaneity, a very sweet gathering, everyone was happy. It's true that we had drunk a little rosé wine from our cellar.

They basically talked about Deligny's work, about what was being done with the boys, how it was being done. Tosquelles was interested because he intended to send us some boys to stay for a spell, to spend time in the country at a moment when farmworkers were badly needed. We did things at a leisurely pace, without much concern for cost-effectiveness, but they had to get done nonetheless, the hay couldn't be left to molder on the ground, and the pastures needed to be watered. A deal was made: we said we would come and pick up the boys, or they would bring them down, and that worked out very well for a time. However, we were on the verge of leaving that huge piece of land.

We were starting to be a little out of breath. It was a property of 135 hectares and we were often eight or ten people. That was few for gathering the hay, irrigating the fields, taking care of fifty goats, three donkeys, with wood to be cut, a small vineyard. One also needed to take on the small building jobs, the cheese making, the big vegetable garden that fed us, the seasonal silkworms—many vital activities, is what I'm saying.

Deligny did the schooling. All the youngsters would go into what was called "the classroom," which turned into a multipurpose studio. A place of invention, a workplace, a contemplation room, because it was very peaceful, always orderly. Nice to look at. At times there would be two or three boys, sometimes a single one. It was a very important place during the day. It had a certain mystery. Tosquelles wanted to go into the classroom with Deligny. They stayed there with the boys for a long spell. Which meant that I, busy with household maintenance, was cut off from what was said that day. Tosquelles had a long-standing familiarity with Deligny's work. He had read *Graine de crapule* [Scoundrel seed] and *Les Vagabonds*. He knew his work at La Grande Cordée.

La Grande Cordée was probably the first clinic for counseling adolescent delinquents *en cure libre*, which is to say they would go back home and would come to the clinic every day for meetings or sessions with the team. There would be a search for places where they could try their hand at social life. This consisted of what was called a "trial stay"—a formula that was implemented subsequently by Maud Mannoni and others. But the first time it was put into practice was at the initiative of Deligny, who was inspired by the networks of youth hostels, represented at the time by Huguette Dumoulin. They did that together, traveling all over France by motorbike, looking for people who would be interested in hosting a young person who was lost, who no longer knew where to go, the idea being to involve them in some sort of work, in community life, and in their own well-being. The hosts were youth hostel people or craftspeople or farmers, but there were also many schoolteachers. And when they would be set up with teachers, the young person wouldn't have much to do, so these teachers would need to have another activity, which was often the case. For example, in the Pyrenees, the teachers were sometimes married to farmers. There would be much to do at the farm of course. I made several visits to the home of a schoolteacher named Labadie. In conversation, Tosquelles took an interest in that network because there were quite a lot of Spaniards. I often went into the Pyrenees, in those border regions that had a certain sense of welcome, of hospitality. Deligny exchanged views a lot with Tosquelles about those historical periods and their traces.[33]

Josée Manenti, in Patrick Faugeras, *L'Ombre portée de François Tosquelles* [The shadow cast by François Tosquelles], 2007

Our pedagogical collectivity in its struggle against enemy forces (that is, the lack of a learning process, the "morals" of rotting classes whose contradictions and philosophies find a privileged terrain, albeit in slangy formulas, among the weakest mindsets) must take inspiration from a more Resistance-type strategy.

The hundred or so kids of the Gorky colony could make a stand in a society that was in the process of organizing its future prospects.

For our young people, making a stand would be to make a target. They increase their chances of doing well by spreading themselves about in a country where all that is seriously intended for them is their exploitation as precarious labor.

And yet they have need of a "collectivity" or, if you like, a supporting milieu that informs them, "inspires" them in a somewhat coherent and steady manner, which provides them with reasons for being because, for the most part, they feel superfluous on an earth where everything takes place as if there was nothing for them to do there. Film gives them a reason for being. They have something to show. They have been treated as disturbed individuals, retards, sickos, wastrels. They can become examples. With the camera, the world looks at them—the world of the Others, who had nothing to do with them, and in a short while will be witnesses to what they do every day.[34]

Ferdinand Deligny, "La Caméra outil pédagogique" ["The Camera, a Pedagogical Tool"], 1955

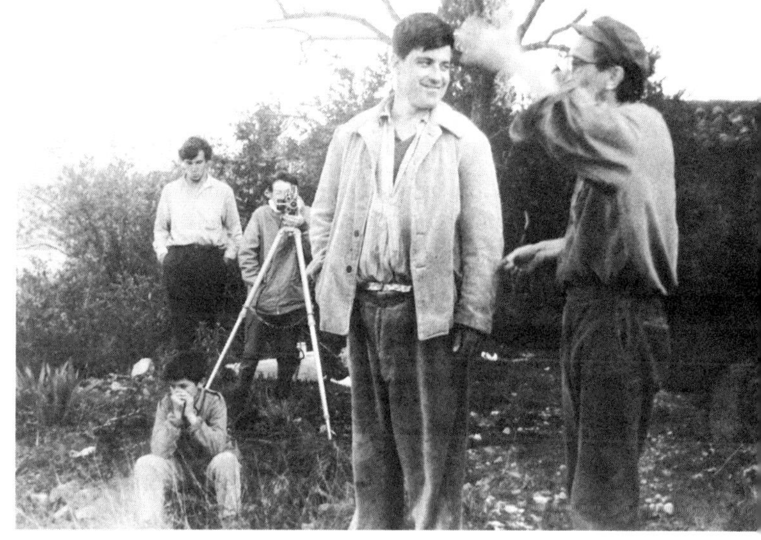

Filming of *Le Moindre Geste* by Fernand Deligny, Josée Manenti, and Jean-Pierre Daniel (who edited the film), circa 1964. *Right foreground*, Deligny and Yves G.; *at the camera*, Josée Manenti; *next to her*, Guy Aubert; and, *seated*, Richard B.

The thing is, it's not an inquiry focusing on "learning impaired" children but on what "milieu" would be capable of sparking some mental liveliness in them and of giving rise to sincere intentions on their part to create projects. To accomplish this, I can't count on any institutional milieus, whatever they may be. So I have to be able to establish somewhere a "milieu" whose participants won't live as children under supervision. Hence the necessity that *Le Moindre Geste* exist commercially.[35]

Fernand Deligny, letter of December 1, 1966, to François Truffaut concerning *Le Moindre Geste* [*The Slightest Gesture*]

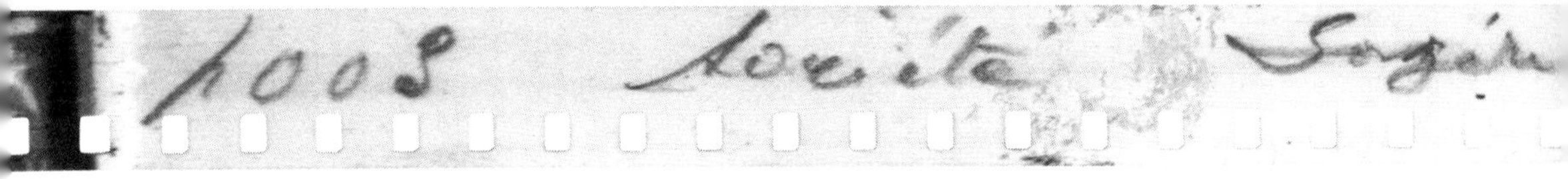

Filmstrip from *Film Tosquelles,* or *Société Lozérienne d'Hygiène Mentale*

A Silent Film That Speaks Volumes

On September 5, 1958, as part of the 4th International Congress of Psychotherapy held at the Universitat de Barcelona, the film made at Saint-Alban was screened. It was the first time that Francesc Tosquelles returned to Catalonia since he went into exile in September 1939. It was also the first time since the start of the Spanish Civil War that a large conference on psychotherapy was organized in Spain, designed to transform the Spanish clinical panorama. Still entrenched in Francoism, this gathering of twelve hundred elite psychiatrists from around the world was a show of the regime's openness. For the first time, psychotherapy was discussed openly in dialogue with the prevailing debates of the time: existentialism and phenomenology; anthropology and the social sciences; psychoanalysis; psychodrama and hypnosis; psychopharmacology; social work and group psychotherapy; and the influence of Eastern psychology on contemporary psychotherapy. For the first time, Jacques Lacan gave a lecture in Spain, along with Jean Oury, Lucien Bonnafé, and Roger Gentis, among many others, in a conference that also featured an exhibition of paintings by patients. For the first time, Tosquelles showed the medical community the institutional work carried out at Saint-Alban, with images filmed over the course of the fifties. He himself had filmed scenes that he would watch with the patients, nurses, and caregivers gathered at special evenings and parties. The film was screened for the international medical community after having circulated, in part, within the Saint-Alban community as a tool both for the present and for collective memory, a tool for relating time with one's own image.

It was a silent film. A film that simultaneously demonstrated what daily life was like in psychiatric hospitals, and Tosquelles's project of transformation at Saint-Alban. It depicted people smoking as they built and demolished walls and wings, sun streaming through

IV
Congreso
DEL 1 AL 7 DE SEPTIEMBRE 1958 BARCELONA-ESPAÑA
Internacional
de Psicoterapia
A. RICARD

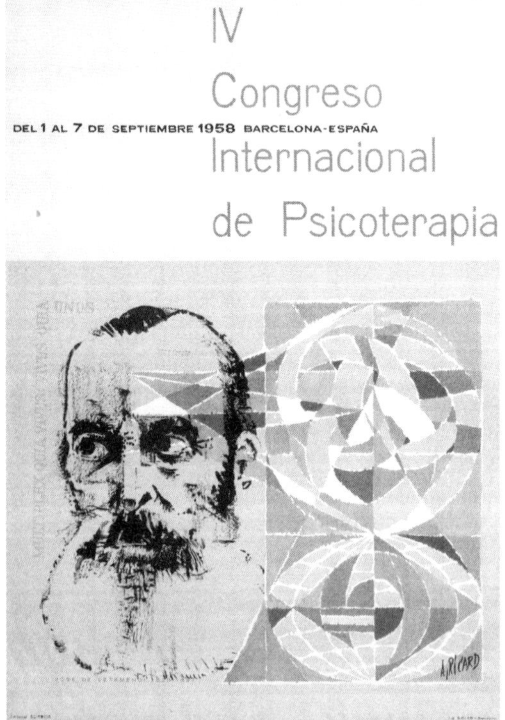

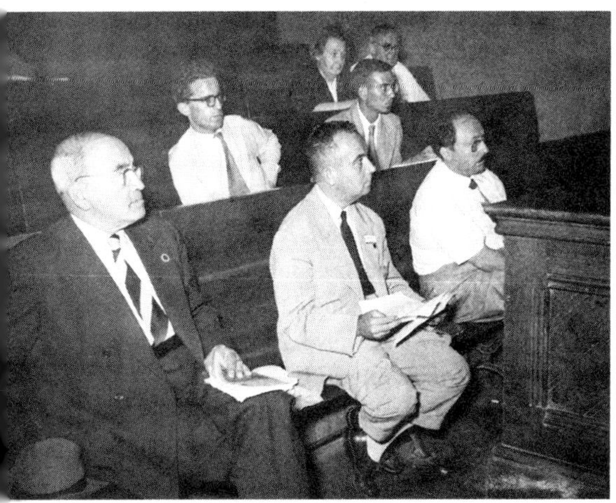

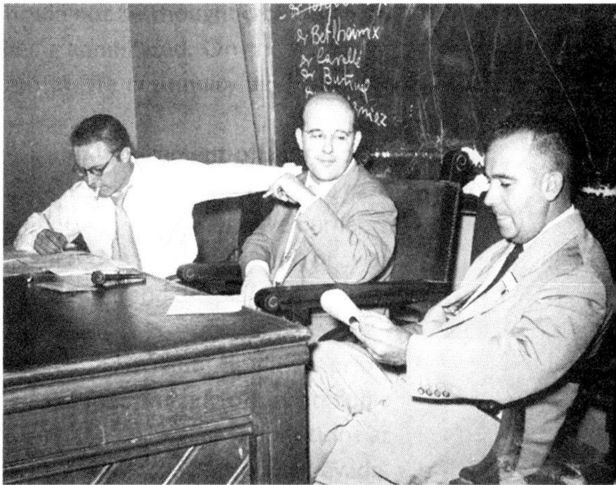

Photographs from the 4th International Congress of Psychotherapy in 1958. *Above, on the left*, Tosquelles seated in the front row in one of the classrooms in the historic building of the Universitat de Barcelona; *on the right*, Tosquelles's name is written and crossed out on the blackboard. *Below*, Tosquelles with Jacques Lacan. *At left*, poster for the 4th International Congress of Psychotherapy.

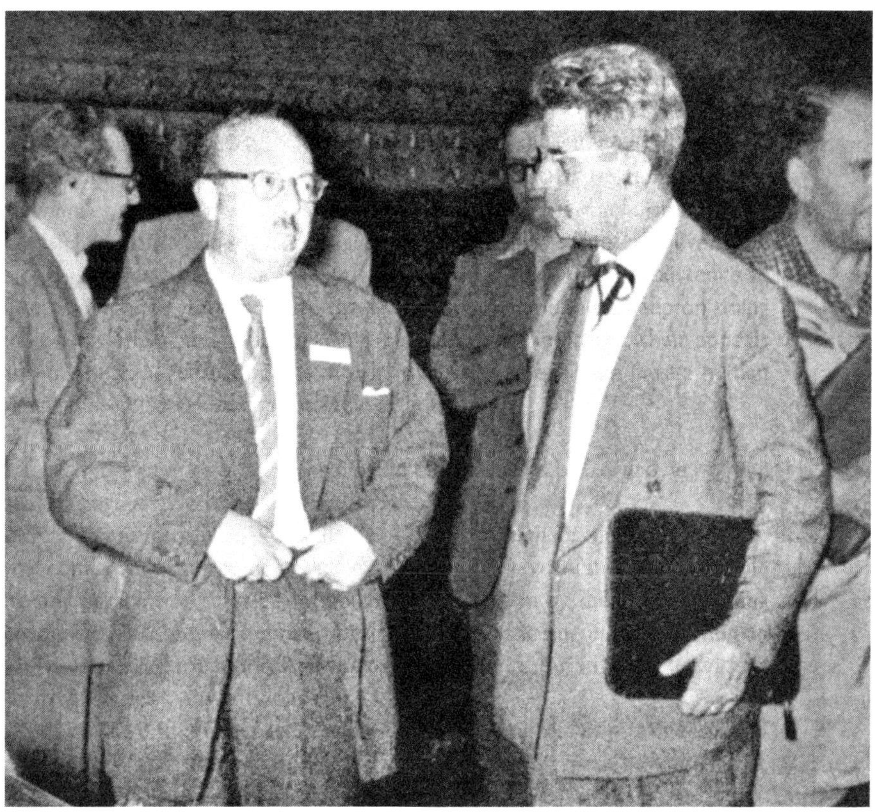

a window and illuminating the daily cleaning activities or the work at the printing press beside the common rooms, creating a living memory of the life of the institution that included festival posters, cinema programming, announcements of the patient cooperative. What all those images conveyed was that, in order to collectively inhabit a space, it was necessary to map out its evolution: *ça va changer* (this will change), says one still of the film. And what would change was not only the place, but what it could become.

As Alejandra Riera has written, this film asks us about places that are worth transforming. It asks us about the places we devote our energy, work, and life to. And it asks us this silently but eloquently. As states one of the posters for one of the versions, it is a "very eloquent silent film." Although we can't hear what they are saying, we see the faces of those participating intensely in a newspaper meeting: Tosquelles is there, with his wife Elena, and other members of the community of caregivers and nuns. It is a long sequence that allows us to glimpse the circulation of spoken and written words, to see their place in the Saint-Alban project. Writing is also present in the intertitles, which offer information and figures and the context and situation of the hospital's transformation. When asked about the most striking part of the congress in Barcelona, Dr. Pigem Serra, from the Girona hospital, responded that what most impressed him was "something practical": the film from Saint-Alban explained that some patients, in a hospital in the south of France, had earned 6 million francs in one year.

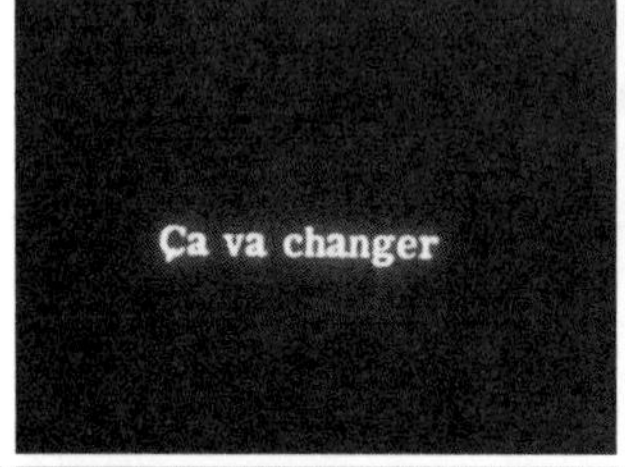

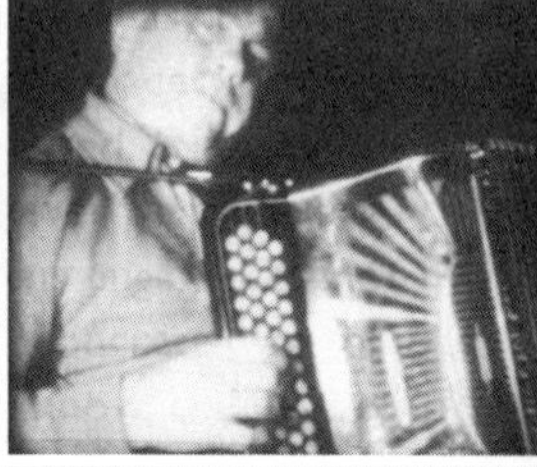
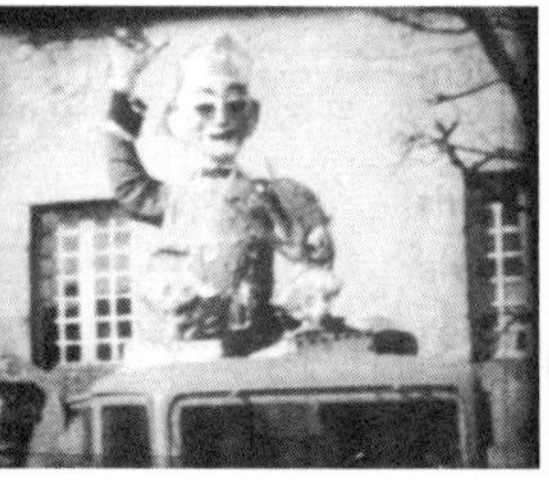
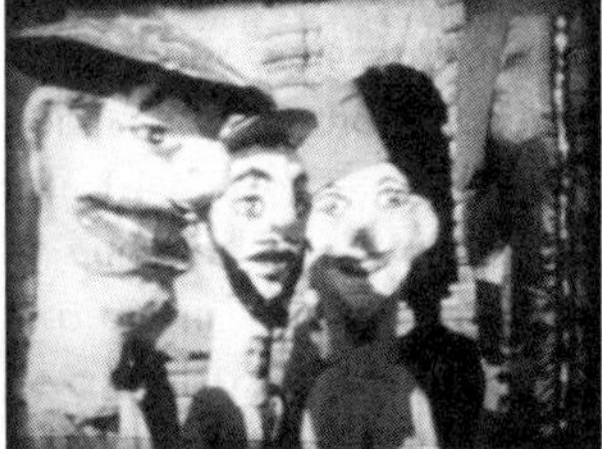
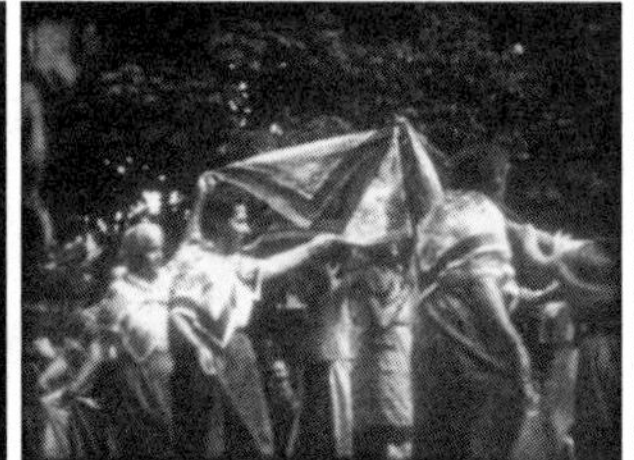
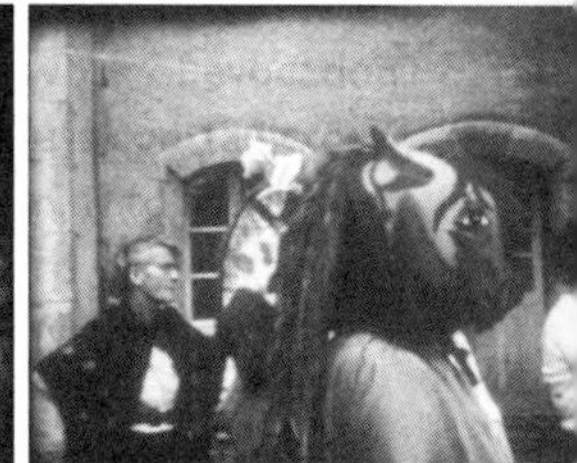

At the congress, in addition to the film, Tosquelles delivered a paper on the possibility of "the encounter" [*la recontre*] during the process of admitting patients to the hospital. He warned against a conception of sociotherapy and ergotherapy understood as techniques designed to produce automatisms of adaptation. What he sought were specific events, gestures of recognition of the other and material gateways into the hospital, in which the words that circulated between the patient and the medical community were never obligatory but always available, and indirectly gave shape to all the actions that took place at the hospital. In the text of his paper, delivered in a roundtable presided over by Henri Ey and devoted to reflecting on "The renovation of psychiatric assistance through existential anthropological thought," Tosquelles spoke on his institutional approach and his unders-

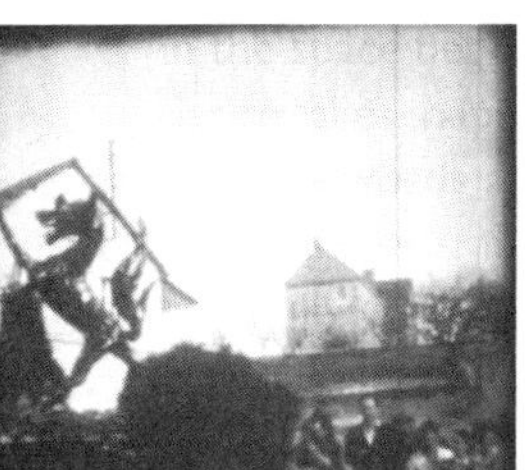
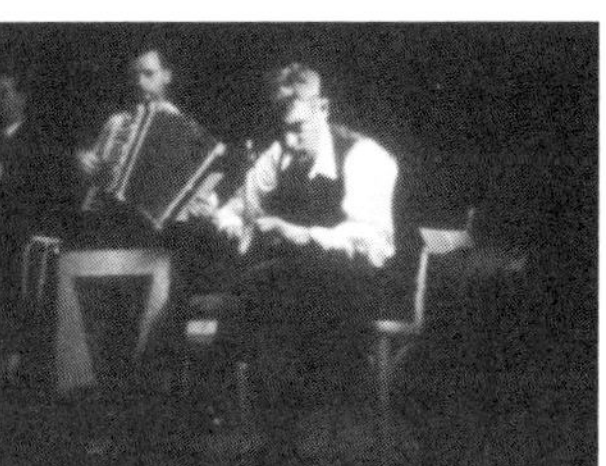
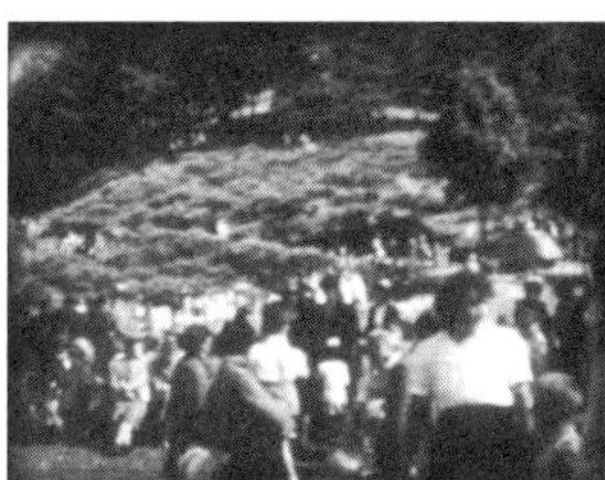
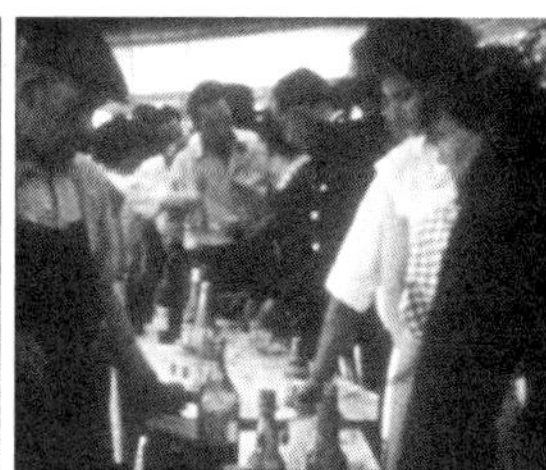

tanding of places as spaces always potentially penitentiary, totalitarian, always potentially closed: no establishment, no organism, no school nor psychiatric hospital, no form of organization escaped the possibility of becoming a prison; that was why institutional work was always necessary and always political, because it introduced concrete forms of the possible.

But the big 1958 conference, which was supposed to transform the space of possibilities in Spanish clinical practice, ended up halting the introduction of psychotherapy, ergotherapy, sociotherapy, and psychoanalysis. The experience of Saint-Alban left no trace in either the collective

With the example and assistance of the other patients, rather than with the personal contact of the doctor, what is medical must be projected, from the first contact to the smallest element of living and of hospital responsibility. It's a matter of teaching the patient to decipher the general sense of the hospital, of stimulating their comprehension and their effort in that respect. One needs to offer them this key upon the initial contacts—even if this appears pointless or unworkable in such circumstances. The welcoming techniques must not be limited to the first act, as my student Dr. Bidault underscores in his thesis. The welcome continues tirelessly throughout their stay and constitutes the basic availability that enables the encounter of patient and institution. [...]

It's not a matter of analytical group therapy that may be organized on a continual basis; such a thing has its place in the institution. By its mere presence in the hospital, this therapeutic method informs, unconsciously as it were, all the other group activities. Numerous and varied, these unfold in a spontaneous and ordinary way, but within the organized temporal and spatial framework, and with their own justification, so to speak. The patient can be invited to take part in them; he must not be pressured to: his free choice is often significant and is always indispensable to the free progress of the therapy.

As they become objects of transference and often havens of resistance, the groups of patients formed around playful or productive activities must preserve their institutional flexibility, a quality without which occurences of therapeutic progress would not be possible. This flexibility is obtained in an institutional setup by means of the democratic and cooperative doings of the club and its organs, so that the institution becomes the pole of ordered security and the concrete activities, the poles of free existence. [...]

I still need to emphasize that the proliferation of group activities within the hospital—including those with a form of group analytical psychotherapy, the psychodrama or the analytical therapies that may be attached to certain weekly meetings of the ward cooperatives, or the internal club newspaper—doesn't eliminate the psychotherapy constituted by the personal encounter between doctor and patient. This encounter is sometimes facilitated even where it doesn't take the differentiated form of the medical-office interview, which can be distorting or inhibiting.

And I need to raise the two theoretical questions which, in my view, the congress should try to clear up a priori:

1) Is it possible to establish and carry through a deep psychotherapy in a closed, indeed a carceral, environment?

2) Must one wait for an end to the acute phenomenon before undertaking a psychotherapy?

As to the first question, the experience of R. Strup with prisoners and our own with patients allow us to respond with a counterproposal. It is possible to bring a psychotherapy to a successful conclusion in any milieu, provided the period of care and the framework of the internal life of the institution are adapted in an appropriate manner, and provided one has a competent supporting staff, or failing that, one can be created. Every life develops within limits or structures that could be called carceral. What makes this framework inoperable to someone in its grip is their experiencing it with feelings of guilt, with reactions of revolt or frustration. The heterogeneity and neutrality of the hospital milieu compared to the past life of the patient are always helpful, whatever the manner in which one gives form to the psychotherapeutic approach.

I would like now to respond to the second question with even more conviction. The fact is, based on my experience and in my judgment, an integrated and integrating psychotherapy is possible only if institutional psychotherapy begins at all levels and on day one of the patient's stay in the center of care. The most serious mistake would be to establish in the closed center an "additional" psychotherapy coming from the outside, not integrated into the life of the hospital. This is especially valid for the schizophrenics. It is indispensable to the reconquest of inner sense that the concretely lived world presents its own cohesion of sense.[36]

François Tosquelles, "L'aménagement de la structure de la rencontre psychothérapeutique en milieu hospitalier psychiatrique" [Structuring the psychotherapeutic encounter in a psychiatric hospital environment], 4th International Congress of Psychotherapy, 1958 imagination or in clinical practice in Spain, and even Lacan's paper, "La psychanalyse vraie et la fausse" (True and false psychoanalysis), which the specialized press had announced as an important event, ended up receiving little notice because it was scheduled at the Universitat de Barcelona auditorium at the same time as a conference on psychoanalysis and religion that got all the attention. And the publication of it suffered the same fate, not appearing until 1992. At the time, the editors of the French text and its Spanish translation, done by Antoni Vicens, talked of censorship, since more than two hundred of the papers were published in various proceedings books during the years immediately following the congress, but not Lacan's presentation. Once again, as had happened in the 1930s under the Republic, the traces of psychoanalysis and ergotherapy in the collective narrative of what had happened in Catalonia and Spain in relation to Tosquelles's practice were erased.[37]

A few years later, Tosquelles would participate in another cinematic experience, this time in collaboration with the Mende film club. In 1961, Tosquelles had met the documentary filmmaker and writer Mario Ruspoli through Ruspoli's uncle, Gilbert de Chambrun, a militant communist who had collaborated with Spanish Republicans and who at that point was the mayor of Marvejols, where Tosquelles worked for the Le Clos du Nid association, which was founded in 1955 by the abbot Lucien Oziol. Ruspoli, close to Chris Marker, Edgar Morin, and Jean Rouch, shot a film in Lozère about the work of poor peasant farmers, titled *Les Inconnus de la terre*. Tosquelles then suggested that Ruspoli film in the hospital—what would become his *Regard sur la folie* and *La fête prisonnière*—and later, along with Roger Gentis, Tosquelles accompanied Ruspoli during the filming. As Michel Tosquellas recalled, his father considered *Les Inconnus de la terre* not a film about poverty in Lozère but a film that showed people with difficulties as a way to speak about people in general. Ruspoli's camera entered the hospital with the *cinéma direct* or *cinéma-vérité* technique, which emphasized direct filming and sound recording of testimonies in situ. And perhaps that was why the hospital's medical community suggested that Ruspoli, at the start of the film, read excerpts from Artaud about the erosion of the soul and *impouvoir* that, as Derrida wrote, was not simple impotence but the power of the void, the total loss of existence.[38]

rédigée par Jean Ravel
Notes et préface de Michel Zéraffa
Voix de Gilles Quéant

—

"LA FÊTE PRISONNIÈRE"

Un film de Mario Ruspoli
Conseiller artistique : Henri Colpi
avec la collaboration des médecins-psychiâtres
MM. les Docteurs Tosquelles et Gentis

Il n'est pas facile de parler des paysans pauvres : ils sont trop misérables pour être romantiques, et comme ce sont tout de même des propriétaires, ils n'ont pas le prestige politique du prolétariat : c'est une classe mythiquement déshéritée.

Sur ce sujet à la fois ingrat et brûlant, Mario Ruspoli, aidé de Michel Brault et de Jean Ravel, a su faire un film juste, qui tout à la fois éclaire et séduit. Son film est une enquête réelle, parce-qu'il a laissé parler ses paysans et qu'à travers leur langage direct, concret, ce sont les problèmes généraux du paysan français d'aujourd'hui qui nous sont immédiatement représentés : la maigreur des revenus, le retard de la technique, l'opposition des jeunes et des vieux, le conflit du groupe et de l'individu, l'exigence du mieux-être liée à celle de la liberté : devant nous, une conscience de classe s'éveille et se parle.

Et pourtant, malgré la tentation du sujet, ce film juste n'est pas un film sombre : une saveur, une chaleur, une clarté circulent à travers les images, les objets, les paroles, une confiance réciproque met une vibration vivante entre la caméra et ces hommes, ces paysages, entre les questionneurs et les questionnés : c'est pour cela sans doute que nous ne sentons ici aucun spectacle et que nous regardons ces images de vérité avec confiance, plaisir et profit.

Roland BARTHES.

Left, press release by Roland Barthes dating from 1962, in regard to *Les Inconnus de la terre* (*Strangers of the Earth*) by Ruspoli: "It's not easy to talk about the poor peasants: they are too impoverished to be romantic, and as they are nonetheless property owners, they don't have the political standing of the proletariat: it's a mythically disinherited class."

In the town of Mende there was an art house, or rather a unique cinema where twice a month, as I remember, they showed an art film in the evening, and the screening was followed by a discussion. Well, the room was always full and almost everyone would stay after the film … to hear Tosquelles, who never failed to do his psychiatrist-psychoanalyst number, but not just that—I think he was keen to give people a sense that what we had just seen concerned us all, more or less, and he was very convincing because he was so concrete. That's how it came about that Buñuel's film *This Strange Passion* was shown. It's the story of a jealous paranoiac, a kind of Mexican Othello, if I remember rightly. In the course of the discussion, someone asked Tosquelles if we had many paranoiacs at Saint-Alban and Tosq answered curtly, in his Catalan accent: "No, the *parranoïaques*, you'll find them sooner in the *préfectourres*, among the police." A general burst of laughter! Obviously, the whole prefecture was in the room, but no one took it badly—on the contrary. Everyone must have thought of this or that colleague. This said, there were in fact a few paranoiacs at Saint-Alban, and not just among the staff.[39]

Roger Gentis, in Patrick Faugeras, *L'Ombre portée de François Tosquelles*, 2007

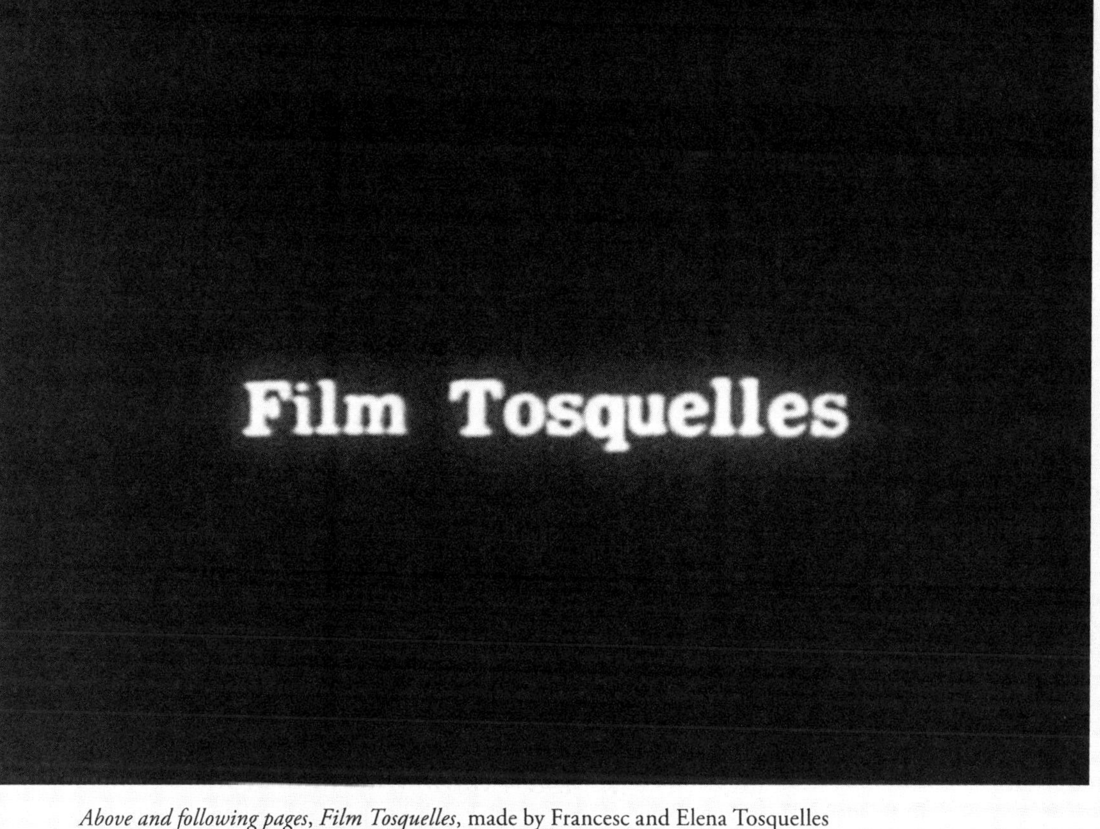

Above and following pages, Film Tosquelles, made by Francesc and Elena Tosquelles at Saint-Alban in the 1950s. The title cards, spread through the film, are placed here end to end and sequenced left to right and top to bottom.

En Lozère

Un vieil Asile
comme beaucoup . . .

Ça va changer

Ça change
grâce à l'effort de tous

Les travaux faits
par les malades dans les
coopératives d'ergothérapie
sont exposés et vendus
en ville

Social Thérapie à l'Hôpital
Psychiatrique de St Alban

Les maladies nerveuses s'expriment et s'organisent au niveau de la vie sociale et psychologique. Ainsi, n'importe quel traitement biologique ne saurait suffire s'il n'était accompagné d'une psychothérapie individuelle ou de groupe.

L'ergothérapie, les distractions, les jeux dans cette perspective médicale, ne sont pas de simples instruments de lutte contre la détérioration et l'autisme.

Permettant de par leur structure <u>coopérative les investissements</u> spontanés particuliers à chaque ma-

Permettant de par leur structure <u>coopérative les investissements</u> <u>spontanés</u> particuliers à chaque malade, ils sont l'occasion concrète de <u>l'engagement</u> d'une psychothérapie en profondeur et en même temps le banc d'essai de la réadaptation sociale.

Le Club Paul Balvet et se organisations coopératives de chaqu unité de soins de l'Hopital Psychia trique de St Alban est l'instrument de cette thérapeutique.

Ce film est fait de morceaux de la vie sociale de l'Hopital

L'imprimerie cotoie
certaines salles de jour
ou même de repas afin de
provoquer l'intérêt et
l'accrochage du malade
à la vie sociale et à
"la communication"

Le "bar", – par ailleurs "bibliothèque" – devient le lieu de "contacts" humains très variés constituant la source la plus importante des revenus du club.

Le souci de sa gestion devient

Le souci de sa gestion devien pour tous un organe thérapeutique de premier ordre.

Les nombreuses serveuses et consommateurs bénéficient ainsi ensemble de cette activité qui n'est

Les mardi, des concours "officiels", et les autres soirs, des jeux organisés ou libres réunissent au club de nombreux malades.

Les séances de psychodrame ne sont pas publiques.

Le club dispose donc de finances autonomes et peut faire face à tous ses frais de fonctionnement : 6.240.000 frs pour 1956. Il paie ainsi toutes les fêtes, les concours le cinéma, la bibliothèque, la discothèque les cadeaux aux malades entrants et la couronne de fleurs pour ceux qui meurent.

D'autres
"sorties collectives"
plus heureuses ...
mélangent les malades
avec la population rurale

Des nombreux problêmes
de comportement
s'investissent dans les
échanges psychologiques
et matériels
créés par la situation

La pratique des échanges
la transformation des
décors, des complets, etc .
constitue et tisse la matière
d'une sociothérapie active

Fête votive à l'Hôpital

pagné d'une psychothérapie individuelle ou de groupe.

L'organisation d'un hôpital psychiatrique en milieu de soins doit permettre une socialthérapie institutionnelle.

Les divers types de psychothérapie de groupe s'inscrivent dès lors naturellement dans les activités sociales de l'Hôpital confiées à l'organisation coopérative des malades eux-mêmes aidés par les infirmiers moniteurs qui coordonnent leurs initiatives

Le medecin peut ainsi anal-

Le medecin peut ainsi analyser individuellement ou en groupe le conditionnement du comportement de chacun à partir des faits, et des conflits sociaux concrets vécus par les malades pendant son hospitalisation.

de la vie sociale de l'Hopital ; simples souvenirs de certaines "Fêtes".

Il a éte tiré pour être passé aux malades eux-mêmes. Ceci explique l'extension de certains passages et l'absence de toute mise en valeur de technique psychiatrique

Le secrétariat du Club
coordonne toutes
les activités sociales
de l'Hôpital

Il est, de fait
un atelier d'ergothérapie

La rédaction
du journal intérieur est
une des réunions du Club
qui se prête le mieux à une
psychotérapie de groupe

premier ordre.

Les nombreuses serveuses et consommateurs bénéficient ainsi ensemble de cette activité qui n'est rien comparable aux typiques ntines".

Le théâtre dans sa forme traditionnelle n'est qu'un aspect des activités de la commission du théâtre et des jeux.

Au-delà des fêtes traditionnelles telles que voici, tous les vendredi, par tour de rôle chaque unité de

Au-delà des fêtes traditionnelles telles que voici, tous les vendredi, par tour de rôle chaque unité de soins offre un spectacle de son choix à la salle du club.

Les mardi, des concours "officiels", et les autres soirs, des

Parfois le Club décide
e se payer un spectacle
origine extrahospitalière.
tel ce Cirque

L'initiative, l'étude, et l'organisation de chaque Veillée du vendredi est un problème vécu en entier au niveau de chaque unité de soins.

Le spectacle est, toutefois, offert à tous au club.

Il s'agit d'un centre d'intérêt

Le spectacle est, toutefois, offert à tous au club.

Il s'agit d'un centre d'intérêt qui engage malades et infirmiers dans son propre milieu de vie concret.

En contrepoint, d'autres fêtes collectives typiques - carnaval, Pâques, Noël, Mai, Armistice, etc.. - élargissent et nt éclater les groupes restreints.

Lutte contre l'égocentrisme et solement des groupes-refuge spontanés s "quartiers".

Une des fêtes collectives les plus

Une des fêtes collectives les plus éfficaces est, à l'image des villages, la Fête Votive.

Un thème général est choisi en réunion du club. Des groupements mixtes s'organisent en vue de sa réalisation

élection d'une Reine du Jour, réalisation de scènes historiques de Fables de La Fontaine, c'est l'occasion d'un rassemblement général des visites et de mimes dans les quartiers de concours, de réceptions, etc.. entourant la traditionnelle kermesse

Les images qui suivent
sont de
la Fête Votive 1954

Film Tosquelles

La caméra surprend
le moment du départ
d'une malade

Ça a bien changé...
voir...

Pendant l'année 1926, par
exemple, seulement 35 malades nou
veaux ont été hospitalisés à Saint-
Alban.

Au cours de la même année,
10 malades sont sortis guéris ou
améliorés. Il y a eu 26 décès.

On peut dire qu'à cette
époque, les malades entrants avaient
à peine 30% de possibilités d'en
sortir vivants.

ONT AUGMENTÉ.
Les statistiques de l'Hôpital
St Alban montrent que les sorties par
guérison ou amélioration ont été:

en 1936 de 42%
en 1946 de 69%
en 1956 de 89%

des locaux de séjour n'ait pas augmenté
depuis 1926 et que les entrées de l'Hôpital aient passé :

de 35 en 1926
à 259 en 1956

FIN

Film Tosquelles

FILM TOSQUELLES

In Lozère

An old asylum like many others …

Which will change

Which changes thanks to the effort of everyone

The craftworks made by the patients in the ergotherapy cooperatives are displayed and sold in the town.

Social Therapy at the Psychiatric Hospital of Saint-Alban

Nervous disorders express and organize themselves at the level of social and psychological life. Thus, no biological treatment would suffice if it wasn't accompanied by individual or group psychotherapy.

The organization of a psychiatric hospital in an environment of care must enable an institutional social therapy.

The various types of group psychotherapy are naturally incorporated in social activities entrusted to the cooperative organization of the patients themselves, aided by the monitoring nurses who coordinate their initiatives.

The doctor can thus analyze individually or in a group the behavioral conditioning of individuals based on facts, and the social conflicts experienced by patients during their hospitalization.

The ergotherapy, the entertainments, the games, are not simply instruments of struggle against deterioration and autism.

Through their cooperative structure, enabling the spontaneous involvements peculiar to each patient, they are the concrete occasion for the engagement of a deep psychotherapy and at the same time for a testing of social readaptation.

The Club Paul-Balvet and its cooperative organizations from each care unit of the Saint-Alban psychiatric hospital are the instrument of this therapeutics. This film is composed of bits of the social life, mere mementos of certain "fetes."

It was made for the patients themselves to watch. This explains the extended length of certain segments and the absence of any highlighting of psychiatric techniques.

Translation of the intertitles from *Film Tosquelles*, or *Société Lozérienne d'Hygiène Mentale*, Saint-Alban, 1958.

The secretariat of the club coordinates all the social activities of the hospital. It is actually an ergotherapy workshop.

Production of the internal newspaper is one of the meetings of the club that best lends itself to a group psychotherapy.

The printshop rubs shoulders with certain dayrooms and even the dining hall in order to draw the patient's interest and engagement in the social life and its "communication."

The "bar"—and library besides—becomes the place for all sorts of human "contacts" and forms the largest source of the club's income.

Concern with its management becomes a prime therapeutic organ for everyone.

In this way, the numerous servers and consumers all benefit from this activity that can't be compared with typical "canteens."

Theater in its traditional form is just one aspect of the activity of the theater-and-games committee.

Beyond the traditional parties shown here, every Friday, by turns, every care unit offers an entertainment of its choice to the clubroom.

On Tuesdays, "official" contests, and on the other evenings, organized or free games, bring together many patients.

The psychodrama sessions are not public.

So the club has autonomous funds available and can meet all its operating expenses; 6,240,000 French francs for 1956. It pays for all the parties, contests, the library, the discotheque, the awards to patient entrants, and the flowers for those who die.

Other, happier "collective outings" mix the patients with the rural population.

Sometimes the club treats itself to entertainments coming from the outside, such as the circus.

The initiative, planning, and organization of each "Friday Evening" is a challenge faced in its entirety by each care unit.

The entertainment, however, is offered to everyone at the club.

The club is a center of interest that involves patients and nurses in their own living environment.

Many behavioral problems are expressed in psychological and material exchanges created by the situation.

The practice of exchanges, the transformation of settings, of sets of people, etc. constitutes and shapes the material of an active sociotherapy.

Saint's Day Festival at the Hospital

In contrast, other typical collective festivals—Carnival, Easter, Christmas, May Day, Armistice, etc.—broaden and split up limited groups.

The struggle against self-centeredness and the isolation of refuge groups on the part of "wards."

One of the most effective collective festivals is, in emulation of the villages, Saint's Day.

A general theme is chosen in the club meeting. Mixed groupings are formed to stage it.

Election of a Queen for the Day, portrayal of historical scenes from La Fontaine's fables, it's the occasion of a general assembly of visitors and mimes in the competing wards, of receptions, etc. ... surrounding the traditional festival.

The images that follow are from the Saint's Day Festival of 1954.

Film Tosquelles

The camera catches a patient's moment of departure.

It has really changed ...

note ...

During the year 1926, for example, only 35 new patients were hospitalized at Saint-Alban.

In the same year, 10 patients were released either cured or improved. There were 26 deaths.

One can say that in this period, entering patients had a 30% chance of getting out alive.

THE CHANCE HAS INCREASED.

Saint-Alban hospital statistics show that releases due to healing or improvement have been:

in 1936: 42%

in 1946: 69%

in 1956: 89%

This despite the fact that the hospital's resident capacity has not increased since 1926 and the admissions have gone from 35 in 1926, to 259 in 1956.

THE END

Inheritances and Legacies: Psychotherapy and Decolonization

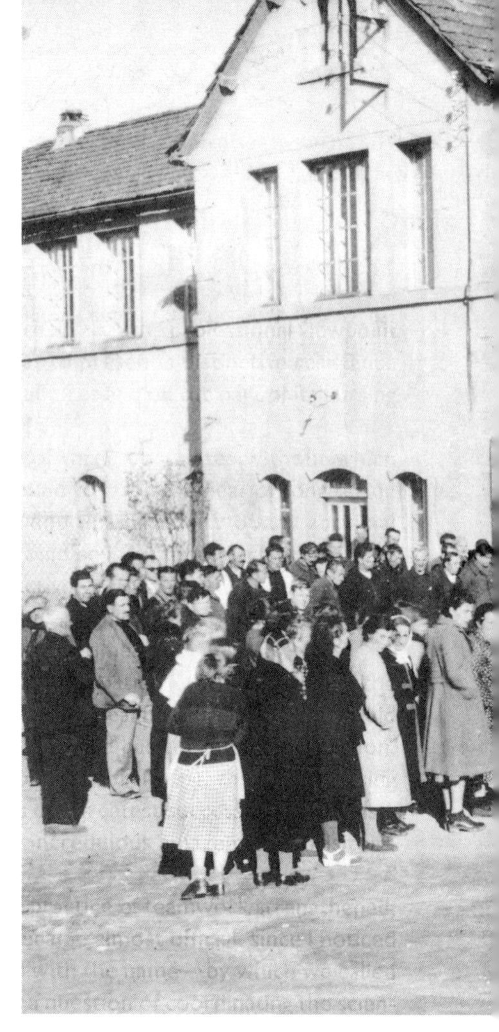

Between the experience of the psychiatric hospital and the experience of the rural world, the trajectory of Ruspoli's films traces the outlines of a landscape that accompanied Tosquelles from Reus to Lozère, as well as the psychiatrist, writer, and decolonial thinker Frantz Fanon, who as a resident doctor was at Saint-Alban with Tosquelles from April 1952 to August 1953, before going to work at the rural Algerian hospital Blida-Joinville. Biographers of Fanon have traced Tosquelles's impact on his work, not only because of the link between psychiatric experimentation and geographic decentralization, but also because of a shared way of interrogating the relationship between psychotherapeutic transformation and political transformation. This relationship materializes in the experience that Fanon had at the Blida hospital between 1953 and 1956, where he developed what he had learned at Saint-Alban while he began his commitment to the National Liberation Front (FLN) during the Algerian War of Independence. For Fanon, the possibilities of revolt in the Algerian revolution for independence and the translation he made in Blida through institutional psychotherapy are based on a concrete landscape: the countryside and the rural masses in struggle. Tosquelles, who always saw peripheral places as having the power for transformation, wrote that, in Frantz Fanon's thinking, the peasant farmers were the true driving force behind the Algerian revolt in the colonial context. When in 1952 Fanon arrived at Saint-Alban to do his medical residency with Tosquelles, he had already written the book *Black Skin, White Masks*—which he gave to Tosquelles—and two plays, and his clinical thesis defended at the University of Lyon the previous year. It wasn't until later, shortly before his death in 1961, that he wrote *The Wretched of the Earth*, the book in which he explained how the

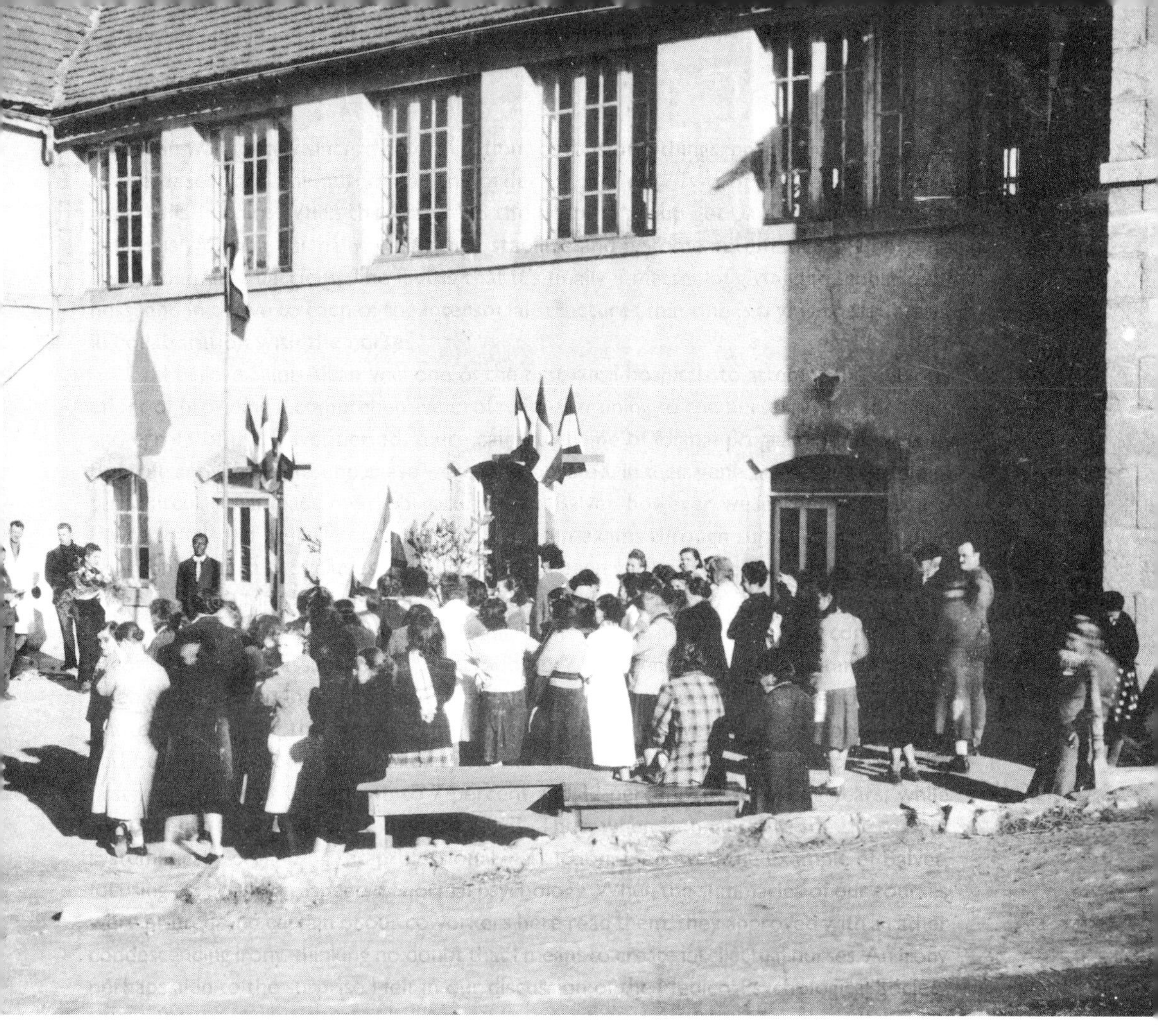

Ceremony at the Saint-Alban hospital commemorating the armistice of the First World War, on November 11, 1952. As a former combatant, Frantz Fanon (*beneath the French flag*) presides over the ceremony.

struggles of the rural masses for independence had been done without the participation of Algerian political parties and why their revolt could be a political revolt.[40]

Nevertheless, the common work of Francesc Tosquelles and Frantz Fanon did not discuss the revolutions they had each taken part in, as Jean Khalfa wrote, in countries where they were forced to think of themselves as other and to wear a mask. Nor did it discuss the forms of colonialism, a question that they both dealt with in other texts, or the decentrality of the places where they worked. The work they wrote together was a scientific contribution on the practice—already denigrated and denounced in that period—of electroshock (called Bini therapy). In July 1953, they together presented three lectures published that same year in which they shared with the medical community their experiences with electroshock therapy at Saint-Alban, always situated in the context of institutional psychotherapy. Those three short texts had one goal: showing the efficacy of that treatment when part of the institutional and therapeutic context, and when fomenting the inter-relational encounter of the patient with others, their implication in concrete actions that allowed them to rediscover themselves and discover the world, forming links with the collective life. For this encounter with life, wrote Tosquelles and Fanon, electroshock could be "complementary but not essential." What was essential was the *encounter* that psychotherapy allowed to happen. During many years, Fanon's psychiatric writings were not part of the understanding of all his intellectual and political work, because they were scattered texts that had only been published in scientific journals, even though his editor, François Maspero, had remarked that those texts revealed Fanon's proximity to the ill patients and the illness of the system that he was combatting. They helped one imagine the world he was fighting against.

Some people close to Fanon, such as Maurice Despinoy, with whom he had worked at Saint-Alban, explained how interested he was in his own research into lithium and biochemistry in general. But this medical part of Fanon's work has rarely been placed into dialogue with his more reflective writing, even with the texts about the experience of rethinking what he learned at Saint-Alban in a situated way in Algeria. As for Tosquelles, his clinical work had even less distribution than his essays, which are very little known. And perhaps the most unexpected aspect of these texts they worked on together in the fifties is that what was allegedly the explanation of a clinical experience ended up taking the form of a lucid presentation of institutional psychotherapy as seen in few of his texts: institutional therapy can only be sustained by maintaining a conscious relationship with the institution, preserving the heterogeneity both within groups of patients and in treatments, limiting the number of patients in each group, and thinking in terms of the scale of the institution and the lived lives that can take place within it.[41]

We emphasize that to treat patients with this approach one needs to give the greatest importance to the hospital framework, the sorting and classifying of patients, and the concomitant setting up of group therapies. The coexistence of the therapeutic workshops and the community life of the hospital as a whole is just as indispensable as is the stage of active, interventionist analysis that precedes the cure. *The Bini cure by itself, outside of this possibility of interlinked therapies, makes no sense to us.* [...]

PAUL COSSA—I would like very much for the author to explain what the expression *institutional therapy* signifies exactly.

FRANÇOIS TOSQUELLES—Yes, there is in fact an annoying confusion around terms: *ergotherapy*, *social therapy*, *group therapy*, and *institutional therapy*. Our general secretary is right to ask that we clarify the meaning of these words. Daumézon imported from America the expression *institutional therapies* to label the form of group therapy that is established, often unbeknown to the doctor, in psychiatric hospitals, due to the material organization—the psychological and social interactions between patients, and between the patients and the staff. It is evident that a therapy, if there is one, can claim to be a true therapy even when it takes place without the doctor's awareness and without his or her directives. Institutional therapy exists, in fact, only on the condition of this *prise de conscience*, and I would say, on the condition of an acquisition of power and control in the medical handling of the "institution" as regards all of its material and living components. So institutional therapy differs in this respect from group psychotherapies, psychodramas, instructional classes, etc., in that those therapies operate by means of "sessions" that are detached from the daily life of the patient. In "group psychotherapies," the doctor must steer the patient in artificial conditions of short duration, with a view to accessing the deepest part of their lived experience. In institutional therapeutics, one starts from a spontaneous, everyday experience and the therapist is at the same time materially absent and present in the clinical institution that in effect represents him. In our communication, we have given a concrete example of the dialectic of this presence and its role in the healing process.

I refer you in particular to the work of Daumézon and Koechlin (*Annales portugaises de psychiatrie*, January 1953); to no. 3 of *L'Évolution psychiatrique* of 1952, on the occasion of the Bonneval symposium; and to the related chapters of *L'Encyclopédie médico-chirurgicale*, in the process of publication. In this last volume, Requet shows how ergotherapy techniques, magnificently developed in the Anglo-Saxon countries, bear no relation to the concept of an institutional therapy.

Ergotherapy can and must often have its place within institutional therapy, just as insulin shocks and Bini therapy do. The same can be said of certain group therapies. But Daumézon often emphasizes, rightly, the fact that what is done in most French hospitals, under the name of ergotherapy, more closely resembles an "unconscious" institutional therapy on the part of the doctor than true Anglo-Saxon ergotherapy.

If we had to draw the conclusions from our experience of fourteen years of "institutional" trial and error at Saint-Alban, we could define the therapeutic requirements of hospital organization from an institutional perspective in the following terms:

1) Have the resources available to organize "life communities and heterogeneous treatments," for ten to twelve patients maximum. These communities should be linked together in the ward (three groups, or four maximum) and moreover—at a different level—should be connected with the whole hospital through the centralization of its shared community life. The life of the group should always offer patients the possibility of expression, and the possibility of therapeutic, psychological, or psychoanalytic utilization of their initiative.

2) Integration of ergotherapy into this living community, using it from the perspective of group therapies and institutional therapeutics.

3) Psychological preparation—by the doctor—"of the group" and especially of the nursing staff in connection with the concrete "case" that one plans to treat or help each other to treat. Ward meetings or the regular meetings of the "cadre" of nurses are the indispensable "organs" of this preparation.

4) Objective limitation of patients in "active" treatment in each group and each ward. The material possibilities of a ward of forty to fifty patients don't permit the "active" treatment or therapeutic assimilation of a large number of new patients—five per month per ward seems to us to be the desirable optimum. In certain cases, it can be exceeded and top out at eight. The physical construction of the hospital needs to take this major requirement into account. The admissions ward is a therapeutic sacrilege. It's a kind of choke point.

5) The classification of patients by "elective affinities," age, education ... etc. prevents any possibility of "progress" in the dialectic of identifications and mythical transferences that the patient establishes with the milieu. As a result, the "milieu" cannot be "manipulated" as a curing institution. On the contrary, the hospital ward tends to "freeze" the patient at pathological levels.

6) Any therapeutic psychiatric work requires medical teamwork ... There need to be at least two or three doctors collaborating closely in the "same life environment" to enable the dialectical play of most developments to proceed in the direction of healing. A single doctor cannot make possible the rapid resolution of most of the oedipal or preoedipal conflicts projected or embodied by the patients in the course of their illness.

7) All the activities—of the hospital—should allow the patient to maintain—indeed, push—their "illness awareness" to the maximum. Gradually demystifying the "approximative" ideas they construct about the morbid event and about themselves, the psychiatric hospital must be a disalienating institution.[42]

François Tosquelles and Frantz Fanon, "Indications de la thérapeutique de Bini dans le cadre des thérapeutiques institutionnelles" [Indications of Bini therapy in institutional therapeutics], 1953

The point of convergence between Frantz Fanon and Francesc Tosquelles was how they both listened to lived experience, which they both evoked through references to the phenomenology that formed part of the contemporary conceptual landscape, *Erlebnis* rooted in culture. Over the years, and unlike Tosquelles, Fanon clearly expressed his suspicions of the hospital and its concentration camp aspect. For example, when speaking of Blida, he explains how the presence in an Algerian hospital of two interpreters, of Kabyle and Arabic, to communicate with the patients who didn't speak French reminded all the inpatients of something they could never forget: that a psychiatric hospital, especially in a colonial context, always evokes the experience of other administrative institutions such as courtrooms and prisons; that a hospital always strives to shed the hierarchical bureaucratic structure inherent in all governmental establishments. As such, if Fanon wanted to make the institutional psychotherapy that he'd learned at Saint-Alban practical for the colonial psychiatric world, first in Algeria and then in Tunisia, it was due to the distrust the hospital institution provoked in him. In the essay he wrote with Jacques Azoulay, in which he presents his attempt to rethink the Saint-Alban experience in Algeria, Fanon situates his failure at the center: none of the institutional actions carried out in Saint-Alban—the newspaper, the theater, the cinema, or the ergotherapy—worked to heal the collective life of the Muslim men committed at the hospital. Western psychotherapy didn't serve Blida and had to be transformed; it had to become other in order to produce transformations in a hospital of colonial inheritance in the midst of an independentist revolt. Frantz Fanon began to implement the Moorish café and the evenings of storytellers rooted in the local culture. His essay "Social Therapy in a Ward of Muslim Men: Methodological Difficulties," written from the experience of failure and from experimentation with culturally situated strategies of transformation, silently formulates the question of ways to transmit and to inherit lessons, experiences, and revolts.

From this unforeseeable attempt at institutional psychotherapy in Blida, Fanon's essay reflects on the difference between an inheritance and a legacy, between receiving an inheritance and leaving a legacy. Fanon had to transform the inheritance received from Tosquelles at Saint-Alban in order to be able to leave a legacy in Blida. The difference between that which can be received and that which can only be bequeathed is perhaps the greatest lesson of the experience of institutional psychotherapy. A legacy that will be revived, intermittently, from Blida to La Borde starting in 1953, and in Reus starting in 1968.[43]

THE FREEDOM SCHOOL (II)

GIOVANNA GALLIO—We're very interested in this aspect of the Saint-Alban experience: the exchanges between the inside and the outside of the hospital …

FRANÇOIS TOSQUELLES—Those exchanges have been very important. There were people from outside who came inside whenever we threw a party, for example. I believe that if it was possible to try new practices at Saint-Alban, it's because there existed a relatively exceptional situation as to the independence of its institutional configuration and the whole Lozére region. Saint-Alban was already an open psychiatric hospital, so to speak, even before my arrival. It's comical, in a way; to go to the fair, the villagers would pass through the hospital grounds with their cows. The patients decided to wait for them and sell their crafts and artworks to the farmers. The so-called nurses, the guardians at the time, in turn would sell wine to the patients: in the middle of the rooms of the different wings, they would set up a barrel of wine and distribute it. It seems surprising, but later I didn't put a stop to this practice. I transformed it into something positive: profit from the occasion to create a bar, which became a site of psychotherapy. But then the bar was no longer between the patients' beds—you understand.

Moreover, for several years the Saint-Alban "guardians" would band together to increase their income by encouraging some patients to slip away. It was a law, in those days, that fifty francs would be paid to anyone finding an escaped crazy. What would you have done if you were one of these rural people? You would have helped the patients to "escape," telling them to come to your place. That's what happened, and then the patient would spend a few days of repose, *en famille*! Thus, in a paradoxical way, at once grotesque and comical, a collaboration between the inside and the outside was already a part of these practices.

I recall a story … At Saint-Alban, we put together a newspaper, and during a celebration someone had written a little article in which they said that things would never go very well till the prefect came to play pétanque [a Provençal game of balls] at the hospital, with the patients. A few days later, the prefect calls me and says: "There's

---

In October 1987, over the course of three days, a group of psychiatrists, psychologists, researchers, and senior officials from Normandy, Lyon, Geneva, and Trieste gathered with François Tosquelles in his home, in Granges-sur-Lot, to talk about the transformative experiences that had been carried out in French, Italian, and British hospitals in their various situated ways: institutional psychotherapy, anti-psychiatry, and therapeutic communities. The recording of this long conversation lasts twelve hours. A shorter excerpt appears in the previous part.

Excerpt from the dialogue between Max Auvray, Maurizio Costantino, Alain Dupont, Jacques Ferrages, Errol Franko, Giovanna Gallio, Max Lafont, and Marie-Noëlle Piednoir with François Tosquelles. "L'École de la liberté," in Giovanna Gallio and Maurizio Costantino, *Per la salute mentale, pratiche, ricerche, culture dell' innovazione*, 1987, pp. 73–100.

one of your people"—as if the patients were my private property—"that treats us like puppets and has no respect for authority." I asked him "But how do you know this?" "I read a paper …" "But didn't you see that it's indicated that this newspaper must absolutely not leave the hospital? It is written by doctors and patients for the patients, for psychotherapeutic purposes!" So it was he that was in the wrong, from a legal standpoint, and in relation to professional confidentiality! And so I told him, more or less, that if he wanted to spy, a true espionage, he should come and play pétanque, maybe bringing along some policemen, but on the condition that he place himself on the same level as the others and that he act a little crazy.

MAURICIO COSTANTINO—So did he come?

FRANÇOIS TOSQUELLES—No. That prefect came to a bad end … But it was to explain to you that people from the outside did come to the hospital, and that those in the hospital went outside. I'm not saying that these comings and goings were selected, but they were aimed-at objectives. For example, we had created a Mental Health Society, later becoming the Croix-Marine Society, which coordinated all the hospital activities (clubs, etc.), as well as the outdoor activities, although its "headquarters" was inside Saint-Alban. The administration of this society was given to a cooperative of patients, the aim being a kind of open psychotherapy. The donating members of this society were people external to the hospital, who paid a membership fee to promote and finance activities independent of the hospital administration, with the liberty to take intiatives that were outside the usual practices.

GIOVANNA GALLIO—In what year did that happen?

FRANÇOIS TOSQUELLES—It was at the beginning of the 1940s. At the heart of these initiatives, there was the tradition of the Catalan workers' cooperatives from which I took my inspiration. One mustn't forget that the Civil War was the outcome of a century of evolution of a social movement whose base was the cooperatives and the unions. But especially the cooperatives. Because in Reus, it was not just a matter of fighting the bosses, but the way in which one becomes a boss oneself. Consequently, I was inspired by my history and by the preceding experience, plus the history of the psychiatric hospital of Reus, which had been established on this basis of cooperation between the different members of the village, associated with each other. Fascism suppressed this experience, but later it reconstituted itself.

Furthermore, this inspiration was also responsible for the origins of the Saint-Alban hospital and the Lozère region, from 1820 onward; in this way, the cooperatives were grafted onto the local culture of a French *département* that was the least French of them all, as concerns the central authority of the state. For example, the prefects sent to Lozère.

There was no state in Lozère and the resident farmers knew it. At the prefecture, there were three office employees, who were the only ones to maintain a continuity and start the education of the prefects over again, since they would understand nothing about the rural inhabitants or Lozère in general. This deconstruction of the French state in Lozère was not the only characteristic of the state of war in those years.

ERROL FRANKO—When you arrived in France, a little more than twenty years old, what was your education, your training?

FRANÇOIS TOSQUELLES—My training before my arrival at Saint-Alban was very eclectic. Up to the age of ten, I would regularly frequent, with my parents, the psychiatric hospital of Reus and I had as my mentor the hospital's director and creator, who introduced me to all the theories. From a very young age, he told me stories meant to teach me tactics. As I was growing up, in contact with this experience and the struggles of that hospital, where I would later become a psychiatrist, I absorbed in Catalonia an international set of notions, including psychoanalysis. But even before 1931, when the first analysts arrived, we learned the different theories and the practice of group psychotherapy. For example, I remember that we would do groups in which one taught the patients not to have hallucinations and not to act out their madness in public. I remember telling a group of paraphrenics: "Hallucinate, go as crazy as you want, so long as we're inside here, but learn not to be crazy on the outside, with your family, with the police! Learn not to act out publicly, otherwise you'll be chased into a hole, locked up!"

My psycho-pedagogy was to teach the patient, in the group activities, to hide their madness in front of people who didn't understand it. "Here in the hospital, we can talk about madness, but on the outside, keep quiet, you're not going to say that you've seen the Virgin Mary …! There are some specialists who will never forgive you." More or less like that!

After the Reus experience, there was the war in Aragon, and in the army I treated more doctors than patients. The reason is that there were not many wounded; the young doctors who joined the army, without any motivation to fight, were worried and I chose, for a year and a half, to do a training course with them. They were general practitioners, surgeons … etc. People who would then have to go treat soldiers on the front. When the "reds" arrived, their decision was to exclude psychiatry from the army. Because, according to them, psychiatry was for the mad, and the mad didn't need to stay in the army but in the psychiatric hospital instead, like all the other—political and religious—deviants. So debates began, very heated discussions between us doctors and them. We, who were also militants, wanted to keep the psychiatric services in the army, not just for the patients but to support the staff of the hospital, to work rescue missions in the ambulances, to select soldiers for the different army units. In point of fact, we saw men assigned to tanks and machine guns suffer epileptic seizures; and others who, because they were ill, would fight in an anarchic and egocentric way, without any sense of the collective. Finally, thanks to a member of the Unified Socialist Party of Catalonia [PSUC], we succeeded in obtaining the recognition of psychiatric services as part of the Spanish Republican Army.

It was then that I was sent into Spain, after winning all the competitions, at a moment when I believed I would not come out of it alive.

It was in fact very harsh to do battle in Andalusia, in Extremadura, at Toledo—in southern Spain. But I was always disciplined, accepting things as they came, while trying to extract all the possible benefits from them. So I went to Valencia. I stayed there a year and a half and, fortunately, I met a political commissar, a farmer by trade, an old socialist from Andalusia. With him, I was able to fit perfectly into things, because he had a natural psychiatric talent, a profound sense of society that led him to tackle problems at their root. This being so, I was able to create a true field practice consisting of therapeutic communities, as it were, mixing soldiers with civilians, on the principle that the hospitals belonged to the people before belonging to the army. This real community structure that we built had its bases in the hospital and its mobile teams. Three or four ambulances would move around the battlegrounds and reach out to the distant bombing zones of the region. We eventually got to that point, and in a few days' time we were doing psychiatry "on site."

This experience was very important to me, because when later I arrived in France, safe and sound, I had developed a deep conviction: with the help and participation of ordinary people—lawyers, country priests, crazies, farmers, painters—in a short span of time, it was possible to create good psychiatric services. Only these people had an innocent position toward the mad, whereas those who had undergone a professional deformation—the "experts," the specialists in madness who had been trained at the school of classical psychiatry—were useless, were obstacles rather. Moreover, during the war, the psychiatric corps was made up of "conflicted volunteers," so to speak, while the civilians were volunteers who had chosen to participate out of a particular affinity. Among these well-meaning folks, I was careful to eliminate those who thought they had any psychiatric expertise, choosing instead those with natural aptitudes for being with others. Because otherwise one wastes a lot of time transforming people into someone who knows how to be with others!

In this sense, there's much less need of a high IQ to belong to a community team than there is of another essential quality, that of knowing how to live, to engage in personal exchanges, to get along with others. However, my psychiatry was something that no one wanted to hear about: neither the socialists, the Army of Catalonia, nor my friends.

And then there was the experience of the internment camp, which I talked about earlier. There, we were truly in a sea of mud and surrounded by wire ... and in spite of that, things happened ... The people were better because we knew what was at stake in order to make a man of a man. I think we had obtained a certain number of results thanks to this awareness of the mechanisms at play in the fabrication of a human being—I mean in their singularity, not in their quest for a social status or a role—as doctor or administrator. So, when I arrived at Saint-Alban, the circumstances were favorable. And then the medications arrived, and I'm not talking about the straitjacket because at Saint-Alban it wasn't used, none of the patients were agitated.

ERROL FRANKO—None?

FRANÇOIS TOSQUELLES—No one. The thesis written by Paumelle in 1946 or '47, done at Saint-Alban, shows this quite clearly.

MAX LAFONT—Agitation is often a carceral psychosis.

FRANÇOIS TOSQUELLES—Yes, exactly! But it's not enough simply to say "liberty," as Lenin said—I'm sorry, but my references are from all over!

So, it was a silly Spaniard, a university professor in Madrid, who in 1923 went to check out the possibility of the Spanish syndicate adhering to the Third International ... This Spaniard was a thinker: "I find that it is lacking in liberty, your system, my dear Lenin and company." And so Lenin replied: "Liberty to do what?" That made an impression on me: Liberty, to do what? Liberty always? Liberty, dear liberty. When I was a student in Barcelona, we would sing "La Marseillaise"; it was a revolutionary song; with those notes one took power. At the hospital we sang "La Marseillaise" to defend our liberty. We were all moved. When I got to France, I discovered that one sang "La Marseillaise" like Gounod's "Ave Maria."

So I have never been a miracles man. I've been a man, perhaps an opportunist, who has tried to do things in catastrophic situations. There are always signs of renaissance or the possibility of doing something. That's all there is to it. But there is a problem—and here I'm in agreement with Basaglia. It is difficult to do something with established social bodies, and especially with the established corps of psychiatrists! At liberation, in 1945, we formed groups in Paris. I was well received, but I was impressed by that whole discussion of roles, the "functionariat," in sum! I often had a chance to destroy the roles—the "private," the "public," "reconstituting the corporation" ... At a certain moment, I saw that for them I was in a bleating predicament and that I had to bleat. I don't believe in that now! Even my "confrères"—a word that gives me goose bumps—Daumézon and Ayme, whom I was very close to ... I think that for them, basically, defending the role, the corporation was more important than doing psychiatry.

I continued to work even afterward, but at Saint-Alban, everything ended in 1952. The death of the experiment coincided with its christening, when Daumézon named it "institutional psychiatry." The fact was that, in that period, we had a certain power, even at the level of the state structures. I even involved myself in visits to the École nationale d'administration [the prestigious French civil service training school]. I gave courses for the training of future prefects, as a way of influencing the apparatus. All that lasted till 1953, 1954, then everything was terminated. That was the occupation of the hospitals and the sector by classical psychiatry and administration. Besides, the sector never took hold in France. There is only a single sector, corresponding to the thirteenth arrondissement, which one can't even define as a complete psychiatric sector; it was formed because a private company financed it and because a team of analysts, led by Paumelle, the Catholic, began to occupy himself with alcoholics. And the state went along with it.

I think there were numerous unfavorable factors, because the reform movement failed. Before anything else, I think it played a crucial role in giving, at a certain point (recall the minister, Thorez), a new status to the civil servants. So when one falls into these statuses of the civil service, and whatever the status, one also falls into a defense of oneself and it's no longer a question of safeguarding the place, the space of psychotherapeutic practice. Because when I do something that can be called psychotherapy, I don't do it in the name of Tosquelles, based on the fact that I am a doctor or director. I am not defending a status. The patient has no effective contact with me as long as they don't forget that I am a doctor, or my social status. When I speak, not as a rich or poor man, but just as a person, they regard me simply as a subject, as a man whom they can deal with freely. From this point of view, the Italian situation seems more favorable to me, because Italy has never constructed a political and administrative entity such as there is in France: it's a state often in crisis, there exists a relative decentralization. In France, there's only Paris and the delegates of Paris. In this sense, I think I'm able to say that Basaglia's effort is rather similar to what I did at Saint-Alban.

ERROL FRANKO—Given what you say, one senses that you have a kind of nostalgia for the war years.

FRANÇOIS TOSQUELLES—Yes, of course. If it were not, unfortunately, that war produces corpses, you should organize at least one or two wars for every generation; in that situation, one understands things one wouldn't understand otherwise. One doesn't understand, for example, why a family is preserved, and why its members are always at war with one another. Because what I'm saying is that every war is a civil war. Now it's no longer the invader, occupation; now it's father against mother, mother against aunt, aunt against children, children against work: all the civil, discreet wars ... But what characterizes man is war.

ERROL FRANKO—For forty years, we can say that we have had the misfortune of living in a time of peace ...

FRANÇOIS TOSQUELLES—That isn't so ...

ERROL FRANKO—What I mean is that one senses how important this disorganization was for creating things ... But now, in the current social and political situation in France, what is one to do in psychiatry? For example, would you take the exam for specialization in psychiatry?

FRANÇOIS TOSQUELLES—No, I wouldn't. Besides, you know that even in my day I had many problems in trying to take the exam. They would do all they could to keep me from taking it and the rigamarole went on for years. I had written a thesis in which I tried to introduce the word Weltanschauung, an essential notion for doing psychiatry: the lived experience in which affect and intelligence are linked, the heart and one's reason ... The original impulse is translatable as Weltanschauung and not as cogito. The cogito eliminates madness and affect. "Madness is a thing I know," says Descartes. He spoke intelligently about it ... This is found, I think, in the "Fourth Meditation"—but the problem is the cogito, a glorious manifestation of the human being ... "Man is reason, reason that lights up the world."

Thus, one of the first things I tried to do at Saint-Alban was to introduce *Weltanschauung* and *Gestalt*. Bonnafé and others liked Gestalt theory very much. But Gestalt psychology results from the work of psychologists on perception that is stable, that doesn't change, doesn't move. As long as the Gestalt theorists remained in Germany, perception remained stable, but when a certain number of them arrived in Barcelona—and especially in the United States—it started to move. And it wasn't only in a single case. Because the Americans had invented cinema, and the Catalans had invented cinema and surrealist painting.

However, this mobile perception gave a lot of difficulty to Bonnafé. There are many people who want fixed, stable things, said once and for all—photographs, in sum. And there are those who prefer, on the contrary, cinema, movement. Bonnafé not only didn't want to listen to the Germans—who were our enemies—but not to the Catalans either.

The word *Gestaltum* (it's what they say in Catalan) is untranslatable: it doesn't refer to form, but to the process of a thing that does the forming, that creates form. Consequently, a movement, a rhythm, if you will. Ultimately, like in Rorschach inkblots, the world is a chaos. The Rorschach inkblots make no sense. And one who looks, one who gives form, overall or in detail, beginning with his or her rhythm, "applies" the words to the blot when they say: "Ah! This is a table." By saying the word, they make a tabula rasa of all the preceding impressions and thus modify it …

Hence the French, when they want to make the children go to school, they say: "You to the right, you to the left … Let's get going …" But all this movement comes from the exterior, whereas the *Gestaltum* comes from a feeling of the child's own activity, which originates in them: the child feels the need to give form to their rhythm. And in this way, for example, when there is a loss of the feeling of activity, as concerns the disturbances in schizophrenia, that doesn't mean the schizophrenic doesn't move about, is not active. On the contrary, it signifies that they move like a dead weight. It means the schizophrenic doesn't perceive their rhythms as the source of their movement, and they attribute them to an external force: "It is the hallucination that makes me do something or is it my enemies that oblige me to …?" In short, we all have inside us the source of rhythms, whether cardiac or those of the nervous system, or … Everything proceeds by way of rhythms, diverse rythms. And these rhythms, which in themselves don't mean anything, are the basis of what will lead to the creation of forms. The Gestalt is precisely the result of your own rhythm.

ERROL FRANKO—Where what matters is not the form, but the action of forming.

FRANÇOIS TOSQUELLES—Yes, it's the action of forming. That eludes Cartesian thought and, of course, the structures of the "Royal" Academy of the French language, which is the way to keep people from thinking, from reflecting for their own benefit. You must think properly, think correctly. That said, you need to think as your professors want you to think and not according to the movement of your creative thought. Only a few poets and a few crazies escape this imposition … The crazy is bound to fail, the poet will cook up some things … and that will be the only more or less tolerated way to protest against the society.

GIOVANNA GALLIO—Speaking of poets, in the 1940s, Saint-Alban became a meeting place and a safe haven for writers, artists, refugees, poets … Would you talk about that?

FRANÇOIS TOSQUELLES—It was starting in 1943, when Balvet left and Bonnafé arrived to replace him, that a profound change became possible at Saint-Alban. That year, the hospital began to take people who were escaping the camps en masse: refugees whom it was necessary to feed and treat with hospitality. During the German occupation, the French fled without food or much else, gradually selling the few things they had, losing members of their family in the rout. During that time, the hospital became peopled with crazies and strangers. The crazies placed themselves at the service of the refugees in the matter of provisions. There were political refugees, there were Jews. That year [in 1944], Georges Canguilhem and his family arrived. It was there that he wrote the last chapters of his thesis on *The Normal and the Pathological.* And Paul Éluard came with his wife, Nusch: a theater person who worked a lot with us, displaying extraordinary gifts with the schizophrenic patients.

Here another chapter opens up, relating to the role of surrealism in my intellectual formation and the life of Saint-Alban in those years, for I am Catalan and surrealism has a Catalan root with Dalí, and an Aragonese root with Buñuel.

The surrealists made an experimental movement of madness, something produced by society, showing the deep ties with sex, the drives, the libido. They brought Freudianism to the gates of the city, before it was transformed into a series of gimmicks for selling merchandise. It was the surrealists who experimented with the ways to make someone crazy, long before the illiterate Americans discovered, thanks to the gravity of psychiatry, that the family is fine with driving someone nuts.

The artists of Saint-Alban were surrealist, therefore, and it's owing to Bonnafé that this surrealist intelligence was put in the service of the practices. As an Occitan, born in Toulouse, Bonnafé possessed the critical strength of surrealism, and at the same time, the discipline, the stability of the Communist Party to which he belonged. Actually, in those years, the forces of the Communist Party were on the side of living things: a natural, authentic, and unique collection of French anti-fascists, the only organized collective force. So it was through Bonnafé that the artists, the surrealists and Éluard, who was his friend, arrived at Saint-Alban. Numerous writers and intellectuals of the French Resistance were connected with the new Éditions de Minuit whose offices were at Aurillac, on the road to Saint-Alban. So everyone stopped off at the hospital, which had become a magnet that received the different wayfarers.

Bonnafé was also a friend of the director of the psychiatric hospital of Rodez, not far from Saint-Alban, where Antonin Artaud was hospitalized, seriously ill. When I met him, Artaud was mute: utter silence, broken only by outbursts, inarticulate cries with which he apostrophized invisible beings. No one at the time still believed Artaud could get well. Even so, I was called in, with a colleague, to do something. To try and unblock him, to enter into some relation with him, we attempted to play chess. In the course of five successive games, I was able to stir him, jostle him, and he ended up telling me improbable things. One day he began to talk using the expressive motions of his hands, then he brought a hand to his nose and said: "Here, this is thought!" And he gave me a completely empty look. As if to say that thought was the death of his brain, which was running from his nose, was snot. When the brain matter starts to melt, the nose runs, and if you can collect the snot, you have thought. That was the only coherent thing that Artaud was able to express. [...]

ERROL FRANKO—So I have this stronger and stronger impression of a state of affairs, always stronger than all the instituted places—

FRANÇOIS TOSQUELLES—All the places are instituted.

ERROL FRANKO—Let's say that now all the places are administered.

FRANÇOIS TOSQUELLES—Ah, that's a different problem. Cooperatives are places that don't get their standing from an institution, at least in the sense of having owners … No one owns a cooperative, apart from the cooperating members …

If we wish to talk about right, it's necessary to make the distinction between right and law … Right is putting something into form. Saying it differently, without the instituting of right, there is no possibility of existence. In Greek culture—which I prefer to the Roman—every isle has its law, whereas in Roman culture power is alienated to the state. That said, there clearly exists the need for a process of social disalienation. In any case, for this social disalienation, no need to do like Saint Francis … to quit everything … But I can, at least as a form of play, try to grasp the circumstances, the possibility of putting my own rhythms into form.

There is one thing I learned from an educator. I said: "Damnation! It serves no purpose to teach mechanics to an individual who will then become a postal worker, who will then work with paper and not with steel …" It serves no purpose to teach them one trade if they will practice another one. So the educator said to me: "What you learn is a law. In all that you learn, it's a law that you're learning." And that's what one does in ergotherapy: learn the rules of apprenticeship. Learn the reasons for the law. The mechanisms of the putting in place of a law. And then applying them; one can apply them to other objects, and to other materials, which in their interrelations create other types of laws. In a word, the kind of laws and exchanges that develop in the bedroom is not the same as in the dining room.

GIOVANNA GALLIO—Unless one only has a single room …

FRANÇOIS TOSQUELLES—Well, in that case we're in poverty. I have never been poor. Utter poverty is a misfortune but if someone doesn't have a room, they invent, they build it in the street, in the woods. They prepare different rooms and behaviors. That poor person has the advantage over the rich ones in that they are not "alienated in the home." They have to invent a social system for themselves in the streets and in the woods. If they don't, they're screwed!

ERROL FRANKO—That brings up the question of spaces: the existence at least of different places to organize, where encounters take place.

FRANÇOIS TOSQUELLES—I think that whether I'm laying the groundwork for institutional psychiatry, or not, one always starts from a blank page: you invite someone to use a sheet of drawing paper. What you do, finally, is to propose limits—the boundaries within which one can project or invent stories in complete freedom. You say: "Draw what you like, what goes through your head." You offer a space that's empty, but limited. So you offer a psychiatric hospital, or whatever open space. And with that you say: "Do what you want." And they see that, in fact, it's true, you don't criticize, one can do a thousand dumb things inside without anything happening. And through what one draws, or not, on the blank page, you speak, or not, and most important, you share a game in the sense of "if you give some numbers, we'll give some numbers together"!

I recall a young psychiatrist who had read a little Melanie Klein. She held that in sessions with children one had to play, but she, the young psychiatrist, had nothing for playing, just some colored pencils. So she suggested those to the boy, an outpatient, and he started playing. And because the psychiatrist remembered that Melanie Klein would say silly things during those visits, that's what she started to do. But they were by themselves, she and the child. At the end of the session, they had had a crazy good time. However, the psychiatrist began to worry about what the parents would think if they heard how the visit went ... She walked outside with him and no one was waiting. The secretary explained that the child lived just a few houses down from there, so the psychiatrist decided to go along with him and, once there, the mother invited her to come in and have some tea. They chatted, but no mention was made of what might have taken place in the consultation. Later, the boy came a second time, a third time, and said, finally: "Don't worry, doctor, I don't say anything to my mother about what we say here!" It's charming, isn't it? The child knows very well that adults live in a state of social alienation, live in nonplay. As for school, one goes there to work, not to play; you have fun only at recess, fun playing. This anecdote may illustrate something that seems fundamental to me: the necessity of creating zones of freedom. I say zones, plural. For example, at Saint-Alban, while we were in a meeting of the work cooperative, someone came to tell stories, partly delirious, partly sensible, about their family, their fantasies, their hallucinations ... So we said to them: "You see that we are listening to you, but we are operational only when we talk about the price of coffee, or whether the cloth should be cut lengthwise or across. But in the club over there, there's another group, there's also a notebook and you can write what you like, over there people will read what you've written; you can say anything that occurs to you, we'll do psychodrama, we'll be able to shed some light on this." That's the freedom of the space of psychotherapy, but if we are to preserve that space, we have to accept that one plays a different game in the cooperative. There is also a superego in the cooperative, but it is not the superego originating in the family, the fantasmatic one, let's say, in the sense of the cruelty of the father and mother who devour you or who say: "If you eat this thing, you die," or something of the sort. In the cooperative there can emerge a "pragmatic" superego. Someone has said that in the treatment of the superego one must find ways to soften it so that it is not a cannibal superego. Soften the superego.

When one says that the goal of therapy is the demand of the patient, well, that absolutely doesn't mean that the patient "demands," but rather that they want to know something. What they ask for—and what you can offer—is your strategy or yours as a team, of whom I would expect attunement to the art of living. Not circumspection or caution. In Catalan the term is clearer: "good sense" [*seny*]. It's that ability to capture the signal, the indications of something that is practically useful in my or our vital strategy. A series of pragmatic combinations of surmised possibilities.

MAURIZIO COSTANTINO—Let me recapitulate a little, but only to restart the discussion ... You said yesterday that if we are therapists we should recognize that there is not one place or specific places in which the encounter "must" necessarily come about, and where it becomes possible to begin to cultivate a concern with foresight, with finding the right direction, with the art of living …

FRANÇOIS TOSQUELLES—In working with a person or a group.

MAURIZIO COSTANTINO—At Trieste—and this is almost a hypothesis—this is linked to a particular situation that we have determined: the possibility of connecting the times of encounter and relation with a transformation of the institution. That is what enables us today not to have places of internment. I mean that now therapists, providers, can share with patients the risk of a path in society, without the coercion of a place where the danger can be hidden.

I'll try to clarify all this because there is a false image of Trieste, transmitted by the media, deinstitutionalization as simply a shuttering of the asylum: a deinstitutionalization that refers to structures and not to persons! For us, on the contrary, it was, and still is, a matter of deinstitutionalizing madness. Hence the necessity of inventing possibilities for encounter on a daily basis, which means—can mean—for both providers and users, the possibility of choosing between different paths, something that was certainly not primordial.

ERROL FRANKO—Me too, I wanted to ask a question that remained up in the air yesterday. All places, with their difference, may become places of encounters, plural, with a psychotherapeutic effect. I think that we agree on that point. However, I wonder: are there places that one must absolutely avoid? How can one recognize them? What can you say about this?

ALAIN DUPONT—I have the same concern, and I would like to know if the places we can offer patients can be "dispersed" in the town or city, places of people's daily life. And further: What places should be considered dangerous for people? Because you've described the psychiatric hospital as a space of freedom.

FRANÇOIS TOSQUELLES—No, I said that the patient had spoken of the psychiatric hospital as a "school of freedom," not a "space of freedom." I talk about a path in order to reformulate the conditions of freedom. In any case, I join you in saying there is no specific space, but a plurality of spaces—each with its own characteristics—through which that school of freedom is realized in different ways. As I said yesterday, each place has what might be called its own law, different from or in opposition to the law of Paris or of Rome. A law that regulates the exchange of places, of space. The placement of those intermediate objects that are pills, or the forty pieces of the game of dominoes …

And next, are all places the same? Even the places spread out over the city? The city is a mosaic, composed of numerous fragments: different places, more or less connected or juxtaposed with each other, and freedom consists in being able to move from place to place, from the center to the other parts, the neighborhoods. In Geneva, the lake, Mont Blanc, a bistro where you eat fondue … So the encounters we can have in different places with different people allow us to say: "That's me." If you fish on the lakeshore, you don't need to identify yourself, because you're alone, isolated. You almost feel like a prisoner of this situation, and if you have a walk around, you're going to say: "Damn, wherever I go, I am me." If you go to different places, then every time you get back home, whenever you reenter the night of yourself, you tell yourself: "This is me, I am the same!" You're defined as a subject, I would say as a *res-ponsible* subject: literally *res*, "the thing"—the placement of the thing. "Responsible" signifies that you identify with the placement of the thing inside you, whence your subject emerges. Isn't that true? At least as a metaphor …

That said, are all spaces equivalent? Could we begin a therapy on the Mont Blanc glacier, then develop it there? I've aready answered that we cannot fully develop a psychotherapy if we are isolated—on Mont Blanc, on a lakeshore. It's the subject that is missing. Despite this variety of spaces, the problem is posed to each of us: Is there a privileged, specific space? It's not a specific space, but there is always a beginning: in our practice, it's the first encounter. Without fail, there is a moment, a space in which you will find yourself with the patient for the first time, and the patient for the first time with you, with you or with a team. Thus, in practice, it's a matter of the first encounter.

The British have declared that psychoanalysis is a *training* and a *learning*. Training, as if one is preparing for a race. But at the same time, the learning of a technique—in short, an exercise. Well, there is a first place where a first encounter occurs, which must consist of a brief welcoming technique—one could say the expression of a certain availability that is not simply that of love: "I like you … you like me." In this encounter a *training* and a *learning* take place, separating the past, marking the past as the past and indicating the future possibilities.

In sum, there is this encounter with the client, their family, and whatever, in which the client provides something from their past—even if they don't say so—and their anxieties about the future—even if they don't put it that way. In which the client does a training and a learning that inevitably end poorly, with the client creating a certain tension … And then unexpectedly they take their leave, or you see them out, to go elsewhere, there where history resumes in historical circumstances and with different physical and human circumstances. But there is always a first locus. For this reason, the first encounter is very important for enabling the patient to return to the same place, rejoin their family, or look for … policemen!

And there is something I'd like to add, about what you were saying—that it is necessary in this place to exclude the blackmail of dangerousness first of all … But blackmail doesn't always have the form of violence. It would be relatively simple if this blackmail, fear, phobia only existed in violence. There is intimidation—doubt, phobia—in the pernicious action, in my view, of capture through love. There are many people … myself in my childhood and later still, I said more than once: "If you do this disagreeable thing to me, I won't love you anymore." My mother probably said to me: "If you don't dress properly …" My wife: "If you don't change this shirt, I won't love you anymore. If you smoke too much, I'll divorce you." Blackmail through love, I'm saying! Which can be even more serious than blackmail through violence, because it is at least as widespread, all but universal … In short, when we are in violence, everyone knows it, whereas love purports to be unique! I can't say no, because without love I would only be left with anguish, and with anguish, the only way out would be violence.

So let's say that the first encounter involves "training and learning," through which one needs to be skillful enough for the patient not to feel the blackmail of violence nor that of love, neither of them. If this first therapeutic encounter, then a second and a third develop with an unavoidable increase of tension, in spite of everything, if it proceeds to love, this provokes the need to go look elsewhere, you understand? On the path to the lake, catching a scent of fondue, you say: "Hmm, I'll stop in, have me a fondue, and go to the lake afterward ..."

There was a good Swiss film that I saw recently on television. This film shows very well that to pass from France to Switzerland, it's necessary to cross two borders ... What happens in the film, and very often in real life, is that, not without a dose of fear or heroism, you manage to cross the first border, the French one: they let you advance, and sometimes they're even nice, sparing you the castration anxiety, the inspections. But there you are, right in front of a second border, and in the film the Swiss police say: "Stop, no passing, go back!" And so you're frozen in place, between Scylla and Charybdis ...

MAX AUVRAY—It's a film by Tanner, *No Man's Land*.

FRANÇOIS TOSQUELLES—There is a "no-man's-land" where there's only one solution: you stay there and wait. You have to prepare some cheap shot to cross at least one of the two borders. In the no-man's-land, important—at times tragic—things take place. Love blossoms in the film. In any event, there's the possibility of passage, a possibility that counts because the unhappiness you experience in France softens in Switzerland and inversely.

To come back to the nonspecificity of space ... There are many spaces but only one is the space of the first encounter; and then there is the need to go elsewhere, and to go into other spaces there is a double frontier. Double, I would say the possible double castration. The customs officer, while he asks what you are carrying—the forbidden, the prohibited—he asks above all for your identity. You think he's asking if by chance you don't have a prohibited something, but in fact he demands to know who you are. At every crossing, he asks who you are. Even if he lets you pass through, you always have a kind of fear, almost obsessional, I would say, at least for me—that's the way it is.

It's the same thing for the patient. The problem that is played out in the encounter is that of their identity. Who am I and what am I doing here? You understand? [...]

GIOVANNA GALLIO—You've repeated several times the word "responsibility," which for us is very important. I have to say that we have used the word more and more over the past few years. I would like you to tell us how you understand this word, what it signifies.

FRANÇOIS TOSQUELLES—Let's speak seriously. I don't take myself seriously but we talk seriously ... To say to someone "freedom," or even to say "I am free or I will be free," means nothing unless at the same time I say: "I assume the responsibility of my freedom." Being free means becoming responsible. Freedom starts with ourselves: freedom and responsibility are the two sides of the same coin. A number of philosophers, of moralists, say that access to freedom coincides with access to responsibility.

All that is in fact serious. Off to the side of that, without denying it, I prefer to play, to do plays on words.

Responsibility; *res-ponsibility.* Now *res* is obvious, it's the "thing" or the "cause," it depends. If you say the "thing," you can think of something purely material. If you say the "cause," that signifies there is a collective judgment, the seat of a tribunal ... There are more people in search of a cause, right? A collective, a discussion team, that *cause*, that talks to see who is right and who is not right. The "cause" and the "thing": to have two versions and be able to play on more translations—French, Italian, Catalan—in Catalan, for example, *res* signifies "there is nothing," nothing objective, if you like—as those against psychotherapy say: what counts are the facts ... But then one is dealing with a nothing, an unconscious nothing ... or a product of discussion, changes of a group, of discourse.

Next, there is *ponsibility*. I don't know, I'm less certain and perhaps I'm getting muddled, but *ponsibility* makes me think of the position of one's body, the bodily attitude: one poses, like for a photo ... prone, seated, with a hand that ... that has to find your physical balance ...

Pons is the "bridge": not the command post, but the strip that links one side to the other, the passage from one space to another. In other words, the position of the body must adapt to the transition from one space to another. You know, the task of the king, of the pope, was "ponti-fical" or "ponti-fiscal," to make bridges, as in Florence the Ponte Vecchio ... In the passage from one country to another, from one space to another, there is always a bridge, with the risk of falling into the gap, there is an indispensable no-man's-land and at the two extremities there are customs agents.

The action of the psychotherapist is not to play pope, but to extend bridges. The client says a thing, then another, and every time, you must establish a connection, extend a bridge. Because the characteristic of the patient—and even of one who feels fine—is to be on one bank, then on another, and to forget the bridging. Women are better at building bridges ... Biologists say that women have a symphysis that makes their pelvis elastic so that the babies can come out of the uterus as if by miracle. So, yes, the gynecologists say there are women who have a "high bridge" and others a "low bridge." Anyway, voilà, that's what I do, a "fool's association," an association of nonsense, of silly shit perhaps, what Freud called "doing free association." I prefer to "fool around together."

FRANÇOIS PIEDNOIR—*Pons*, isn't it also *pondre* [to lay eggs], or *peser* [to weigh]?

FRANÇOIS TOSQUELLES—Ah, yes, weighing. Gravity, being gravid, pregnant. Producing a new birth ...

So we've already found three words, *pont*, *position*, *peser* ... You see, then, if one associates words and the contours of words, one is no longer fascinated by the one, equivocal meaning given by Richelieu's Royal Academy. That's why I say "fool's associations," there are not just things we freely associate with each other, but also the fact that each word itself is free: free to be serious or not, or to be a piece of foolishness. And so I say: "We give numbers, we say bullshit, we babble, we speak nonsense together!" And instead of "psychiatry" I suggest saying "foolaboutry"!

Actually, our listening should always be of at least two types because language always has a sound and always has a dual determination. What will be related about what I am saying—if something is related—will be the sound—that is, what you will be left with will be my sounds. The residue of my sounds that touch you …! Or something like that. […]

GIOVANNA GALLIO—I think that these things you've said constitute key points concerning the conditions for the practice of psychiatry … and yet, we seldom find them in the organization of the services. On the contrary, you're aware that today many services are restricting their boundaries in order to defend themselves from the demand: selecting, compartmentalizing, dividing up …

FRANÇOIS TOSQUELLES—In that regard, there was almost a war between Sivadon and me. At the Maison-Blanche hospital, one was obliged to receive everybody, but one day Sivadon decided it was more convenient for him to provide a service in which one would admit, after prior selection, only a certain group of patients, in this case, teachers. I told Sivadon all that was very bad because by placing together patients who had a shared background, no one would be cured. In fact, in order to heal, it's necessary to be in contact with someone of a different character and structure. Now, if we bring together all the teachers in France, or all the military people …

If Saint-Alban enjoyed a certain success, it's because there were people of every sort there: there were intellectuals, refugees, farmers. A dangerous limitation of the sector could well be that of bringing into the system of care equals among equals: the same work, the same education, the same affiliations. At Saint-Alban, there were people who came from a deeply heterogeneous region, characterized by a kind of permanent civil war between Protestants and Catholics, which corresponds to two completely different ways of being crazy [*délire*], of reading [*de lire*] the world, of reading spaces, God, the father, and death. The Protestants of the Cévennes had flowery schizophrenias, very beautiful deliriums, paraphrenia, paranoia, hallucinations in abundance, whereas the Catholics of the north were sick with what we call *schizophrenia simplex*—the thoughts of imbeciles, in sum; they neither said nor did anything worthwhile. Lazybones, there was no way to get them moving. You can easily confuse simple schizophrenia with stupidity, with the slowness of idiots, while the Protestants knew the value of speech, the creation of speech—they had auditory hallucinations. I have to say, if there was anyone who healed spontaneously among the Catholic peasants, this happened thanks to the Protestants of the south.

GIOVANNA GALLIO—So there was a diversity.

FRANÇOIS TOSQUELLES—A difference in the way of reading the world!

FRANÇOIS PIEDNOIR—"Liberty, difference, fraternity": that's what we should promote.

FRANÇOIS TOSQUELLES—I'm not sure. You know, I'm rather wary of moral values. The freedom we've spoken of is the counterpart of responsibility or something of that ilk.

And then, there is a freedom defined in relation to the particular law of each space, in concrete relation with the concrete law of exchanges that you can have. But, for example, when we speak of equality, I'm no longer in agreement because that always implies a uniform (black, khaki, blue). As a defender of diversity, I can't help but be against all that. There is tendency to put the uniform on, even onto this certainly more acceptable equality, including in terms of the equal opportunities offered to the different individuals, so that no one is locked into the fatality of their destiny, although this equality has produced its armies of occupation: the armies of functionaries, the "instructors" sent by the state to colonize the countrysides.

FRANÇOIS PIEDNOIR—Actually, I said: "Liberty, difference, fraternity."

FRANÇOIS TOSQUELLES—Ah, yes. I'm okay with fraternity, not without a certain reservation, because brothers are always liable to tear each other apart. As an only child, I didn't kill my brother, but I often dreamed of having killed my twin brother before his birth, so as not to have to do so later. These fantasies are more common than you think. They have, moreover, a scientific basis, for one of the tasks of the fetus in formation is to prevent other fetuses from forming.

In psychiatry, conflict between brothers is a pertinent topic: it's often a painful conflict, as it was for Basaglia, for certain French or Catalan psychiatrists. I tend to reach for the rifle in disputes with my colleagues ... So yes, fraternity, provided we readdress the inevitable violence between brothers.

ERROL FRANKO—I thought that we had come expecting farmlands and instead we get a hotbed of the French Resistance, the Maquis. We're going to leave here with that word: *Maquis*.

FRANÇOIS TOSQUELLES—The Maquis is very important and scary at the same time. You could say it in another way. During the Spanish Civil War, a union of anarchist barbers had a poster that made you laugh. There was a drawing, a caricature of a barber, and below it was written: "Let's organize indiscipline." In short, it said that the first thing to do is to create an atmosphere of indiscipline, to disarm the army, to take to the Maquis.

So, that's about it. There are pearls everywhere: pearls applicable to the core of our activity. Everything is not so amusing, but it's also by laughing that one finds the truth. A truth that doesn't even make you laugh is false ... Well, you've made me laugh a good deal and I think I've made you laugh at least a little.

ERROL FRANKO—That's for sure!

FRANÇOIS TOSQUELLES—Then you're in good shape for organizing our indiscipline.

WHAT IS TO BE UNDERSTOOD BY INSTITUTIONAL PSYCHOTHERAPY?

[…] Throughout my presentation, I will place the accent somewhat carelessly on a few theoretical aspects as they have been revealed to us with the passing years, and which were more or less clarified through the efforts of a large number of French establishments with various orientations and impacts. As you'll see, my aim on this point is not to define the practice in a dogmatic way, since I'm fond of saying that institutional psychotherapy exists nowhere and that there only exists an institutional psychotherapy *movement*, born and repeatedly reborn in the classical psychiatric establishments. Thus, if one only considers this already lengthy experience, one can say that the institutional psychotherapy movement results from the internal contestation of the psychiatric establishments and what they support. It ends up laying bare its original and concrete contradictions—those that are hidden and sterilized by the *immobilism of the establishments*, those that are solidified by a deliberately segregationist practice, aiming to create barriers, as artificial as they are artificially insurmountable, between the inside and the outside, between the social life of the city and asylum life, between the normal and the pathological, between the somatic and the psychic, between frozen statuses and accidental roles, between the individual and the group, between the family group and the therapeutic group, between the past and the future, between adaptive (ideological, scientific, or delusional) rationality and so-called unconscious irrationalism, between structure and history.

If one is not to spoil the therapeutic anchoring that one has a right to expect for every patient grappling with their own contradictions, such a movement in situ, as Moreno would say, cannot rush or evaporate into the aerial drift proposed a priori and abstractly or intellectually by a clever psychiatric *willfulness* that is obsessively predictive, benevolent, and oppressive in degrees that are carefully distribued by the scientific and social authority of the *leading* therapist.

Such a movement in situ can't result from an abstract baring of contradictions with no connection to the doings of daily life. Such a movement is above all—if you will—the precondition and effect of a *clinic* that, as Daumézon would say, can only be a *clinic of activities*—insofar as this action is connected, or at least *connectible*, to the hospital as a whole. Or I should say instead, more exactly (to avoid an idealist misconstrual, the trap of the totalitarian or pseudo-Gestaltist imaginary), that what is necessary first of all is to create action: the activities that break the artificial rigidity of classical establishments. All the more as we know that in and through this classical structure of the establishments, what one establishes is *silence* at every level, notably by creating and facilitating fragile refuges in silence, in the symptom, or rather in the

---

François Tosquelles, "Que faut-il entendre par psychothérapie institutionnelle," *L'Information psychiatrique*, no. 4, 1969, pp. 377–384. A communication of the 3rd International Congress of Psychodrama, Sociodrama, and Institutional Therapy, Baden, September 1968. (This text was written in French for the Baden conference, but it was not discussed there.)

silence of the symptoms, where the patients take shelter if not with deference, at least with an attitude of compromise, if it's not with an attitude of resignation. This is what is rightly called "hospitalism" and less aptly "institutional illness," since in these cases it's not at all a question of institutions but rather of anti-institutional establishments organized so as to prevent the emergence of the life of true institutions. [...]

To be clear, at our site we've opened things up to encourage the spontaneous actions of groups that pulsate and institutionalize themselves in the devolution of the establishment. For us it's a matter of the actions of and reactions to this tendency, embodied sometimes by the doctors, sometimes by the nurses, sometimes by the patients, or by everyone together, in a way that is discontinuous and dependent on spontaneous, chance combinations. However, in themselves such events are only anecdotal since what matters, what makes the mattering possible, are *the effects of breaks in the quotidian*, which becomes diversified and receptive to the permutations that enable the dialectizing of desire—through the play of the meaningful oppositions that are unveiled.

So one mustn't understand, as some have, our *push* for action as a desiderative will—to transform the care establishments in accordance with some more or less justified reformist "ideal." Our goal is neither a reform, nor a specific revolution of public assistance that would immobilize it once and for all in a new anticipated structure, thought to be the best. Our goal is *movement* itself, by which something of the patients' desire, overcoming its distortions and its occasional blockages, may gain access to speech. This obviously goes by way of its participation in the life of the institutions that come to light inside the care establishments or elsewhere. This is only possible through a certain availability and openness to changes in the constituted therapeutic milieus.

One sees, from my last remark about desire—more than an insinuation—that the institutional psychotherapy movement, at least in France, aims to constitute itself in reference to the Freudian corpus—but without sacrificing to a naturalism or a non-dialectical primitive materialism that would fail to acknowledge the process of humanization of nature in every human being. We believe, along with Freud, more radically spelled out by Lacan, that *the field of psychotherapy is the field of speech*. However, access to desire, to speech, is always mediated, indeed barred—if one understands "barred" not to signify a prohibition, but rather a hindering caused by social constraints but already at the start subsequent to the split, the gap or division—known to us via Saussure and the work of other linguists (this is a good place to pay homage to the Prague school)—that exists precisely between the *signifier* and the *signified*.

The whole problematic of psychotherapy places itself and develops within the field of speech, not so as to retrench into affective and even genetic positions—as one would say of military strategies, in positions prepared in advance, positions that the psychotherapist would help the patient get back to, the patient gone in search of lost time; it's more a matter of an approach that, given the lure of speech, of the welcome reserved for the signified, aims to reengage the play of permutations, of semantic shifts, which through the well-known mechanism of condensations and displacements (metonymies and metaphors, if you prefer) put the signifier at stake, so that it is through the saying that we must expect and hear that *it* is speaking, that *id* is speaking. So it's through the sometimes noisy silence of the symptoms that one can expect and hear *it*; one must hear *it* in its project, in its process of humanization through the laws of language that, at the end of the day, will enable an always more or less mystified verbal expression. [...]

There is no field of speech secreted by an abstract and solitary individual—themselves a social non-product, a historical non-product detached from *the others*. Delimiting domains of speech with *the others* is perhaps the essential task of institutional psychotherapy, perhaps that of preparing the terrain or placing non-constraining paths, paths that psychotherapy can go down.

But speech can never be simply an event of me and you, isolated from the social context and from any preformation ex nihilo. In the field of speech, one is never just a duo; there is at least a reference to a third, to a mediator, and ultimately to something that must be given the name of *institution* by contrast precisely with all the institutional qualities that are stifled for the sake of the established, be it the establishment or the state: nothing less than the subjectivity of desire.

One of the important theoretical tasks of our group was the one handled by Mademoiselle Michaud, who set to examining what we meant by "institution," and on that score, make no mistake: when we employ the word "institution," we have in mind the *process of institutionalization*—that is, the existence of those middle terms, or mediators, that institutions are; an apparatus, so to speak, likely to favor the dialectic of exchanges at all levels. Thus, one must not confuse whatever establishment with the system of institutionalization of certain of our services, most especially that of Saint-Alban, and the one that, with more internal coherence and with a more thoroughgoing theoretical development, was forged by the psychiatric team of the château of La Borde. So one must not confuse institutionalization in the sense that I have just specified with the bureaucratic setting in place of activity centers; whether these involve ergotherapy or even group therapy techniques or those of classical psychiatry in an establishment where everything is designed to prevent the kind of speech I've laid out. Despite appearances, these latter attempts can constitute impassible defenses that, if the need arises, prevent the development of, or divert into impasses, the process of institutionalization that is underway. That development has to proceed as the third term operating through mediation in the dynamic of exchanges where some element of desire connects and dialectizes with the other.

On the other hand, one is already on the institutional psychotherapy road when one facilitates, in a care establishment, the *different places* that may become veritable fields of speech created by the institutionalization of various activities. Among these diverse activities, I won't fail to include, of course, ergotherapy, ludotherapy, and perhaps especially the therapy that addresses and engages the level of the body: organo- or somatotherapy. [...]

Let me say in passing that the system of exchanges called occasional includes, however, an institutionalization where the doctor, if they play a major role, must do so in the cinematic sense of the word, instead of in the sense of hierarchies. Such a role will be played by them, properly speaking, as a "representative of representation" rather than as a "representative presence."[1]

It's only then that in this field of speech—through the symptoms, through the articulations of contacts and the interferences of the personnel and the patients as well, through the conscious demand, and above all through the mantles and coverings of language—something of desire comes to light and the position of the subject in the face of it can be reoriented in the direction of psychotherapy. [...]

In reality, the human being has always been caught between various processes of institutionalization. It is in terms of this coexistence between groups—where something heterogeneous at times, or often and happily heterogeneous, pulsates—that there is established (by the grace of instutionalization, I would say) the human being in their humanity.

It follows from what I've been saying that the concrete history of institutional psychotherapy can only, by definition, attend closely to the historical and concrete modifications of psychiatric assistance—I mean that of the care establishments. This is done and can only be done thanks to the actions that link together in time, and that do not have their consistency solely in the all-powerful imaginary of the doctor or the director of the institution or even some cutting-edge team. It develops through the joint, coordinated—which doesn't mean identical—actions of the care personnel, who for some unknown reason continue to be called "auxiliary"—auxiliaries of whom?—and the actions of the patients themselves. This conjunction of actions comprises, in fact, the elaboration of a strategy in situ. I'm not at all personally alarmed or scandalized, as was Madame Abraham, for example, two years ago, at Barcelona, during the last psychodrama conference, if I remember correctly, who exclaimed—in an aside, yet very audible by the plenary gathering—when faced with what was revealed in a convention speech to be a sort of conspiracy by French doctors: "But that is politics!" Yes indeed! That is politics, meaning that action of the human animal that, as we've known since Aristotle, is a political animal. We are not scandalized because in fact the conjunction of these actions can properly be called a political action, which obviously is not mechanically congruent (far from it) with the traditional models of the "politicians" by profession or vocation. However, "technical neutrality" cannot be based in its obliviousness. That supposed technical neutrality would then also be a politics, and of the worst kind: that of denial, the politics of the ostrich or that of Pontius Pilate. Refusing to see the political aspect of human beings, the real problematic of everyone's connectedness in the system of exchanges with the others, leads to catastrophes.

To us in any case, this appears self-evident, and we believe it is precisely through the articulatory play of these exchanges, as they come to light to some extent with others—through the creation of institutions and by means of those—that the human in its becoming sets itself dialectically apart from biological animality. We think that the so-called neuroses and psychoses are above all failed attempts or more or less heroic or more or less imaginary successes at recapturing such a process.

We don't refuse to draw all the consequences of such a self-evident fact. Especially given that our profession of psychiatry, grafted, if you will, on that of a more or less biologizing, more or less "veterinary" medical practice, consists precisely in facilitating the resumption, the reshaping, the repair, or the revision of the processes of institutionalization that are peculiar to every human being: that ill human being who comes to us with their symptomological offer by which they let us know something about their failures, their evasions, or insurmountable [?] hindrances in their process of humanization.

Now, for us this practical dependence is neither a secondhand empiricism nor an adaptive relativism. On the contrary, this dependence on contingency and events makes it indispensable that the therapeutic team can avail themselves of a very precise and coherent conceptual panoply. Without such a theoretical tool kit—*assembled in place, moreover*—psychotherapeutic activity would risk being bogged down at any time in a passivity of the "accept-everything" or 'nondirective" type, or getting involved in escalations of acting-out, brought on by hasty "academic" or "divinatory" speculation. Further, most often these two dangers appear in tandem. This is doubtless at such a level that one can say in advance that all institutional psychotherapy becomes possible only at the cost of creating, in the hospital, meetings with the care staff as a whole, where analysis of the countertransference of the various participants in the therapeutic enterprise can produce the desired results—with all the slowness and technical precautions that such an enterprise requires. However, one should not forget that such an action in situ with the care personnel can never be instituted in a magical way and certainly not in isolation from the overall movement of the nurses—as a professional grouping in the country or the region. There too, participation in an external politics in relation with the so-called professional training of nurses becomes indispensable. It's not a coincidence that all the doctors engaged however little in the "institutionalist" movement in France have in fact been very active on the outside in the nurses' organizations, notably in the long history of internships and activities of the CEMÉA [Centers of Training in the Methods of Active Education].[2]

The maturation that has resulted in France, in this respect, is not negligible. One can get some indications of this from the proposals that have been reported pretty much everywhere, when during the political-social movement that surged last spring, in many regions and without any coordination or password, the big problem of teaching psychiatry was raised anew. Very often, this problem has not been limited to the universities. Indeed, the proposal that appeared with a certain insistence was that of establishing "regional colleges," or even sectors where the training of psychiatrists would be connected with that of nurses. People almost everywhere talked about a core curriculum for caregivers, even of the opportunity for a certain nursing practice to produce psychiatrists. Recently still, Dr. Daumézon pointed out that practical familiarity with patients on the part of the psychiatrists of the "mental health centers" could be brought more in line with the real knowledge—often unformulated—of the nurses. [...]

Actually, if our movement presents distinctive practical characteristics, there is no doubt that it results, in a direct line, from an activity that has centered around the systematic creation in all the French *départements* and in accordance with a well-defined model of all the psychiatric asylums originating after the law of 1838.

We shouldn't be surprised, then, that behind the relative convergence that one can easily see, up to a certain point, between our movement and what are called "therapeutic communities," indeed between us and the anti-psychiatry communities of Cooper and Laing and others, one also finds numerous divergences, resulting above all from the real initial conditioning by their own classical history and—it goes without saying—by the cultural aspects peculiar to the period and to the place where they developed. It should be added that we don't mean to defend here everything in France that claims an affiliation with institutional therapeutics, but only what a good number of us, by accentuating the words or the label "institutional psychotherapy," would like in this way to mark a cleavage and distinguish it from the mere humanitarian modifications or improvements in the life of the hospital that seem to be deserved by today's patients. We would also like to note the ways that psychotherapeutic effects cannot be expected from institutions simply by a training in—so-called correct—community life.

Similarly, we must not neglect to say that insofar as the "psychoanalytic mode"—notwithstanding the special conditions of practice that are well-known—has modified the customary orientations of a large number of young French psychiatrists, a large number of them—in America as well—either have been led to reduce Freudianism to an adaptive rose-scented culturalism, or else been led to note, sometimes in consternation, the purely negative dissolution of care establishments and of any collectivity. That is, to be sure, when they have not been the contented victims of a simple narcissistic and counterphobic reattachment to their proprietary technique, sometimes going so far as to block any purchase on this purely negative destruction for the sake of a utopian, not to say delusional, individualism that is utopian or delusional, in fact, because it is focused on the image or rather the imaginary and the splendor of the ideal ego. Such psychotherapists often hold that an institutional psychotherapy is possible only because the only analytic science is based on the dual relations of doctor and patient. Even if on occasion they yield to the unfortunate [?] demands of our times, often by engaging in a few group therapy sessions, or even psychodramas, or staff training sessions, they can only do so on the model of a dualistic group psychotherapy, excluding without a real critical examination group activities centered on the groups, whether these be of Kleinian inspiration, or in the style of Bion and the school of Pichon Rivière, or of Morenian inspiration, or others. [...]

We don't miss the implementation of suggestive practices, any more than Freud himself did, but we hope as he did, saying this in so many words at the Budapest Congress, that someday soon the psychiatric institutions will be directed (but not commanded) by psychoanalysts and that—I'll say in passing—the patients inside them will get free care. One could conclude with Freud that there's nothing wrong with doing psychoanalysis in such institutions, or suggestion, depending on the case, provided one always knows what one is doing—always knows that what is in question, in so-called mental illness, whatever its origin, is the subject faced with desire.

We're not far from believing that Freud's discovery of the fundamental rule only becomes operative from the fact that it brings to light breaks in the classic discourse of the face-to-face in its "raw" state, or rather in *statu nascendi.* We don't mean to say as some do that discourse is always an act that surpasses the individual in the field of care establishments and elsewhere as well, in the patient's family, or in the free clinic, or elsewhere. This discourse, however individual it pretends to be, is sustained by language, which is always a collective reality; and in every institution a language develops conjointly with group development, with exchanges of every sort and the activities of that group.

Psychoanalysis, even individual or dual psychoanalysis, can only take place by working through this particular language created by the group. It's only by the occurrence of interruptions, crossings-out, repeated Freudian slips, that this analysis of discourse gains access to the unconscious. The analytical attentiveness of an institution or an institution as a whole must be practiced in the same manner. Such an analytical attentiveness cannot help but be collective itself, therefore—that is, the work of what Dr. Torrubia in one of our conferences called, perhaps in an approximative way, "analyzers of the institution," which certainly did not mean, should never be interpreted as, the work of a chief analyst, the possessor of a presumed expertise.

This is the direction that an institutional psychotherapy appears to be heading, albeit haltingly, undergoing in the course of its progress all the conditioning and all the vagaries of history. And yet it's a considerable advance that these vagaries can now be analyzed and recognized through analysis at the very level where they are produced.

THE LIVED EXPERIENCE OF THE WORLD'S END IN MADNESS: THE TESTIMONY OF GÉRARD DE NERVAL

[…] No project of transformation of the social apparatuses of assistance and cure in psychiatry achieves a coherent implementation solely on the basis of the "liberatory" impulses of certain psychiatrists. In any case, young or old, we were more or less disoriented or rendered passively inactive, before and during the generalized social upheavals that, all over Europe, as in other eras, were the daily bread of us all between 1936 and 1945. The uncertainty, the anxiety, and the questioning of the quality of lived human relations are of a piece with these situations of generalized open crisis.

An attentive examination of the various theories and concrete situations, which are found throughout the history of psychiatry, was incumbent therefore on all those who, like us, found themselves in the midst of or buffeted by extremely tragic situations.

I don't hide the fact that despite my young age, in 1940 I had a certain experience of psychiatry, indeed a relatively extensive familiarity with its international "variations," which in fact contrasted somewhat with the current habits of French practioners. However, it's fitting to say here, on the occasion of this work on the "tragic lived experience" in psychopathology, that my arrival at Saint-Alban corresponded to a staging for us all, but in a special way for me, of true phantasmagoria that, beyond a certain "end of the world" perspective, brought shimmering possibilities within one's reach: those of a renaissance, whereby one could become other, without ceasing to be oneself. This is doubtless what made more relevant our search for more or less analogous phenomena in the patients, and also made reflection on their scope more effective. It became evident that the catastrophic experiences of the world's end, often recounted by the schizophrenics, were not specific to those patients.

At the end of the war, certain members of the Saint-Alban team, Bonnafé in particular, motivated by the psychiatric as well as political issues there, drafted a series of seven communications, addressed to the Societé medico-psychologique. They summarized certain "critical reviews" written by the Saint-Alban group, of which I was the secretary. […]

In spite of the reservations we formulated with regard to work that called for the observation of the "concrete lived experiences" of patients, as they are expressed in clinic or in psychotherapy, we considered that in any case it was a matter of the advisability that all concrete relations beween the care staff of every category and the patients be established on the basis of acceptance of and respect for the unknown in human beings, whatever that otherness might be. This did not have to do with—or not only with—a moral value to be defended, but above all with the possibility of

---

François Tosquelles, *Le Vécu de la fin du monde dans la folie: Le Témoignage de Gérard de Nerval* (1948), published by Éditions de l'AREFPPI in 1986; republished by Jérôme Millon in 2012. Despite the oddness of certain formulations, we haven't made any changes to the AREFPPI text.

recognizing the narcissistic factor that is quite obviously so poorly integrated into the practical life of the patients in our care, indeed into the system of their conscious manifestations. Said differently, as caregivers, it's a matter of a basic receptiveness to some fumbling, around transference, that they always display when they, like all human beings, strive to establish relations with others, as they constantly do. However, the clinical problematics that privilege thought, speech, or acts don't exactly reflect all the vital dynamic architecture of each flesh-and-blood person in their concrete interconnection with others. Beyond the mobility and the shiftings of thought, speech, and acts, *it* exhibits the signs and impulses of a different, nether reality that is not always transparent.

There is not just exclusion or social isolation, indeed repression, that creates insurmountable obstacles to the cure. The more serious, diabolical temptation that presents itself to the "mad" is the temptation of so-called normality, paid in advance by the crushing of the subject of unconscious desire: it's the risk of social alienation of all men and women into the "cultural" machinations of the various societies to which they belong. Obviously, our own offers a good "consuming" caricature—with the objects of desire trapped in a role reduced to that of fetishes and thus scarcely capable of aiding the process of curing. Morever, our culture offers everyone the enticements of the ego, questing for power and independence. These are some of the true "discontents of civilization." The difficulties generated by this social alienation doubtless contribute to all the forms of madness as human existence. Further, if madness and the lived experience of the so-called patients cannot possibly be reduced to the "scientific" notion of mental illness, on the other hand, what comes to light at the level of the *vécu* [the existential] can open up the operational field of our work. From the start, the so-called *vécu* comprises complex structures, always in play, even beyond speech and thought—that is, assemblages that are actually "logical" rather than rational, at multiple levels. Consequently, it's on the basis of a receptiveness to the other so defined that the therapeutic treatment of madness seems to us to still be possible.

There's no doubt that medical discourse—in the wake of religious discourse—has had an opportune say, and must continue to be present faced with the complexity of the human phenomena of madness. However, the latter always go beyond the limits of mental illness. It's only from the radically singular and singularizing perspective of each human being that one can make sense of the pathological event. [...]

The frequency of catastrophic reactions in madness and the special dramatic character of these are consequences of the persistence of the struggle, of the defense of the person who previously got themselves into a position of inferiority through a partial or total isolation at the level of their structure as a social being. It's *under these conditions alone that the catastrophic reaction can become a failure for the person*. The effects of isolation on the general condition of the organism and its neurology in particular have been so thoroughly studied by Goldstein that there's no need to dwell on them here. But when one does this analysis in clinical psychiatry, *one must specify the frame in which the isolation is manifested*. The social isolation described by Follin and Bonnafé toward the end of the Bonneval Conference is best understood and registered in connection with the catastrophic reaction.

Hence the *Erlebnis* of the end of the world should not be thought of as an *image* reflecting *supposed real phenomena* of a psychism being annihilated. On the contrary, this lived event is the pure and simple manifestation of the continuity and even the surfeit of human efforts.

We have seen what there is in the way of image and movement of approach in our understanding of irritability as it appears in Heideggerian transcendence. We have also seen how psychoanalysis, while enabling a comprehension of certain developments and clinical manifestations of the existential experience of the world's end, proved contradictory and ambivalent on the subject of its human value and the place it occupies in the pathogenic event as a whole.

In reality, these ideas are based on an intuition of "non-value" applied a priori to the catastrophic manifestation. Goldstein's biological understanding of catastrophic reactions opens up an entirely different perspective. While enabling investigations at the level of classical medical biology, which psychiatry cannot and should not evade, it reveals in addition the human presence in madness. Apprehending pathological attitudes only as a non-value threatens to drown our scientific and human research, our therapeutic action, in preconceived ideas such as those of "padding" or automatism or even "morbid mental subduction." In this way, the freedom, the responsibility, the sensibility, and the energy peculiar to the deranged would disappear.

We believe, on the other hand, that the personal effort of the deranged remains invariable in quantity and intention. The normal human and the mad one are beings that construct themselves by taking heed of their being. In the drama of existence, one is born of one's own manifestations. Whenever the curtain falls we raise it up again, perhaps with anguish but not without energy. What *unveils* the human drama is not *constituted* by the picturesque succession of events but above all by the existence of the hero who, sweating with anguish, lifts the curtain to appear and be born into life. *The mad person continues this action without stopping.* Their efforts, their anguish increase, at least at certain moments of their pathological existence. They sometimes even take cognizance of this, something we do without noticing it (give ourselves existence as persons). Our body and society facilitate the task. The mad one must keep on doing it against their body and against society. Whence their thousand *tricks*, their appeals to myths and to the exaggerated forms of primitive existence. These have a human meaning. *Madness is a creation, not a passivity.*

I envisaged furnishing a new version of the life and poetic works of Gérard de Nerval, written from the perspective of psychoanalysis.

That boat was to remain happily in the harbor, even though for me psychoanalysis, or rather what comes out of its practice, constitutes a productive watershed, indispensable nowadays to any psychiatric practice, when this latter is seen by therapists as being inserted in complex processes that constitute the characteristic singularity of all human phenomena. The so-called mentally ill always testify to this … but in fact—as with all humans—in an ambivalent way, if one is to be honest.

In any case, beyond any occasion to broaden the space of comprehension of phenomena where the question of the identity of each human is raised, psychoanalytic practice clarifies certain concepts that are spun out into a clever confusion by a large number of popular cultural products. Among them, there appears the glaring fact that in the practice of relations with the other, which psychoanalysis deals with in its way, the sui generis character of every element or set of elements that enters into the games and issues of people with each other is reaffirmed. Namely, their specific character—in no way reductive—of *representation* of any element one may consider. Representatives of the drives, representation of words, and representation of things, as Freud said. In the functioning and structure of the psychic apparatus, it's never a matter of the "things" in themselves. It's the shifting movement of the "representatives" that form themselves into a subject with its occasional and lasting appearances and disappearances.

Psychoanalytic practice itself becomes "representation" that gradually unveils, within very precise limits, the linking in segments of the products of the art of memory that come up against its own impasses rather than the threats that would come from elsewhere. Under the weight of momentary impossibilities, more or less easy to overcome, certain "representations" double back toward and with other spaces, or else are abandoned in a loss that is more or less disconcerting and regretted. Experience of the consequences of classical psychoanalytic sessions shows however that in every case, these diversions and setbacks are actually temporary: *it* remains engaged in the situation in question—that is, engaged in a *re-elaboration in place*, that concrete place of the psychoanalytic encounter which continues for a long time, as we know, and where one aims always to reinsert hang-ups into the texture of the desiring subject. Whatever may be said about the gratuitousness and disinterestedness of the work of evocation that is pursued, while the objective remains confused and more or less contradictory, the specific thrust that forms the subject opens up the paths of becoming to the subject always in question. Every completed stage only constitutes a record of the passage, relative to the movement itself. Every transparency and every denial, indeed every occlusive coagulation, derives, fortunately, from the original precariousness.

The dramatic character of the events sometimes evoked in the course of psychoanalytic narratives, as well as their progression interrupted by different kinds of difficulties, the very content of certain misfires identifiable as symptoms, even what lies beneath the manifested symptoms, *only constitute more or less calming islets* of a troubling movement that surges forth without any real beginning or detectable end. One seems to be faced with a real catchall that braids and unbraids, ties and unties lengths of string without head or tail. The metaphor suggestive of braiding and unbraiding [*de la tresse et de la détresse*; *détresse* means both "unbraiding" and "distress"] seems apt for clarifying and sustaining *the setups, maneuvers, nets* for fishing, or ropes and sails hoisted in the face of winds, nothing more nor less than a real assemblage capable of transforming the energy and the blind dynamic of the winds that blow—the air of passing time—into the operational detours of a navigation that carries our corporeal boats, always marked and traversed in this way by language that is being inscribed there. This is what Freud meant by psychic apparatus.

It's true that the sound of the winds and the goings-on of men, the voice itself, often arrives muffled or stifled by the turbulence of the waves, and by our own fears. But it is just as true that speech always reawakens even when it has cuddled itself and nodded off on the smooth sands of happiness. Speech stays ready to resume upon the encounter with other men affected by their own vital suspenses. It's the same with all the thematic variations and all the awakenings, where everyone's activity and passivity make a nice couple, precisely by swinging together with the oscillations, with the changes in tone of saying and listening.

Often, in the course of psychoanalytic sessions, the impact of *various representations*—indeed the surprise of accidents along the way—fashions spaces and times whereby the discourse opens to the variations of meaning that the other throws in. It's there again that a certain meaning comes to the foreground, detaching itself from the many blanks and silences where it is rooted, and from which it seems to draw precisely from what the narrative is attesting. An amazing space of personal creativity, where the partners in the psychotherapeutic labor, conjointly and separately, never reject a priori that which the silence and even the blanks—that is, the sometines willful erasures—actually accentuate: the rhythmic pulsations that resonate all the more as in the space between the two and in the empty space, the subject of the unconscious desire takes shape, disappears and reappears, or else hides itself. It's in this very situation that the words addressed to the other, proferred in an ambiguous approach to the other, always traffic in a certain concrete representation of the desiring subject, which hopefully does not fall on deaf ears.

Without the attentiveness and possible interventions of the therapist, events evoked by the client or patient would risk looming up in discourse like fixed megaliths erected on an archaic desert plateau.

Perhaps it is in this sense that nearly everything we've recalled here about the formulations of Gérard de Nerval, or his friends, scarcely goes beyond the structure of the islet, without ever reaching the moving ensemble that could break forth in a true psychoanalytic evocation and follow-up.

Obviously, I've never held a couch session with Gérard de Nerval, at my home or at the hospital.

Even if I had, it's not just my respect for professional confidentiality that would make it impossible to reproduce point by point what that supposed ill person—or any other—might have expressed on the couch, with its procession of silences, changes of tone or rhythms, and account taken of my own interventions, and even those supposed as such by the patient in question.

As in other "cases" mentioned in the psychoanalytic literature, I could only formulate a few remarks about a theory of practice in which I had in fact been embroiled. The explication of our selected excerpts, reformulated in "scientific" terms, becomes above all an illumination of our effort to theorize. This is not to completely deny their value and the level of effectiveness of the theories in question, though I have to recognize that the function and practical effects of these theories, often formulated from an orthodox perspective, are welcome, perhaps especially for how they help save us from the temptation to abandon our faithful, and often dogged, insistence on persevering in the practice of a therapeutic relation, where the depressive oscillations and the after-effects of more or less divisive and persecutory impacts get to us. The purview of the psychoanalytic therapeutic relation never guarantees us a radical asepsis in advance, or even protects us from a reduction in prestige or in our expected recognition. In every theoretical reframing of practice there is a pause and a recharging of batteries, indispensable to the pursuit of our engagements. A shifting, too, of our own need for recognition, indeed of our displaced agressivity toward our colleagues in the service of an "idealized, even sacred" cause. There is a satisfaction in the very act of couching in a formal, logical, and conscious discourse something that apparently escapes our practice and thus becomes retransmissible and verifiable by other experiences of the same kind.

So I can't really report anything here in response to the structure and dynamism of the psychoanalytic narratives concerning our poet in his suffering and his singular existence.

The transparencies and deformations voluntarily formulated by Gérard de Nerval according to the requirements of his poetic calling, as well as the "gossip" of his friends, are inevitably insufficient for furnishing a coherent if discontinuous system that might be compared to a true text produced in the course of analytic sessions. The inadequacies and stereotypes that one could formulate under the cover of psychoanalytic "science" would border on the ridiculous, rather than constituting real scandals. How could one not sympathize—it will be said—with the sorrow of a child whose mother and father abandoned him, or even vice versa? Why would one not bear the vestiges of these separations, these wounds, dragging them through the years?

Perhaps it is less affecting and more technical to consider various differential thrusts, fixed in place by certain stoppages and suspensions cataloged in the distribution of the libido over the *corps propre*, one's own body, and on the body of eventual partners, more or less predetermined by our hero's labile and reiterated projections.

Some of these possible aspects have been addressed in the preceding chapters, and with the help of certain "scientific studies" of certain psychoanalysts, I have found it advisable, especially in the absence of information that only Gérard de Nerval could have supplied us on the couch, to forgo any discussion concerning for example "the poet's oral anxieties." And for the same reason, I haven't taken up the possible dynamic of his oral anxieties that, with their nuances, constructed a system of withdrawal or defense for itself, a real line of escape or a refuge from his own—masochistic or obsessive—anal anxieties, about which in fact we know nothing. And that goes as well, of course, for what the range of sexual relations, platonic or otherwise, might have been, coated with a semblance of how-to, of supposed adults, who would have reached the phallic stage? Besides, what would that have had to do with his poetic creation?

At what moment would Nerval have sought to reinvent his libido—which is always thought to be maternal—to spread it out if necessary on the symbolic plane, whose turnkey would perhaps be signaled by the father, no less invested with libidinal urges, which in the name of the mother, and acting as her "affects," would give a very *adhesive* quality to the more or less frustrated relations established between Nerval and his father?

Moreover, by putting aside if possible a certain "adhesive," "clingy" aspect, very helpful in fact, and organically dependent basically on biological relations established with his mother, is it not true that Nerval, like so many others, confused the symbolic plane, which links together interhuman collectives, with the splendors of the imaginary, or even with the more or less nightmarish "chimeras," that figure in his impotent, disillusioned reveries, hyper-idealized to boot?

Isn't it rather along this line of analogical transformation that displacement toward the distant absolute finds in Nerval's poetry an ideal, flawless blanket that might—now or someday—welcome him into its folds?

At what moment, then, and from this same perspective, do the "remnants" of a largely enshrouded culture, always in fragments and always taken up again by those pieces with some gleam to them, create in Nerval a new flesh for himself? Isn't it in this way that a certain magic—not just brought about by the cultural mood—operates in Nerval, in the form of those "pieces" of suffering flesh that he links and themes in his poetry? Doesn't *adhesion* to the mythical traces have the same adhesive structure in him that we have remarked on above? What representation is there in the drive-based and narcissistic economy, with its imprints of archaic culture?

Moreover, it's in this connection that I came to reverse myself in turn when reading Gérard de Nerval with pleasure. I started tracking the same myths he touches on, always in a sporadic and understated way. As a result, I found myself drawn more to the work of Jung than that of a Freud. And in this my attitude, which many analysts would consider as countertransferential, may reveal something about the basic problematic of Gérard de Nerval, which I couldn't do justice to with other "positions." With the evocations of a Jung often laid bare in his famous *Transformations and Symbolisms of the Libido*, I was gripped by emotions that probably correspond, as it were, to the effort Nerval must have made to accomplish his own "personalization."

Jung, as we know, talks about the work of personalization that we all have to do.

With that, however, I believe I'm distancing myself from the concrete work that only the practice of the couch—where Nerval never appeared—might have led me to. Too bad.

The erudition of a Jung in the area of myths and legends pulls its strings on the one hand from libidinous problematics in search of more or less fixed and unitary *representations*; but also and in contrast it pulls its strings from what occurs simultaneously and out of phase, in the order of *active narcissism*. As a matter of fact, it is the narcissistic problematic that is foregrounded in Jung, and we know about his groping practice with the psychotic patients of Zurich, labeled schizophrenic, more or less autistic, and in the old Freudian nomenclature, afflicted with "narcissistic neuroses."

The retreat into the mystical or mythical egg, propelled to the first origins—the omnipotent hatching of the egg that incubates and produces itself, appearing in I don't know what Indian tale Jung called our attention to—points up the narcissistic project that emerges as it were and acts as an obstacle to the fluidity and the opening to the other in the form of an erotic relation, conceived in its singularity.

The fact that Nerval is present in his way, like everyone, with anxiety, at the intersection of the narcissism in question and his own moves toward the amorous or sexual quest, should not surprise us. Besides, a certain quality of his suffering in these situations of intersection doubtless becomes the specific possibility of his poetic elaborations. It's for this reason that his poems, whose expressive tone seems so right, go in quest of a reception and a new sharing with all those who wish to accompany him with a certain attentiveness oscillating between fascination and lucidity.

There is some degree of a voyeur's real regret in me, in not having found the exhibitionist manifestations of the poet, to be frank—nothing that would allow us to detail the erotic geography of his body, which one sees, however, thickened and weighed down by time or else by undetermined metabolic problems.

Placed in the sphere of a psychoanalytic type of theory—as was already the case when one considered clinical cases defined as analogues of the aesthetic existence described by Kierkegaard—we can venture that in Gérard de Nerval, there is also a real arrested persistence, endlessly revisited, of the typical problems of puberty, which, one can say in passing, shrouds in forgetfulness the infantile conflicts of the past.

In any event, on the surface what presents puberty with a difficulty, or rather what is difficult in the so-called puberty crisis, is the challenging conjunction of awakened narcissitic dilemmas with the particular uncertainties about the chosen or possible sexual object. This double determination often turns the two problem sets into the opportunity for a deadly, self-destructive escape, since it's not always easy to construct satisfactory enveloping shelters under that menace. One has reason to wonder, in these critical stuations, what the mournful mirrors are, and what are the mirrors broken by the echoes of the nymph on the water's surface. We know nothing about the concrete lived experience of Gérard de Nerval. Nor about the succession of hopes often shelved, as in puberty, for later and later.

One sees, then, that an excursion on the terrain of a presumed knowledge deriving from psychoanalysis has contributed nothing that would have added more coherence to the fragments already gathered in the previous chapter. One could have saved the ink and the paper. However, I don't want this promised chapter with its relative emptiness to serve as a simple negation of the value and significance of psychotherapeutic practices based in that discipline.

What I've said is little, and perhaps a lot at the same time, seeing that in this way we have come to imagine a Nerval who would have gone awry, not in his poet's activity, but rather in what on other occasions I have called the "second coming out," into the social domain of men in process: the event that is the thing at stake in puberty, but that comes to restage in another context the crisis of opposition and the attempts at independence, or rather, already, at self-affirmation, that asserts itself between the third and fourth year, give or take a few months. This would be the "first coming out," from the family context, which even as a failure leads to different, very positive, developments. We don't know anything about this period in the life of Gérard de Nerval. And thus our references to the so-called Oedipus complex in his case could only constitute bookish add-ons. It's true that the Oedipus that comes into play around the first coming out in question furnishes the representative elements of an organizing myth, with variable but universally valuable advantages, very useful for fitting out our boats. It's much later that the overtures, the adventures, and the pubertal consequences push everyone beyond their own mythology and beyond the family conflicts experienced in childhood.

Let's recall that we have retraced in the preceding texts a few general lines characterizing an exit from pubertal problematics in the often-exaggerated form of aesthetic existence, which one encounters in our clinical practices, in the fleeting between-time from childhood to puberty. It is there that the arts of memory, seduction, and reverie—rather than dream—spin their spider web where one often traps oneself with the sweet honey of fine words. [...]

For us psychiatrists, this makes it possible to understand the human value of madness. The pathological events confront the man turning crazy with the collapse of the world, where, for him, it's a matter above all of saving existence. The mad one will do what he can, on the aesthetic, ethical, or religious plane. It is mainly this effort that the "psychological" symptomology registers and takes hold of in such a person. And it is *also* in this journey that we, in our task as caregivers, must follow him and assist him.

It goes without saying that the doctor must be something more. But before going into a study of structural and biological aspects, the psychiatrist must understand the dialectic that is peculiar to man's spiritual structure, as we say, as it is present in each of his patients, even if one runs the risk of a mystifying, identifying fascination with it. Not only that, or even in a more clinical language, as in the final page of *Aurélia*:

> "Why," I asked him, "don't you want to eat and drink like the others?"
> "It's because I am dead," he said. "I was buried in such-and-such
> a cemetery, at such-and-such a place ..."
> "And now, where do you think you are?"
> "In purgatory. I'm doing my expiation."
> Such are the bizarre ideas that these kinds of illnesses produce.

In this way, the mad person will cease to be deranged to himself, and this will enable the doctor and the caregiving team to guide the rest of their scientific and therapeutic efforts down less overgrown paths.

It's not through a mere superfluous, accidental metaphor that we have come to consider the existential experience of the world's end—sometimes that of time's end, indeed of the apocalypse—as being the *annihilation* or withdrawal of attachments to the "external" world and also the possible revelation of a different existential space. *Annihilation* with its violence, even with a return to a mythical chaos presupposed to be original, was already ascribed a positive function in Hegel's *Phenomenology of Spirit*, and for that author, it forms an episode or a passage regarded as indispensable to the constitution of new figures of desire always defined as *desire for a desire*, engaging in this way the fight to the death for one's recognition by the other, in every given context—and this, it goes without saying, operates especially in family contexts, where it's not so simple as it appears to get oneself recognized as a son by a mother or father, and so on, without talking about the difficulties of getting recognized as a being of desire by a father, a sister, etc. It's not simply a question of "family roles," but rather of *changeable positions relative to libidinal distributions in human groups*. The fight to the death was bound to remain hypothetical due to the simple fact that if the other dies, they will no longer be able, alas, to recognize us, which is the real objective of such a fight. The whole domain of the family becomes a heavenly green pasture rather rarely.

In narcissism there is a pole of negativity that simply expresses the withdrawal of attachment, indeed of libido, from social objects. Doubtless one can't define narcissism by this negative pole alone—although sleep notably represents what emerges as restorative satisfaction in the beyond of the withdrawal in question. The fight to the death against the objects and "their" desire, which we desire, even their possible capture in the nets of the imaginary, includes in the worst instance its replacement by a veritable void rendered narcissistically full of nothingness whose satisfaction lies in the very *desire for the vagaries of the desire in question.* It's in this way that all retreat into the devitalized shell could prove dangerous, as Baudelaire says, in the possible case of not awakening, or from the fact of waking up in an unimagined elsewhere. Therefore, the function of *annihilation* is inseparable from that of *transcending more or less closed situations or those thought to be such.* This is the context in which the so-called transcendence of the philosophers appears to be always at work in everyone in their specifically human functions. Without transcendence one could not even pass from one social group to another—even if these movements do call into play, at a minimun, a certain "annihilation," for the sake of narcissism, of the things actively at issue in the group one belonged to before.

It seems that the fluidity and, if you will, the capacity to exile oneself, the attraction of travels to and explorations of elsewhere, is the precondition of a certain health, but without denying the dangers and risks of this type of fundamental adventure to human development.

It is true that in the psychiatric clinic we sometimes note manifestations of *rigidity* and phobic reaction that appear to explain all sorts of displacements and changes in the spaces and the systems of interhuman and habitual relations. The same holds for adhesive and clingy tendencies, which it seemed correct to highlight in the case of Gérard de Nerval. It is probably in this case that the acting out of man's transcendent function becomes catastrophic, given the destructive potential of our system of defense against the fluidity of the libido.

The defensive withdrawal—agoraphobic in fact, in the broad meaning of the word—that the transcendent function produces attains its most extreme levels in the asthenias and in invasive boredom, which led to a true psychoanalysis in the raising and lowering of the curtains where all the scenes of life play out. This is how the obsessive or positively satisfied experience, once and for all, of the world's end was found to play a primary role in all psychopathological manifestations, *normal or not*, resulting from certain disturbances of the nervous system and its ancillary endocrine functions.

THE RESISTANCE: SAINT-ALBAN

LUCIEN BONNAFÉ—For me, Saint-Alban is placed at the beginning of the story of the OPHS [Public Office of Social Hygiene]. It is necessary to leave Paris. There are extraordinary anecdotal aspects. This has nothing to do with the story of sector psychiatry, but I still have to tell it because it's interesting; and it says a good deal about the climate of that period and about the existence of a certain combativeness in spite of everything. One fine day, we take the competitive exam; it's a residual or vestigial exam. This happens in 1941 and most of the people who entered psychiatry on the threshold of the war scatter, finding a way to make a living somewhere, or they are Jewish, like Lubtchansky. Follin, also in my graduating class, is of Swedish origin. He is not of a French father, so he doesn't have citizenship, he can't go into public service, so he assembles his clientele in Paris ... Anyway, we take this exam in 1941 and one day in the on-call room of Sainte-Anne, where most of the class is waiting, the news arrives that we've been appointed. One guy is sent into the ministry, where he learns how things stand: the postings are completed. At that point a movement of resistance expresses itself with vehemence, saying: It's unacceptable that the ministry appoints us like that, without regard to our rights, etc., so we'll do a demonstration. We all go to the ministry and say: We're not playing a game here! Mignot, who wasn't at Sainte-Anne, and who is an ex-employee of the AP [Public Assistance], which is not connected with our profession, was appointed to Saint-Alban, and me to Prémontré, a detail I remember. At the time, I wanted to go into the southern zone.

And then, I had good reasons for loving Saint-Alban, where I had been raised. I had been nurtured with the milk of the Beast of Gévaudan. When I was little, I played with toys made by the Saint-Alban patients and my images were the images of the Beast of Gévaudan. During the war of 1914, my grandfather, who was a retired alienist, had been called back into service as the director of Saint-Alban. And as a little boy, I had been fed on the spirit of Saint-Alban—it's something extraordinary! It's at Saint-Alban that my antiestablishment grandfather had once published a reflection on a reform of the law, saying that since he had heard talk of a reform of the law concerning the mad, his blood had begun to heat up and he was waiting impatiently for the moment when one would think to pass a law *for* the mad. When he was at Saint-Alban, he wrote savage reports in verse to the prefect of Lozère. I remember verses I read when I was little:

> one thousand meters up
> in this rough and untamed land
> the cynical administration
> sends us its mad from Africa

An interview with François Tosquelles, together with Lucien Bonnafé and Georges Daumézon, "La Résistance: Saint-Alban," *Recherches*, no. 17, 1975, pp. 80–95.

This was the big struggle against the deportation of the deranged (Daumézon and I made it a specialty later with our focus on the traffic in slaves: the deportations of the mad). So I had excellent reasons for going home to Saint-Alban. For me the Lozère in 1941 was perfect, it was marvelous.

We all went to the ministry, then, and said: Let's get serious! So they made a bombastic speech, a Pétainist speech: "It's finished, the good times when the French took it easy, smoked fat cigars, etc." You know, the talk one hears every day now, like in 1940: penitence, the consumer society, the love of pleasure, and all that. "And now it's over! Now the state is in control and will do as it pleases!" We said: "No, the state will not control, will not do as it pleases!" We carried the day, in fact, and imposed our choice on the new order of things, and that is how I went to Saint-Alban.

FRANÇOIS TOSQUELLES—Saint-Alban was founded in 1821 by Tissot, among twenty-five psychiatric hospitals in France and Belgium. He spoke a line that in many respects resembles that of the current anti-psychiatry. At the time of Saint-Alban's creation, Tissot recruited supporters, for example two locals, Gauzi and Rousset; he sent them to Paris to see Dupuytren, a guy who was anti-doctor as some people speak now of anti-psychiatry, because he was fighting against the bloodlettings, the baths, the purges, all the barbaric therapies that the psychiatrists administered. And this Tissot sent Gauzi and Rousset, Lozère countryfolk, to work for a year with Dupuytren, to learn what there was to learn of a clinical practice that was valuable from a therapeutic point of view. They were France's first psychiatric nurses ... The years went by, and when I got to Saint-Alban, I found the head nun of the convent, who was of the Rousset family, and a few months later there was a Gauzi offspring who was hired on at Saint-Alban.

[...] All this was a rumbling that had long preceded the law of 1838, which was already a way of integrating, of hijacking, this anti-psychiatry. Tissot was an anti-psychiatrist who would say: Hospitals like Saint-Jean-de-Dieu are completely absurd, new things have to be done. All the hospitals he created are anti-Saint-Jean-de-Dieu, with a discourse about the basic work to be done on the population; public charity, but often oriented toward the participation of users. The law of 1838 would co-opt this movement, but everything would depend on the way it would be utilized.

LUCIEN BONNAFÉ—So I arrived at Saint-Alban, where there was Balvet, who had been appointed at Lyon but had not yet departed. I succeeded Balvet, who had presented to a Montpellier conference in 1942 a very significant, very extraordinary communication: "Asylum and Psychiatric Hospital: The Experience of a Rural Hospital." It's one of the seminal discourses of hospital institutionalism, an amazing communication about the unity of the hospital, the process of the hospital as it dissolves, divides, fragments: each service is autonomous, there's no unity, etc. It has to be noted that in that period Balvet was still a Pétainist and had an ambiguous discourse, imbued with a certain ideology of the chief, which Balvet never completely lost; it's complicated, complicated!

FRANÇOIS TOSQUELLES—You ask me about Balvet. Your question, while not impertinent, presents something of a risk. What I'm able to say is very subjective, and I think Balvet won't hold it against me that I can't get out of your trap! Balvet, if one were to place him in the sort of ideology that identifies everyone, or rather hides them, had seen his way of being in the world. He walked through life (and I say this advisedly—even at Lyon, he would walk around barefoot!) oriented by a culture revolving around Proust on the literary plane and a political culture centered on a left-leaning Catholic ideology that produced the MRP [Popular Republican Movement], alas. As you know, many people of that persuasion fell into Pétain's trap, a masochistic one, if you will—all the more so since a brother of Balvet's died gloriously as an aviator in the war of 1914, which immediately caused Balvet to become preoccupied with the German language. As he gathered flowers at Saint-Alban, he would walk barefoot with his head full of Proust and his brother's airplane falling from the sky ... His wife, who was a psychiatrist, worked at Saint-Alban covertly and played a big role there. Already in her dissertation, Madame Balvet dealt with the social relation established between nurses and patients during insulin treatments, and this was long before I arrived at Saint-Alban. But at the asylum, she concentrated on botany, cultivating flowers in the garden scientifically, perhaps an interest she inherited from her father. So actually, I should admit that I don't know if Balvet walked barefoot inside, or outside, looking for flowers at Lyon. Basically, my point is that, whatever his political profile may be, it's quite possible that something essential in the perception of madness passes between Balvet and me.

Balvet received me at Saint-Alban in 1940, through a convergence of rather extraordinary circumstances. I found a man who was both anxious and open, bent on transforming that mess of a hospital, which had six hundred patients. When I arrived, I explored with Balvet how I could be useful in this transformation of the hospital, and he put the emphasis on the trouble he had meeting with Hermann Simon. He didn't know the man and asked me if I knew him. After the plane called France went down, in June of 1940, Balvet got necessarily busy during the exodus organizing a charitable welcome ... more than charitable, because it had major impacts on the hospital. It was the reception of refugees into the hospital that brought in this life from the outside, a teeming life, an atmosphere of catastrophe and universal suffering, which made the most authentic madness look almost trifling given the general panic. Balvet was enrolled in the Pétainist drama, but he was aware of that. I don't think I'm revealing any secret that might hurt him by saying that as Darlan was disembarking in North Africa, at the same time Balvet was writing a silly text to the interns, who were Gaullist, saying there was nothing to be happy about, he gave me an urgent call for a meeting, where he said: "You're not from here. With you I can say things. I don't want the French to talk this way, but since you're a foreigner, with you I can: What bullshit are we involved in now? Where are we at with this?" And from that moment—obviously it is very hard for anyone of us to leave the path they've traced out, to leave a sense of belonging, let's say—and starting from that moment, he calmly prepared his departure from Saint-Alban, and when he arrived in Lyon, he was not a Pétainist, but an active Resistance member. His case is not the only one, of course. Many have traveled the same road.

LUCIEN BONNAFÉ—When I arrived at Saint-Alban, Tosquelles was already there, and he had played quite a revelatory role. When I say the Popular Front, for us, especially for the Toulousian student that I was, it's the Spanish Civil War. The Popular Front and the Civil War are one and the same adventure, and the discourse of the people who lived through that is always our reference. The war was our school. During that period my work was with the Centrale Sanitaire Internationale—border crossings, the problem of solidarity, supplying medicines, doctors, etc. I handled on-call services in Cerbère at the time of the retreat from Spain, and did what revolutionary doctors do—which is to say, under the umbrella of health, I did a bit of anti-police work at Cerbère. It was an extraordinary experience to see how the hospital trains arriving at Cerbère station were greeted by the cops. It was a demanding job to deal with the cops, a really extraordinary load of crap. This experience of the Spanish Civil War was our fundamental experience, and as if by chance, in the Resistance, what is not common knowledge is that the whole military system was actually articulated and structured on the basis of the veterans of that war, something that shows very well that this whole ensemble of Popular Front–Spanish Civil War clandestine combat, etc., represents the continuity and fidelity that I mentioned earlier. So I arrive at Saint-Alban, where I find Balvet, whom I was succeeding and who had gone to pick up Tosquelles at the Caylus refugee camp, if I'm not mistaken[1]—following I don't know what contact with I don't remember which Catalan psychiatrist, who must have been Àngels Vives, I think. Vives had told Balvet there was a psychiatrist in the Spanish refugee camp. Listening only to his courage and his big heart, Balvet will go to get Tosquelles, will liberate this violater of nuns, this red psychiatrist placed in a camp by the French authorities of that era. It was a concentration camp, in fact; those Spanish camps were frightful things.

So Tosquelles joins the Saint-Alban staff and contributes many, many things to the asylum, including a deep knowledge of German psychiatry. Catalan and Spanish psychiatry in particular was a psychiatry instructed in part by books translated from German. German psychiatry exerted a huge influence on Spanish psychiatry, and that explains why Tosquelles would add Hermann Simon in German to Saint-Alban's library. It was a book titled *Aktivere Krankenbehandlung in der Irrenanstalt* [A more active medical treatment in the mental hospital], which Balvet's sister, a teacher of German, translated with the help of the Saint-Alban psychiatrists.

FRANÇOIS TOSQUELLES—I had crossed the Pyrenees on foot, with a briefcase in which there was an English grammar, the book by Hermann Simon, and the reports that I had to write every month on the psychiatric services of the Army of the Republic. With other colleagues (Peña, Sauret, and Marín) and associates, we had created a kind of therapeutic community for certain patients, during the war. I was in charge of the army's psychiatric service—not just the hospital, and that was a success: for two years, I took care of many other things besides the hospital—for example making modifications in the services of neurosurgery, where the clinical observations would be collected with a view to a future psychiatric research (perhaps in the style of what was done during the war of 1914 by Kleist, in Germany). Or further, I oversaw professional selection, and not only for the health services: it would be stupid to assign a tank or a machine gun, or give an army officer appointment, to someone who would fuck everything up. We tried to do something positive in this respect. As a psychiatrist, I was part of the General Staff, not for deciding if a particular battle should be launched here or there, but for articulating problems of mental health. For example, as an anecdote, the military chiefs would ask me whether in such and such a sector, they ought to accelerate the leave permissions, or if they should replace, for psychological reasons, a particular sector of the front, or whether they should decorate certain men or replace them ... We can call *that* sector psychiatry! And this sector psychiatry had a center at Almodóvar del Campo, where there was a psychiatric hospital of which I was also the director, although I rarely set foot inside. That hospital was entrusted to one of my comrades. It was a place for the trepanned, the mute, the reactive schizos, or cases of that sort ... But this made my action possible on several points of "prevention" or mental health in the sector.

Consequently, when I arrived at Saint-Alban, I was bearing something different than those I encountered there. Me, I came from a foreign land, from Catalonia, from the Catalonia of the Spanish Civil War. And in spite of my youth, I was already a veteran in psychiatry. The force of circumstances had it that since the age of seven, I was concretely involved in the services of psychiatry. It's a constitutional vice. When the Spanish war began, I was twenty-four. That included the four years that I was a psychiatric doctor at the Institut Pere Mata in Reus. It's rather exceptional, I believe, that in French history there is only Daumézon who found himself in the same circumstances: for some time when he was very young, he was a chief physician. I was more or less internal-external, since the age of sixteen or seventeen: hence, despite my young age, I was highly experienced. Experienced especially because I had had the good luck to have as my introducer, teacher, and friend an exceptional man named Mira. He wasn't a classical psychiatrist, nor a classical teacher—instead often a psychologist, particularly in his school of work, at Barcelona. He had said that if I intended to pursue my interest in psychiatry, if I was to deal with the mad, it was necessary first to understand "normal" men, so I would go every evening with the workers into the apprenticeship centers, doing professional orientation and studying the organization of work. Based on that practice preparatory to psychiatry, I rid myself of the notion of the basic strangeness of the mad ...

There was also German psychiatry, it's true. I had learned from Mira that there was a guy named Bartz who had conceived and realized a series of services that weren't centered on the hospital. That is, behind a hospital appearance, it would enable different forms, spread throughout the city or region, according to a staggered system of differentiated care structures. This informed our work in Catalonia, which had an autonomous government, so that in 1934, we had the opportunity to organize health services as we saw fit. The Generalitat de Catalunya had created a "psychiatric council" for studying the problems of organization, and the perspectives, both legal and functional, of psychiatry. I was a rapporteur to this council along with a guy who's still living, Fuster, for the organization of what was not called a sector at the time: in Catalonia we called it a *comarca*. The *comarca* was a geographic and sociological structure that had a very long existence. It was a very lively form in Catalonia, especially given that while the process of industrialization was centralized, if you will, in Barcelona, we can say that there was no *comarca*, no agricultural region, that did not have one, two, or three factories. The *comarca* was a Catalan tradition that only became administrative again with the Generalitat de Catalunya. However, after the political collapse at the end of 1934, over the course of a year, our Catalan leaders were thrown into prison by the Castilians and the right-wingers; and for a year, we weren't able to work as we had planned. So I lived through the first political failures of sector psychiatry.

It was by accident that I arrived at Saint-Alban. For me, another happenstance was the events of June 1940 and those that followed: the arrival of Bonnafé, of Paul Éluard, of Tristan Tzara, of refugee patients, of doctors that we hid ... The hospital continued to be maintained as an open place, truly open: whether a place is open or closed doesn't just depend on its walls. Open to the sector, to real life. Apart from the rural inhabitants, this openness was also a piece of good luck, somewhat. I wrote a little article about this with Gentis (Gentis spent five or six years at Saint-Alban).[2]

There was also the surrealist connection, which was a real factor: it enabled a mutual understanding to be created between Bonnafé and me. There were very ambiguous relations between surrealism and psychoanalysis, and even between surrealism and politics. One of the slogans of surrealism speaks of placing a sewing machine in a wheat field. It so happens that the Catalans had done this by putting factories in the fields, something that Monsieur Allais didn't manage to do in France after he said that cities should be put in the country and the country put I don't know where ... The problem is how to integrate madness into the city. It's obvious that madness automatically entails phenomena of exclusion, not just social repression, but I would almost say, paraphrasing Freud, primary repression. Certain people are tolerated so long as the madness is masked as art. I'm thinking—why not say it—of Dalí, and others. If a doctor leaves the hospital with the notion that he's leaving madness behind, well, he's mistaken; he can't leave madness behind even if he leaves the hospital; he goes into the sector, into the fields of wheat ... There was a fondness for the word *secteur* in France, a shared conspiracy by the administration of the establishments and quite a few of the psychiatrists who are deathly afraid when faced with the problem of madness. For them madness cannot be what is precisely at issue in a limit situation for each of us in fact, in the process of a man's singularization, to speak like Lacan. Naturally, this doesn't mean that all men are fit to be tied up or hospitalized, but that madness is constitutive of man. The mad that are said to be ill, are people who, for very diverse reasons, don't "make something" of their madness. Without this prior analysis of madness, sector politics, or to use the Anglo-Saxon blather, community psychiatry, construes the problem of madness as a simple mechanics of the inside and the outside. That seems less than serviceable to me, and even dangerous: for me, it's even comical that some have been able to speak of institutional psychiatry as an effort to "keep" the mad "inside"!

LUCIEN BONNAFÉ—Tosquelles is probably the main booster of the patients' club of Saint-Alban, but actually it's a collective enterprise. There existed a Saint-Albanese collective: Balvet stayed a month or two before leaving for Lyon. We cohabited with him. He occupied one floor, me the other. Tosquelles lived on the top floor, and there was Chaurand who arrived a short time before (after having mishaps with the good sisters of Puy, which was his home, where he had his family and everything). That adds up to a very collegial group. Balvet leaves us, but the collegial work at Saint-Alban becomes an astonishing reality, at least in hindsight. We form a learned society, so to speak; we call the Saint-Alban meetings "réunions de la Société du Gévaudan." The Société du Gévaudan produces and produces, and it becomes impossible to say who came up with what or vice versa, the collegial work is so intense and engrossing. The producer is in fact the Société du Gévaudan. It's truly a very collective producer. I was twenty-nine. We were more or less contemporaries, practically the same age; we were already seasoned combatants who had spent our youth that way.

FRANÇOIS TOSQUELLES—At Saint-Alban, our meetings (doctors and others) were almost nonstop. It was often necessary to wait for parachute drops of arms, or a clandestine visitor. So we talked psychiatry. Those almost daily encounters, or nocturnal ones, were what we called, with Bonnafé, the "Société du Gévaudan" ... In order to prepare for brighter days to come, we would talk psychiatry, we would review the basic concepts critically along with the possible types of action. In this way, we would analyze the psychiatric hospital, and we said, half joking, half serious, that it was a marquisate, the territory of a marquis. The chief-doctor structure was that of the castellan, with its tiered social classes, the nurses, the patients ... The paternalism of the psychiatrist looked to us like a self-defense that effectively ruled out any serious attempt at psychiatric therapy.

LUCIEN BONNAFÉ—The teamwork didn't just involve the group of psychiatrists. One can regard as a benefit of the Occupation the very thorough reorganization that was produced within the body of caregivers, the doctors and nurses. The Occupation played an extremely important role in that mutation from the *I* toward the *we* of the caregiving team. Under the Occupation there was an experience of fraternity that is essential, and not only at Saint-Alban. At Ville-Évrard, for example, that experience was sometimes tragic—when a nurse is deported, that hurts—and this created a very strong bond that marked people like Follin, Lubtchansky, Duchêne. Daumézon is emphatic about this: we have been among the killers of the *I*, of those against autocrats. We've engaged in a constant battle against the personalization of things. Of course, this process of democratization, of fraternity, has taken very diverse forms at the level of practical reality. We noted this very late at the time of the Sèvres symposium on the participation of nurses in psychotherapy.

Ontogenesis recapitulates phylogenesis, and psychiatry outside the asylum is the daughter of psychiatry inside the asylum. Historically, psychiatry was formed inside the walls of the asylum and would leave it to "do clinic" at Aubervilliers. It's the same at Saint-Alban. In the reports about Saint-Alban, the aspect that stands out as if by chance (and this is an effect of ideological pressures, which is quite remarkable and significant) is the *intra*-hospital work, whereas the other aspect of the Saint-Albanese investigations is unacknowledged, namely the *extra*, the external work of Saint-Alban. Saint-Alban was a leader in France of research into this kind of work: the work of disalienation from the hospital system as such went hand in hand with work *outside* the hospital—a development of consultations, a development of medical-pedagogical relations, a kind of migratory work that we called "geopsychiatry." At a certain point, the Société du Gévaudan had christened it as a psychiatry that exists only in relation to its insertion in human geography—in the raw. We referred back to a mountain-dweller tradition: in line with that mountain tradition, it was the asylum that would go and pick up the crazies when a notice came from the mayor saying there was a crazy to be locked up. In this wild land, a thousand meters high, with the Margeride to cross at fourteen hundred meters (in winter this was not easy, and often even in the spring, or in May, what with the snowdrifts on the summits), it was necessary to go get the new patients from the other side of the Margeride. And so it was that an amazing person who had preceded Balvet, by the name of Agnès Masson, had bought one of Citroën's tracked vehicles so as to be able to go pick up the said patients! It became a member of the Saint-Alban car lot. This tradition was put to good use in the sense of a new conception of public service provided outside the hospital, and we continued to go pick up the crazies where they lived. We would go as a team, and we would use the occasion to stop along the way for some ambulatory aftercare of certain patients. We would stop at a farm where there was a patient who had been out for a month or two, to do "bread and salt" together—that is, sausage with red wine—and talk about things. There was a whole activity of contact with the patient in their living space. It would happen, for example, that there was a patient to pick up at such and such a place, and a healed patient to drop off at home on the same route, things of that sort. We called that geopsychiatry. It was, if you like, the first naming, the first verbal identification of what a sectoral type of practice was, let's say.

FRANÇOIS TOSQUELLES—To Saint-Alban, then, I brought this active notion, let's say, this action project, into the *comarca* ... into the sector, let's say. It's obvious, as Bonnafé says, that the war events did much to help this idea take root at Saint-Alban: the work with the farmers, the gendarmes ... There were many gendarmes who had participated in the Resistance. We conspired together, to say nothing of some priests, notaries, etc. We also worked with the village doctors, the cinemas and film clubs, the families, we made home visits. For example, I taught courses to the gendarmes. There was a captain of the gendarmerie who had discovered that the first article of his gendarmerie manual said that it was a corps created to prevent the raving of the mad, following a tradition of the custodians of the hospital. He had been touched by that and had me come in order to try and change the systematic attitude of repression ... So I would talk with the gendarmes. Class collaboration! Why not? In a concrete situation, I need to consider what's adjacent to this institu ... to this situation. I just committed a *lapsus*: I said "institution," because at bottom the dialogue centers around that. What is an institution? If one calls "institution" that which one has involved oneself in as a psychiatrist, through inheritance—namely, the hospital establishment—then one doesn't know what it means, an institution. Institutions, there are some, or one makes sure there aren't, in the hospital establishments, just as sometimes one makes sure there aren't on the outside; many families are not institutions, but are establishments: one gets established! An institution is a locus of exchanges, with the possibility of exchanges with what presents itself. If you will, we can say it is a place where commerce—that is, exchange—becomes possible. From another angle, there is no singularity, or process of singularization, brought into being without the context of a group, of an institution. Hence the problem for me, at Saint-Alban, was simply to make it possible in the hospital for institutions to exist, which explains the accent placed on the club as a device that would enable us to shatter the classical establishment and facilitate its replacement by an ensemble of institutional places. So it was relatively easy to institute something like what came to be called the sector. When Bonnafé left, he was the paladin of the sector. We had already talked about geodemography, about the sector, but in my view that risked being understood as a mere administrative division, or even being used, I don't mind saying, by psychiatrists to escape the problem of madness.

ON COLLECTIVE PSYCHOTHERAPY

[...] A rural psychiatric hospital, traditionally regarded from the professional viewpoint as a starting and transitional post, Saint-Alban was to present a distinctive resistance and transformativity in both its administrative structures and on the part of its nursing staff, and this ensured its historical continuity.

With Balvet, Saint-Alban became aware of three postulates without which any attempt at organizing a social therapy was bound to fail in the near or long term.[1]

a) Holism of the hospital: impossibility and unadvisability of any artificial dichotimization between medical services that would be ignorant of each other in the social framework of hospital life. Really and objectively a single entity.

b) An informed life, through an indispensable medical direction—attentive to intersocial life, at present and sufficiently spread over time.

c) A clear awareness that one can't "heal" the patients without healing the hospital structure. Healing a ward, orienting the staff, healing oneself (Balvet would say), this is our task. In this way, we took up one of the basic aspects of H. Simon, who is almost never talked about. The healing of the Morel wing, the ward housing the agitated patients of the women's service, was our greatest success; it still persists for the greater good of our patients and to the incredulous amazement of visitors, especially if they are psychiatrists.

With Chaurand and Bonnafé, the idea and practice of teamwork strengthened, and the frequently broadened doctors' council became almost official, since I noticed Bonnafé's mention of it in *L'Évolution psychiatrique* with the name—by which we called it, ironically—Société du Gévaudan. It wasn't just a question of coordinating the scientific research, but of the whole politico-administrative life of the hospital, so to speak. We had found the formula that could be easily accepted by French doctors opposed to any intra-medical hierarchy, as well as one conforming to the "unity" thesis that Balvet seemed to propose, and even resembling certain foreign preferences. However, experience would show that it was possible and even quite useful to make this group medical direction not a closed circle at risk of being engulfed by ideological views or wishful fantasies, but a circle open to heterogenous contributions. Actually, since the disappearance of the Société, the incorporation of the directives of Gallavardin and especially of the current doctor-director, Despinoy, has proven to be very effective, or in any case it has been translated into the hospital's living reality with the most coherence and continuity. I'll say nothing about a period of administrative direction through which the essential has been saved.

I still need to talk about the relations between doctors and nurses, without which nothing that was done could have been done, and above all, about two mistakes

François Tosquelles, "Symposium sur la psychothérapie collective," *L'Évolution psychiatrique*, no. 3, September 1952, pp. 537–545.

that lie in wait for any sincere determination to transform things: prophetic sermonizing in the desert and the authoritarian "order of service." Two opposite sides of the paternalistic coin. While they can help the hospital group get past a hang-up, albeit deliriously or phantasmally, when they stabilize and become automatic they become insurmountable barriers. The fact is that it's finally a matter of giving life, consciousness, and initiative to each of the intersocial structures that one is trying to structure, in collaboration with the nurses.

I believe Saint-Alban was one of the first rural hospitals to attempt the quixotic effort of providing a comprehensive professional training to the nurses. After the trials and errors of the Balvet period, there came the time of formal programs drafted with Bonnafé and Chaurand, and these were incorporated, in their general lines, into a ministerial circular that made them obligatory. With Balvet, however, we learned how absurd it was to try and prepare our nurses for written exams through summaries that could only contain a litany of names. I admit that I had been very surprised to see Balvet spend three months, the three months of the first food restrictions, explaining in front of an assembly of farmers who were the guardians of that period the most complicated theories about the assimilation and metabolism of nutrients, about alimentary balance. Then I got it, when I witnessed the creation of a "cooking council" and especially when I noted that during the restrictions, which were quite severe, but comprehensibly laid out for everyone, the mortality rate at Saint-Alban reached only 14 percent the first year and went back down to 7 percent and 12 percent the following years, while the patients elsewhere were dying like flies. Thus, when Bonnafé gave me the task of systematically organizing the professional instruction, I followed the example of Balvet, focusing especially on aspects of normal psychology. When the summaries of our courses were printed, and certain of our coworkers here read them, they approved with a rather condescending irony, thinking no doubt that I meant to create intellectual nurses. An irony perhaps akin to the surprise I felt in our discussion of the Medico-Psychological Society tests, since our nurses are not brilliant test takers! Moreover, it was in spite of the more or less concealed hostility of our audience of nurses that we succeeded in creating the first little group of advocates of hospital reform, with whom the whole hospital would effectively become aligned. On the first day, I had begun to explain the elementary facts of analytic psychology. Well, the head nun of the community made an official visit to Bonnafé to convey her indignation and Chaurand saw himself denounced to the Vichy ministry because he had taught this "smut about love" to the nurses and children of our school of reeducation. And yet, it's this same mother superior and this same community that now constitutes the most active, the most devoted core of our social therapy … It's true that ten years have gone by, and also that on the very day of the first protest, I did my second course in psychoanalysis, Bible in hand and with the help of Saint Thomas and Saint Caesarius of Arles, whose birthday had just been celebrated. While I'm no longer doing courses, at least temporarily, I still bring together the heads of wards every Friday in an assembly that deals with practical facts, and sorts out the most classical and accessible techniques of group psychotherapy.

After this long wait for our main collaborators to find their footing and their place in the process, after the victory constituted by the elimination of the agitated ward, and the agitated themselves, and the successful organization of the common room that Balvet created and where in 1940 the "manageress" invented a group psychotherapy of the same style as that of the Americans, we ended up, to our great surprise, discovering that a series of little "tumors" had been created within the hospital. The living organism that it is had detected them before us and logically, or rather biologically, regarded them as malignant cancers. Bringing in "external" psychological technicians, while technically very useful, had only deepened this clan warfare, of which we were the attentive spectators. When I understood—due to the aggressive contacts of these "parties"—that the enemies of our gains were so pervaded by the positions they thought they were fighting, we didn't hesitate to liquidate and sacrifice our first victories in favor of a coherent organization of the whole. This ebb and flow is doubtless familiar to you from your personal experience. In any case, it caused me to understand the practical role of psychologists and work monitors, from an angle somewhat different than the experience of big-city hospitals leads one to imagine. We'll come back to this later on.

The whole current setup of Saint-Alban can't be understood, moreover, without being informed about the existence of the Lozére section of the Mental Health League of the Central Region, the private organism on which a number of our projects are constructed. In reality, in the time of the Société du Gévaudan, Bonnafé, Chaurand, and I concluded that some therapeutic activities of a social type, in which our patients ought to be involved, were predicated not only on the exercise of the patients' initiative, but on a large freedom of basic handling incompatible with the traditional hospital organizations and the normal administrative functioning of the establishments. Futhermore, we were also believers in what is now called outreach psychiatry, or rather in the need to interest a fairly extensive public in the problems of mental health—not only to sell them on personal preventive practices, but to enable the extramural creation of that atmosphere of tolerance and understanding of psychopathic disturbances that is indispensable to any reform, even internal reform ... This is why we worked in the Lozère *département* to create that movement. In 1944, these initiatives resulted in Dr. Clément managing to create, with the support of Monsieur Le Préfet,[2] the Mental Health Society of Lozère. Then, when Dr. Doussinet, of Clermont, developed a regional organism, our society dissolved and became an autonomous section of the Society of the Central Region, within the framework of its statutes.

We made an effort to assure it of an active participation of the leading administrative figures of the *département*, but also to preserve its complete independence and a real involvement in the region. It would make possible both the internal operation of the hospital apparatus planned by the Gévaudin team, and the indirect but effective control of the necessary funds. Similarly, the liaison with the hospital proper was established through the active participation of certain members of the oversight committee, that of the doctors, it goes without saying, and that of nurses voluntarily enrolled as active members of the society.

As to the interior life of the hospital, the central problem lay in being able to ensure a "personal and autonomous" life for the former common hall and then to establish a certain number of ergotherapy workshops based on the cooperative formula. This alone would allow us to go beyond, within very specific limits that I'll explain later, the stage of ergotherapy as distraction or utilitarian ergotherapy for the establishment as a whole. It was this whole that would open the doors, by means of organizations, to a group psychotherapy and a social therapy. The oversight committee, at the request of Dr. Gallavardin, approved the provisions of the new common hall to be called the "Club Paul-Balvet," which would be linked financially to the league and placed under the dual control of the two head doctors of the service. The hospital would lend, as it were, a parcel of its territory, the clubroom, to this external organism that would be in liaison, however, with the general administration and that of the hospital. This historically revolutionary act is a transcendent thing for us, the key element not only of "our system" but I believe of "any possibility" of resolving a priori the unavoidable difficulties of adapting "new needs" to an administrative and hospital system that has its traditional rights and a legitimate experience to defend.

The club is largely the self-expression of the hospital as a whole, due to the fact that, although it has many specific activities, these activities transcend the life of the wards, as we shall see. For us doctors, it's the source of practical problems, the scene of concrete interhuman conflicts, of the "spontaneous" activities of numerous groups, and of the establishment of vital relationships between various patients, nurses, and the staff in general. It's often the therapeutic opportunity that the doctor welcomes and analyzes more or less publicly. It's always a new life that creates "new needs" and with these needs there is the chance for that *neutral* and *social* group psychotherapy needed by schizophrenics in particular.

As a matter of course, the club is managed by an assembly of patients called ward delegates who are elected inside the wards. The election doesn't follow a strict protocol. Thus, the doctor will determine the right method, depending on the living standard of each ward, and will proceed to organize particular subgroups, not for the stated purpose of elections, but for that of fostering and exercising such contacts between patients. While in my experience there are wards for which the elections are an occasion to meet together as a group, where the doctor can orient the session toward a discussion of personality disorders, or the dispute of a paranoiac in a form that is typically democratic, there are other wards where the patients can only be convened in groups of ten to twelve, and one is surprised then that the mere presentation of candidates and the ensuing discussion can provoke the most unexpected reactions in the doctor, and take spectacular turns in behavior. It goes without saying that with no need to "rig" the outcomes, it is always possible for a government worthy of the name—and the doctor must be one—to get all its "candidates" through, by bending the electoral system to its aims. In any case, whenever I've been witness to a failure of one of my "favorites," kept secret moreover, the real problem I faced was not a possible error in electoral technique but in psychiatry. I examined my opinions of that patient's characterology and social life; I realized my error, then, and I was led to partly correct my diagnosis. For example, there was an obsessional neurosis whose simple-schizophrenic base had eluded me and whose true nature was exhibited subsequently, on the occasion of a typical processual psychotic flare-up. I could cite here a whole set of results of observations of patients that only our type of hospital life could have revealed. But this aspect of clinical analysis and revision of our scale of "symptomology" would merit several sessions, and besides, our studies are still not solid enough to make public.

Let's return to the structure of the club. These ward delegates form, therefore, the general assembly that meets every second Wednesday of the month. They have elected a board among themselves that gets together every Wednesday. Each member of the board is the reporter to a section, which meets in turn to prepare the work, etc. These meetings always take place in the presence of a different nurse, appointed for that and called a "social adviser" for a given concrete committee. They take place at a scheduled hour, so that the doctor himself can attend and send there—as auxiliary members with the right to speak but not to vote—patients who stand to benefit. In this way, there's not a day when the doctor doesn't have one, two, or three groups available where he can try to integrate patients, or personally attend their meeting to give the session the psychotherapeutic direction he desires.

The club connects with the life of the wards in other ways as well. For instance, it organizes parties and competitions, it awards prizes, oversees and distributes work in the wards. This work maintains a collective goal for our ergotherapy workshops and offers countless practical possibilities: posters, garlands, paintings, stage sets, cloakrooms, decoupages, programs ...

For two years running, every ward has been offering a social event to the others in the clubroom. It's unpredictable: a theater play, dances, songs, etc. The competitive spirit of the delegates and social advisers is activated; the variety is a constant stimulation and explains an activity *in the ward* that goes well beyond *public performance*. Often, moreover, at the close of the circle a choice is made, and the society gives a public performance that helps to increase its funds.[3]

And since we're talking about funds, this is how we give an economic life to this whole endeavor. One of the sections of the club is a canteen that is run, naturally, by the patients, like all the other projects. The patients, the visitors, the staff all pay, and though our prices, set by the assembly, are lower than in town, there are profits. There are also a few gifts, 10,000 francs projected out of an annual revenue of almost 2 million. I repeat that there is continuous economic control by the league, but the initiative of everything belongs to the patients themselves, the doctors reserving only the right of veto, something I don't recall ever exercising.

To give you an idea of the volume of these activities, I'll say something about the hospital's internal newspaper. Starting in 1940, the common room had its wall-posted newspaper. Since then, like many of you, we've tried out various things. Little by little, and after I understood the importance of Daumezon's audio journal, at Fleury-les-Aubrais, I came to the following conclusion: there are three different problems in our attempts to establish newspapers:

1) It's partly a question of creating an activity like any other such ergotherapy workshop: to occupy a certain number of patients, enable them to express themselves ... Not that this goes very far in that respect ... We've noticed pretty much everywhere that this effort doesn't involve the whole group of patients.

2) It's a matter of using the paper to change the entire hospital environment, by giving it a sense of its own existence. This seems to occur sometimes with the emergence of *history*; the newspaper is the *written history* of the hospital. Here one aims, then, for both a collective psychotherapy of the hospital understood as a patient itself, and a therapy of one or several patients in particular.

3) It's also a matter of creating external "propaganda" addressed to the country's doctors above all, in order to change their ideas concerning the hospital and nervous disorders, but also in relation to the authorities, the regional councillors, etc.

Consequently, along with Gallavardin, our Mental Health Society decided to put together a journal for the outside, an organ of the society, with the Club Paul-Balvet participating in the writing, but the general target and orientation being entirely "external." Incidentally, these first issues of *Le Chemin* and our patients' participation in an exposition of the general activities of the department facilitated the unanimous vote by the departmental assembly of 10 million francs for certain urgent repairs to the hospital.

Thanks to Despinoy the logical solution was found. What we needed was not one but two publications: *Le Chemin* (external) and *Trait d'union* (internal). To get there, we would have to consider the problem of professional confidentiality. If the newspaper was to be lively, and if was to become of real interest to the patients, the latter would need to sign their texts; one would have to be able to name this one or that one, etc. After many hesitations, we decided to authorize this type of newspaper, which was what the patients wanted in fact, and to *absolutely prohibit its being taken outside the hospital*. The said newspaper is printed at roughly eight pages every eight days. It will soon have been in existence for two years. It owes its life to the patients who buy it and to a subsidy from the printshop club that the Mental Health League created (we'll talk later about these league workshops). The newspaper staff meets every Saturday; it gathers up and discusses the texts that the patients in each ward write in a notebook delivered for that purpose. It also discusses general news from the outside that will appear in print or not, depending on the need for "papers." Generally, the first page is reserved for the doctors to deal with problems of the moment. The paper devotes a lot of space to the activities of the club, with a delegated member presiding over the editing. The administration of the paper, on the other hand, is handled by the printshop itself. The newspaper comes out with almost an eight-day delay but it seems to us that nothing can be done about this. The doctors have a chance to look over the texts on Fridays, thanks to the ward notebooks. This means that their intervention—or not—in the editors' meeting on Saturdays is a question of appropriateness.

So I'll open up this collection of newspapers more or less at random to speak to you about the life that the club contributes to the whole hospital.

I chance upon this issue of August 31, where I see a program of the week's soirees with a particular Sunday's contest of sketches and improvised declamations—an offer of prizes to the contestants. For Monday, I see a board game session completely organized by the patients of the "Games and Entertainments" section. On Tuesday, a session reserved for the ladies of two wards, relatively unskilled socially, with games, a blackboard drawing contest, mimes, Kim games, and a game of blind man's bluff featuring two opposing teams named ahead of time. On this Wednesday, six groups belonging to different wards enter into collective competition, asking each other spontaneous questions about "surprise projections," and then there is imitation of the scenes and attitudes shown in these images. On Thursday, and this is the subject of an article by Dr. Despinoy (addressed as much to the patients as to the staff): "I see that the organizers of this usual club soirée were asking the patients to demonstrate their know-how in everyday life … healthy living …" And, I will add, the miming by the contestants reminds one very significantly of the sessions of Moreno's sociometry … but emerging in a spontaneous way so that the doctor and his auxiliaries only have to channel the unfolding of it. On Friday, it's as usual—a session offered by one ward to the others. I note, for this week: a danced minuet, a one-act play, a song, a sketch, and collective singing; thirty or so patients onstage, sometimes fewer. Saturday, a movie, and so on. And so it goes, regularly, every day—it's already a firm habit with us.

DISABILITY AND WORK: ON THE WAR DISABLED

Faced with the perspective of returning to Catalonia, our condition as doctors and as socialists leads us to consider the problem of the mutilated. Among the numerous cases of social inadaptation that we will encounter once the tragic parenthesis opened by fascism has closed, the case of the war mutilated, due to its number and importance, will force us to take a series of urgent measures. It is in the interests of both the mutilated and the collective that these measures are not exclusively dictated by simple emotional reactions. That would limit the efforts society owes to the mutilated to mere economic support.

The mutilated, victims of their functional limitations, are at risk of surrendering, sometimes unconsciously, to psychosocial reactions of discouragement, in very different and often paradoxical forms.

In the most recent meeting of the Association of Catalan Doctors that took place in Toulouse, we defended, and approved, a presentation in which we requested the immediate creation, in the heart of the Ministry of Health Care and Social Aid, a secretariat for the victims of war and fascism, devoted in large part to the study and solution of the problem of the mutilated. Here we must insist on one of the driving thoughts: as much or more than economic aid, *which is naturally indispensable*, the real problem is the mutilated's readaptation to the world of work.

It is not about establishing a cold, bureaucratic percentage of incapacity. What must be done is a personal study of each mutilated person, not only from a physical perspective, but also from economic and psychosocial points of view. One mustn't lose sight of the fact that a mere financial compensation does not solve much, but rather this partial measure can often even lead to greater social maladaptation. The mutilated's exercise of their remaining capacities is an indispensable condition for their reencountering their balance within society.

The reintegration of the mutilated into social and economic life is not only an act of social justice, but a biological necessity for each individual and an economic and political necessity for society. Furthermore, it responds to the socialist conception of the world, to the appraisal of work as a primary element of progress for peoples and individuals.

The economic problem of the mutilated is no different, in and of itself, from the incapacity brought on by a work accident or following an illness. The volume, urgency, and patriotic character of the problem of the war mutilated highlights the misery of health care policy in regard to the incapacitated.

Many chronically ill people are victims of a series of prejudices that must be banished. Medicine must begin a policy of social recovery that most of our medical organizations are unfamiliar with.

Excerpt from Francesc Tosquelles and Jaume Sauret, "Invalidesa i treball: A propòsit dels mutilats de guerra," *Endavant: Òrgan del Moviment Socialista de Catalunya; Federació, democràcia, socialisme*, no. 9, October 1945, no pagination.

Too often work is still thought of as a yoke, that the ill should all rest. In hospitals and within families, the chronically ill, stabilized in a limited lifestyle, are victims of their treatment and end up in social and organic exile. This is the case, above all, for a large number of the tuberculose and psychopathological, not to mention those who use their wounds as a means of earning a living by arousing public charity.

Prejudices are very entrenched. We have seen families urging the ill to abandon the work their doctor has recommended. We have seen unions opposing allowing the ill to work. The root is merely a misunderstanding, and a lack of social organization. Which is why, in 1936, one of us urged the Generalitat to pass a law declaring the right and duty of certain ill people to work.

There are very few medical-educational organizations directed to social reeducation. Nothing is being done to this end, not in hospitals, not in sanitoriums, not in health centers. The traditional organisms come up against an invincible resistance and often doctors accustomed to treating the ill based on their anatomical wounds generally do not have a clear awareness of their social tasks.

Traditional policies for social readaptation [*sic*] of the war mutilated are limited to reserving them, blindly, some administrative posts, which are often inferior and sometimes superior to the mutilated's capacities. There is no personal discernment of each case, nor is there reeducation.

Catalonia must break with this deficient tradition. With a focus on the problem of the social readaptation of the mutilated, along with the creation of specialized reeducation centers, the organizational conditions must be created to allow for the treatment and social recovery of other sick people.

The American and Russian examples allow us to demand such policy. In 1912, in the USSR, where for some time the prevailing idea has been that an invalid should and must work, the Cooperative Union of Invalids, an organism dependent on the Ministry of Social Provision, organized 1,772 "artels" allowing more than two hundred thousand invalids to work at home, without counting those who, thanks to the special reeducation services, have been able to have a complete recovery.

PERSPECTIVES AND MIRAGES

When we examine the problem of Spain—we do not believe that the Catalan litigation can find an isolated solution to the general problem of the Peninsula—we must distrust our tendency to daydream. Desires always play a large role in "scientific" ideas we come up with for the future. But the special situation of the exile—woven of hopes—even further distorts the objective realities. The party leaders are not exempt from this general rule.

In the history of all exiles one can see that the exiled often make mistakes. In any case, when they return to their country, even their supporters soon express some disagreement with the repatriated's point of view.

The disorientation and discrepancies between the exiled are natural outgrowths of the exile life itself. The ideas that we come up with about "down there" are distorted by the prism of our current lives. Our constellation of desires is too strong. The desire to return to our land and the desire to affirm our victory. For the exile it is not only about the victory of the Republic for which he fought. It is, above all, an intimate, personal victory, that of his political group. "We did not err," we secretly tell ourselves every day. It is pride and the consolation over our situation. Getting past this self-deception is difficult if not impossible. It is our spiritual bread. The isolation of exile, however, contributes to separating us from our own compatriots and comrades. The personal satisfaction of *having been right* costs us an increase in the isolation inherent in exile. To the two aforementioned desires we add another, secret, hope: we wish that our future life, that of our children, never knows the horrors we've seen and suffered over these years.

Due to those hopes and desires, objective reflection is elusive and we often deceive ourselves. It is with sorrow that we rediscover that politics and the country's future are only very superficially linked to our desires. We realize more than ever that our country is an inseparable part of Europe and the world. And here a new mirage awaits us: the victory of the Allies. It seems that *ideologically* it is impossible that Francoism can continue. We forget that the ties that bind various peoples together have a fundamentally economic basis. We forget the semi-economic colony nature of our people. We forget that the victory of the democracies is, in a way, a threat to capitalism. We forget that no people has ever yet been liberated from its economic chains. That larger capitalism has no country.

The socialist perspective on the world is merely a perspective. The struggle on a world scale has not even been proposed in a clear manner. Quite the opposite: the "national" victory of each of the Allies awakens a certain nationalism that perhaps will be exploited by the bourgeoisie. We must not forget that they must search for a solution that allows them to adapt to the new political conditions. The bourgeoisie is primarily trying to avoid the economic transformation that the circumstances demand. [...]

Excerpt from Francesc Tosquelles, "Perspectives i miratges," *Endavant: Òrgan del Moviment Socialista de Catalunya; Federació, democràcia, socialisme*, no. 6, June 1945, no pagination.

It is a study that deserves the attention of all those who take a vague and ineffective interest in the problems of the Peninsula. The horrors of the war are present in everyone's memories and no one can unscrupulously again take up the idea of a civil conflict within their country. [...] Is there no way to move toward socialism without further bloodshed? ask the workers. Is there no way to avoid socialism without further bloodshed? asks the bourgeoisie.

In the face of the international indecision of the working class, the states in hands of the bourgeoisie are treading water. The years pass. But we, who have not forgotten that history is woven on the loom of class struggle, can suppose there is an interest in maintaining the current confusion. One knows the role played by smoke screens in military strategy. Behind the smoke, a policy of attack or of defense is being prepared. There is an interest in clouding the Spanish problem in smoke. Spain is a semicolony, as are others. Without a socialist organization of the world or at least of Europe, the Iberian Peninsula dances and will dance to the tune of its masters.

Before starting the great world massacre, they waited for our war—the dress rehearsal—to end. Or, perhaps, they ended the war in Spain in order to be able to begin the world war.

There is no Spanish problem. There is a worldwide problem. Outside of a worldwide perspective, the solutions proposed to the Spanish litigation are a mirage. That does not mean that we Spaniards should stop fighting—inside the country and beyond—against Francoism. The fight for freedom is never barren. Not even when lost. A people exists as a summarized expression of their struggles. We have to fight for the existence of the Catalan people and for the existence of the other peoples of Iberia.

A unanimous cry cuts through the fog: Avoid civil war! This is said in Spain and everywhere. It is thought, and rightly so, that the war criminals must be punished. The traitors of each people die and thus, by shedding that tainted blood, we will avoid the creation of the organism that opposes, through weapons and blood, the forward march toward socialism. Thus there would be no new civil wars. What is humanly horrible about civil war is not *its* dead, but the deaths of innocents.

The bourgeoisie when cornered—by its own sins—will sacrifice some of its men, but while searching out other options. The leaders of the workers' movements have the difficult duty to guess them in time. They must be able to strip away the mirages and see the true perspective in which the current problems are situated. The exiles are quite poorly prepared for that. Their emotional and vital needs condemn them to live too much through illusions and desires. Their personal point of view plays too important a role. It cannot be any other way.

Our comrades who fight from within Francoist Spain, despite their isolation from the democratic world, can see these things more clearly, more dispassionately.

Longing is a poor guide. It looks back at the past more than at the present and at the future. The men "down below," the heroes who are able to, despite the dangers, keep up the fight against the police state, will end the divergences of the exiles. We needn't do anything more than try to understand them and work with them. Leave the mirages behind. Fight in accordance with those who remain in the country, striving to establish a true concordance of thought and objectives.

THE LIMITATIONS OF LIBERAL STRUCTURING IN MEDICINE

The subject of our article is not one of purely professional interest, since it is not related only to the medical sector, but rather of general interest.

The fact that medicine is not a private affair for doctors is proven by the existence of the ill and that, within this qualification, all men can presume that they could be ill. While one could object, claiming that to be true of all professions, everyone will have noticed that in matters of medical aid, the acceptable minimum coincides with the maximum aid that current medical knowledge allows for each ill person. All doctors agree on that, and since they know better than anyone what quantity and quality of care must be given to each patient, it seems that, on the face of it, they can be trusted and allowed the independence necessary to structure their own profession.

We believe this trust will surprise no one and arouse no suspicion. Before being a technician, a doctor is by—definition and tradition—a trusted man. Medicine has only developed its techniques on the fundamental principle of the trust the patient places in his doctor, to the point that any attempt to rationalize the profession that ignores that principle of trust is headed for inevitable failure.

This is the basis of liberal medicine and the doctor has become a nearly exceptional being within a society that increasingly limits individual freedom with each passing day. Thus, the medical profession remains a model for liberal professions, while its public power is limited to intervening in these two aspects: free medical assistance for the poor deemed as such and the organization of a reduced network of preventive medicine and health control of the general population.

Therefore, it seems paradoxical that the doctors themselves come to propose to the public powers, and to all citizens as a whole, the problem of their freedom being limited. In effect, one could thus interpret the health-structuring plan presented by the Association of Catalan Doctors for the Renewal of Medicine, written by us and our colleagues Martí Feced, Sauret, Llambies; but the paradox vanishes when it is acknowledged that the liberal medical structure gives doctors complete freedom to earn a living, but not the freedom to exercise their profession with the proper efficacy. So, if it is the doctors who address this problem, they are merely showing themselves worthy of that trust that the patient and society more generally places in them. In other words, at a moment that could be decisive for medicine, they are trying to save that which is essentially indispensable.

On the other hand, transforming the profession consciously can avoid the blind, progressive transformation imposed on it by the needs of the economic order. Man demonstrates his qualities and his freedom when, while recognizing

---

Excerpt from Francesc Tosquelles, "Els límits de l'estructura liberal de la Medicina," *Quaderns d'estudis polítics, econòmics i socials*, no. 11, November 1945, pp. 22–24.

the needs in time, he foresees them and, instead of merely tolerating them, he directs them.

***

The progresses of medical techniques are determined by two new factors, both in the act of diagnosis and in the therapeutic realm: first, the frequent necessity of collaboration with other professionals who are able to handle difficult devices that are economically inaccessible to the rural doctor and any patient below a certain level of privilege; secondly, the urgency of these acts, which oblige the rapid transfer of the patient or of the doctors with their tools.

We do not refer here, as one might think, to a generalization of the already traditional habit of calling "an expert" in for a consultation. This Catalan middle-class custom is a good custom, but it is insufficient. First of all, because the "meeting of doctors" often happens too late; almost always when there are grave symptoms, when things have taken a bad turn, sometimes when the patient is dying. On the other hand, that custom remains economically limited to well-to-do families.

In reality, the problem of medical collaboration—or of group medicine, as it is now called—occurs in every phase of illness and even in the exercise of specialties. Thus, for example, we neuropsychiatrists often cannot make a true diagnosis without certain examinations by an ophthalmologist, or a phthisiologist or an internist, not to mention the collaboration of the laboratory and radiology. The same thing occurs with treatments; while sometimes we can establish them ourselves, other times we must resort to a surgeon or a specialist in physical therapy. In our professional lives we've often discovered too late, after years of evolution, an illness that, if we had initially applied the good, expensive diagnostic techniques to it, would have been discovered and treated in time.

Even in the field of research and discovery, the lack of true group medicine is harmful. A telling example is in the history of penicillin, which is so often spoken of. The antibacterial properties of the *Penicillium* mushroom were discovered by Fleming in 1928. The first clinical trials could not be done until 1938 and it wasn't until 1942 that a concentrated and manufacturable penicillin was obtained for therapeutic application.

Sir Fleming worked at St Mary's hospital and was unable to extract the penicillin from the *Penicillium* (that was achieved in 1929 in Oxford). Why? The wise Englishman tells us himself in a recent lecture, published in this year's February issue of the *Journal of the Royal Institute of Public Health and Hygiene*: "At Oxford they [Drs. Chain and Florey] had a complete team of chemists, bacteriologists, and experimental pathologists. At St Mary's I had been short of chemical help, and at the School of Hygiene, Raistrick [another of the researchers who worked with *Penicillium* without managing to extract the penicillin] had lacked complete bacteriologic co-operation. The success of the Oxford workers is a great argument for teamwork in a detailed investigation of this sort."

Thus the organization of group medicine at the service of the general practitioner seems indispensable.

That is not possible in the framework of strictly liberal medicine, for economic reasons; nor is it possible for the patients themselves to pay for this medicine, since it is very expensive; nor is it possible for doctors to exercise it while their economic lives remain based on competition, while the patient continues to be a "client" and the doctor colleague a "competitor." That is why we propose this organization in the national plan of health centers in Barcelona and the primary regional hubs.

These "health centers" would not only serve as outpatient clinics but would become the health care unit for the region, so that, in addition to coordinating the specialized technical team, they would be organs of a truly social medicine. Not only would their services function as consultants on demand for the general practitioners, but their services of detection would alert the doctors each time when they discovered a new ill person when examining en bloc a school full of students, or the staff at a factory, or the members of the youth centers, etc.

It remains to be discussed whether, as in the English project, doctors are free or not to enter into the "National Service." This is a relatively secondary aspect of the matter because what is important is creating the service. In the sessions in Toulouse of the aforementioned Association of Catalan Doctors, we proposed that first and foremost the Generalitat limit itself to coordinating a good number of the already existing (but disconnected) services into "health centers." These first steps would give us experience and guide us in the future.

* * *

Another aspect of the limitations of liberal medicine, and one that is of interest to a greater number of doctors, is that of the general practitioners or family doctors. Here the limitation is related to the development of social security insurance coverage. We have already explained in the pages of *Quaderns* (the June issue, "Social Insurance and Medicine") what needs to be considered.[1] The most essential is that an insurance system makes it possible for each and every citizen to have their family doctor and be able to choose that doctor. The other aspects of the question are unrelated to the efficacy of the medical assistance and are merely of a social nature.

Lastly, a final limitation of liberal medicine lies in the fact that the private doctor, no matter how private he is—for example, in the case of a specialist who doesn't form part of the "National Service"—cannot be considered detached from his regional health center, especially in regard to the collaboration of all the doctors in the sector's services of general hygiene and prevention.

We have seen that, at the heart of it, two main problems in the new medical organization revolve around social security insurance and the health centers. These two institutions have equal importance. If the social insurance is organized without the parallel creation of the health centers, patients will suffer the consequences. The health coverage would be a swindle, because while it would ensure the presence of a doctor capable of curing tonsillitis or the flu, it wouldn't ensure any patient received the medical assistance that is indispensable in most cases.

The health care presentation given by the Advisory Board of the Presidency of the Generalitat de Catalonia included most of the solutions proposed by the

Association of Catalan Doctors in exile; we celebrate that but we also must say that they, with a perhaps exaggerated discretion, did not want to take any position against the perspectives of limiting doctors' traditional freedom. The speakers and spokespersons do not seem to have understood the utmost importance of organizing the "health centers," Perhaps they have confused this work tool—that is indispensable to the practice of good medicine—with excessive bureaucracy; perhaps they have let themselves be led astray by two highly influential tendencies, Catalan individualism and the fear of socialism.

The Association of Catalan Doctors for the Renewal of Medicine had foreseen that their propositions would not find an easy path. Which is why they agreed to not limit their action and propaganda to the medical profession, nor to political circles. Which is why they decided to invite all citizens, as such and as potential patients, to reflect on these problems that affect us all individually and, above all, affect the collective interest.

We wrote this article in order to promote this reflection.

FRANTZ FANON AND INSTITUTIONAL PSYCHOTHERAPY

Today the call came from Algiers, to reminisce for a meeting of psychiatrists—and various actors in the field of psychiatry—about that other encounter that joined Frantz Fanon and institutional psychiatry.

I won't dare assert that in every human encounter the stakes are predetermined, the dice always loaded. I want to say, however, without any ill-intended slyness on my part, that there are no words that circulate between people that are not themselves a real amalgam—a montage—of numerous events that gave form to previous encounters, and that have straddled the time and space traversed by human beings. The short duration of our lives doesn't encapsulate in a single bloc the movement of knowing and forgetting—of the registered and the unperceived—that turn up superimposed in all the turns of discourse that humans deliver in their concrete encounters. This is why the life and the life story of Frantz Fanon—engaged in his real presence at Saint-Alban, where I played the role of catalyst among the many actors caught up in the gestures staged in the local psychiatric practices—came to light only in a sporadic way during the three years of his stay among us.

Instead of answering straightaway, in an overtly meaningful way, the request from Algiers concerning what Frantz Fanon contributed to Saint-Alban and gleaned from it, I'll limit myself to sharing three or four anecdotes whose use value is still unresolved, making them worthy of several retellings.

First, I'll call back to mind what constituted my first encounter with him. This will be followed by other anecdotes gathering various caregivers—indeed friends and familiars—around meals where the mood was more joyful than not. Obviously, to end it, I'll briefly recall some truly professional anecdotes.

Straight off, I'll say that in the spring of 1952, when Fanon came to meet me at my home, at Saint-Alban, no one was talking yet about institutional psychiatry. It was only around that time that Daumézon and Koechlin used the term for a certain number of discontinuous, but coherent, activities that we'd put in place at Saint-Alban starting in 1940.

Here is my account of the first meeting between Frantz Fanon and myself, at Saint-Alban.

Useless to conceal here my surprise—indeed the awakening of my curiosity—on noting the radical difference there was between the color of his skin and that of

---

François Tosquelles, "Frantz Fanon et la psychothérapie institutionelle," *Sud/Nord*, no. 1, 2007, pp. 71–78. This text was written at the request of the National Institute of Public Health of Algiers, which intended to organize, on December 4 and 5, 1991, a psychiatry conference on the occasion of the thirtieth anniversary of Frantz Fanon's death. This conference did not take place, due to the political context and for lack of Algerian psychiatrists' participation. But Francesc Tosquelles asked that it be published in the proceedings of the second Journées de psychiatrie de Dax, *Histoire et histoires en psychiatrie*, under the direction of Michel Minard, Éditions Érès, in 1992.[1]

most of the other men I was used to having concrete relations with. I minimized my first reactions of surprise by inquiring as to what he expected from us. I think I told him that we were favorable to his wishes, which were actually obscure to me. Being relatively well mannered, I shook his hand, invited him to sit, and asked him, "What can we do here to serve you?" At Lyon, he replied, the word was that at Saint-Alban we had implemented a psychiatric practice attentive above all to the complexity of differences—maintained and sometimes tragically accentuated—that bound men together and that we were determined to treat with care.

I remember having said that in fact his statements corresponded rather precisely to what guided our professional actions at Saint-Alban. Nevertheless, I agreed with him about the fact that the differences were still numerous and complex in what every person brought to their encounters with others. There was also, in the background, a host of similarities, analogies, even identical processes active in all men.

No difference can appear between men—or between things—without one's at the same time factoring in their resemblance, indeed their sameness.

The abstract character of these first exchanges didn't fool him or me. The discreet reference to the contrasting color of our skins, on the other hand, migrated to the center of our conversations. The thing in question was immediately understood that way by Fanon, since he immediately gifted me his book *Black Skin, White Masks*. Then he told me about his pain exacerbated quite recently in the street, at Lyon, while he was walking with his (white) fiancée. He was violently accosted, taken away, and mistreated for hours in the police station by cops who accused him of trafficking or enslaving white girls.

In this first conversation, rather than dwelling on his conflict with the Lyon cops, I directed my interest to the use of *masks* in human relations, which he had addressed in his book. I said to him: "Whatever the color of the face or skin of this one or that one, we go masked to meet the others. The mask is a staging of the personality, but what enters back into the challenges of encounters is actually the person the mask has covered with artifacts, always made of social conventions."

I believe I said that beyond the masks, it was necessary to credit the other with a diffuse complexity.

I thought of the two presents that Fanon blessed me with in that encounter as being his formal credentials. He had presented himself to me as the ambassador of the *singularity* of his history.

Years later, I met with Fanon again, in Paris. He was already involved in Algeria's war of liberation. [...]

For something close to our daily professional life, I recall another occasion when Fanon's historical line and mine intersected, this time in the concrete space of our clinical practices at Saint-Alban.

I have to say that Frantz Fanon had chosen in good faith to hew almost blindly to the gospel distilled from standard clinical practice; that is, by psychiatrists focused on the objective constants of mental cases.

He had followed, without being personally engaged, the life of a patient who had greatly improved. She appeared almost cured, after several sessions of insulin therapy.

Myself and a number of nurses took advantage of her awakening from the insulin comas to bring back the language connections of a hesitant speech. She relived retrospectively her own birth and entry into the world of grown-ups. In anticipation of her release, this patient—very improved, socialized, sophisticated, attuned to the vagaries of culture—had changed wards, in order to stay in an open wing (the Terrace) whose walls were characterized, among other things, by the number and transparency of the bay windows.

Now, one day—I was still at my home, discussing one thing and another with Fanon and Dr. Koechlin, who was passing through—someone telephones us, demanding the resident Fanon for an emergency at the Terrace. When he returned to us, he was very angry and very disappointed, since this patient, quite unexpectedly for all of us, had broken almost all the window panes of the ward. This was very serious in itself … However, what Fanon also complained about was that one of the ward's caregivers—a nun, Sister Carmen—didn't want to transfer the patient to her original ward, against the opinion of Fanon. He said, like any good doctor, that this patient had relapsed, miserably, and it would be necessary to recommence the insulin treatment. Sister Carmen had gotten wind of the existence of what was called, with Kretschmer, fake psychoses, an unfamiliar concept in the classical psychiatry of Lyon. She thought that often patients, faced with the anguish of rejoining their family and social normality, would engage in spectacular demonstrations of madness that no longer corresponded to a biological constraint. The nurse, Sister Carmen, demanded authorization to continue in place the uncertain trajectory of a long therapeutic intervention by calling out the designs of the patient. I had to quickly arbitrate this conflict between Fanon's expertise and the knowledge of the nurse. Crediting this nurse with a certain confidence, I thought she could try and unravel the threads of this relapse.

As it turned out, there followed forty-eight hours of efforts between the patient and the nurse, without a break, day and night. Based on her practice of drawings and comments that always had a clear sexual connotation, notably with autoeroticism, the patient regained her footing in altogether correct social behavior. A month later, she left, and I can report that our heroine married normally and had two children without any recurrence of her rowdy paranoid schizophrenia.

The recollection of this spectacular and dramatic professional anecdote is offered simply to underscore that, whatever the right approaches taken by a therapist may be, draped as he is in his knowledge, when a certain number of catastrophes occur in the course of the treatment of a psychotic, we all revert almost automatically to our old objective ideas about the so-called mental illnesses. One can say that everyone is the dupe of these traps that appear in every more or less institutionalized psychotherapy. The same goes for psychoanalysts of the first order.

Still connected in my memory with the activity of Fanon at the club, I recall that, just before leaving for Blida, he occupied the podium of the Literary Society at Mende, where he delivered a lecture on the space of scenic performances of human comedies and tragedies. […]

Actually, what my text is reporting apropos of Fanon constitutes "episodes" very analogous to what is evoked during any concrete psychotherapy, when the latter is conducted to term in a discontinuous way, but artfully crocheted together.

Unfortunately, institutional psychotherapy has been understood solely as being reduced to the intra muros *of classical psychiatric hospitals.*

In contrast, my account here, which concerns the reception and certain encounters that Fanon experienced and arranged at Saint-Alban and its environs, testifies to this reach that always far exceeds the hospital enclosure.

Fanon's lecture, at Mende, the administrative center of Lozère, in the course of which he laid out the theoretical development of his practice at Saint-Alban, already attested to the reach of its social services aimed at awakening and focusing the interest of a few cultivated individuals rooted in the regional "peasantry." The form of the discourse he delivered at Mende corresponded to a certain level of cultural expectations among the group he was addressing that evening. As a matter of fact, the development of the human networks that appear in towns marked out for industrialization takes its energies and resources from the soon-to-be abandoned countryside. The least that one can say, without any nostalgia for nature, is that the resource of rural collectives is more easily identified than what is formed in the mastodonic cities that grind people to dust.

The accent that Fanon placed after the fact, during his stay in the Algiers region and his participation in the FLN [National Liberation Front], on the peasant as driving force in political change, was also an echo of his experience both in Martinique and around the hospital of Saint-Alban.

SOCIAL THERAPY IN A WARD OF MUSLIM MEN: METHODOLOGICAL DIFFICULTIES

Frantz Fanon and Jacques Azoulay

[...] Let's call to mind some particularities of the Blida Psychiatric Hospital. Upon our arrival, our four colleagues were in charge of the medical surveillance of more than six hundred patients each. So any attempt to orient their services around a social-therapeutic perspective was impossible for them. The arrival of a fifth doctor, however, relieved these four colleagues of four hundred patients and only then did the possibility of performing real social therapy arise.

At Saint-Alban we had observed a type of organization that, overall and in detail, we thought measured up to a maximal type of sociotherapy in the current conditions of psychiatric care in France. So we took our ward as a point of departure that would in a sense serve as an experimental milieu. We sought to implement biweekly ward meetings,[1] as well as staff meetings, newspaper meetings, and bimonthly celebrations. In our ward of European women, results appeared before long. [...]

In the meantime, we had studied our ward in-depth, the character of the patients who resided there and, on the outside, their background. We had naively taken our division as a whole and believed we had adapted to this Muslim society the frames of a particular Western society at a determinate period of its technological evolution. We had wanted to create institutions and we had forgotten that all such approaches must be preceded by a tenacious, real, and concrete interrogation into the organic bases of the Indigenous society.

By virtue of what impairment of judgement had we believed it possible to undertake a Western-inspired social therapy in a ward of mentally ill Muslim men? How was a structural analysis possible if the geographic, historical, cultural, and social frames were bracketed? Two explanations could be put forward.

1) First, North Africa is French and, when one does not look, one really cannot see how the attitude has to be different from one ward to another. The psychiatrist, reflexively, adopts the policy of assimilation. The natives do not need to be understood in their cultural originality. It is the "natives" who must make the effort and who have every interest in being like the type of men suggested to them. Assimilation here does not presuppose a reciprocity of perspectives. It is up to one entire culture to disappear in favor of another.

In our Muslim ward, leaving aside the need for an interpreter, our behavior was completely unsuited. In fact, a revolutionary attitude was essential, because it was necessary to go from a position in which the supremacy of Western culture was evident, to one of cultural relativism. And again it was necessary to return to Piaget: the notions of adaptation and assimilation are very important and far from having been fully developed.[2]

Frantz Fanon and Jacques Azoulay, "La socialthérapie dans un service d'hommes musulmans: Difficultés méthodologiques," *L'Information psychiatrique*, vol. 30, no. 9, October 1954, pp. 349–361. This English translation, by Steven Corcoran, is excerpted and reprinted with permission from Frantz Fanon, *Alienation and Freedom*, edited by Jean Khalfa and Robert J.C. Young. London: Bloomsbury Academic, 2018, pp. 353–371.

2) Lastly and above all, it must be said that those who preceded us in trying to divulge the North African psychiatric fact remained somewhat too focused on motor, neuro-vegetative, and so on, phenomena. The works of the Algiers school, while they revealed certain particularities, did not, to our knowledge, proceed to the functional analysis, which nevertheless appeared to be indispensable. It was necessary to change perspectives or at least supplement the initial ones. It was necessary to try to grasp the North African social fact. It was necessary to demand that "totality" in which [Marcel] Mauss saw the guarantee of an authentic sociological study. A leap had to be performed, a transmutation of values to be achieved. Let's say it: it was essential to go from the biological level to the institutional one, from natural existence to cultural existence.

The biological, the psychological, and the sociological were separated only by an aberration of the mind. In fact, they were tied indistinctly together. It is for want of having integrated the notion of Gestalt and the elements of contemporary anthropology into our daily practice that our failures were so harsh.

For a period of six months, the Muslim women had regularly attended the celebrations held in the European wards. For a period of six months, they applauded in the European way. And then one day, a Muslim orchestra came to the hospital, played and sang, and our astonishment in hearing the applause of the Muslim women was great: short, acute, and repeated modulations.[3] Thus they reacted to the configuration of the ensemble, in line with its specific demands. It became evident that we had to try to find ensembles that would facilitate reactions already inscribed in a definitively elaborated personality. Sociotherapy would only be possible to the extent that social morphology and forms of sociability were taken into consideration.

What were the biological, moral, aesthetic, cognitive, and religious values of Muslim society? How did the Native react from the affective, emotional point of view? What were the forms of sociability that rendered possible the various attitudes of this Muslim? We were faced with certain institutions that astonished us. To what did they correspond? It was necessary to carry out a functional analysis that ought to facilitate the task. In a work in preparation, one of us intends to show the complexity of North African society, which is currently undergoing extremely deep structural modifications. Here we limit ourselves to recalling a few characteristic elements of this society.[4]

Traditional Muslim society is theocratic in spirit. The Muslim religion is in effect, apart from a philosophical belief, a rule of life that strictly regulates the individual and the group. In Muslim countries, religion impregnates social life and gives no consideration to secularity. Rights, morality, science, philosophy—all mingle with it. Alongside the properly religious, Islamic imperative, tradition forcefully intervenes, as bequeathed from the ancient Berber customs, and this is what explains the rigidity of the social frames.

It is also a gerontocratic society. The father is the one that steers the life of the family and he—or in his absence the eldest brother or even the uncle—must be consulted for all decisions of some importance. The family is incidentally very ramified, and sometimes an entire douar shares the same patronymic name! It tends to be identified with the clan, which is the true natural group of Muslim Algeria. Decisions are taken by the djema'a, a sort of municipal council at the head of which there is a president—and whose importance the civil service has, incidentally, recently recognized. There did not in fact exist, at least not until in recent years, a veritable national community, but instead a familial, clan community.

It is also necessary to emphasize the region's ethnic complexity, since the Kabyles form a large minority among the rest of the Arab population. If both groups [are] united by the Muslim religion, their separation is clearly marked by differences of language, tradition, and culture. The Kabyle, of Berber origin, inhabit the mountainous regions. Their villages, perched on the hilltops, constitute the elements in which the tribal organization remains the most solid. The Arabs live in the plains and the cities. Farmers are to be found there, but so also are traders and petty artisans. We can obviously not expand upon the other local particularisms: nomads, Arabs of the South, Mozabites, Chaouis—of much less importance for our aims. So it is that in our ward, out of 220 patients we had 148 Arabs, 66 Kabyles, and 6 Chaouis, Moroccans, and Mozabites.

Lastly, we ought to say a word about the Muslim patients' usual living conditions, which by and large explain their state of ignorance, their traditional primitivism. Prior to French conquest, land was the property of the collective and the notion of wealth was linked to the notion of useful land, arable land, and as a result to the possession of a yoke or a plough; people who owned such things were the real property owners.

French settlement led to the transformation of land ownership and a redistribution of wealth. The old collective property was subdivided between owners, and then private proprietors. The members of the old tribe led a poor life, but it knew no proletarians. Today there exists, outside of a minority of large landowners, whether European or Muslim, a mass of small proprietors, of fellahs, who find it hard to make a living from farming a small patch of land with primitive techniques, however much such patches are still an object of envy for those who did not benefit from the carve up. These latter people became destitute, their sociological bond with tribal collective identity loosens daily and they began trying to hire out their labor as *khammès*[5] or day laborers. There is, thus, a movement of dissociation of that once homogeneous society, between on the one hand small proprietors and on the other shepherds, sharecroppers, or day laborers.

Furthermore, as a result of the extension of modern farming techniques to large properties, today we see taking shape a mass of unemployed farmworkers, whose hunger draws them to the towns, but who are forced by the absence of industrialization into the condition of the proletariat—and even the subproletariat—further heightening the social disequilibrium. And it must be underscored that, above all among the population of Berber origin, many go to France for an indeterminate period, to seek either a job that they cannot find at home or a supplement to their meager harvests.

This development among sedentary peoples results in the group's splintering, and in this sense merges with the development of nomads. Today, we struggle to picture the importance of ancient nomadism in North Africa: the tribes of the south went as far as the littoral edge, like a periodic tide rising up from the steppes and the sands, surging up through the high plateaus. But the French occupation naturally led to a constant regression of this nomadism, resolving it into two terms: sedentarization, and renting of labor. But the seasonal workers remain outside the sedentary grouping that they come to support. Ancient nomadism strictly maintained traditional forms of authority and group cohesion; the individual movements that can be seen now proceed outside of any tribal rule and greatly contribute to hastening a dangerous detribalization: the decline of nomadism is ineluctable, but it is being replaced by proletarianization.

These factors, which foster the dissolution of the groups, whether sedentary or nomadic, explains the formation of sizeable shanty towns at the entrances to large cities, thus constituting not only a challenge to aesthetics or even to simple urbanism, but also a serious danger from a health and moral point of view.

By way of example, we studied the social composition of our ward of Muslim men. Out of 220 patients, we had: 35 fellahs (that is to say, individuals with a piece of land that they cultivate themselves); 76 agricultural workers, sharecroppers, or day laborers; 78 workers (bakers, painters, etc.); 5 intellectuals; 26 without profession. But these figures call for interpretation. It might be thought that there is a relatively high number of workers: seventy-eight out of 220. In actual fact, we were most often dealing with precisely those elements that had been torn from and who had managed to find some manual labor in the city, of whatever kind. Ultimately, out of 78 "workers," only 20 had at least some form of job specialization. Concerning the 5 "intellectuals," let's note that they are indigenous primary school teachers with something like the equivalent of a school leaving certificate.

These problems have considerable resonances: the individuals who escaped traditional society on their own are too numerous to count, but their number is constantly growing. These elements are the forces, still poorly analyzed, that are in the process of breaking the domestic, economic, and political frameworks. This society, which is said to be rigid, is fermenting from the base.[6] These few notions, although all too brief and each being in need of a lengthy elaboration, are enough to explain the specificity of Muslim Algerian society that we had to take into consideration in our efforts to create the fundaments for social therapy among Muslims.

We can now understand the reasons for our failure. We said that the ward meetings had turned out not to be productive. This is essentially because we did not speak Arabic and had to make use of two interpreters (for Kabyle and Arabic). This need to have an interpreter fundamentally vitiated doctor-patient relations.

In normal circumstances, a patient may have encountered the image of the interpreter in his relations with the administration or the justice system. Within the hospital, the same need for an interpreter spontaneously triggers a distrust that makes all "communication" difficult. Incidentally, when the patient's trust had been won, his speech was filled with enthusiasm, such as when explaining vehemently that he was cured and had to leave quickly, often forgetting the presence of the third person and addressing us directly: he felt that the other could not say all that he wanted to express with the same "warmth." It is not hard to see the extent to which a study of this three-way dialogue would reveal a disruption of the phenomenon of the encounter.

The interpreter does not only bother the patient. The doctor, especially the psychiatrist, makes his diagnosis through language. Well, here the gestural and verbal components of language cannot be perceived in synchronous fashion. While the face is expressive and the gestures profuse, it is necessary to wait until the patient has stopped talking in order to grasp the meaning. At which point, the interpreter sums up in two words what the patient has related in detail for ten minutes: "He says that someone took his land, or that his wife cheated on him." Often, the interpreter "interprets" in his own way the patient's thinking according to some stereotyped formula, depriving it of all its richness: "He says that he hears djinn"—indeed, one no longer knows if the delusion is real or inferred.

Going through an interpreter is perhaps valid when it comes to explaining something simple or transmiting an order, but it is no longer valid when it is necessary to begin a dialogue, a dialectical exchange of questions and replies, alone able to overcome reticence and bring to light abnormal, pathological behaviour. But as Merleau-Ponty said, "to speak a language is to bear the weight of a culture."[7] Unable to speak Arabic, we did not know the elements of affective or cultural patrimony apt to awaken interest. Among the European women, it was easy to engage a conversation about a record by Tino Rossi or a film with Fernandel. With the Muslim men, meetings soon came to an abrupt end because one no longer knew what to talk about.

Similarly, with a little hindsight, our first attempts at organizing celebrations appeared rather naive. The very notion of having a celebration outside of family or religious events appears rather abstract to a Muslim. Moreover, the content of collective festivities seems to us to be essentially different from Western festivities. It was difficult to form a choir, because the Muslim loathes to sing in a group. In the house, one does not sing because one respects the father or the eldest brother. And among the Muslim nurses of our ward, we could get no one to consent to sing or to perform on a stage. In the same way, putting on a theater play is impossible, firstly because the theater as we understand it does not exist among Muslims, and secondly because one does not play a role in front of others. It is true that an Arab theater does exist today, but its existence is a recent thing and it only reaches the populations of the big cities. The actor or the singer is a professional who remains outside the group. In the villages, in the douars, this figure will be an itinerant "storyteller" who goes from place to place spreading news and telling folktales accompanied by a rudimentary lute or a darabukka, thus evoking the troubadours of the Middle Ages.

Abandoning our plan to have a celebration, the brief evening meetings had no further success. Going through the reports of these sessions, we see that initial accounts mentioned the games of hide-and-seek or *pelote cavalière*. Indeed, we had strongly impressed upon the nurses, whom we chose randomly from among the Europeans and the Muslims, that they should find activities apt to awaken a team spirit: the games of *pelote cavalière* and hide-and-seek in effect require each person to act by taking into account the reactions of his companions. One cannot ignore them.

But Muslims rarely play such games. At school is where you learn to play hide-and-seek or cops and robbers, where you acquire a team spirit. But at ten or twelve years of age, the young Arab boy is a shepherd or else he helps his father with small jobs. If we had wanted to have daily evening meetings, it would have been necessary to take inspiration from reality: after work, the Muslim gathers together with other men at the Moorish café. He remains seated around a table playing cards or dominoes, or else lies down on a mat to discuss daily events or listen to music for hours while drinking a cup of coffee or a glass of tea. And this is indeed what experience has shown us: after some weeks, the nurses in charge of the evening sessions had lost all sense of initiative, and the few patients who still consented not to go to bed did nothing but listen to the radio.

Outside of these attempts at active resocialization, the entertainments organized by the hospital were not for the Muslim patients a practically "vital" need as they were for the Europeans. Thus, apropos of the cinema, most of the films able to be seen did not generate any emotional engagement in the Muslim patient. We list here some of the titles of recently screened films: *Little Women*, *King Solomon's Mines*, *Les Noces de sable*, *La Duchesse de Langeais*, *Crisis*, *Rio Grande*, *Teresa*, etc. Obviously, the only films that were somewhat followed were the action films without great psychological or sentimental complications. But more than to a certain "primitivism," this disinterest can probably be attributed to its not being possible for the Muslim to understand the Western characters' reactions, which are completely foreign to him. The example of the film by Jean Cocteau, *Les Noces de sable*, is particularly telling. The film relates the adventures of an Arab prince who goes to find his fiancée among the nomads of the Sahara. Although the costumes and the setting were in principle specific to North Africa, the psychological framework remained Western. It did not interest the Muslims, because they were unable to participate fully in the action or identify with the personages. And what are we to say concerning the other films? The schema in "action films" is simple, the picture speaks for itself, language is unnecessary.

Similarly, for the celebrations in the European wards: if a fashionable tune was sung, if one played *Les Précieuses ridicules*, *Le Médecin malgré lui*, *Cyrano de Bergerac*, put on a play by Courteline or by Colette, then a whole section of the audience in the room would remain completely unmoved: at most it would indistinctly emerge from its torpor on the occasion that an actor threw a glass of water into someone's face or struck someone with sticks.

As for the journal, the failure was even more pronounced: as the journal only reflected more or less faithfully the social life at the hospital, it was rather uninteresting for those who remained excluded from it in practice. This is why even the few patients who knew how to read and write never sent any articles. However, the failure is due above all to the fact that most of our Muslim patients are illiterate. More exactly, out of the 220 patients in our unit, only 5 knew how to read and write in Arabic and 2, how to read and write in French. The others were illiterate. And again, let's say that out of the 7 "literate" patients, only 6 had passed the level of school certificate.

At the start we considered the possibility of having the articles written by a nurse, as we did with the Europeans when they did not know how or want to write. But the uniform use of this procedure is practically useless. In actual fact, it can be said that in the conditions of illiteracy prevailing currently in Algeria, culture is more oral than it is written: teaching is essentially carried out through speech. Each group in general has one or several literate individuals tasked with reading and writing for the rest of the group: this is why we were easily able to recognize the writing of the same *taleb* or public writer in the letters that we received from the parents of all patients that hailed from the same douar. We have already noted the important role of the itinerant "storyteller," who goes from village to village spreading news and stories from folklore—that is, sorts of epic poems relating the events of previous centuries—and thereby ensures a cultural liaison between the different regions.

To end this explanation of our first failures, we must speak about ergotherapy. In a heavily industrialized Western country, it is easy to organize a patient's readaptation on the basis of already existing possibilities. On the contrary, for the Algerian Muslim, who lives in a framework that is still feudal in many respects, this readaptation is much more difficult. A man works the land, he has no specialization. He is sometimes able to perform rather rudimentary handicraft work outside of the major urban centers, but he loathes to work with wool or raffia, because that is feminine work: baskets and mats are produced by women.

In a psychiatric hospital, one might seek to organize workshops for raffia, weaving, or pottery. But it would be better, it seems to us, to entrust this work to women patients. For the men, you must set out from the most general dispositions and from those most strongly rooted in the patient's personality: we conducted this experiment with delusional patients and even catatonic ones. All you need to do is give them a shovel or a pickax to get them to work and start digging up earth and hoeing without having to push them to do so in the slightest. These peasants are close to the land; they are one with it. And if you succeed in getting them hooked on a particular patch of land, in getting them interested in the yield gained from farming, then work will genuinely be a factor of re-equilibration; such ergotherapy can be embedded within a specific social activity.

Ultimately, we see why our first attempts at undertaking social therapy among Muslim patients ended in failure. We nonetheless believe that this failure was not worthless, to the extent that we have understood its reasons. Since then we have altered the direction of our efforts and have seen certain accomplishments crystallize. The establishing of a Moorish café. in the hospital, the regular celebration of traditional Muslim feasts, of periodic meetings around a professional "storyteller" are already concrete facts. With each new event, the number of patients engaged in these activities increases. This social life is only in its beginnings, but already we believe that we have eliminated the methodological errors.

IV

THE RETURN.
A FOREIGN BODY

REUS
1967–1994

> I think I must point out here something that, for more than a century, has characterized French psychiatry and that isn't really found in Spain: nothing more and nothing less than the long history of psychiatric practices as the concrete exercise of a public function.
>
> FRANCESC TOSQUELLES

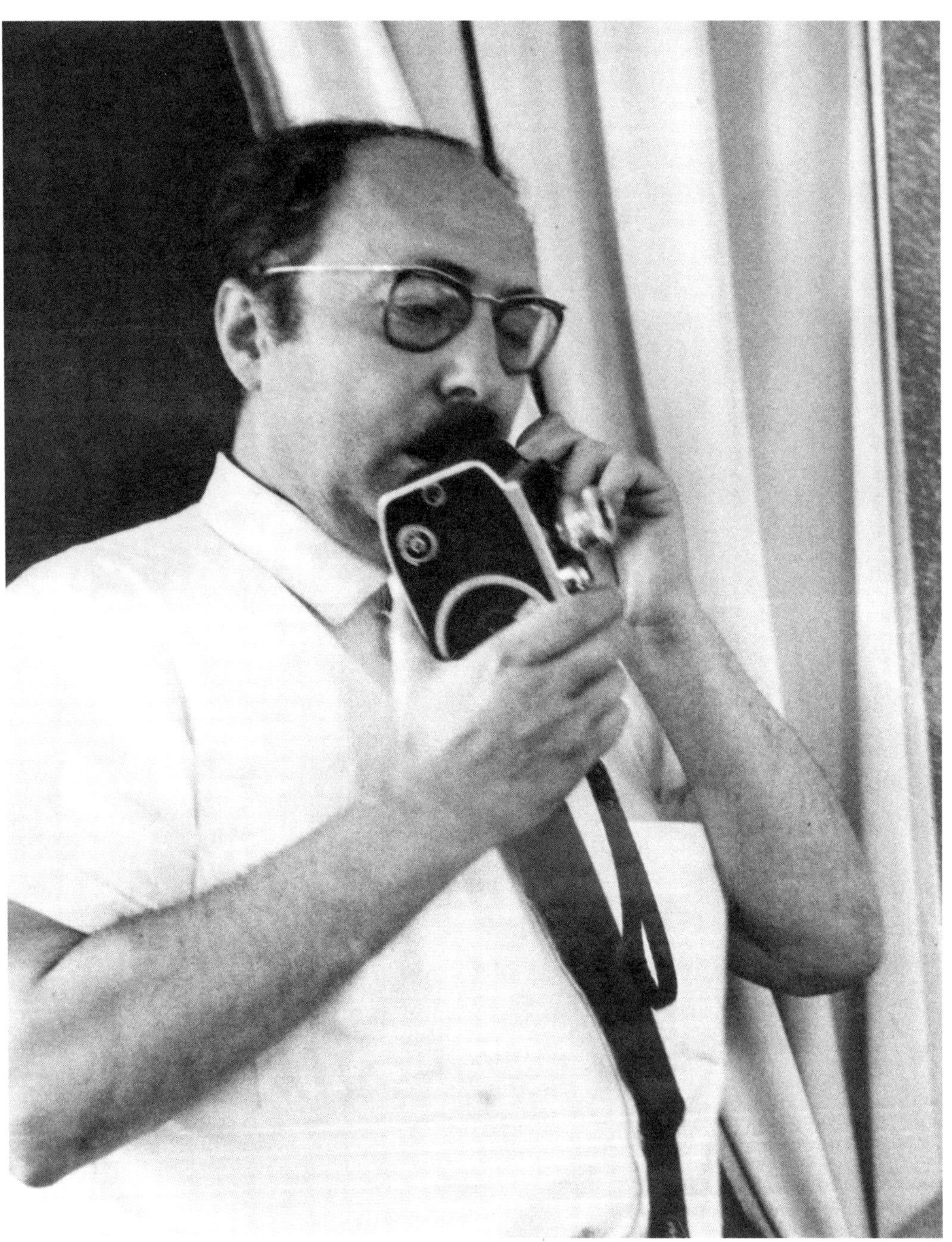

Francesc Tosquelles, circa 1970

Transmitting Tosquelles

In 2011, in *Déconnage*, the video-essay that Angela Melitopoulos and Maurizio Lazzarato made about Francesc Tosquelles, the psychiatrist and psychoanalyst Jean-Claude Polack said that the life of institutional psychotherapy had only been possible in wartime. These times of war could be specified, in Tosquelles's case, as the fight for the Republic, the Spanish Civil War, and the Second World War; in Fanon's case, it was the Algerian War of Independence; and in the case of the La Borde therapeutic community, it was having to hide Algerians when the colonial power was weakening and the French national hegemony went into crisis. But the question of what war Tosquelles had to face when he returned to the Institut Pere Mata in 1967 with the intention of initiating a situated psychotherapy there is a question that perhaps needs more than one answer: a dictatorship that would continue for almost another decade; a hospital system debilitated by three decades of Francoism, and that was only sustained by the long and poorly remunerated shifts of caregivers; a hospital life designed to drive people crazy, to make people sick; institutions to die inside; and a system of pharmaceutical companies who were preparing for the arrival of psychopharmaceuticals that would produce a new therapeutic society, inside and outside of hospitals, increasingly dependent on the fabrication of normality.

His desire to transform the Institut Pere Mata was what made Tosquelles return to Reus in the late sixties, after Ramon Vilella and Francesc Mateu went to France to offer him the direction of the Institut, which he refused. What he did agree to was forming part of a new phase in the life of the institution, although intermittently while mostly remaining in France. For the following twenty-five years, Tosquelles would visit Reus for a week or ten days each month.

He not only returned to Reus with the knowledge he'd acquired at Saint-Alban, but he returned there with his experiences and his failures, with pasts that could inspire possible presents, and with a world of reading and role models. The new institutionality allowed him to recover the extensive psychiatry of the Civil War that Francoism had interrupted, to incorporate the practices of sector psychiatry from Saint-Alban, as well as other centers where Tosquelles continued working after 1962: Marseille, Melun, Longueil-Annel, and Agen. In Reus this legacy took shape as the adoption in 1968 of situated forms; the dissolution of the figure of the director into leadership by committee; the obligatory exclusive devotion of the medical community, renouncing private practice; the reduction of the length of the workday for caregivers from twelve to eight hours; the regulated training for the nuns in the infirmary and other spaces of responsibility; the creation of the Club Emili Briansó—following the experience of the Club Paul-Balvet at Saint-Alban—that included twelve sections managed by the patients: cinema, field trips, theater, music, parties, café bar, soccer, baths, ping pong, a library, tennis, and the internal newspaper *Club*, which like *Trait d'union* at Saint-Alban allowed Tosquelles to gather incomplete, informal, and disjointed words of the inpatients. In this context they also organized an annual psychiatric conference, the Jornades d'Interès psiquiàtric, which dealt with questions such as the problem of space in psychiatry, the narrative of daily life in medical records, the organization of collectives, training for treatments, and the experience of freedom, legislation, and justice in psychiatry.[1]

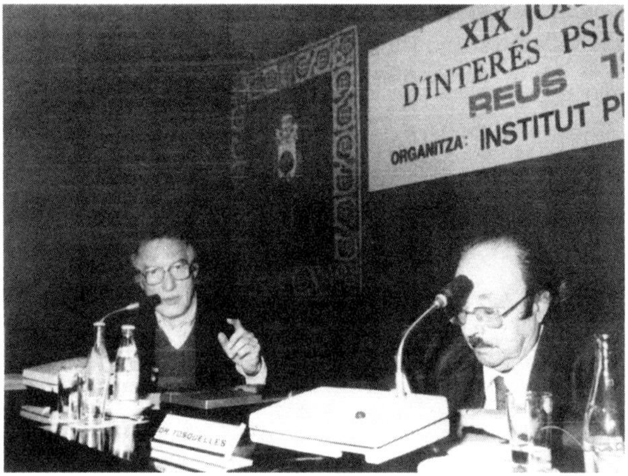

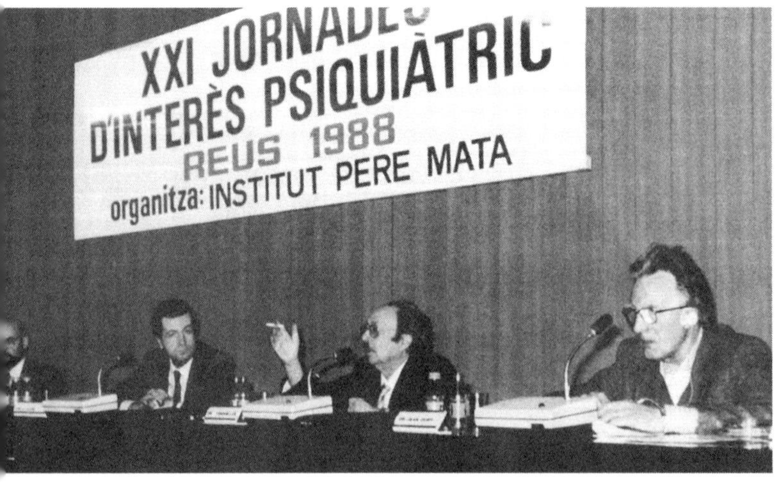

Tosquelles and Jean Oury with other speakers at the XXI Jornades d'Interès Psiquiàtric de Reus in 1988

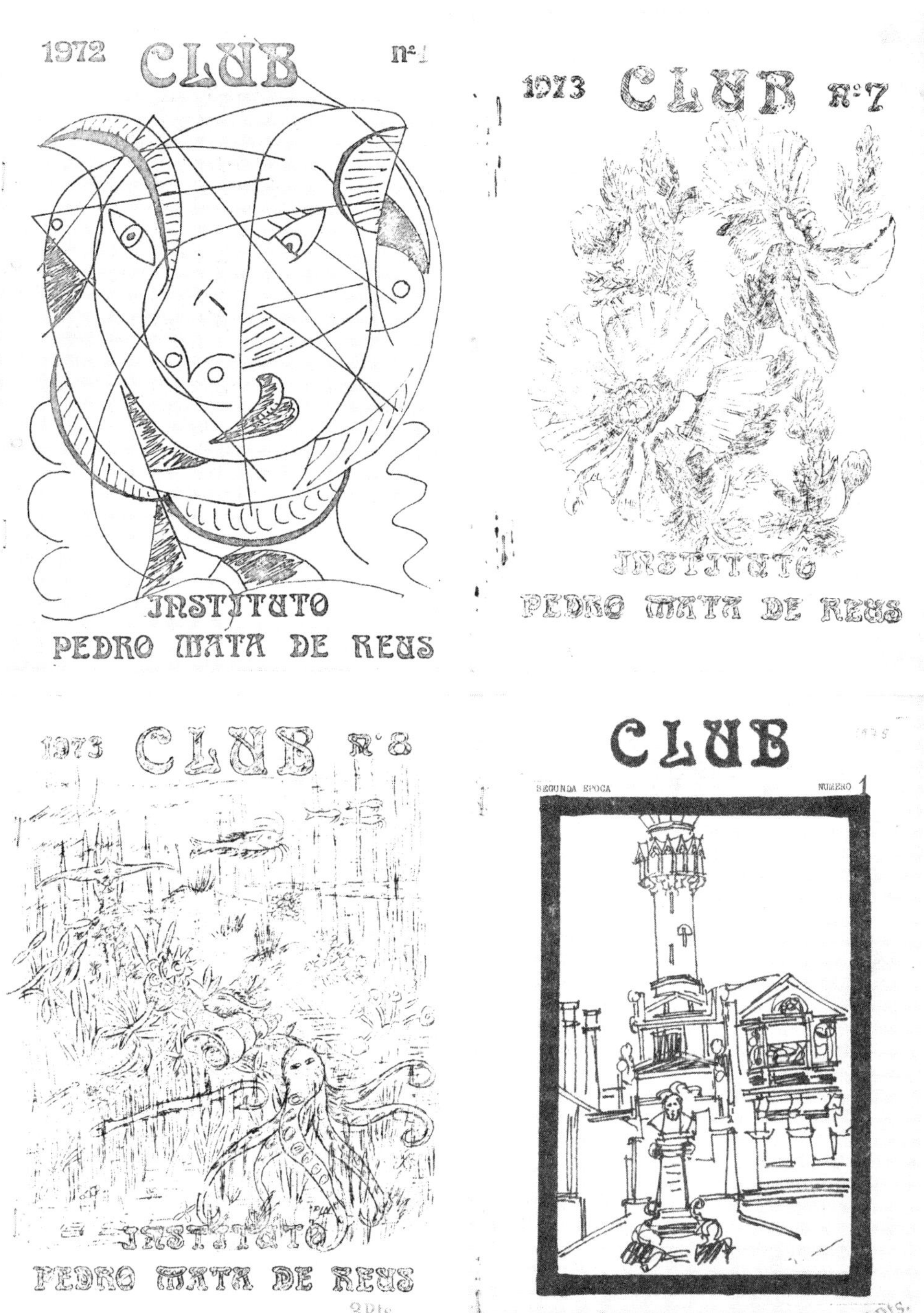

The magazine *Club*, published by the Club Emili Brians, at the Institut Pere Mata between 1972 and 1979

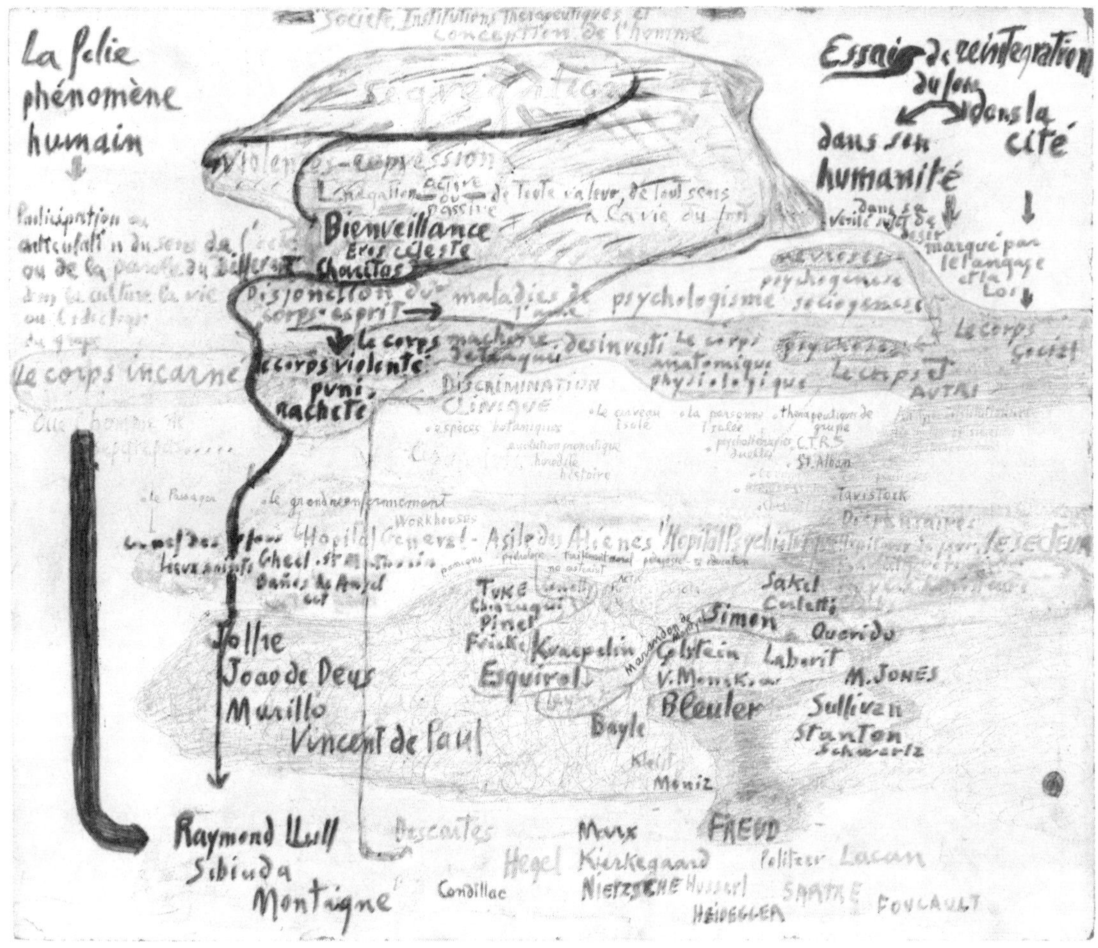

Querido, who organized the psychiatric service in slums with ambulances. Esquirol. Sakel—insulin—and Cerletti.

Below are the neurological and integrational problems: Goldstein. Von Monakow. Bayle. Kleist and Moniz. Jones, for the therapeutic communities. Sullivan, first therapeutic community for schizophrenics in 1911. Saint Elizabeths Hospital. Stanton and Schwartz's study, first article on the functioning of a hospital.

Further down, madness as a human phenomenon. First of all is Ramon Llull, without whom nothing can be understood. Sibiuda, who modified Ramon Llull, only somewhat, although he introduced Montaigne to Ramon Llull, an entire volume that talks about Sibiuda, which is a way to depict the problem of Ramon Llull: language, pedagogy, *ars magna*.

While, over here, on the path of the negation of all meaning in the life of the insane person, is Descartes. Below is Condillac. Then come Hegel and Marx. Kierkegaard and Nietzsche. And below the psychiatrists: Freud, Nietzsche, Husserl, Heidegger, Politzer, Lacan, Sartre, and Foucault.

Transcription of a recording at the Institut Pere Mata where Francesc Tosquelles talks about his two "wall paintings," map-diagrams he made with marker on wood (reproduced on these pages), which show a trajectory of his influences in his clinical practice

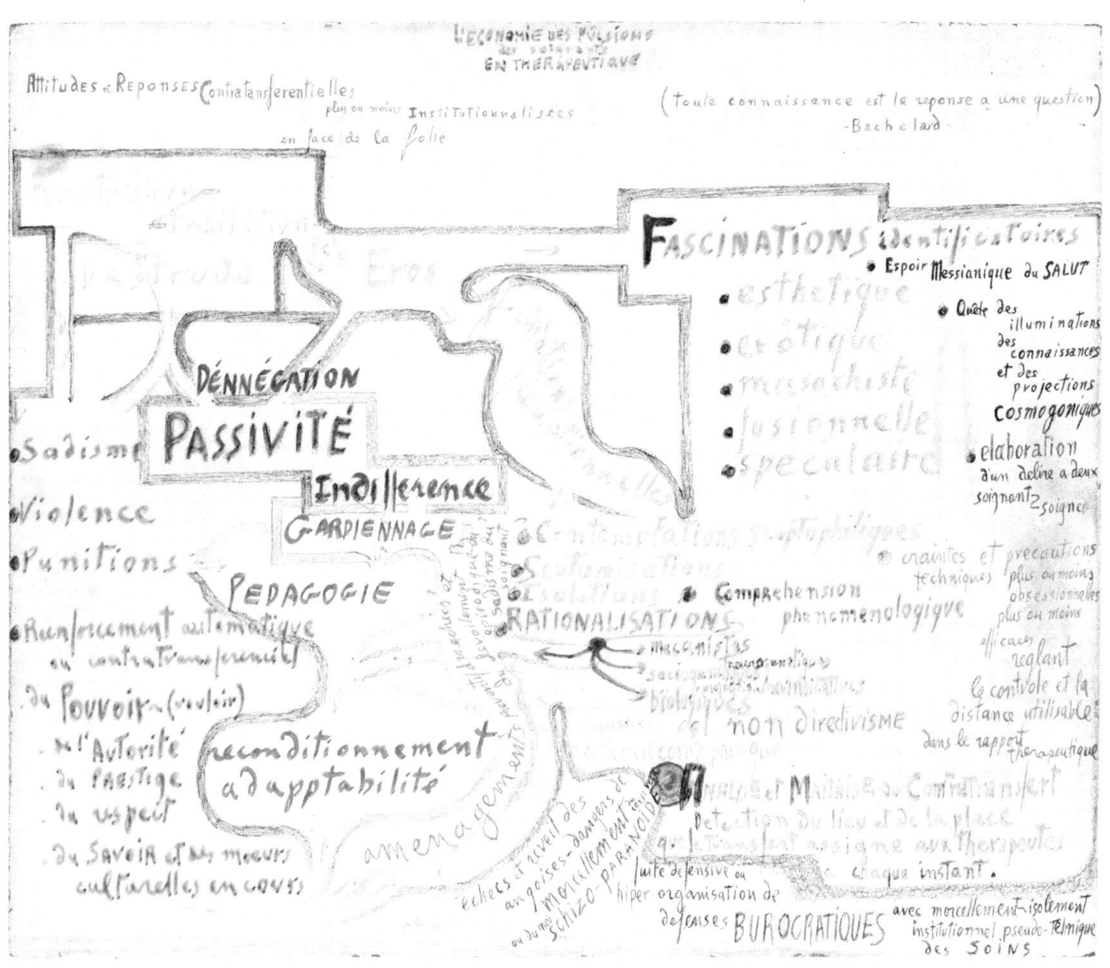

At left, above, and following pages, diagrams made by Tosquelles, in color and on paper, held at the Institut Pere Mata

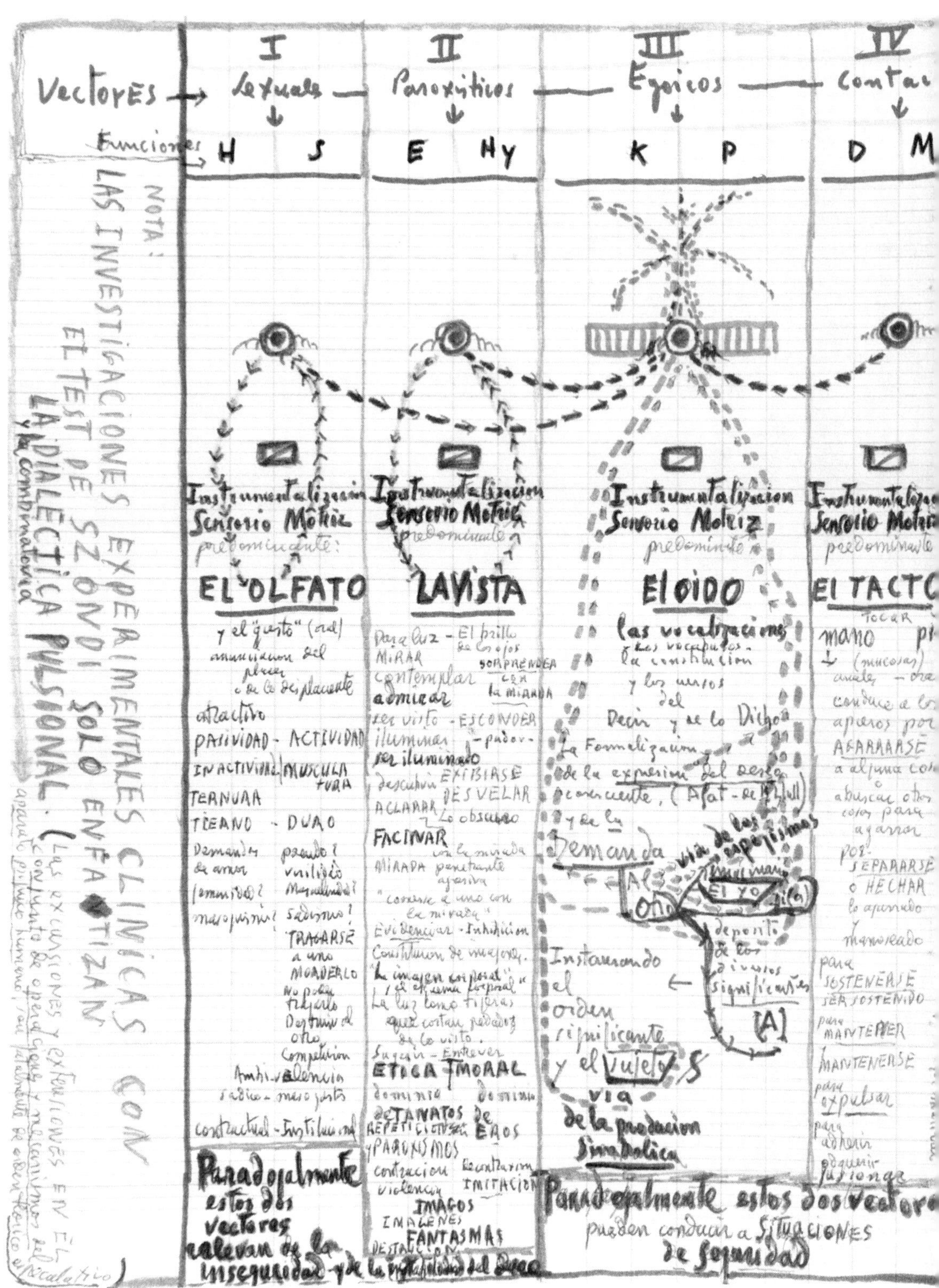

Vectores
I
Sexuale
II
Paroxíticos
III
Egoicos
IV
Funciones
H S
E Hy
K P
D M
NOTA: LAS INVESTIGACIONES EXPERIMENTALES CLINICAS CON EL TEST DE SZONDI SOLO ENFATIZAN LA DIALECTICA PULSIONAL
Instrumentalización Sensorio Motriz predominante:
EL OLFATO
PASIVIDAD - ACTIVIDAD
TIERNO - DURO
Ambivalencia
Paradojalmente estos dos vectores relevan de la inseguridad
LA VISTA
MIRAR
contemplar
admirar
ESCONDER
EXHIBIRSE
DESVELAR
ACLARAR
FACINAR
ETICA MORAL
TANATOS
EROS
IMITACION
IMAGOS
IMAGENES
FANTASMAS
El OIDO
las vocalizaciones
Decir y de lo Dicho
Demanda
EL YO
el orden significante y el sujeto S
VIA de la producción Simbolica
[A]
Paradojalmente estos dos vectores pueden conducir a SITUACIONES de seguridad
EL TACTO
TOCAR
mano
AGARRARSE
SEPARARSE o HECHAR
SOSTENERSE
SER SOSTENIDO
MANTENER
MANTENERSE
expulsar

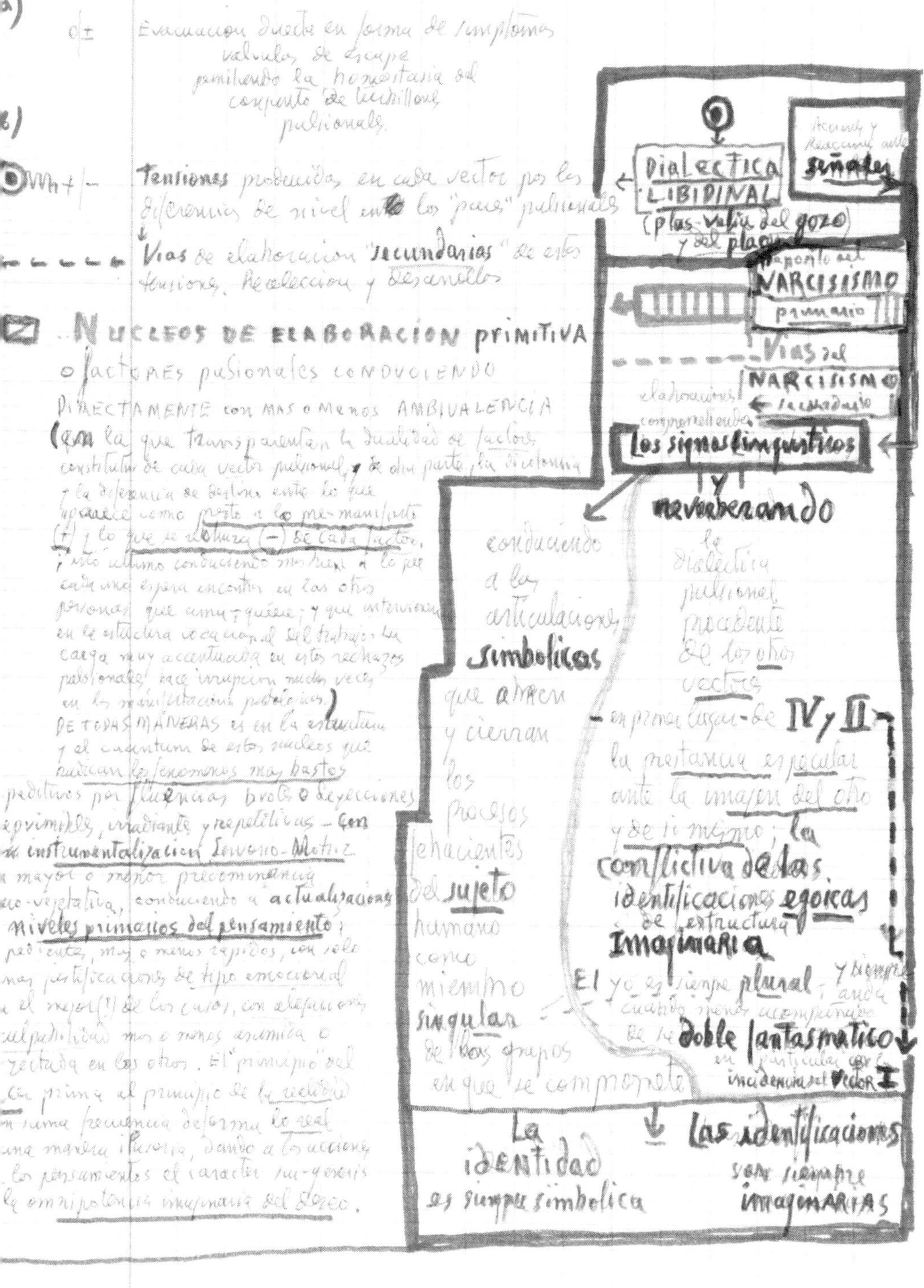

Tensiones producidas en cada vector por las diferencias de nivel entre los "pares" pulsionales
Vias de elaboracion "secundarias" de estas tensiones. Recoleccion y Desarrollos
NUCLEOS DE ELABORACION PRIMITIVA
o factores pulsionales conduciendo
DIRECTAMENTE con mas o menos AMBIVALENCIA
DE TODAS MANERAS es en la estructura
niveles primarios del pensamiento
DIALECTICA LIBIDINAL
(plus-valia del gozo y del placer)
señales
NARCISISMO
primario
Vias del
NARCISISMO
secundario
Los signos linguisticos
y
reverberando
conduciendo a las articulaciones simbolicas
que abren y cierran los procesos fehacientes del sujeto humano como miembro singular de los grupos en que se compromete
la dialectica pulsional procedente de los otros vectores
en primer lugar de IV y II
la prestancia especular ante la imagen del otro y de si mismo; la conflictiva de las identificaciones egoicas de estructura Imaginaria
El yo es siempre plural
doble fantasmatico
incidencia del Vector I
La identidad es siempre simbolica
Las identificaciones son siempre imaginarias

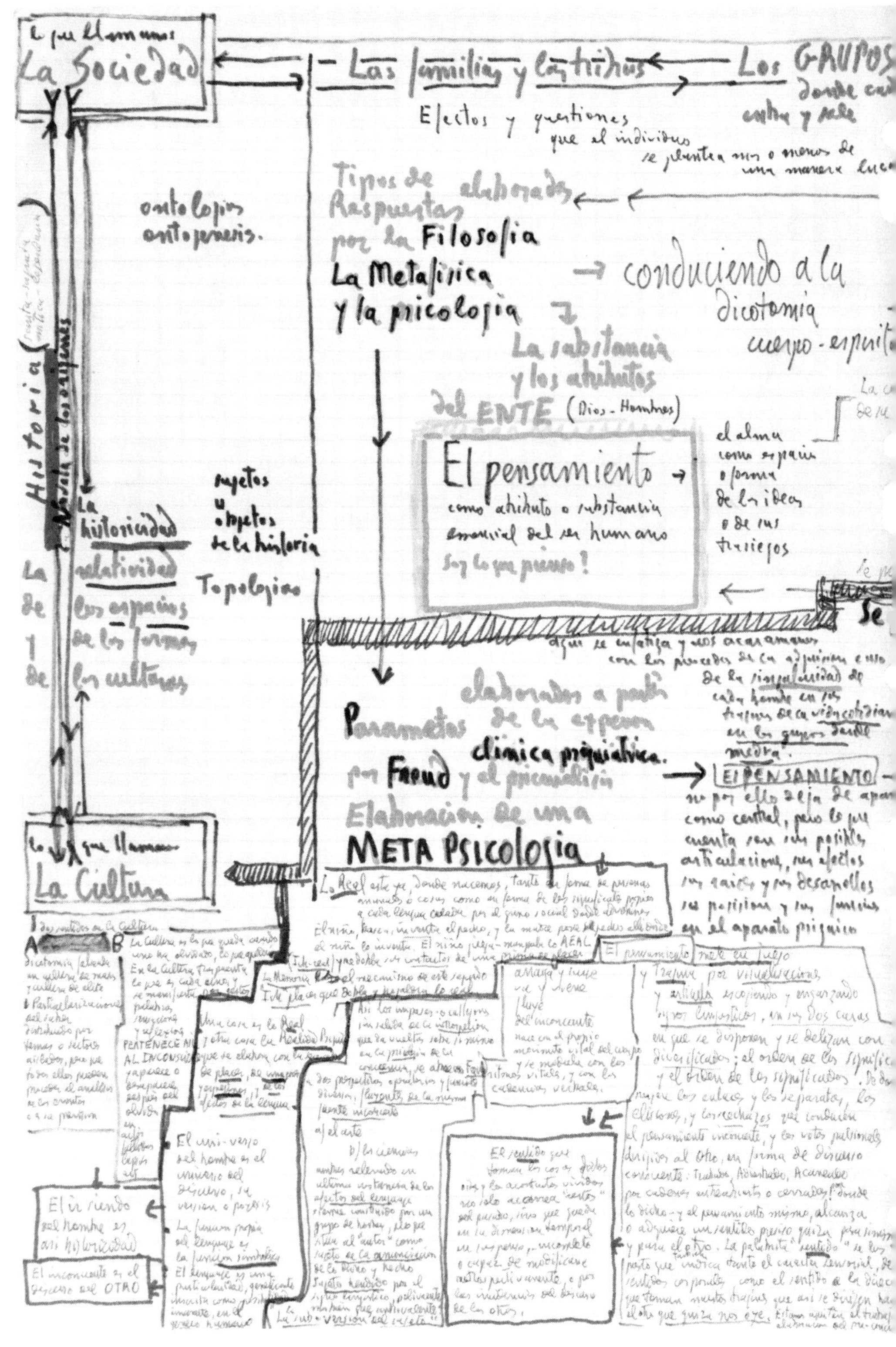
Lo que llamamos
La Sociedad
Los GRUPOS
Efectos y cuestiones
que al individuo
se plantea más o menos de
una manera
Tipos de
Respuestas
elaborados
por la Filosofía
La Metafísica
y la psicología
conduciendo a la
dicotomía
cuerpo-espíritu
La substancia
y los atributos
del ENTE (Dios - Hombres)
El pensamiento
como atributo o substancia
esencial del ser humano
Soy lo que pienso!
ontologías
Historia
La
historicidad
relatividad
Topologías
sujetos
u
objetos
de la historia
Parametros
clínica psiquiátrica.
por Freud y el psicoanálisis
Elaboración de una
META PSICOLOGIA
EL PENSAMIENTO
Lo que llamamos
La Cultura
El inconsciente es el
discurso del OTRO

Las instituciones y los procesos de institucionalización

¿Quién es uno? ¿Quién une? ¿Quién separa? Quien me aísla – me abandona – me excluye
Que es lo que se une o se para? ¿Quién soy yo? ¿Que me falta? ¿Quién es el otro? Quien soy yo para el otro
Que me falta para ser mi mismo. Que me dan, Que me quitan. A que tengo derecho. Que me da la gana de hacer o de no hacer! La conducta explícita releva o revela – esconde o manifiesta este vasto y complejo tipo de preguntas

a su relativismo sociológico

La pseudo síntesis del hombre y la circunstancia

La solución a estos problemas "de cada uno en los grupos de convivencia, o a pertenencia... QUEDA en suspenso este enigma y misterio o se cosifica en problemática sociológica

...mentalismo psico-físico

...estos fantasmas inconscientes, surgen o se destapan poco a poco durante el curso de la cura. (muchas veces en forma de interpretación del propio analista) y su aparición entonces en la transferencia, es utilizable en el proceso de la cura) o surgen espontáneamente de súbito sea quien sea, La sorpresa entonces es grande, y las acciones o conductas de la gente son entonces difícilmente elaboradas o contenidas. (Conviene mantener un distingo, estructural y en el orden de las consecuencias entre fantasma inconsciente y fantasma consciente)

El fantasma inconsciente surge pues de súbito y por sorpresa, a pesar que sus trayectorias subliminales pueden poder incidir modelando numerosas conductas, en particular las conductas lúdicas y placenteras

El fantasma inconsciente releva pues del propio movimiento pulsional y aparece como en una válvula de escape de las "energías" pulsionales poco o mal traducidas en las "acciones" diversas tales como pueden vislumbrarse con el SZONDI. Aparece pues según la dialéctica pulsional del vector de sorpresa (P) y contribuye así paradójicamente a la homeostasis pulsional del conjunto, escapando a las vacancias de la elaboración y a los efectos funcionales del vector (Sch). El sentido que aquí protagoniza la escena; es fundamentalmente la visión

La lógica del fantasma supone tres tipos de actos

a/ El momento (el instante) de ver
b/ El tiempo de reelaboración (inconsciente) donde los destinos de las imagos, de los "otros" pulsiones y de los significantes, en su disponibilidad elemental persiguen sus movimientos, sin tener acceso a las conductas explícitas
c/ El momento, de la decisión, ineludible, de su objetivación escénica, dramática comportando "otros" en una...

...el desarrollo de la apetencia verbal, o de su personificación organizando actos fabulantes y actitudes diversas ante los otros humanos y las cosas

El lenguaje surge misteriosamente el verbo recibido de Dios, se encarna y modifica, o determina los pensamientos en la... de los efectos de una... los propósitos. ...

...n dos hipótesis nuevas míticas

Las instancias pulsionales
El narcisismo (P + S)

... circunscribe una "otra escena" radicalmente inaccesible a la elaboración consciente

y que no obstante, sostiene los procesos de elaboración preconscientes y conscientes

A esta escena, se le llama:

El inconsciente

No puede haber ni psicología ni metafísica del inconsciente

Los "elementos" del inconsciente son de diverso orden:
a/ las pulsiones y el narcisismo
b/ los significantes
c/ Las imagos

d/ los restos y los residuos de los traumas... pulsionales del pasado

Identificaciones producto de las... en la captación especular por la imagen del otro

El yo y el otro relevan de esta estructura imaginaria

En el inconsciente NO HAY Objetos sino representaciones de objetos – imagos y representaciones pulsionales – repetitivas y representaciones de palabras, o mejor dicho de significantes. La organización móvil e inestable del inconsciente, conduce a la elaboración ...nudos relacionales, o funciones operativas, en forma de ...anismos más o menos característicos...

el acceso a esta escena se deja entre-ver cuando en el proceso de la cura analítica surgen ciertos fantasmas

EN LA FORMULACION EN ACTOS O PALABRAS de lo que se dirige y pide al otro,
Hay dos líneas de desarrollo a considerar:
a/ la línea del deseo que se dirige del yo al otro imaginario
b/ la línea de la demanda simbólica que paralela a la primera, pasa por la cadena de los significantes. En uno de los extremos de esta cadena, situamos el OTRO, depósito de los significantes y en la otra punta yo, pues el sujeto ... por el ...

That moment coincided with other projects of health care sectorization that failed to come to fruition, like that of the hospital in Oviedo, in 1966, inspired by Hermann Simon, Francesc Tosquelles, and Maxwell Jones, among others. As Manuel Desviat and Anna Moreno pointed out, it also coincided with community mental health practices conceived as part of various processes of psychiatric reform in which institutional psychotherapy emerged as one of the historic attempts most deeply invested in saving the psychiatric hospital.[2] In a context in which in the national conferences of the Asociación Española de Neuropsiquiatría there were discussions of whether it was necessary to reform the asylums, coinciding with the end of the dictatorship, between 1966 and 1967 the Institut Pere Mata incorporated a group of young doctors from the Universidad de Zaragoza—Antonio Labad, Jesús Otín, José García Ibáñez, Antonio Vergós, and Eduardo González—with whom Francesc Tosquelles developed a new way of introducing dialogism into the psychoanalytical listening within the institution. Starting in 1970, they introduced "cassette groups" through which, to avoid individual psychoanalysis, a series of small groups were created. They began to carry out collective supervisions that were recorded and regularly sent to Tosquelles in France and discussed when he was in Reus. Antonio Labad and José García Ibáñez described them as groups of *contre-transfert*, or countertransference, in which they analyzed the meetings and the responses of the medical collective regarding the patients. In polyphonic form, each person's individual words had a place as they wove together with the institution's fabric, since the framework of those twice-weekly meetings was the collective discussion of the cases at the Institut. In his contemporary writings, Tosquelles barely mentioned the cassettes. He would speak of the device itself, recording at the meetings over the years.

Despite Tosquelles's intermittent returns over numerous years, today we feel that he was a foreign body because he left so few traces in our collective imagination and in the history of psychiatry and psychoanalysis in Catalonia and Spain in the late Francoist and post-dictatorship periods. Just as he'd left few traces during the Second Republic in the 1930s. The French exile of

The first phase is gathering, without yet recording, to reveal the first anxieties. There is only one rule: everyone has to put forth a question; all of them, except for one, will be addressed. There is one that remains frustrated. One person has to live with the frustration—today it's my turn and tomorrow it'll be yours. Two sessions each week. An hour and a half each time. Outside of regular work hours. You pay with your time for the right to be here, with the others, as part of a flagship group, the place to bring your burdens to, your concerns, in order to be able to, slowly, gradually, glimpse to the jumping-off point for the unconscious reaction to transference. Entering into the work that allows one to go beyond their own complexes and their own internal resistance. Not head-on, but always through an anecdote, a situation, a meeting, a dialogue, etc., with the patient, with their family. [...]

During all these years there have been various phases. The first, with only four or five doctors fully committed to the process of change, apparently focused on the analysis of attitudes, and introduced the tape recorder after some time. Obviously, the interruptions are anxiety producing and paranoiac reactions begin to appear, suspicions, fears over the use of all that is said. By the third phase, people from all professions and trainings are participating, as well as elements foreign to our center (teachers from centers for the mentally deficient, social workers from the Guardianship Court for Minors, doctors and caregivers from other hospitals, etc.) This is the current phase, with five cassette groups and forty-five people. [...]

In the formal aspect, the cassettes constitute an institutionalized meeting that is repeated in an almost liturgical manner and that has two objectives: the training of scattered attention and the participation in the collective production of a discourse. [...]

The cassette practice is like a lived experience of polyphonic verbal productions.[3]

José García Ibáñez and Antonio Labad, "Experiència viscuda de les produccions verbals polifòniques: El mètode dels 'cassettes' en la formació professional de l'Institut Pere Mata," 1986

Cassette recordings of the *contre-transfert* groups that met at the Institut between 1970 and the early 1990s

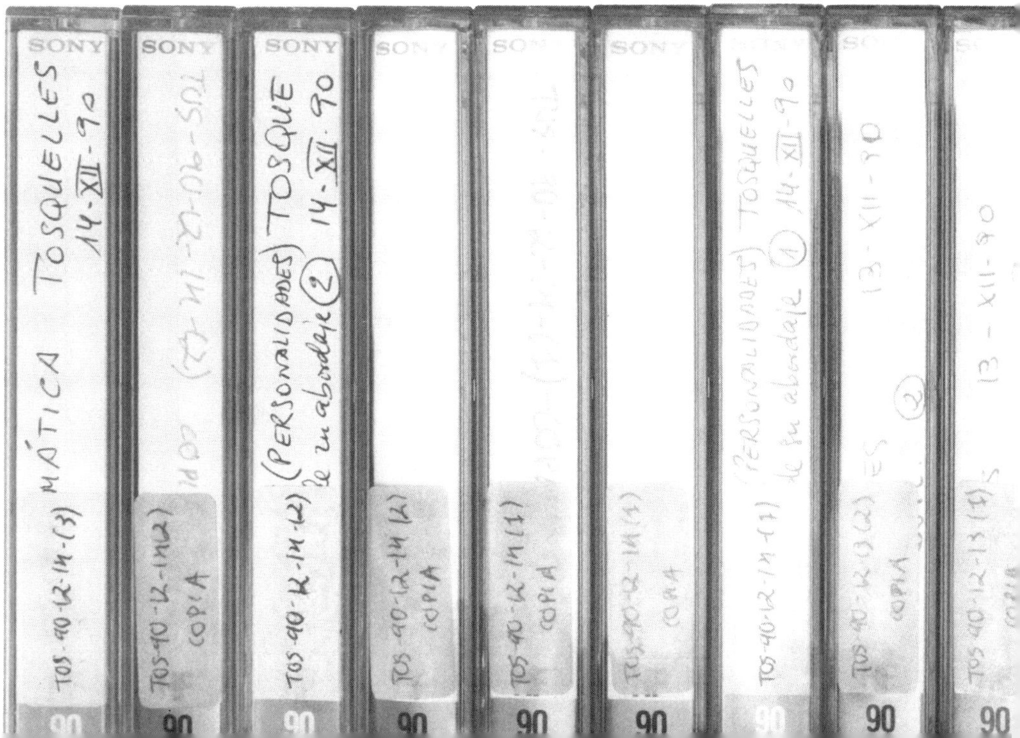

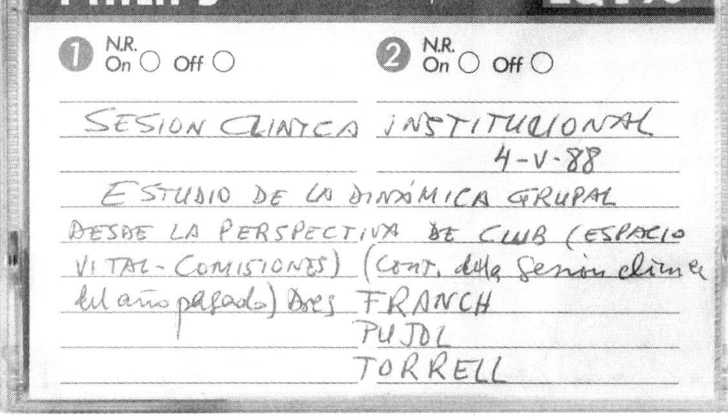

INSTITUTIONAL CLINICAL SESSION
May 4, 1988
STUDY OF GROUP DYNAMICS FROM THE PERSPECTIVE OF THE CLUB (PERSONAL SPACE—COMMISSIONS) (cont. of the clinical session of last year)
Drs. FRANCH, PUJOL, TORRELL

Institutional Psychotherapy
Comments regarding space, intermediary objects, relationships, etc.
TOSQUELLES
June 21, 1989
COPY

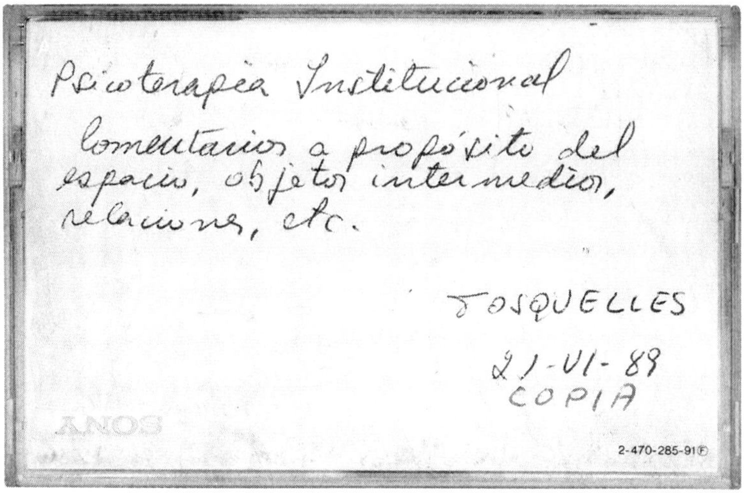

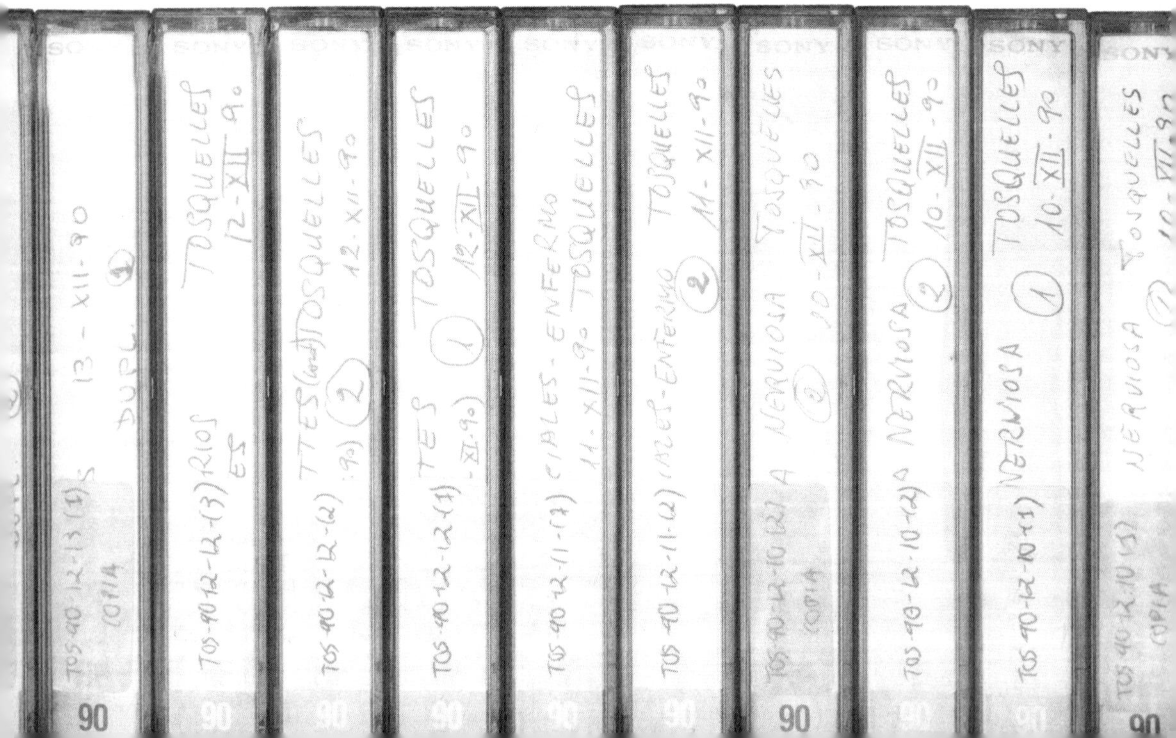

The language of the cassettes is filled with metaphors and metonymies.

We recall that Bion used to say that a group is like a schizophrenic and a schizophrenic is like a group. Both positive and negative relationships can be established between them. Negative ones are established when what someone says increases tensions, when they display hostility or antagonism, as well as when they air personal grievances.

The neutral areas of intercommunication are the most useful; they lead the group toward the objective, which is knowing how to listen and respond to a patient.

It is quite possible that 50 percent of the patients participate in the cassette sessions out of discipline and, as such, get no benefit whatsoever from their participation. The secretary must know how to listen to the group and, later, re-elaborate what took place within it. Furthermore, only one session a week is insufficient.

In order to participate in a group, even when not saying anything, you must give the others the impression that you are giving them a personal gift. It is not an easy exercise at all; much time must be devoted to it.[4]

Francesc Tosquelles, "Els sentiments (29 d'abril de 1986)"

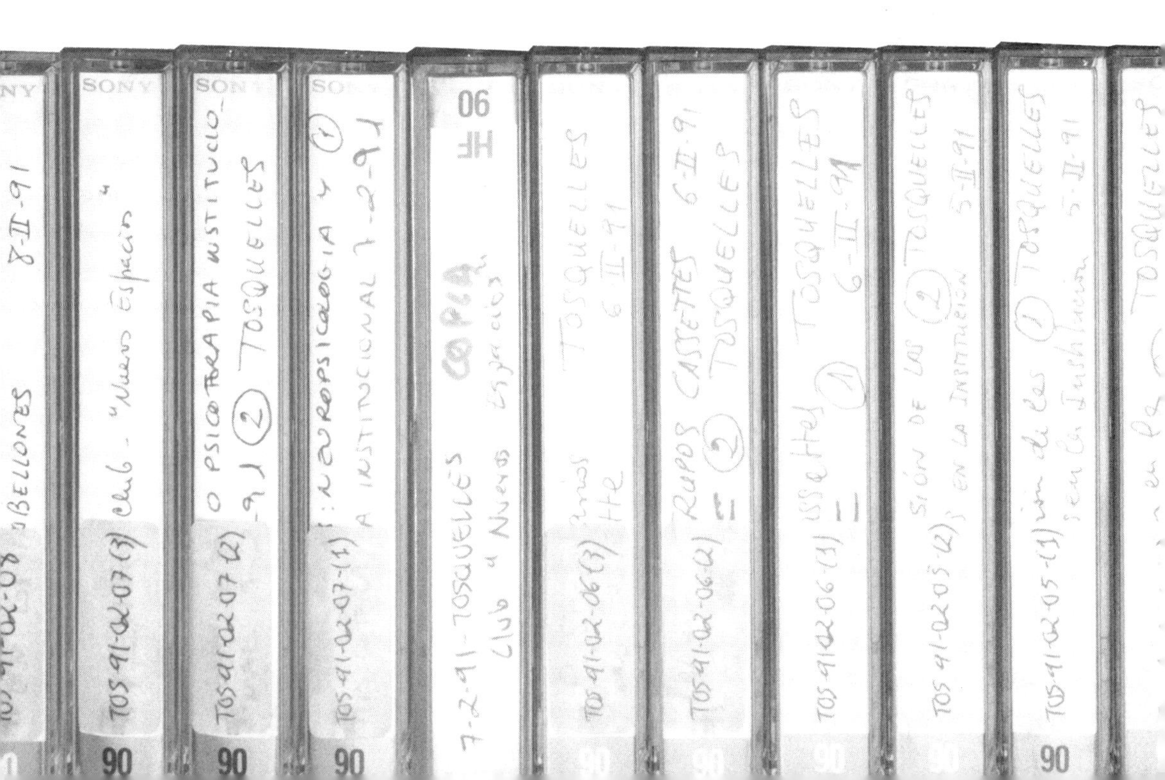

TOS-92-04-09
TOS-92-04-08
8-4-92
TOS-92-04-07-(1)
TOS-92-04-07-(2)
TOS-92-04-07-(1)
TOS-92-04-06-(2)
TOS-92-04-06-(1)
TOS-92-12-17-(1)
TOSQUELLE
17-XII-92
TOS-92-12-16-(2)
TOS-92-02-11-(2)
COPIA
11-2-92
COPIA
TOS-92-02-11-(2)
en las Calles
TOSQUELLES
ATS
11-II-92
TOS-92-02-11-(2)
Comas 11-II-92
TOS-92-02-11-(1)
COPIA
TOS-92-02-11-(1)
en las Calles
TOSQUELLES
ATS
11-II-92
TOS-92-02-11-(1)
e Comas
11-II-92
TOS-92-02-10
COPIA
TOSQUELLES
10-II-92
COPIA
TOS-92-02-11-(1)
COPIA
ACION A DOMICILIO
29-I-92
TOS-92-01-29-(2)
(Unió Catalana d'Hospitals)
ACION A DOMICILIO
29-I-92

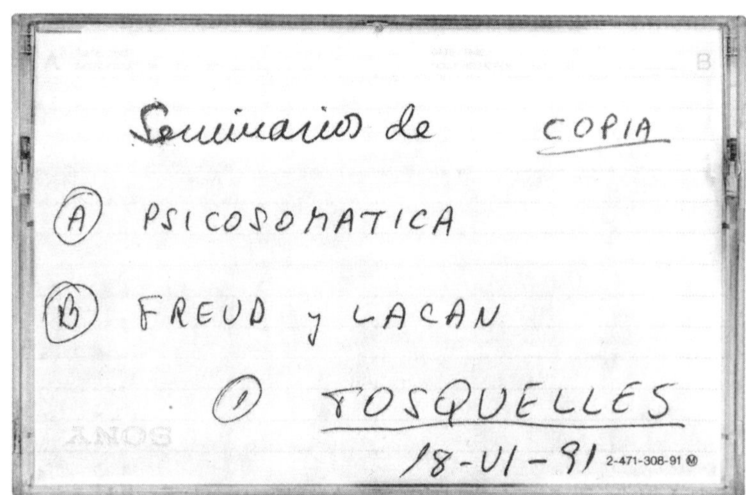

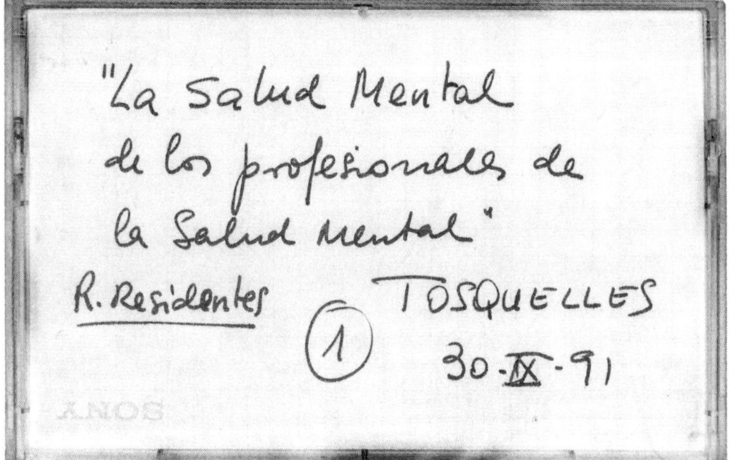

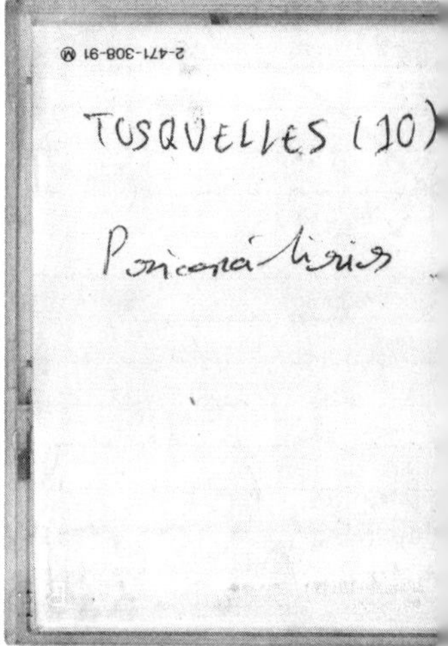

COPY
SEMINARS ON
A PSYCHOSOMATICS
B FREUD AND LACAN
1 TOSQUELLES
June 18, 1991

"The Mental Health of Mental Health professionals"
R. Residents TOSQUELLES
September 30, 1991

The cassettes are an anxiolytic. Anxiety is the sole basis of freedom; without anxiety no one searches for anything. One of those who attended one of the cassette sessions says they've been disillusioned, since they thought they would acquire the knowledge necessary to be able to lead a group. One is disappointed; you search for one thing and you find another that might be better. We must manage to shift anxiety; there is no therapy without pain or without handling anxiety.[5]

Francesc Tosquelles, "Sessió del 30 d'abril de 1986"

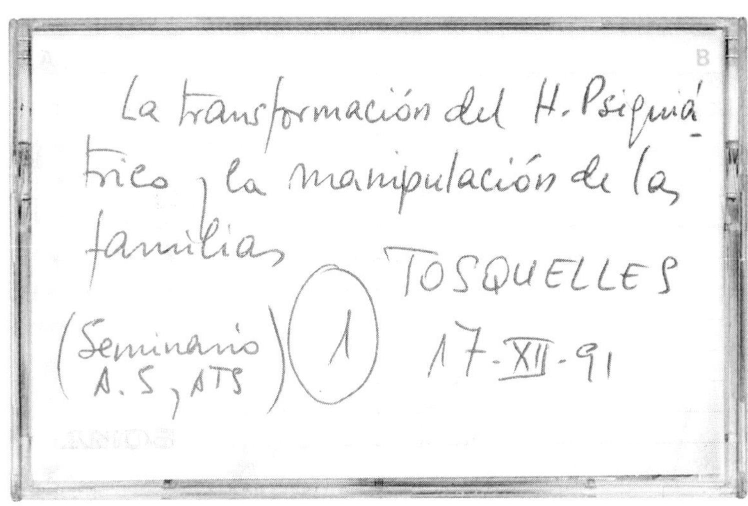

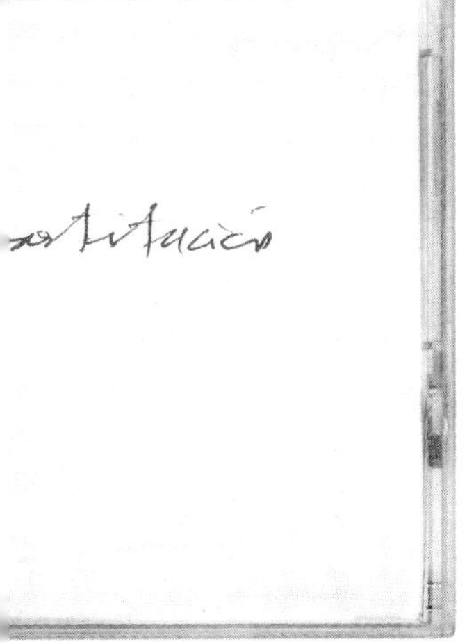

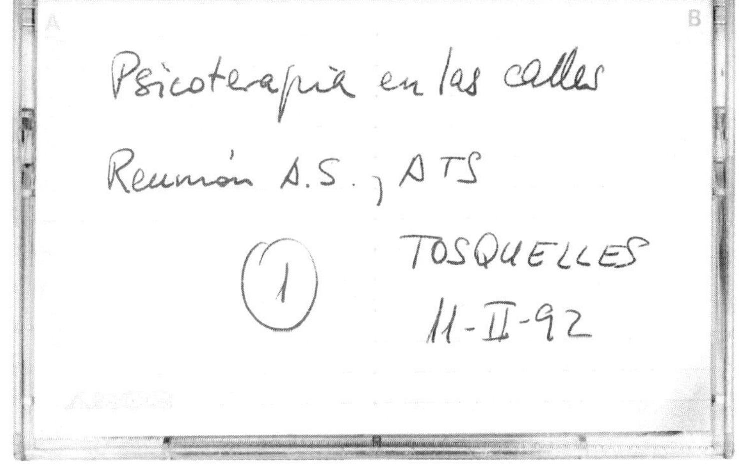

TOSQUELLES (10)
Psychoanalysis and Institution

The transformation of the
Psychiatric H[ospital], the
manipulation of families
TOSQUELLES
December 17, 1991
(Seminar A.S., ATS)

Psychotherapy in the streets
Meeting A.S., ATS
TOSQUELLES
February 11, 1992

Tosquelles, like that of other psychiatrists including Julián de Ajuriaguerra in Switzerland and Félix Letemendía in England, created an interruption to Spanish institutional therapeutic practices, which the transition to democracy did not restore. Even though in the late sixties and early seventies Spanish translations of books such as *Folie et Déraison: Histoire de la folie à l'âge classique* by Michel Foucault (1967), *Asylums: Essays on the Social Situation of Mental Patients and Other Inmates* by Erving Goffman (1970), *Psychiatry and Anti-Psychiatry* by David Cooper (1971), and *The Negated Institution* by Franco Basaglia (1972) were published, and soon after magazines like *Ajoblanco*, *El Viejo Topo*, and *Ozono* situated anti-psychiatry (and the resistance to becoming "therapeutic subjects" in times of democracy) within the collective debate, institutional psychotherapy did not form part of that critical space, which had to also be a political and cultural space. Although in Spain anti-psychiatry resonated politically, interpreted as a critique of the repression and censorship of Francoist society, of its prisons, its schools, and its concept of family,[6] institutional psychotherapy—which critiqued precisely those institutions—was not received as a critical practice. Anti-psychiatry, which sought the disappearance of institutions, spread throughout Spain along with deinstitutionalizing approaches; these didn't make legible a psychotherapy that wanted to cure ill institutions instead of making them disappear, because it was the world that was ill. The institutions were only a sign of that, and a sign of where the work needed to be done. However, anti-psychiatry traveled better over borders and, in Catalonia and in Spain, along with the tendency to close asylums, concealed the return of situated psychotherapy rooted in place.

The *return* of Tosquelles and of the institutional psychotherapy that had begun in Reus in the thirties would have been able to articulate, in Catalonia and Spain, the links between psychiatry and psychoanalysis. But in a country and a time period that failed to link psychiatry with psychoanalysis, or institutional with political practice, or psychoanalysis with literary criticism, perhaps the work of Francesc Tosquelles was condemned to be illegible or anecdotal. Perhaps because the new democratic space didn't weave links with the radical experiences of the Second Republic, a legacy like Tosquelles's was left untransmitted. Even though Tosquelles wrote a lot during the seventies and eighties—the book about Gabriel Ferrater and the numerous papers of the Jornades d'Interès psiquiàtric are just some examples—and despite his presence at the Catalan Summer University in Prades and his receiving distinctions during those years—recognition as an Illustrious Son of Reus in 1985 and the President Macià Medal in 1994—the lived experience and collective practices associated with Tosquelles today scarcely evoke a world, a legacy, a genealogy.[7] In the twenty-first century, there have been programs at the Museu d'Art Contemporani in Barcelona and the Fundació Antoni Tàpies that, along with some film productions on the figure of Tosquelles and his work,[8] allow us to glimpse his experimental legacy from various, quite different perspectives.[9]

On the other hand, in France, Tosquelles's legacy at Saint-Alban occupies a central place in the history of sector psychiatry. François Fourquet and Lion Murard devoted a special issue of the magazine *Recherches* to him in 1975. It is a compendium that constitutes an authentic living archive of sector psychiatry, with accounts by Tosquelles—who at the time was working at the Institut régional de psychothérapie et de rééducation de Longueil-Annel—and by Eugène Aujaleu, Pierre Bailly-Salin, Lucien Bonnafé, Georges Daumézon, Félix Guattari, Robert-Henri Hazemann, Mrs. Laurenceau and Mrs. Mamelet, Hubert Mignot, Jean Oury, Danielle Sabourin-Sivadon, Paul Sivadon, Horace Torrubia, and Charles Vaille. These testimonies evoke the creation of institutional groups and networks that Tosquelles was involved in: the Batea group in 1945; the Lozerian section of the Société d'Hygiène Mentale in 1947; the Fédération des sociétés de Croix-Marine in 1952; the Sèvres in 1957; the Groupe de Travail de Psychothérapie et de Sociothérapie Institutionnelles in 1960; and the Fédération des groupes d'études et de recherches institutionnelles and the Société de psychothérapie institutionnelle, both in 1965.

The French history of sectorization is inseparable from the projects of institutional transformation that Tosquelles conceived as a network. The hospital is linked to a territory and the collective life it houses, but most of all the network is articulated, for Tosquelles, on the work that everyone must carry out in order to "create their network [...] to tie things up." The legend of Saint-Alban, in France, evokes Tosquelles's Catalan past. That past, which he apparently never transcended, allowed him to implicate himself in places that history had condemned to be like concentration camps, through a work that mixed disciplines, clinical and psychoanalytical traditions, languages, popular culture brought into the hospital, and an artistic practice that should not have been called art brut. He was always working to "create anchors." Contemporary art traces a path for all those institutions that wish to transform. This unexpected legacy of Francesc Tosquelles in artistic practices is a form of transmission that reveals the always-unfinished project of becoming an institution. Not in order to change the institution, but rather to change life.

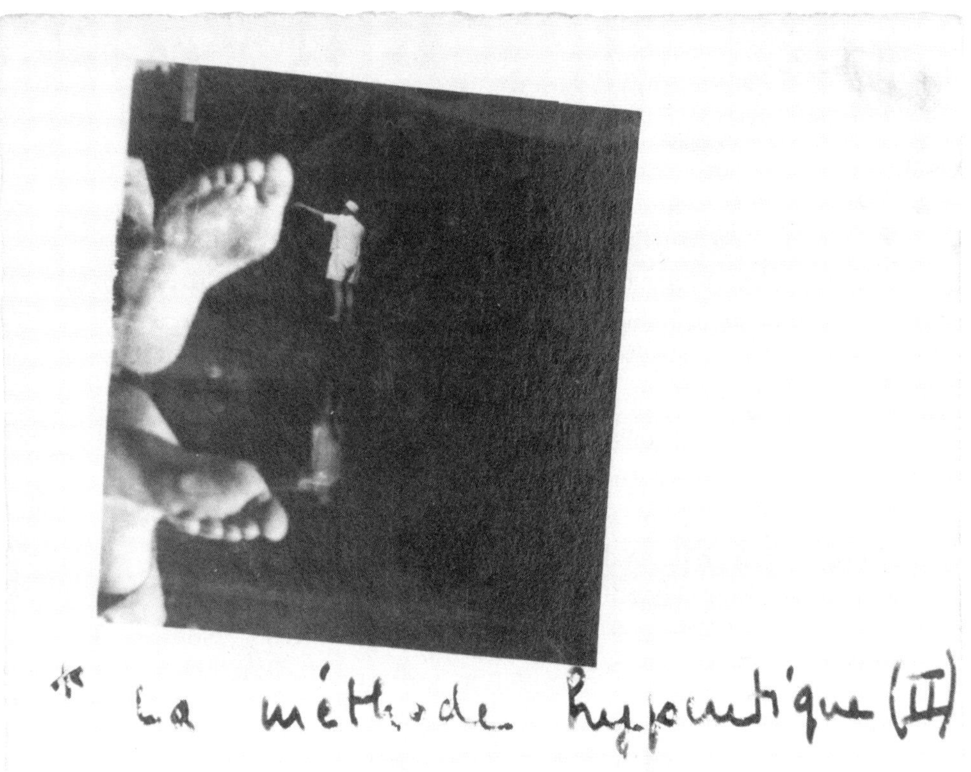

Photomontage of Tosquelles from the series *La méthode hypocritique*, made by superimposing several photographs. Tosquelles is in the background, fishing near Saint-Alban. Bare feet form part of Tosquelles's self-representation in many of the photographs taken at the hospital, such as the ones in which he appears holding up Auguste Forestier's boat, or the group images with the Bonnafé family. They reflect his vision of therapeutic practice in which it is our feet, and not our heads, that take us places.

JEAN-CLAUDE POLACK—Wouldn't that allow one in fact to redefine what is called institutional therapy?

FRANÇOIS TOSQUELLES—It's to take the networks into account. And most networks, like the first one that I formed in my life, based on the net, the labyrinth, on my mother's pathways, in the end it was an Ariadne's thread—brilliant, it was light to the eyes, a star. So it's not just any network. Freud, who saw the matter quite well, but didn't see it while seeing it because he was blind, he was focused on this one man: Freud's local culture was Arthur Schnitzler, the man who described for the theater—like Sartre in a way—the networks of women amongst themselves, the women's market of Vienna, the exchanges of Vienna's women, *La Ronde* and the other plays in which one sees better and more concretely than Deleuze and Guattari when they talk about networks. Read *La Ronde* and you'll know what network is in question. In describing my own life, when I place my mother somewhere, along with the nanny, my grandmother, and the two little girls across the street, it is clear that what one does, finally, is to lay down anchor points for constructing a network.

JEAN-CLAUDE POLACK—Is the network simply a network of persons?

FRANÇOIS TOSQUELLES—Person is a legal, Roman concept that bothers me a good deal. As to the person, with the Greeks one knew at least that it was a mask, with a loudspeaker in front of the mic. The crazies aren't dying simply from the social constraints, they're dying or not dying according to their difficulty in constructing the net or not. And in that net, it's not a myth of inner life, but pragmatic stories of man's going about living. Man is his going about. That's why I've emphasized the fact that I walk with my feet. [...]

JEAN-CLAUDE POLACK—That's still too complicated. A more naive definition of institutional therapy?

FRANÇOIS TOSQUELLES—One can be naive, but not as much as the Americans, who believe it's a matter of human relations: Give me a cigarette; if you give me a cigarette, I'll give you a light. If you give me a cigarette, how much will that cost me? One of the quite fundamental stories of the Lozère in this regard is that apart from the song "La Coupo Santo" they also sang another song: How much do they cost, those shoes, those "esclops, quant costaven els esclops"? How much do they cost, those things we put on our feet, the same as now whenever they release a television commercial for a car, how much does that cost? That whole motley assortment of things is why it is hard to follow what could be called my thought, because I go from one level to another with extraordinary ease, which is not hypomaniacal. Apparently it suggests hypomania, but it's not hypomania. It's going with the net to look for the fish where it's at. Saint-Alban was a pool with a lot of half-alive fish in it. [...]

As for work, not the schoolwork of learning the mountains and the rivers, but the work that every child has to do, must do, to constitute his or her net, to connect things there, like all the spiders do. [...] What they do, the spiders, is to stick one thread to the right and another to the left. Without that, there would be no web. The intimate work, as Freud would say, is a work of attaching the string ends to something that looks more or less solid, which may be the corner of a house, the father, the dog, the cat, the horse, or the car—that's all. But it's this intimate work that one doesn't do at school. And when they say that one has to consider the personality of children, one is screwed because the personality is a legal concept, connoting property.

François Tosquelles and Jean-Claude Polack, rushes not included in the film by François Pain, *Une politique de la folie* [A politics of madness], 1989

REGARDING THE DIFFICULTIES OF THE PRACTICE AND TEACHING OF PSYCHIATRY (AN ORIENTATION THAT COMES TO US FROM THE PAST: ARNAU DE VILANOVA)

I will not mention Freud. In my harvest, I will gather wheat sown here, using what was written by one of the doctors rooted in teaching here, about his own clinical experience. As I said, my second topic will be Arnau de Vilanova. I first learned of him at this academy: he was introduced to me by Jaume Aiguader and the *Monografies Mèdiques*.

However, do not think that I bring him up now and suggest a new take on the manner of his time—of sword and nest, as Fuster would say—out of some desire to pull out a museum piece covered in Catalan cobwebs. It is his timelessness, and the lesson he offers us on practice and method, his teaching that is often focused on the issue of "dreams and visions" [*sic*].

There is no need to shift his harvest much for my contemporary reading. Clearly, our world is not the same as it was in the thirteenth and fourteenth centuries. But the seed of what he says has not changed much, nor has the land where it took root.

Let us say that what he writes is an elaboration of the practice of his time, of a concrete practice, which is truth and will lead him especially to answer the uncertainties of his clientele: a clientele that we would now call rich, and not always "psychiatric." In fact, they were people in the royal court here and in Sicily and occasionally even the pope. People often preoccupied by the mere fact of their collective responsibility to comprehend and determine the opportuneness of their decisions and attitudes, both in the disposition of their private and family lives and in the political disposition of their tasks.

As such, it is an elaboration of concrete "clinical" experience of dreams and visions—which to a certain extent would be ludicrous if we were to consider only the care invested in the prospection, or in reading the future of the clients, or even the efforts made to not seem too heretical in a world such as his that was so tied up in religion, or in a sociocultural religious apparatus that was gradually waning. The end of the world, of "his world," he would say, happened in 1343.

The text we wanted to comment on was published in Toulouse in 1485. I don't know when he wrote it; I suppose if you have the time and are so inclined you can find it at the Library of Catalonia. I held it in my hands in 1933 and I hope it hasn't been lost.

But it is important, for us and for the subject at hand, that he says that many books like his must be written, because to date everything that is known and said about dreams and visions has only been retransmitted through the word, *through practice*, and he even adds that "it has been done without *method*."

And it is the "method" that he speaks of in his book, offering us a vivid example. A method that goes from *practice to teaching*, always in relation to clinical fact and observation. But don't think that his book is a bunch of anecdotes: he deals with

---

Excerpt from Francesc Tosquelles, "A propòsit de les dificultats de la pràctica i de l'ensenyament de la psiquiatria: Una orientació que ens ve de lluny; Arnau de Vilanova," *Annals de Medicina*, 1978, pp. 1108–1115.

clinical facts "worthy of mention"; above all, we will focus on "*those facts of which teaching will give us the general and particular reasons*"—in other words, *a theoretical philosophy.*

"First"—he says—"I will propose theoretical aspects." More or less what we would today call the philosophy, explicit or implicit, of what he describes, less about things than about how to see them. Something that one often forgets to do when explaining, for example, the works of a Bleuler or a Clérambault and one takes clinical anecdotes from each and puts them together, without first explaining the meaning of the research of the author in question.

Furthermore, what we truly need is to glimpse the author's "position." Our task always refers to the relationship between doctor and patient. One cannot separate the therapeutic activity or even the theoretic activity of a doctor from his personality. The psychiatric clinic brings two or more "subjects" into play.

"After this theoretical explanation, I will show"—says Arnau—"*the things that can be deduced through 'reasonable' speculation*, and thus *I'll be able to teach 'a general method of prognostication.'* Finally"—he says—"I will end by teaching each of these aspects in *particular.*"

Who, today, could speak better of the mutual relationships of clinical practice and teaching? Who? Arnau de Vilanova, he himself; of whom one can say he kills two birds with one stone. The same birds still fly over psychiatric settings.

So, look: "Thus"—he says—"we can *move forward the science of the knowable,"* and he underscores that among people of science—in his era, of course—"many were irritable and disappointed because"—says Arnau, literally—"they didn't find in my text the divisions and *subdivisions* of a nice philosophy" (and a cheap one, I would add).

The people of science he discusses in the same sentence "are the people who applaud science's *function to comfort ignorance*" (who cannot tolerate—I say—their ignorance).

With Arnau de Vilanova we have to tackle the teaching of "the art of prognostication" (interpreting dreams and visions) with method, moving from practice to theory and from theory to practice without making our heads spin, and avoiding the *divisions and subdivisions of a philosophy or a science used to comfort ignorants*: and, at the start, we are all ignorants.

This is a difficult task—undoubtedly—for any doctor and especially for those of us who have a more or less "seminal desire" that blooms in sublimated activities: pedagogy.

How indeed can we teach others, when precisely what we teach serves, with the science Arnau speaks of, to conceal and comfort us in our ignorance? Aren't the patients and our pupils coming to us precisely because they believe that we "know" what in fact we do not know?

So how can we bear the loss of prestige that, in any case, comes with our dealings and treatment of the other, if that pupil or client gradually realizes that the therapist or the professor—while not a fool—is fumbling his way through? And in such a way that, both in the course of the teaching and in the treatment of the patient, the client or the pupil finds their own path, if moved to and if they have the balls.

I won't apologize for using a vulgar term. I can't find a better one, one that better expresses what many psychoanalysts formulate as access to castration. Although we must remember that other analysts don't turn this distressing problem into a real "ballbuster." For them, "castration" is the true entrance and *parcours* of each person along the paths and labyrinths of language. I agree.

When I was a little boy, there was a song that said "The Holy Virgin, as a girl, went to school to learn to read and write." The girls' school was called *costura* because they also learned to sew there, and to cut pieces of discourses that come from outside, from the fair, from others, and to sew them to make clothes that fit the dimensions of our bodies: cutting, choosing, giving letters shape and sewing them to dress the body. Indications or signs of castration. Call this cutting and sewing, if you wish, a useful and necessary "narcissism" … and let us not confuse narcissism with the egocentrism we sometimes dress ourselves in or wrap ourselves in, sometimes presumptuously. Clothes that haven't been sewn or cut by us ourselves; that have been bought or stolen from the shops frequented by the "ego." This "ego"—a place of imaginary identifications, as Lacan would say—that "courted and primped" when some boys and girls said "farewell, dark carnation, farewell star of life," real metaphors of narcissism from another song that ties us to the heavens and the earth, and perhaps carries us to yet another song. "I've turned toward a bad life": "bad life," which goes from neurosis to certain behaviors that are called characterial—and are always egocentric—with significant collapses of the "primary" narcissistic wound. With greater efficacy than the mere aesthetic evocation of our "Cançó del lladre" [The song of the thief], Kunkel, among others, offers us techniques for treating egocentrism.

Let us now please return to Arnau de Vilanova's text and we will see what pieces we can sew together to make a work outfit for psychiatrists—at least as far as dreams and visions are concerned.

In the same theoretical part of his text, there are many concepts that have only been rediscovered centuries later, and many that are still forgotten. For example and as a starting point, the one that leads him to point out *the place and function of ghosts* in dreams and visions, but not only in what we could say breaks ground or a page of writing in the telling of a dream.

In order to situate this concept, Arnau de Vilanova needs to, as we need to, try to see more clearly what could be called the topology of *inside and outside*. Like Bion in our time, literally, Arnau finds himself with the—let's call it theoretical—need to establish first and foremost a theoretics of the "content" and of the "continent," in his relations of mutual "coincidences." And it is not a matter of simply establishing well-defined limits once and for all.

In few words, Arnau ridicules the abusive simplifications with which, frequently, the concepts of both "man and his circumstance" and Heidegger's "being in the world" are understood. Nowadays, following these simplifications and schematic presuppositions, many people, even Federn—who has treated so many schizophrenics—think that the insane and the sane are a product of the "social continent." Widely considered a mechanical determinant and even alienated in essence and contingence. In fact, Federn speaks of and works with the concept of impact on the peripheral self. Arnau de Vilanova says, of course, that many changes develop out of *the fact of the "continent"* that is each one of us. But he begins by considering that there is no *"singular" continent*; that it is always a *"plural" continent* and, furthermore, that "*all continents are also contents.*" If we were able to say it in today's language, we could declare, with him, that "these continents and contents function in a dialectical manner," so that "the last continent"—the fourth in his division of things—"is in fact the first cause."

Between us, we find the cliché of the Möbius strip more appropriate to the "thing" and to the structures of the living word.

But Arnau must work to avoid magic and heresy in his essays and thus he offers us a very suggestive "image" of what he means. For instance: he says that four forces are always combining, in this dialectics of the continents … "*in the same way as manifested in art.*" In a work of art *that integrates* "*artifice, fantasy, hand and tool*" [*sic*].

And clear as a bell, he says that it is possible only because in the art object they form this chain:

> "It is the working tool that divides, cuts or trims the figure, toward which the hand travels …"
> "and the hand moves toward the image of the fantasy"
> "… the fantasy takes the form of artifice."

And, finally, that through this dialectical chain of the four forces, we find ourselves "*leaning or stirred up in multiple ways while awake and dreaming …*"; as soon as we are led to imagine that, and then led "even to capture it or create it"; "desiring it and phantoming" (his word) "it until it is achieved" (take note here of what he says) "*if we are not led by intellect and allow ourselves to be distracted by outer movements.*"

Arnau then alludes *to what becomes, in certain moments of passion or inebriation, "in which the intrinsic inner movement"*—he says—"*is so strong that outer events have no 'entity.'*"

Therefore, we are with Arnau de Vilanova at the very threshold of the experiential—which is not to say necessarily therapeutic—situations that began at the turn of the century with psychoanalysis: a path opened up for the researcher who wanted to be a therapist who was attentive to "dreams and visions."

Then Arnau said, as today's neurological studies and electroencephalograms have proven, "that dreams at the break of dawn" are, to put it one way, richer and more fertile and more explicit; richer—he says—in "significant phantasmagorias." These dreams occur "after the first and second digestions and, furthermore, according to the suitability of the weather"—spring or autumn, for example.

That would almost be enough. Yet we must—and I will be brief—remark that, loyal to what he termed "the method," he establishes that once the abstract theories have been expressed, explicit reference must be made to the range of diverse mechanisms or forces that intervene in dreams and visions, in order to be able to conceive and work with reality: forces that *move and move us* according to the diverse ways that "we prepare ourselves to be moved" [*sic*].

I will underscore some concepts that show up in this range. On the first rung, *he situates the act*, the driving impulse, "*the motive virtues*"—he says—"*that act independent of 'any sign'*" (the word *sign* is also his); a sign that would be received by the "virtues" or the cognitive elaborations—as we would say. And that happens, not without paradox, "*more often during the day, when awake, than when sleeping.*"

And now Arnau can speak of and situate another mechanism that those who have psychoanalytic experience have also gradually discovered. He speaks verbatim when he describes the second rung, which "happens after the first": "This second step *is a result of what has been imprinted"—imprinted* is his word—"*by the motive virtues onto the cognitive virtues.*" But—he quickly adds—do not think that this "impression" takes the form of a "suitable metaphor" (the expression *metaphor* is also his and I will discuss it later on). Now, whilst we are on this second stage—on the level of *the impression of the motor drives on the cognitive forms*—this "mark" is made, "*is represented"*—he literally says—"*by the opposite form*" (!!).

This "*representation by the opposite*," while we sometimes grasp it easily at the clinic, is very difficult to accept and to incorporate into our practice when we are preparing to listen and intervene in what patients do and say. Rather, we make a "moral" judgment when we speak of "negativism" in symptomatology.

Often, if we believe we understand the mechanism at work in every process of humanization when it manifests this "second stage," we interpret it as inauthentic, as a dissimulation or ambivalence, or even that the patient—sane or insane—is trying to deceive us.

We have already mentioned that in a third ring of Arnau's chain, visions and dreams that diversify the existential project of the future in multiple ways, as we would say now, "are not always formulated in a confusing manner"—he says—"like the driving forces of the first stage."

Now what is drawn, what appears or, more precisely, what is spoken "*is designated through an adequate metaphor*" [*sic*]. And it is precisely here where Arnau de Vilanova speaks about the "*metaphoric variability*" that is formulated "according to the properties of the time and of the concrete conditions in the lives of men" [*sic*]. It cannot be said more directly: the metaphorical constitution of our discourse, the plasticity of the cultural verbal material that nourishes the metaphor and takes on meaning, sliding and moving, affected, clinging if possible to the concrete conditions in the lives of men, makes up the third stage, which in any case presupposes and does not cancel out the other two.

Therefore, the path of the interpretation, based on the gathered metaphors, becomes—says Arnau—"artificial." I suppose, in any case, that he believed it to be indispensable, even though one can assume, from what he's said up until now, that he was never able to reduce the therapeutic action to some simple magic of the word or of "interpretative" knowledge. However, I believe that is what justifies what comes later with the concrete clinical examples that he relates. In any case, Arnau de Vilanova does not explain precisely the artificiality of the interpreter, which makes doctors always—whether we admit it or not—men of art more than men of science. Especially if we employ the ironic perspective he alludes to regarding certain "scientists" of his time.

We are clearly men of art because we intervene with our own subjective metaphorical elaborations, and we more or less commit to dialogue or "dialysis" with what patients say or do.

Arnau also mentions another concept that is key to the examination of discourse and use of language. In the fifth stage he uses the same word as Freud, "displacement." As we've mentioned previously, it travels along the same path as metaphor.

People, said Arnau, "do not see, in visions or dreams, the object itself—of the project or of the impact—directly"; Arnau says that people designate "*this object through another thing*; and not always in a clear manner *but rather in an atmosphere of enigma and metaphors that have some similitude to the thing in question*." This is "often how prophets speak."

I find it extraordinary that all this was written in the thirteenth century, and that now, today, we struggle with and play at our profession, I don't know how or in what way, but Arnau de Vilanova returns in his writing, and with other precisions, to the *problem of the body in visions and dreams*. Now he is not referring to the "motive forces."

Arnau does not suggest eliminating the body from visions, as it often seems we psychiatrists do in practice. It truly is not that difficult to envisage, incidentally and between us, and without the need to know much more, with the indiscreet practice of didactic analyses—to find, I say, and I apologize—many cases of "true phobias" of corporal contact that are poorly hidden or transformed into practical attitudes in psychiatrists: that of exclusively psychological or phenomenological exams, for example.

The body intervenes in visions, says Arnau, on one hand according to its "complexion"—by that I assume he means constitution—and on the other by what results from "accidents." Here I must say that I find that Arnau de Vilanova, in this highly important chapter of his work, introduces a maneuver of saying without saying, perhaps because of the risk of his text being tossed onto a bonfire. Not only was he not obtuse, but he knew how to run with the hare and hunt with the hounds while saying everything that needed to be said, because for him it was the truth and the condition of his efficacy.

Before explaining his cases—and notice that this also forms part of his method—Arnau sums up what has been said and done with visions and dreams both in India and in Egypt.

In India, there was interest in interpreting dreams and visions particularly through the "disposition" of the body's parts, "especially the head and neck, the kidneys and the penis."

And Arnau then says what we struggle—yet succeed—to forget today: that "the disposition of the head, kidneys, and penis is not the result of a simple consequence of the muscular ligaments, but that it results more from the fact that"—listen carefully, please—"*the holes* of these parts of the body have a notable preponderance in the person." They already knew how psychoanalytic experience has led us to take "holes" into consideration, the rims of the body's orifices in the theory of the "drives."

And what did he say about Egypt? He simply reminds us that all art deriving from dreams and visions "always refers to desire."

Body and desire, this is the double problem that in a way Arnau tackles beneath the mantle of historical evolution, yet without forgetting that, regarding the body and illnesses, as he goes on to say, this derived art is a "prognostication"; he says that "*only doctors can deal with visions and dreams, because they have experience of illnesses*."

Often—and he cites numerous examples—substantial changes—illnesses of the body—manifest themselves in dreams and visions "when the clinical signs of the illness have yet to appear" [*sic*].

MAKING A CLUB

In order to create a club, one needs anthropology and sociology: knowing the customs, habits, and traditions of a people. In Algeria, Fanon was unsuccessful until he built a mosque. One must be familiar with the traditions and customs of the patients: knowing, for example, what the Andalusians in Reus do and think.

In the concentration camp, good psychiatry was done without money. Sometimes, little girls throw away the dolls their parents buy them. Toys have to be made by the children; the rest can't be played with. What does it mean to buy a kettledrum? It makes no sense, and it doesn't last long. You can make one with a tin can. Trucks get ruined, but children can play with pieces of wood and make things. For those who have lost their capacity to play, the club is the best place.

I've always said that, even when things are done systematically, the patient speaks. There is a double game: of matter and of the word. It may seem that the patient is talking to himself, but he is talking to someone else. Sometimes the skirt doesn't match the jacket, nor the hairstyle with the shoes. If something doesn't match, there is a conflict. The patient is not the same in the club as he is in the ward or with his family.

In a congress of psychoanalysts, I asked an Italian bachelor: "Why is it, as a psychoanalyst, that you have never married?" And he replied: "I've never met the woman with the right qualities. I will marry when I find one who knows how to be a good wife and cook." Everything in its place, including the club. An insane person can be well behaved in a workshop, where he is well adapted, and criticize everything in the club. A person can play different roles.

It is said that, in the commission of assistance for patients, one of the things they do is charity. That is a Francoist discourse. According to Marx, money is the alienated ability of mankind. A rich man can never get to heaven. "Blessed are the poor in spirit." Charity consists of seeing others' desire in their faces. Man always desires what he does not have, be it money, tobacco, or other things. Charity is discovering that lack.

There is a very ancient game: chess. It is played more here than in France. I learned to play at a recreational club that was located at Carrer hospital in Barcelona. There were only workers there. In France no worker plays chess. A minister of education said that chess could make people think too much. People shouldn't think so much, they might dry out their brains. In this game there is a board with no institution, no fanfare, nothing; there are limits within which a conflict between blacks and whites—speaking of symbolism—is played out. The king and the queen are fundamental pieces. Everything consists in avoiding our king being killed, and he can hardly move. The queen, however, can go anywhere. In the social life of many peoples, women are trapped at home. The king is, therefore, the fundamental piece, followed by the queen. The rooks barely move. The bishops and the crazies move diagonally. The knights leap, but not far, and the pawns move in slow little steps: they are the peasants, with their picks and shovels. The king symbolizes the father, and the queen is the mother. The

---

Francesc Tosquelles, "Fer un club" (December 18, 1986), in Josep M. Sánchez Ripollès (ed.), *Algunes conferències inèdites del Doctor Francesc Tosquelles i Llauradó (1912–1994): Escrits periodístics del Doctor Leandre Cervera (1891–1964)*. Tarragona: Universitat Rovira i Virgili, 2000.

bishops represent the nobility. The pawns are the infantry. In a game there are three phases: the opening, the development, and the conclusion.

The opening is the same as what you all did when you were small and mobilizing the impulses and representations of society. The idea is to put all of the pieces—the representations (as in psychic life)—into motion and have them support each other; to organize the inner freedom of the player, the freedom of their representations, as is done in therapy (helping the patient organize his freedom, so he has representations of his own story).

When I started playing chess, I would attack quickly to try to kill the father (king); and I did so with the queen. But I would lose the game, if the other player wasn't an imbecile. I neglected my inner freedom. As we get older, we see how important that is. The game is won by the person who, after twelve or more moves, acquires more inner representations in freedom. This is the same freedom one must have in psychotherapy: one mustn't want to win at all costs; one must know when to retreat, if necessary.

WHAT TO SAY? HOW TO SAY IT?

One of the practical problems of our professions consists of measuring the distance between people who are speaking. In order to be able to speak, we need to know to whom we are speaking. I've been told that today in the classroom there will be medical students from the psychiatry class.

Our profession has three legs: we've got one in the middle of the doctor's pot, another in the teachers', and the third ... I can't recall. Maybe there are only two legs.

The medical model that looks for symptoms and makes various diagnoses may not be valid in psychiatry. The separation between medicine and psychiatry is stupid. There is no examination without words, just as there is no prescription given without words. The words that the doctor addresses to the patient, and his family, do him good, but could also hurt him. Sometimes what doctors tell their patients has serious consequences. There are illnesses produced by words. We don't take words into consideration because we put more trust into medication. A slight exaggeration: at least 50 percent of the chronic ill are ill because their doctors don't know what to say to them.

How can we grasp what the patient says in silence? There are silences that speak volumes. The psychiatrist and the caregiver often do not know what to say to their patient. And the same thing happens in psychosomatic medicine. I do not know what that term means. I do not know what it means to place the spirit to one side and the organs to the other.

I read an issue of the club newspaper. A patient wrote a warning that he would commit suicide, that he could no longer stand living without love. Once it was written, it wasn't listened to, it wasn't again elaborated in group before it was published. You tell me that this patient had already said similar things some time ago, that alcohol was no longer any help to him, etc. That is a cry for a help, a request for love. There are suicides that are caused by a sudden impulse, but most of the time the cause has been brewing inside for a while. Sometimes they visit a lawyer or a priest in the weeks beforehand.

A caregiver tells me that she has just spoken with a boy who is unemployed and who asked for her help. Many people come to us over just such problems. In any case, every crazy person finds themselves stuck in some way. Was he a civil servant? Being a civil servant means they pay you for doing nothing. His family didn't want to have anything to do with him. He was a new kid at the house. The activities helped them to get to know him. He didn't know the caregiver either, but he sensed there was something there.

Many years ago, here at the Institut Pere Mata, a schizophrenic invented a procedure to keep the race of male doctors from reproducing. In those days there were no female doctors. According to his invention, the couples would only have daughters.

Francesc Tosquelles, "Què dir? Com dir-ho?" (December 18, 1987), in Josep M. Sánchez Ripollès (ed.), *Algunes conferències inèdites del Doctor Francesc Tosquelles i Llauradó (1912–1994): Escrits periodístics del Doctor Leandre Cervera (1891–1964).* Tarragona: Universitat Rovira i Virgili, 2000.

I hadn't yet returned from the war; otherwise, I would have been doomed to only have daughters. For the schizophrenic, the fact that his doctor was a man or a woman was important; he speaks and behaves differently depending on whether the doctor is a man or a woman. One day I was introduced to a woman in Paris, at Sartre's house, at a bar filled with existentialists. She was old and ugly. She was sitting and smoking. She looked at me with disdain. "Oh, gosh! You and I could get along because you are neither one part masculine nor feminine." Her phrase struck me deeply. By that I mean that when you meet a patient, he examines you, he looks you up and down and gives you a diagnosis. The Balint groups have proven that when the doctors arrive in a town for the first time, they begin to receive visits from patients who've come just to see if they are good doctors. I remember the case of a patient who, after I had examined him, said to me: "I can see that you are a good doctor, tomorrow I'll send my wife here to you."

The examination is nothing more than giving the patient time to speak. Examining means listening, making the other's body speak. When we examine the McBurney's point to confirm appendicitis, we have to give the patient the opportunity to speak. It is the ABC's of the art of medical examination. We have to ask questions of our patients: about the most recent movie they saw, about the books they read, about their parents. And that has to be done in a certain way, as if we didn't see them and they didn't see us. Psychiatric examination has another dimension, because the patient's attitude depends on the words the doctor says to him. And these young doctors seem to be unconcerned about the patient's answers. I don't understand that. When I was a general practitioner, I realized the importance of the doctor's contact with the patient, having dealings with them person to person: their social and erotic body. There is no man nor woman who is not simultaneously an erotic body and a social body. When a drunkard complains about a part of his body, his social body is also suffering.

Medical student and doctors in training are surprised when they hear the language of the patients for the first time. The meaning things assume there is ambiguous and mysterious. Man has trouble understanding another man. With the insane there is a simple solution: if you don't understand them, you remove them from the conversation and that's that. The silences of the dimwits and the nonsense of the delirious cannot be understood.

There are doctors who don't know what to say in the face of death. The same thing happens when the patient asks you if he is crazy. The phobias of death and madness are very common. Everyone dies and everyone is crazy, thanks to God. Man is born of insanity and eliminating it for the benefit of the body of the man leads to the creation of good veterinarians, but not good doctors. We have already said it: one must take into account both the erotic body and the social body, as well as the material body. There is nothing more foolish than saying: You are crazy, but we will cure you. In the face of the aforementioned question, the response is conditioned by the idea they have of madness. If they have a negative idea, they will only increase their resistance to being crazy. Being a psychiatrist can be comfortable and serene: "I'm not crazy, my client is." The first contact with the patient has to lead us to search for how one can live while making the most of madness.

Accepting the human condition and one's own death is difficult, because the existence of those two phobias makes it difficult; and until we release them there can be no progress. Bravery serves to deny that one is scared to death. That is seen in war, where many terrified soldiers run forward. Actually, that lessens the chances that you'll be hit by a bullet.

In Switzerland, Bleuler wrote a book about schizophrenias in which he said that alcoholism is a type. One day he received a visit from a Protestant bishop, who told him that the patients in his asylum seemed like the people he saw on the street, and that he thought that the life they led inside the institution was how one should live outside, in squares and on the streets.

The social life inside asylums is well organized; there are hardly ever any fights. The best treatise on madness is *Don Quixote*, when he explained to Sancho Panza that he had to choose between the two types of melancholy in order to be able to live in the world, while he searched crazily for the ideal woman. As you know, they had a thousand adventures. They came to Barcelona, where they encountered the struggle between the farmers and the landowners. Don Quixote was healing more and more, and finally the time comes when he returns home saying that he was no longer Don Quixote but Alonso Quijano el Bueno. And he died, cured. Freud said that Don Quixote was a paranoiac, but that has nothing to do with it.

HUMAN LIFE CRISES EMERGENCIES

INTRODUCTION

We all know that in the course of each person's life, and undoubtedly also in human groups, "moments" of crisis emerge. Their manifestations are surprising; they contrast with what we have all grown accustomed to. They are often unexpected; other times a certain angst or uncertainty precede their sudden outburst and warn us of the danger each crisis can drag us into. In any case, it is not true what they say about "a stitch in time saves nine." Prevention and knowledge of the critical manifestations often do not keep them from arising in rather precise periods of development. Each crisis has something that suggests its inevitability. For example, the oft-mentioned pubertal crisis or the forgotten crisis of opposition at four years old, the depression at eight months or the violent rupture that is birth itself.

Crises are often repetitive, and they all have a certain expansiveness that propagates with various triggers. That happens with both a boil on the nape and an appendicitis in septic shock. This also occurs when a social crisis erupts—for example at the Renault factories in Paris, people there would say that "when Renault coughed, all of France caught a cold."

In a family with a very coherent and closed structure, we see for example that a brother suffers a serious traumatic accident, and then another brother wakes up with a endogenous psychotic crisis. Not to mention the violent and lethal delusions of certain vindicative, passionate love crises. And epileptic crises and hysterical crises, etc.

Many human crises, surprising as they may be, facilitate new developments and fruitful changes, or they herald them amid obscure uncertainties. Here there is the opportunity for prior awareness of many possible new arpeggios that crises can lead us into.

Crises, everywhere and on every level of human life, reveal the generally *invisible complexity* of the elements and lines of development that precede their eruptions. We might realize it afterward, often thanks to *later* reflective analysis; although it is not indispensable that it be led in a methodical and conscious way. Invariably, some elements and lines of force that precede the crisis emerge and are experienced then. Unfortunately, they are often assessed as errors of the past or as guilt. It is true that, in crisis, we become aware of the *coexistence of tensions* due to the concrete opposition of some of their vital parameters. It is the *unbearableness* of these tense oppositions where the crisis erupts. It is not pure magical coincidence that certain disparate factors in the crisis lead to differences of perspective and primarily to differences of the *procedures* that are then articulated regarding that which compares differently in *public life* and that which corresponds to *private life*; their differentiation has a highly varied impact on

---

Francesc Tosquelles, "Introducció" and excerpt from "Comentaris sobre les diferents exposicions," in *XXVI Jornades d'Interès Psiquiàtric: Emergències de les crisis vitals humanes; Urgències en el seu tractament social, mèdic i psiquiàtric.* Reus: Institut Pere Mata, 1993, pp. 7–9 and 171–176.

crises. Their limits change and lead to phenomena that surprise us and sometimes shock us, because they are uncommon. What is private becomes evident (visible) in public ambits and, I would almost dare to say, vice versa, since what then becomes evident tries to hide itself, willingly or not. Exhibition, in crises, is not a behavior exclusive to true exhibitionists.

Crises do not merely highlight the changes of limits between the public and the private, as is clearly seen in social crises, which also have surprising disjunctions between the plans of the *justice* system and those of the *politics* of a group, nation, or state. But also, in the course of personal, intimate events, the disjunction arises between what is perceived and conceived of as a *law* of action and the same course of the development of each person's impulses, intentions, and objectives. The strategies followed by games of proximity and distancing suffer, during crises, changes in rhythm and in substance. We are all surprised by this disjunction regarding crises. It is not an exaggeration to say that there is no correspondence between the law and the comings and goings of the politics pursued or manifested by each person. The same dichotomy appears and surprises us when crises make evident that which belongs, on one hand, to the arpeggios of the *political economy* and that which corresponds, on the other, to the *private economy* that organizes each person's body-ego. In both cases we experience economic crises with anxiety and often they appear interrelated; one echoes the other.

As such, I repeat that individual and collective crises reveal the fact of disarticulations, which drive the variability of the original parameters and aspects. They never obey the apparent safety that, prior to their eruptions, was considered to have been definitively acquired. The best discourses, when attempting to give an account of the various objective parameters pursued or achieved in order to *placidly* obtain each person's or each society's development without conflict, fail. They even often lead to giving the *oppositions and structural dichotomies* a violent aspect, increasing the subjective weight of gravitas or narcissism then called into question. Serene analysis is substituted for the struggle for prestige and spectacular, dramatic parrying between the various *opinions*. This further aggravates the *tenor* of the crises. Every crisis provokes anxieties and fear.

The professional training of the teams called to offer assistance to people in crisis—both in the field of psychiatry and in the field of reeducation—makes one realize that it is not enough for each member of the team to follow their own sensibility awakened at the dramatic critical appearance of the crisis, nor is their desire to help enough. They would do better learning about the various possible connections and outcomes prompted by all the human manifestations of a critical nature. Unfortunately, often, members of these teams—like nearly everyone—prefer to deceive themselves with approvals and illusions that presuppose the existence of a peace with no nicks or accidents. Even worse is when they rush into dramatic scenes with the sole perspective of finding a *guilty party* for the crisis, and rest from their own dissatisfactions and personal tensions.

Our attention to the discomforts produced by the crises, first of all, can help us avoid the roles of *avenger* or even *arbiter* that we are often encouraged to assume.

The *responsibility* of each person who articulates their relationship with us is, by its very nature, *inalienable*. Nothing erases the responsibility of that person, not a lack of information, nor supposed silly stupidity, nor human folly. It is precisely here where the opportune respect for human dignity lies. It is this respect that presides over all of our therapeutic practices. There is never freedom without prior recognition of this. The prisons we live in take many forms. They are not merely the social spaces called prisons. "In any case," in our professional tasks, it is convenient to comprehend that the arabesques of *guilt* almost always impede the examination and production of reliable remedies during the critical events that punctuate each person's vital development. The pressure, for each person, of assuming his responsibility is not the same in he who considers himself guilty.

COMMENTS ON THE DIFFERENT ADDRESSES

First, I'd like to say that not one particle of psychic life ever arises simply in the mental process of an isolated individual. For psychic life to take form, there have to be several others, more or less collected together and of different kinds, in fact—often of different generations. It takes *moving encounters*, *displacements* in space and in time—which coalesce however into *a single dance* through ensembles that develop at different levels.

Here the meeting of many friends attests that each and all are mindful of the psychic suffering called into play by those in one's care. Of course, that doesn't fail to provoke various resonances in ourselves, more or less analogous to those set off in their entourage, before our encounter.

Here and now, we're trying to rearticulate accounts that can illuminate and orient our practices, where we cannot pretend to be engaged in an innocent role, When one thinks he is neutral, it's because one has chosen to be *neutralized*, indifferent, disengaged, and in fact *irresponsible*.

—How do things stand with psychopathological crises?

—How do things stand with all sorts of human crises?

If we were not ourselves situated at the intersection of numerous *critical convergences*, I would be surprised to find that we're together here trying to get a handle on things! In any case, every time we meet, especially in the small working groups, what the critical phenomena involve, what we have experienced in our contact with patients and their social entourage, the very different elements joined together in our encounters, *make sense*. It's only when ensembles take form that sense is produced in us and in each member of the encounter with some efficacy. *The category of sense is introduced in all our activities*.

You may have read, and I urge you to reread, the brief note appended to the program of our sessions. However, after having heard what has been said here and having noted the pertinence of many of the presentations, I can't help but mention what seemed to me to be an excessive caution on the part of the presenters. I don't believe this caution was due only to the *fear of compromising oneself* in a large number of conflictual assessments. I believe that above all it is the *catastrophic character* of many psychopathological crises that has made the evocations of what we do very cautious. The fact is, we're afraid of crises … of dying … and of the *je ne sais quoi that the crisis may reveal*.

Often we are much less ashamed to publicly evoke *our anxieties*—or our hesitations—than to evoke *our fears*. But any critical state, in its psychological, social, economic, and political manifestations, triggers fear. The little that remains vivid of our childhood memories—or even the relatively recent life experiences—shows that what one lives in fear *cannot be shared*, even though the fear is contagious. Fear encloses us in an incommunicable opacity.

In a crisis, it may be in fact that one doesn't always see what's involved. Moreover, the urgency it gives rise to ... often causes one to hurry and supply some supposed elements of survival, rather than a thoughtful, effective, and differentiated aid. Further, the crisis protagonist is not necessarily in a state to share, in a critical and lucid way, the production of *the way out of it*.

Each one of us, whatever their professional training, finds themselves at sea and disoriented before most of these critical phenomena, even when they are not that spectacular. Moreover, the light that one can shed on the critical events that one perceives cannot be offered as objective truths either, although it's intensified and made more penetrating by our subjective delivery. This may be why our interventions in what we regard as crises of the other—indeed of society—can hope to benefit from reformulations gradually arrived at in small groups of professionals from various disciplines, which may occasionally be assembled into the same caregiving team. It's in these encounters, which most of you know firsthand, that one deals with situations and *concrete elements* whose consideration can give a coherence to our activities.

I've sometimes compared our small-team encounters to *the multipart goings-on of circuses*, but you'll understand why I've spoken with much more idealized interest of the fact that the caregiving teams *dance sardanas*. Actually, in the series of sessions that bring together so many people, the tone and the concepts risk being too abstract, as much in the formulation of discourses in Catalan as in French or Castilian. It's not really a matter of speaking together, of talking—a sardana is danced. It's a fully engaged activity: speaking is not enough.

The language of humans operates with metaphors and parables everywhere. It's important to consider an efficacy of language and speech. It's important to consider the large precedence that is indispensable to the concept one uses, but one should be wary and distance oneself from it in a critical way, so as not to slip into sterile and sterilizing systematizations.

Here, in these daily sessions, in the face of psychopathological crises and urgencies, we're all engaged in metaphorical and parable-like formulations that, at every moment of our concrete work, on the occasion of the encounters with patients, their families—in fact with the social entourages of their life milieus—*need to be interpreted afresh*. It's at the level of their revisiting and updating in the course of subsequent evocations in our meetings that our interventions can *successively and progressively rearticulate* some efficacy. The urgencies, whose justification I don't deny, lead in fact to errors that are never fatal, seeing that they can be corrected in the course of the therapy. The post hoc work in small groups, the retrieval of what we have experienced rightly or wrongly as *blows*, can thus be separated from the necessity of certain mechanical adaptations to the circumstances. No one can deny the usefulness of these, as long as one is aware that real therapeutic work doesn't depend on mechanics, and not even on technical relations. *It depends on the real creation in situ—where the encounter takes place—of the sensations and rhythmic feelings that occur and develop on occasion*, so it's not just fear and caution that have led our encounter today into a certain number of impasses in *response* to our meetings. Here one could not even dream of concretely becoming a dancer of the sardana. Without becoming a prisoner of the contradictions in which we are often trapped, I would say that we are too numerous to address and reformulate through progressive interpretations that which each of us contributes. We know how what flows, swirls, and often invades the concrete person of the patients—indeed the friends with which one is working—can only emerge with an apprenticeship like that of the sardana dancers.

There is nothing recondite or inaccessible, really, if I have sometimes evoked—in France especially—the history and techniques of the sardanas; it's not out of nostalgia or in a romantic spirit. Interpreting with others what *comes forth* and *pulsates* from the sounds of a few musicians, placed together in certain conditions like a family group, playing different instruments, *urges and leads one to dance* a corporeal engagement that doesn't come from an a priori knowledge, but from a poetic type of movement, from a mute and diversified poetry that pours out in the place of the other with whom we are playing without their inevitably assimilating our rhythms, or without their being repulsed by what we are making explicit in our words … Perhaps it's for this reason that I have evoked instead *the pleasure of encountering the other,* a pleasure that one experiences at different levels in our trade and even that one gets right here, for example, in the sessions of our psychiatry conference. I've already said now that I had almost regretted not hearing more said about the fear of what one is going to say, of what we may receive in a violent way. When this fear takes the disguise of pain and violence, it's like in many carnivals where love plays cat and mouse … that is, where the evasion is hidden behind numerous scenarios and at variable speeds.

I have to admit that in the course of my slow and persistent participation in the professional training at the Institut Pere Mata, I have not had the occasion to introduce the marks of and remarks on the form of mise-en-scène of the groups that *the theory and practice of the sardana dance* can suggest regarding the movement of a large number of our therapeutic projects.

Often one attempts everywhere to understand and copy the *letter* of a sardana, rather than shaping and giving a new tempo to a *music* to be drawn from the very sources of the person and the group … and to be *danced together.* Said more simply: many caregivers—some of whom are present here—who speak Castilian in the small groups doing real work around the suffering that arises from the psychological crises of the persons in their care *dance veritable sardanas* of which they are completely unaware. Their daily praxis follows that rhythm.

I've already said that it's not just a matter of an egocentric nostalgia that has led me to install in France my singular experience as a young "former dancer" of the sardana. If I have often spoke of it openly, paradoxically more often than here (the thing seemed to go without saying), the way the various theories overlooked the practice of *dancing* in the caregiving teams in psychiatry struck me as a revealing echo of the illiteracy transmitted, alas, in most of the professional training dealing with the radically human activities and constructions. Yet it was a French poet and philosopher—Paul Valéry—who described something of the basic ties that constitute both "the soul and the dance." I'll move on …

In Greek, *krinein* signifies "to choose," "to decide," "to judge," as well as "to separate." "Choose and separate," in possession of the facts, or without that, because of the urgent jolt where the subject—always in formation and in question—often finds themselves wiped out by the heartbreak, or pushed to transform themselves by a kind of leap into the void. As Weizsäcker said in *Der Gestaltkreis*, "the subject is not an unchanging possession …" It doesn't always stay in the same position … "the unity of the subject is only constituted in its tireless restoration beyond the variations and crises." Here "variations" should be understood as those that can be formulated with the same musical theme. Being pushed to a position displaces and in fact transforms us. There is a *continuity* and diversity of the themes, indeed of the persons encountered, when one dances sardanas.

In the same work, Weizsäcker said that "the subject's recovery following each crisis doesn't prove their inconstancy, but their strength and their energy."

I emphasize like this author that it's not a matter of the inconstancy of the subject dealing with discontinuous crises, variable in time, but of their *energy*, of the potential force that flows from the deployment of the well-known steel spiral of the mechanisms of clocks, but also of what springs forth in the life of each person … The crisis actualizes, re-represents *objects* or *sketches* of events already lived through. Indeed, in the course of the crisis, *extracts* or ex-traits crop up again, reformulated in musical themes that call for new *interpretations* when one plays with others and in front of different publics. What one sees then is not the same thing as what one hears on the other hand when the music becomes dance and song. The lived experience emerges from the crises in the form of tableaux that come into view and touch us with their keystrokes. From touch to touch, from nascent vital rhythms—of which one sometimes only hears the distant echo—*something* hits home, repeats, and passes vibrations from person to person that are difficult to identify. And yet the nascent, muffled rhythms are the background of numerous effects of the unforeseen all through the epochs. There have been and there are discreet or spectacular leaps in the human aims awakened in our encounters. There are awakenings and different resonances in everyone. Pounding heart rhythms alert each one of us, even before our movement toward the other takes visible forms.

Thus, we are never placed immediately in front of the other by a movement of the cogito. In advance, one doesn't know anything at all about the other when something about them touches us and nuances the *contact* and gives rhythm to the sequences of successive touches, awakened by the orchestrations that play one's own vital fibers.

I'm not saying that the product of the cogito, of knowledge—of lucid cogitation—serves no purpose. I'm only saying that the activities and formulations of the intellect appear afterward—if they appear. Such a model—if one can regard it as one, although I don't like the term—justifies the meetings *après coup* of what we call the caregiving teams. The *concrete recognition* can then emerge apart from the wild rollout into which the thought of the so-called cogito often leads us. This is the case with a *disinvested* expertise, blindly projected into the supposedly scientific discourses that concern humanity. One can never elide the *subject* and its vagaries of the cogito.

In our crises, in their constitutive shifts that are always at play in the best of cases, as occurs in most of the social and scientific activities of our time—alas!—it's not so much the *misdeeds of the bureaucracy* that prevent the greatest number of vibratos and human developments. It's above all the *strict quantified abstraction of the statistics that the political and scientific bureaucracies favor, disregarding the contingencies of the subject that manifest in our professional work.*

The keys touched by the other *touch us* before we grasp their possible lucid representations. Artistic activity has played its role and still does, in man's process of organization, a major role that preexists and subsists relative to the movements of a complete consciousness of one's own process: things have shifted before anything can be said. It all leaps and pushes.

In any case, what is *it* all about? That is the question ... I proceed here as others have done. In most of my activities as a clinician I have returned to the evocation of two levels of things at play and things at stake, where one apprehends diverse elements of our lives and their transmission to other human beings. There are always *two* levels of construction and reconstruction at work in tandem when *it* leaps and pushes.

Here again, there is a distant echo that shapes all the *dances* of humans, and in particular that open circle of the sardanas. [...]

NOTES AND REFERENCES

THE LIVES OF FRANCESC TOSQUELLES

A selection of photographs from the Tosquelles family albums (pp. 16–35). The quotes reproduced as captions are all by Francesc Tosquelles and from the following sources: pp. 16 and 35, François Pain, *François Tosquelles, une politique de la folie*, 1990; pp. 19, 22, 29, and 32, Angela Melitopoulos and Maurizio Lazzarato, *Déconnage*, 2011 (these two films offer different edits of the Tosquelles interview conducted by Jean-Claude Polack and Danielle Sivadon, recorded by François Pain in 1987 at his home in Granges-sur-Lot); p. 25, *Història de la psicoanàlisi als Països Catalans*, 1986.

I. THE INSTITUTIONS IN LITTLE VIENNA

The quote on p. 41 is from *Història de la psicoanàlisi als Països Catalans*, 1986.

1. François Tosquelles, "Que faut-il entendre par psychothérapie institutionnelle," *L'Information psychiatrique*, no. 41, 1971, pp. 377–384. See p. 266 of this volume.

2. Francesc Tosquelles, "A propòsit de l'anàlisi d'una personalitat anormal," *Fulls clínics*, May 1935, pp. 5–13.

3. Letter dated May 15, 1979, written in French.

4. Salvador Vives i Casajuana, *L'organització de l'assistència pública dels psicòpates a Catalunya*. Barcelona: Fundació Salvador Vives Casajuana, 1979, pp. 106–110.

5. Josep Maria Comelles, "Catalanisme, salut mental i avantguarda: Les polítiques públiques de salut a Catalunya (1883–1938)," in Montserrat Duch Plana (ed.), *La II República espanyola: Perspectives interdisciplinàries en el seu 75è aniversari*. Tarragona: Publicacions URV, 2008, pp. 51–84; Josep Maria Comelles, "Forgotten Paths: Culture and Ethnicity in Catalan Mental Health Policies (1900–1939)," *History of Psychiatry*, vol. 21, no. 4, pp. 1–18; Carles Hervás i Puyal, *Sanitat a Catalunya durant la República i la Guerra Civil*. Barcelona: Institut Universitari d'Història Jaume Vicens i Vives, Universitat Pompeu Fabra, 2005, p. 28. [Doctoral thesis.]

6. Josep Solanes, *Com se surt dels frenocomis*. Tarragona: Gràfiques Fores, 1935.

7. François Tosquelles, *De la personne au groupe: À propos des équipes de soins*. Toulouse: Éditions Érès, 1995, pp. 34–35.

8. See the image on p. 322 of this volume.

9. Antonio Labad, "La psiquiatria pels volts del 1900," in Jordi March (*et al.*) (eds.), *L'Institut Pere Mata de Reus, de Lluís Domènech i Montaner*. Reus: Ajuntament de Reus, 2004, pp. 205–220; Josep Poca Gaya, *Institut Pere Mata: Cent anys d'història (1896–1996)*. Reus: Institut Pere Mata, 1996.

10. Hermann Simon, *Tratamiento ocupacional de los enfermos mentales*. Barcelona–Buenos Aires: Salvat Editores, 1937. On Simon's biography and the reception of his work, see: Joseph Biéder, "Les faux-semblants: Hermann Simon (1867–1947)," *Annales Médico-psychologiques*, no. 164, 2006, pp. 451–453; Bernd Walter, "Hermann Simon: Reformer of Psychiatry, Social Darwinist, and National Socialist?," *Der Nervenarzt*, vol. 73, no. 11, pp. 1047–1054; Mary Seeman, "Mental Health Reform Not Always Beneficial," *Psychiatry*, vol. 70, no. 3, 2007, pp. 252–259; Franz-Werner Kersting, "Der Psychiater Hermann Simon im Erinnerungskulturellen Kontext," in Matthias Frese and Marcus Weidmer, *Verhandelte Erinnerungen*. Leiden: Ferdinand Schöningh, 2017, pp. 209–229; Münster Fraktion Bündnis 90 / Die Grünen im LWL (ed.), *Hermann Simon: Reformpsychiater oder Sozialdarwinist? Die Eugenikdebatte—historische Aspekte und aktueller Bezug*. Lippe: Bündnis 90 / Die Grünen, 1999; Christine Teller, "'Ich muss wirken, solange es Tag ist'—Biographische Anmerkungen zu Hermann Simon," *Werkstattschriften zur Sozialpsychiatrie*, no. 41, 1986; Theo Payk, "Hermann Simon: Aktiver Therapeut und überzeugter Sozialdarwinist," *Krankenhauspsychiatrie*, vol. 14, no. 2, 2003, pp. 67–72; Angela-Maria Grütter, *Hermann Simon: Die Entwicklung der Arbeits- und Beschäftigungstherapie in der Anstaltspsychiatrie; Eine biographische Betrachtung*. Herzogenrath: Murken-

Altrogge, 1995; Bernd Walter, *Psychiatrie und Gesellschaft in der Moderne: Geisteskrankenfürsorge in der Provinz Westfalen zwischen Kaiserreich und NS-Regime*. Paderborn: Ferdinand Schöningh, 1996, pp. 253–296 and 387–414.

11. François Tosquelles, "Essence et place du travail thérapeutique dans le dispositif de soins psychiatriques," in *Le Travail thérapeutique en psychiatrie*. Toulouse: Éditions Érès, 2009, pp. 25, 33–47, 106–107, and 81–82.

12. François Tosquelles, Jean Oury, Roger Gentis, Georges Daumézon (*et al.*), "Les échanges matériels et affectifs dans le travail thérapeutique," *Bulletin technique du personnel soignant de l'hôpital psychiatrique de Saint-Alban*, December 1961, pp. 46–47.

13. Isabel Fernández i Carramiñana, *Escola del Treball: 75 anys d'història*. Barcelona: Institut Politècnic de Formació Professional, Escola del Treball, 1989; Alexandre Galí, "1917: Institut d'Orientació Professional," in *Història de les institucions i del moviment cultural a Catalunya: 1900–1936; Llibre XV*. Barcelona: Fundació Alexandre Galí, 1985, pp. 100–126.

14. Francesc Tosquelles, "Maestro y amigo," *Revista del Departament de Psiquiatria de la Facultat de Medicina de Barcelona*, vol. 1, no. 1, 1973, pp. 54–55.

15. Emili Mira, Alfred Strauss, and Jeroni de Moragas, "Un any de treball a l'Institut d'Observació Psicològica La Sageta," *Revista Catalana de Psiquiatria i Neurologia*, vol. 1, no. 2, 1937, p. 230 and following; Manu Valentín, "El exilio judeoasquenazí en Barcelona (1933–1945)," *Entremons: UPF Journal of World History*, no. 6, June 2014, p. 28.

16. François Tosquelles, *La pratique du maternage thérapèutique chez les débiles mentaux profonds*. Paris: Jean-Louis Aupetit, 1966. See also Pere Anguera, Albert Arnavat, and Xavier Amorós, *Història gràfica del Reus contemporani: 1803–1939*. Vol. I. Reus: Ajuntament de Reus, 1986.

17. Francesc Tosquelles, "Seminari per a metges i psicòlegs (14 de diciembre de 1987)," in Josep M. Sánchez Ripollès (ed.), *Algunes conferències inèdites del Doctor Francesc Tosquelles i Llauradó (1912–1994): Escrits periodístics del Doctor Leandre Cervera (1891–1964)*. Tarragona: Universitat Rovira i Virgili, 2000, pp. 36–37.

18. Josep Coll, "L'Ateneu Enciclopèdic Popular," in Josep Coll and Josep Pané, *Josep Rovira: Una vida al servei de Catalunya i del Socialisme*. Barcelona: Ariel, 1978, pp. 24–28; Joan Navais i Icart and Frederic Samarra i Sancho, "La bandera roja del comunisme dissident: El Bloc Obrer Camperol i el Partit Obrer d'Unificació Marxista," in Joan Navais i Icart, *Tres banderes i una revolució: Anarcosindicalisme, separatisme i comunisme dissident a Reus*. Reus: Edicions del Centre de Lectura, 2001, pp. 103–156.

19. Francesc Tosquelles, *Funció poètica i psicoteràpia: Una lectura de "In memoriam" de Gabriel Ferrater*. Reus: Institut Pere Mata i Centre de Lectura de Reus, 1985. See pp. 126–127 of this volume.

20. Joaquim Molas, "Salvador Dalí, entre el surrealisme i el marxisme," *Tele/eXprés*, April 22, 1974; Félix Fanés, *Salvador Dalí: La construcción de la imagen; 1925–1930*. Madrid: Electa, 1999.

21. Jean Oury and Florent Gabarron-Garcia, "Psychothérapie institutionnelle et guerre d'Espagne," *Chimères*, no. 72, 2010, pp. 12 and 16.

THE FUNCTION OF THE STATE IS TO AVOID INSTITUTIONS

1. A magazine created in the 1930s by a group of doctors in Reus to disseminate various medical and clinical aspects of their activities. It was founded by Francesc Abelló Pascual, Jaume Sabater, Antoni Oriol i Anguera, Pere Cavallé Pi, Jaume Roig, Josep Solanes Vilaprenyó, Josep Maria Ibarz, Lluís Grau Barberà, and Enric Olesti, and they were the most active collaborators. Other contributors included Josep Briansó, Salvador Vilaseca, Francesc Tosquelles, and Antoni Escolà.

2. Emili Mira i López (1896–1964), psychiatrist, head of the psychology section (1919), director (1927) of the Institut d'Orientació Professional de Barcelona (1919), and, along with Strauss and Moragas, founder of the Institut d'Observació Psicològica La Sageta. In 1933 he taught psychiatry at the Universitat Autònoma de Barcelona and held the first chair in psychiatry there. He was director of the Institut Psicotècnic in Barcelona (1931–1939), the Institut Frenopàtic Pere Mata in Reus (1935–1939), and the asylum in Sant Boi (1936–1939). Exiled, in 1945 he settled in Brazil, where in 1947 he founded and led the Instituto de Seleção e Orientação Profissional (ISOP) in Rio de Janeiro and the journal *Arquivos Brasileiros de Psicotécnica*. He is the author of the first popular text on psychoanalysis published in the Catalan language: *La Psicoanàlisi* (1926).

3. Here Francesc Tosquelles mixes up his dates. He is actually referring to the XXIII Congrés de

psicoanalistes de llengües romàniques, held in Barcelona in 1962, devoted to "Problèmes cliniques et techniques du contre-transfert." It was organized by Pere Folch Mateu and Pere Bofill, members of the Associació Psicoanalítica Internacional in Barcelona.

4. Institut d'Observació Psicològica La Sageta, founded in Barcelona by Emili Mira in collaboration with Strauss and Moragas.

5. Edmond Ortigues (*et al.*), *Infancia alienada*. Madrid: Editorial Saltés, 1980. This volume collects the translated papers delivered at the Journées d'études sur les psychoses de l'enfant, Paris, October 21–22, 1967.

6. Francesc Tosquelles, *La pràctica del maternatge terapèutic en els deficients mentals profunds*. Barcelona: Nova Terra, 1972.

7. The Saint-Alban hospital is a crucial institution in the history of psychiatry. Founded in 1821 by Hilarion Tissot, in 1824 it became one of the first departmental asylums in France, open first to the patients in the Lozère region. In 1990, it became the Centre hospitalier François Tosquelles.

8. Cotard's delusion is a hypochondriacal melancholic delusion that Jules Cotard (1882) deemed "délire des négations," described as a self-certifiable delusion, unlike persecutory delusion, which is derived from states of moral hypochondria, as described by Jean-Pierre Falret.

9. L'Enseignement de la folie. François Tosquelles, *Funció poètica i psicoteràpia: Una lectura de "In memoriam" de Gabriel Ferrater*, op. cit.

PSYCHOANALYSIS IN CHURCH, SCHOOL, OR THE CIVIL GUARD

1. See p. 347 of this volume.

II. THERAPEUTIC EXPERIENCES IN WARTIME

The quote on p. 91 is from "Lleis, violència, fantasmes, ètica i moral," 1992.

1. François Tosquelles, *L'Enseignement de la folie*. Paris: Dunod, 2014, pp. 59–60.

2. François Tosquelles, *Funció poètica i psicoteràpia: Una lectura de "In memoriam" de Gabriel Ferrater*, op. cit., p. 135; Patrice Hortoneda, "Préface à François Tosquelles," in Jacques Tosquellas (ed.), *Archives complètes: Chantier I, Sardanes—1928 à 1943*. Cour-Cheverny: Institutions, 2014, pp. 16–17; Pere Anguera, *A bodes em convides: Estudis d'història social*. Reus: Edicions del Centre de Lectura, 1987, p. 18; Pere Anguera, *Menjacapellans, conservadors i revolucionaris*. Reus: Centre de Lectura, 1991; Joan Navais i Icart and Frederic Samarra i Sancho, "La bandera roja del comunisme dissident: El Bloc Obrer Camperol i el Partit Obrer d'Unificació Marxista," op. cit., pp. 103–156.

3. Pere Anguera (dir.), *Història General de Reus: Entre dues dictadures; 1923–1975*. Vol. IV. Reus: Ajuntament de Reus, 2003, p. 221.

4. *Llibre d'actes del Comitè de Control Obrer de l'Institut Pere Mata*. Reus: Institut Pere Mata, 1936.

5. Luis Arcarazo, "El hospital militar de Sariñena (1936–1938)," supplement of *Armas y Cuerpos*, no. 413, May 2018, p. 2; Manuel Grossi, *Cartas de Grossi*. Sariñena: Sariñena Editorial, 2009, pp. 35–48; Moisès Broggi, *Memòries d'un cirurgià (1908–1945)*. Barcelona: Edicions 62, 2001, pp. 137–174; Joaquín Ruiz, "El hospital militar de Sariñena," available at https://osmonegros.com/2015/12/15/el-hospital-militar-de-sarinena/; Arturo Morera, "La guerra civil en Sariñena," *Quio: Boletín informativo de Sariñena*, no. 21, 1992, pp. 14–15; no. 22, 1992, pp. 16–17; no. 27, 1992, pp. 12–13.

6. François Tosquelles, *Le Vécu de la fin du monde dans la folie: Le témoignage de Gérard de Nerval*. Ligné: Éditions de l'AREFPPI, 1986, pp. 67, 74, and 79. See Laure Murat, *La maison du docteur Blanche: Histoire d'un asile et de ses pensionnaires, de Nerval à Maupassant*. París: Folio, 2013; Albert Béguin, "Misère de la psychiatrie," *Esprit*, no. 197, December 1952, pp. 777–788.

7. François Tosquelles, *Le Vécu de la fin du monde dans la folie*, op. cit., pp. 101–102.

8. Letter by Francesc Tosquelles sent from the psychiatric services of the Extremaduran Army on August 25, 1938. See François Tosquelles, "La psychiatrie militaire dans la zone gouvernementale pendant la guerre d'Espagne," "Hygiène mentale dans l'Armée: Une enquête psychologique chez les auto-mutilés de guerre," "Remarques sur les postcommotionnés," "Extrait de la note 'La psychiatrie militaire dans la zone gouvernementale pendant la guerre d'Espagne,'" in Jacques Tosquellas (ed.), *Archives complètes: Chantier I, Sardanes—1928 à 1943*, op. cit., pp. 107–120.

9. François Tosquelles, *L'Enseignement de la folie*. Ligné: Éditions de l'AREFPPI, 1986, pp. 61–62.

10. Unedited interview with Bernard Favre by François Tosquelles, 1983–1985, Archives Jacques Tosquellas.

11. Javier Montejo, "En un lugar de La Mancha ... Francesc Tosquelles y Max Hodann, creadores de las primeras comunidades terapéuticas durante la Guerra Civil Española," *Intersubjetivo*, vol. 14, no. 1, 2013, pp. 46–66; Cándido Polo, "La confusión de Babel: Una controversia psiquiátrica sobre las Brigadas Internacionales," in Manuel Requena Gallego and Rosa María Sepúlveda Losa (coords.), *La sanidad en las Brigadas Internacionales*. Cuenca: Ediciones de la Universidad de Castilla–La Mancha, 2006, pp. 101–130.

12. Max Hodann, "Consideraciones sobre el problema sexual en el Ejército," *La Voz de la Sanidad de la XV División*, no. 20, December 7, 1937, p. 7.

13. Geneviève Dreyfus-Armand, "Survivre et résister dans les camps: Artistes, intellectuels et activités culturelles," in *Septfonds 1939–1944: Dans l'archipel des camps français*. Perpignan: Le Revenant Éditeur, 2019, pp. 293–317; Jean-François Gomez, "Traces vivantes de Tosquelles et de quelques autres: Chronique à propos du camp de Septfonds, de la Retirada, et d'une paire d'espadrilles usées jusqu'à la corde," *VST-Vie Sociale et Traitements*, no. 105, 2010, pp. 123–128.

14. François Tosquelles and Antoni Subirana, "Un nouveau cas de calcification intracérébrale visible radiologiquement chez une hémiplégique de l'enfance avec crises épileptiques jacksoniennes: Aspects encéphalographiques," *Revue neurologique*, no. 6, December 1934, pp. 1–5.

IN MEMORIAM
Gabriel Ferrater

1. Gabriel Ferrater, *Les dones i els dies*. Critical edition by Jordi Cornudella. Barcelona: Edicions 62, 2018, pp. 23–33.

III. MATERIAL LIFE: A PSYCHIATRIC REVOLUTION

The quote on p. 151 is from *L'Enseignement de la folie*, 1986.

1. Letter from Lucien Bonnafé to Paul Bernard, *L'Information psychiatrique*, vol. 79, no. 7, September 2003, pp. 621–626.

2. Jordana Mendelson, *Revistas y guerra: 1936–1939*. Madrid: Museo Nacional Centro de Arte Reina Sofía, 2007.

3. Francesc Tosquelles, "El Club (26 de juny de 1986)," in Josep M. Sánchez Ripollès (ed.), *Algunes conferències inèdites del doctor Francesc Tosquelles i Llauradó (1912–1994): Escrits periodístics del Doctor Leandre Cervera (1891–1964)*, op. cit., p. 40.

4. François Tosquelles, *Trait d'union: Journal de Saint-Alban; Éditoriaux, articles, notes (1950–1962)*. París: Éditions d'une, 2015; Óscar Martínez Azumendi, "La revista Club en el contexto de la psicoterapia institucional, promovida por Tosquelles, en el Pere Mata (Reus, Tarragona)," in Óscar Martínez Azumendi (*et al.*) (eds.), *Psiquiatría y cambio social, apuntes para una historia reciente: XI Jornadas de la Sección de Historia de la psiquiatría de la AEN*. Madrid: Asociación Española de Neuropsiquiatría, 2013, pp. 45–56; Mireille Gauzy, "L'effervescence saint-albanaise," in *Les chemins de l'art brut à Saint-Alban-sur-Limagnole: Trait d'union*. Villeneuve-d'Asq: LaM, Lille Métropole Musée d'art moderne, d'art contemporain et d'art brut, 2007, pp. 13–25.

5. Louis Gauzy, "Cinéma et télévision dans l'Hôpital Psychiatrique," *Bulletin technique du personnel soignant*, August 1958, pp. 30–32; "Une expérience de vente à l'extérieur," *Bulletin technique du personnel soignant*, December 1962, pp. 30–33.

6. Hervé Bazin, "Le tour d'Europe de la folie," *France-Soir*, April 25, 1959.

7. Various authors, "1838: Un nouveau partage de pouvoirs," *Recherches*, no. 17, March 1975, pp. 22–33; Michel Foucault, *Moi, Pierre Rivière, ayant égorgé ma mère, ma soeur et mon frère ...* Paris: Gallimard, 1973.

8. Report drawn from the archives of Tarn-et-Garonne.

9. Unsigned article, "Pour guérir ses malades l'alieniste Agnès Masson les fait danser," *Samedi-soir*, March 22, 1947.

10. Lucien Bonnafé and Georges Daumézon, "Perspectives de réforme psychiatrique en France depuis la Libération," in *Comptes rendus de la 46e session du Congrès des médecins aliénistes et neurologistes de France et des pays de langue française*. Paris: Masson, 1947, pp. 584–590; Georges Daumézon, "Les aliénés pendant la guerre," *Le malade mental: Qu'en avons-nous fait? Présences: Revue trimestrielle du monde des malades*, no. 54, 1956, pp. 65–66; Isabelle von Bueltzingsloewen, *L'hécatombe*

des fous: La famine dans les hôpitaux psychiatriques français sous l'Occupation. Paris: Aubier, 2007; Max Lafont, *L'extermination douce: La mort de 40.000 malades mentaux dans les hôpitaux psychiatriques en France, sous le régime de Vichy*. Ligné: Éditions de l'AREFPPI, 1987.

11. Marie-Rose Ou-Rabah, *À l'ombre des poiriers: Hélène et François Tosquelles; Un secret de famille*. Paris: Edilivre, 2014, p. 129.

12. Georges Sadoul, "Portraits du poète à plusieurs âges de sa vie," *Europe*, no. 91–92, July–August 1953, pp. 47–49.

13. Georges Canguilhem, "Ouverture," in Élisabeth Roudinesco (ed.), *Penser la folie: Essais sur Michel Foucault*. Paris: Galilée, 1992, pp. 39–42.

14. Georges Canguilhem, "Entretien de Georges Canguilhem (avec François Bing et Jean-François Braunstein)," in Camille Limoges (ed.), *Œuvres complètes: Histoire des sciences, épistémologie, commémorations (1966–1995)*. Vol. V. Paris: Librairie philosophique J. Vrin, 2018, p. 1283.

15. Georges Canguilhem, "Observation à l'hôpital psychiatrique de Saint-Alban (Lozère) (Juillet 1944, maquis), Mme C. Observation proposée et contrôlée par le Docteur Tosquelles," in Camille Limoges (ed.), *Œuvres complètes: Résistance, philosophie biologique et histoire des sciences (1940–1965)*. Vol. IV. Paris: Librairie philosophique J. Vrin, 2015, pp. 183–189.

16. Paul Éluard, "Le génie sans miroir," *Les feuilles libres*, no. 35, January–February 1924, pp. 301–308.

17. Paul Éluard, *Souvenirs de la maison des fous*. Paris: Seghers, 2011 [1945].

18. Paul Éluard, "Les Sept poèmes d'amour en guerre," in *Œuvres complètes*. Vol 1. Paris: Gallimard, 1943, pp. 1181–1187; *Souvenirs de la maison des fous*, op. cit.

19. Cécile Agay (Cécile Vulliamy), "J'ai visité des femmes enfermées dans leur propre univers," *Les Étoiles*, October 9, 1945, p. 3.

20. Tristan Tzara, *Parler seul*. Paris: Maeght, 1948–1950.

21. Letter from Tristan Tzara to Michel Leiris, Saint-Alban, August 20, 1945. Bibliothèque Littéraire Jacques Doucet, Paris.

22. Jean Dubuffet, *L'art brut préféré aux arts culturels*. Paris: Galerie René Drouin, 1949; *Asphyxiante Culture* (1968), *Asfixiante cultura*. Jaén: Ediciones del Lunar, 2011.

23. Valérie Rousseau, "Révéler l'art brut: À la recherche d'un musée idéal," *Culture & musées*, no. 16, 2010, pp. 82–85; Michel Thévoz, *L'Art Brut*. Ginebra: Skira, 1975; Lucienne Peiry, *L'Art Brut*. Paris: Flammarion, 1997; Sarah Wilson, "From Asylum to the Museum: Marginal Art in Paris and New York, 1938–1968," in *Parallel Visions: Modern Artists and Outsider Art*. Los Angeles and Princeton: Los Angeles County Museum of Art and Princeton University Press, 1992.

24. Michel de Certeau, Dominique Julia, and Jacques Revel, "La beauté du mort: Le concept de culture populaire," *Politique aujourd'hui*, December 1970, pp. 3–23; "La belleza del muerto," in Michel de Certeau, *La cultura en plural*. Buenos Aires: Nueva Visión, 1999; Michel de Certeau, *La invención de lo cotidiano: I, Artes de hacer*. Mexico City: Universidad Iberoamericana, 1996, p. 9.

25. *Trait d'union: Journal intérieur*, March 1956.

26. Jean Oury, *Essai sur la conation esthétique*. Orleans: Éditions Le Pli, 2005, pp. 59–60.

27. Ibid., p. 21.

28. Unpublished text by Éric Fassin and Joana Masó.

29. Antonin Artaud, *Le Théâtre et son double*, in Évelyne Grossman (ed.), *Œuvres*. Paris: Gallimard, p. 505.

30. Gilles Deleuze, "Introduction," in *Instincts et institutions*. Paris: Hachette, 1953, pp. viii–xi.

31. Ginette Michaud, *La Borde … un pari nécessaire: De la notion d'institution à la psychothérapie institutionnelle*, with a preface by François Tosquelles. Paris: Gauthier-Villars, 1977, pp. 54–55.

32. François Pain, *Félix Guattari sur un divan*, 1986, 20 min.

33. Josée Manenti, in Patrick Faugeras, *L'Ombre portée de François Tosquelles*. Toulouse: Éditions Érès, 2007, pp. 165–167.

34. Fernand Deligny, "La Caméra outil pédagogique," in *Œuvres*, edited by Sandra Alvarez de Toledo. Paris: L'Arachnéen, 2017, p. 407.

35. Fernand Deligny, letter of December 1, 1966, to François Truffaut, in Bernard Bastide (ed.), "Correspondance François Truffaut—Fernand Deligny," *1895*, no. 42, February 2004, p. 97.

36. François Tosquelles, "L'aménagement de la structure de la rencontre psychothérapeutique en milieu hospitalier psychiatrique," lecture given at the

4th International Congress of Psychotherapy, Barcelona, 1958.

37. Anne-Cécile Druet, "La psiquiatría española y Jacques Lacan antes de 1975," *Asclepio*, vol. 66, no. 1, 2014; Jacques Lacan, "La psychanalyse vraie et la fausse," *L'Âne*, no. 51, 1992, pp. 24–27; Jacques Lacan, "El psicoanálisis verdadero y el falso," *Freudiana*, no. 4–5, 1992, pp. 23–34; "La psicoterapia se avecinda en Sarrià," *Destino*, May 10, 1958, p. 28.

38. Jacques Derrida, "La palabra soplada," in *La escritura y la diferencia*. Barcelona: Anthropos, 1989, p. 242; Roland Barthes, "Les Inconnus de la terre," press release for *Les Inconnus de la terre: Une enquête cinématographique*, by Mario Ruspoli, written by Jean Ravel, for Argos Films, Paris, 1962; Raymond Bellour, "Ruspoli au pays des hommes," *Cinéma 63*, no. 76, 1963, pp. 25–27; *L'Express*, February 22, 1962, p. 27; Mario Ruspoli, "Remarques sur le cinéma direct, dit: 'Cinémavérité,'" *Cinéma 63*, no. 74, 1963.

39. Roger Gentis, in Patrick Faugeras, *L'Ombre portée de François Tosquelles*, op. cit., pp. 56–65.

40. Frantz Fanon, *Les Damnés de la Terre* (1961), *Los condenados de la tierra*. Tafalla: Txalaparta, 1999; Mohammed Harbi, "Fanon et le messianisme paysan," in Sonia Dayan-Herzbrun, "Vers une pensée politique postcoloniale: À partir de Frantz Fanon," *Tumultes*, no. 31, 2008, pp. 11–15.

41. François Tosquelles and Frantz Fanon, "Indications de la thérapeutique de Bini dans le cadre des thérapeutiques institutionnelles," "Sur un essai de réadaptation chez une malade avec épilepsie morphéïque et troubles de caractère grave," and "Sur quelques cas traités par la méthode de Bini," in *Comptes rendus du Congrès des médecins aliénistes et neurologues de France et des pays de langue française (51e session, Pau, 20–26 juillet 1953)*. Paris: Masson, 1953, pp. 363–368, 539–544, and 545–552; Jean Khalfa, "Soigner les pathologies de la liberté: Fanon psychiatre," *Les Temps modernes*, no. 683, 2015, pp. 229–255; Jacques Tosquellas, "Entretien avec Maurice Despinoy," *Sud/Nord*, no. 22, 2007, pp. 105–114.

42. François Tosquelles and Frantz Fanon, "Indications de la thérapeutique de Bini dans le cadre des thérapeutiques institutionnelles," in *Comptes rendus du Congrès des médecins aliénistes et neurologues de France et des pays de langue française (51e session, Pau, 20–26 juillet 1953)*, op. cit., pp. 363–368.

43. Frantz Fanon and Jacques Azoulay, "Social Therapy in a Ward of Muslim Men: Methodological Difficulties." See p. 309 of this volume.

WHAT IS TO BE UNDERSTOOD BY INSTITUTIONAL PSYCHOTHERAPY?

Notes by Francesc Tosquelles

1. See on this subject the discussions of the various French schools of psychoanalysis on the translation of the Freudian term *Vorstellungsrepräsentanz* [ideational representative].

2. An article by Catherine Sachot-Poncin gives an overall view of these activities. The *Revue de psychothérapie institutionelle* published it in a special issue. [Catherine Sachot-Poncin, "Les CEMÉA et le perfectionnement des infirmiers des hôpitaux psychiatriques," in Danielle Sivadon (ed.), *Psychothérapie institutionelle*, special issue of *Recherches*, no. 10, May 1970.]

THE RESISTANCE: SAINT-ALBAN

1. In reality it was the Septfonds camp.

2. François Tosquelles and Roger Gentis, "L'Accueil des malades à l'hôpital psychiatrique," *Revue pratique de psychologie de la vie sociale et d'hygiéne mentale*, no. 2, 1957, pp. 18–27.

ON COLLECTIVE PSYCHOTHERAPY

Notes by Francesc Tosquelles

1. Balvet: Montpellier Congress, 1942.

2. The prefect was perfectly tuned in to our movement because of his own personal experience as an "active school" pioneer, and because he'd had the occasion to experience our interior efforts at Saint-Alban during a short stay that he made secretly at the hospital in the course of the German occupation.

3. Here's an example of these interrelations. It's already been years that I've expounded to the nurses on the usefulness of organizing "beauty treatments," this with the support of accounts of visits to certain American hospitals, and of a more or less far-fetched theory on the subject of depersonalization. This sermonizing produced very limited results. However, since the regularity of the evening club events obliges patients and nurses to get ready for a social self-presentation, there's a spontaneous rush of patients to the village coiffeuse—a much better solution, moreover, than the "in-house beauty

salon" that I had advocated before. Now it's a matter of a "need" that's actually felt instead of a "theory" or "charitable" act. One such patient, quite agitated for the moment, would willingly undergo a permanent and start a conversation with another customer from her village on the subject of certain childhood memories. I can't affirm anything about the real significance of these occurrences, but a few days later she was made responsible for regular tasks at the patients' library. It should be said that this took place in the course of an insulin treatment ... The nurses who accompany patients are no longer in the traditional facile and sterilizing master-slave relationship. They must manage to invent a psychotherapeutic contact that stabilizes the patient's social behavior, at least at the hairdresser's salon. In short, they are no longer "on duty" at the hairdresser's, as Bernard would put it.

THE LIMITATIONS OF LIBERAL STRUCTURING IN MEDICINE

1. Francesc Tosquelles, "Les assegurances socials i la medicina," *Quaderns d'estudis polítics, econòmics i socials*, no. 6, June 1945, pp. 14–17.

FRANTZ FANON AND INSTITUTIONAL PSYCHOTHERAPY

1. Michel Minard (ed.), *Histoire et histoires de la psychiatrie*. Toulouse: Éditions Éres, 1992.

SOCIAL THERAPY IN A WARD OF MUSLIM MEN

Notes by Frantz Fanon and Jacques Azoulay. Editors' notes by Jean Khalfa and Robert J.C. Young.

1. At Saint-Alban, the collective psychotherapy meetings mostly take place within the club meetings or the journal-committee meetings. But as we were at the experimental stage, we were obliged to group everything in the pavilion.

2. As Gusdorf showed so well in his *Traité de l'existence morale*. [Georges Gusdorf, *Traité de l'existe morale*. Paris: Armand Colin, 1949.]

3. Called "you-yous."

4. [The following pages take up long passages from a book by André Leroi-Gourhan and Jean Poirier, subtly modifying them toward an indictment of colonialism: *Ethnologie de l'Union française*. Vol. 1, *Afrique*. Paris: PUF, 1953, p. 121.]

5. *Khammès*: sharecroppers who work for a fifth of the crop. ["A kind of sharecropper who received only a very small share of the crop, usually a fifth." Pierre Bourdieu, *The Logic of Practice*, translated by Richard Nice. Stanford, CA: Stanford University Press, 1990, p. 127.]

6. [The initial dilemma of this paper will thus be solved by understanding "Indigenous" patients against the historical backdrop of the progressive colonial destruction of traditional structures. Here again Fanon replaces a substantialist approach, that of the Algiers school of psychiatry and of the hospital nurses, with a temporal perspective, as he had done in his analysis of the relationship of the neurological and the psychiatric.]

7. [In *Black Skin, White Masks*, Fanon simply wrote, without the reference to Merleau-Ponty: "To speak a language is to take on a world, a culture." *Black Skin, White Masks*, translated by Richard Philcox. New York: Grove, 2008, p. 25.]

IV. THE RETURN. A FOREIGN BODY

The quote on p. 317 is from "A propósito de los modelos de asistencia en psiquiatría," 1984.

1. Antonio Labad, "El periódico *Club* y el libro de actas de la *Comisión periódico* en el Institut Pere Mata," in Óscar Martínez Azumendi, *Psiquiatría y cambio social: Apuntes para una historia reciente; XI Jornadas de la sección de historia de la psiquiatría de la AEN*. Madrid: Asociación Española de Neuropsiquiatría, 2019, pp. 57–66; Antonio Labad, "Papel de la Revista Club (1972) en la terapia institucional del Instiut Pere Mata de Reus," in Silvia Esteban (*et al.*) (coords.), *Historias de la salud mental para un nuevo tiempo*. Madrid: Asociación Española de Neuropsiquiatría, 2016, pp. 117–135; Josep Poca Gaya, *Institut Pere Mata: Cent anys d'història (1896–1996)*, op. cit.

2. José Rodríguez Reyes, "El departamento de terapias colectivas en el Hospital psiquiátrico de Oviedo," Oviedo, 1966; Josep Barceló-Prats, Josep Maria Comelles, and Enrique Perdiguero-Gil, "Las bases ideológicas y prácticas del proceso de regionalización de la sanidad en España (1955–1978)," in María Isabel Porras Gallo, Lourdes Mariño Gutiérrez, and María Victoria Caballero Martínez (eds.), *Salud, enfermedad y medicina en el franquismo*. Madrid: Catarata, 2019, pp. 146–167. See also Manuel Desviat and Anna Moreno, "La reforma psiquiátrica" and "Principios y objetivos de la salud mental comunitaria," in *Acciones de salud mental en la comunidad*. Madrid: Asociación Española de Neuropsiquiatría, 2012, pp. 21–27 and

28–36; Manuel Desviat, "El devenir de la reforma psiquiátrica," in Andrés Blanco de la Calle (ed.), *Manual de rehabilitación del trastorno mental grave*. Madrid: Síntesis, 2010, pp. 29–49.

3. José García Ibáñez and Antonio Labad, "Experiència viscuda de les produccions verbals polifòniques: El mètode dels 'cassettes' en la formació professional de l'Institut Pere Mata," in *Història de la psicoanàlisi als Països Catalans*. Perpinyà: GAIRPS, 1986, pp. 87–88.

4. Francesc Tosquelles, "Els sentiments (29 d'abril de 1986)," in Josep M. Sánchez Ripollès (ed.), *Algunes conferències del Doctor Francesc Tosquelles i Llauradó (1912–1994): Escrits periodístics del Doctor Leandre Cervera (1891–1964)*, op. cit., p. 44.

5. Francesc Tosquelles, "Sessió del 30 d'abril de 1986," ibid., p. 46.

6. Federico Menéndez Osorio, "Veinte años de la reforma psiquiátrica: Panorama del estado de la psiquiatría en España de los años 1970 a los 2000; De un pensamiento único a otro," *Revista de la Asociación Española de Neuropsiquiatría*, vol. 25, no. 95, July/September 2005, pp. 69–81; Patricia Mayayo, "Creatividad artística y psiquiatría alternativa en la transición española: La experiencia del Hospital de Día de Madrid," in Rafael Huertas (ed.), *Psiquiatría y antipsiquiatría en el segundo franquismo y la Transición*. Madrid: Catarata, 2017, pp. 105–123.

7. Various authors, *Història de la psicoanàlisi als Països Catalans*. Perpignan: GAIRPS, 1986.

8. Angela Melitopoulos and Maurizio Lazzarato, *Déconnage*, 2011, 100 min.; Jean-Christophe Montferran, *Traces*, 2012, 60 min., https://videotheque.cnrs.fr/doc=3740; Sonia Cantalapiedra, *Saint-Alban, une révolution psychiatrique*, 2016, 60 min.; Martin Deyres, *Les heures heureuses*, 2019, 77 min.; Mireia Sallarès, *Història potencial de Francesc Tosquelles: Catalunya i la por*, 2021, 135 min.; Enric Miró, *Oblideu Tosquelles*, 2022, 110 min.

9. Montserrat Rodríguez Garzo, *Esquizofrenias y otros hechos de lenguaje: De la clínica analítica del Macba (2002–2013)*. Madrid: Brumaria, 2015; Gabriela Berti and Carles Guerra, *Práctica política, arte y clínica: Entre Tosquelles y Guattari*. Barcelona: MACBA, 2012; Jean-Claude Polack, "François Tosquelles i Fernand Deligny: Psicosis i experiències de l'espai," lecture delivered as part of the seminar *Fernand Deligny: Permetre, traçar, veure*, Barcelona, MACBA, 2009. In 2008, Gabriela Berti coordinated the reading group *La penya Tosquelles*, with sessions by Antonio Labad and Jorge de los Santos, at the Fundació Antoni Tàpies in Barcelona.

BIBLIOGRAPHY AND FILMOGRAPHY

TEXTS BY FRANCESC TOSQUELLES (1925–1994)

1925

Tosquelles, Francesc. "Sospirs," *Joventut Catalana*, vol. 2, no. 32, July 1925, no pagination.

1928

— "L'afer de Glozel," *Letras: Revista escolar mensual*, no. 1, January 1928.

— "Vides adelerades," *Letras: Revista escolar mensual*, special end-of-school-year issue, no. 5, May 1928.

1929

Tosquelles, Francesc; Vilaseca, Salvador. "Interprétation analytique du Syndrome de Cotard," in Emili Mira (ed.), *Congrès des médecins aliénistes et neurologistes de France et des pays de langue française: XXXIIIe session, Barcelone, 21–26 Mai 1929; Comptes rendus*. Paris: Masson, 1929, pp. 371–374.

1931

Tosquelles, Francesc. "Estructuració de la societat i la follia," Barcelona, Ateneu Enciclopèdic Popular, May 31, 1931. [Unpublished lecture, text has not been found]

1933

— "De la cultura," *Estudis*, vol. 1, no. 1, December 1933, pp. 27–28.

1934

Tosquelles, François; Subirana, Antoni. "Un Nouveau cas de calcification intracérébrale visible radiologiquement chez une hémiplégique de l'enfance avec crises épileptiques jacksoniennes: Aspects encéphalographiques," *Revue neurologique*, no. 6, December 1934, pp. 1–5.

1935

Tosquelles, Francesc. "A propòsit de l'anàlisi d'una personalitat anormal," *Fulls clínics*, May 1935, pp. 5–13.

— "La col·laboració de la joventut," *Estudis*, vol. 2, no. 21, September 1935, pp. 351–352.

— "La psicologia del treball," *Estudis*, vol. 2, no. 21, September 1935, pp. 398–399.

1936

— "Les multituds i la guerra," *Estudis*, vol. 3, no. 25, January 1936, pp. 454–455.

— "Bécquer-Centenari," *Estudis*, vol. 3, no. 26, February 1936, pp. 478–479.

— "A propòsit de la visita a l'Institut Pere Mata," *Estudis*, vol. 3, no. 28, April 1936, p. 515.

— "Valoració del congrés local per a la millora de l'ensenyament i contra l'analfabetisme," *Estudis*, vol. 3, no. 30, June 1936, pp. 551–552.

1937

— "Sentit de les consignes del POUM," *La Torxa: Portantveu del POUM i de les JCI de Reus*, no. 4, January 30, 1937, p. 3.

1939

— "Hygiène mentale dans l'Armée: Une enquête psychologique chez les automutilés de guerre," in Jacques Tosquellas (ed.), *Archives complètes: Chantier I, Sardanes – 1928 à 1943*. Cour-Cheverny: Institutions, 2014, pp. 107–112.

— "Remarques sur les post-commotionés," in Jacques Tosquellas (ed.), *Archives complètes: Chantier I, Sardanes—1928 à 1943*. Cour-Cheverny: Institutions, 2014, pp. 113–120.

1941

— "Examen des questions théoriques qui sont à la base de toute classification psychiatrique (Société du Gévaudan)," in Jacques Tosquellas (ed.), *Archives complètes: Chantier I, Sardanes – 1928 à 1943*. Cour-Cheverny: Institutions, 2014, pp. 147–166.

1942

Tosquelles, François; Balvet, Paul; Chaurand, André. "Considérations techniques et statistiques sur 60 malades traités par électrochoc," in Pierre Combemale and Paul Hugues (eds.), *Congrès des médecins aliénistes et neurologistes de France et des pays de langue française, XLIII session, Montpellier, 28–30 octobre 1942: Comptes rendus*. Paris: Masson, 1942, pp. 347–352.

Tosquelles, François. "Sur les changements survenus chez quelques malades au cours de l'électrochoc: Contribution à l'étude des structures psychotiques." [Unpublished paper for the Congrès des medecins alienistes et neurologistes de France et des pays de langue francaise, Montpellier, October 28–30, 1942]

1943

— *Cours aux infirmiers de Saint-Alban (1943–1945): Psychologie, psychiatrie, soins à donner aux malades.* Paris: Éditions d'une, 2018.

1944

Tosquelles, François; Bonnafé, Lucien. "Expérience onirique: Début d'un accès maniaque," *Annales médico-psychologiques*, vol. 1, January–May 1944, pp. 168–171.

— "Au sujet du test de Rorschach," *Annales médico-psychologiques*, vol. 1, January–May 1944, pp. 171–174.

1945

Tosquelles, François. "La fascination au cours du Rorschach," *Rorschachiana* vol. 1, no. 1, 1945, pp. 108–114.

Tosquelles, François; Bonnafé, Lucien; Chaurand, André; Clément, André. "Premières notes sur la notion de structure: Ambiguïté du terme," *Annales médico-psychologiques*, vol. 1, no. 1, January–May 1945, pp. 89–93.

— "Structure et sens de l'événement morbide," *Annales médico-psychologiques*, vol. 1, January–May 1945, pp. 174–180.

Tosquelles, François. "Perspectives i miratges," *Endavant: Òrgan del Moviment Socialista de Catalunya; Federació, democràcia, socialisme*, no. 6, June 23, 1945, no pagination.

— "Les assegurances socials i la medicina," *Quaderns d'estudis polítics, econòmics i socials*, no. 6, June 1945, pp. 14–17.

Tosquelles, François; Sauret, Jaume. "Invalidesa i treball: A propòsit dels mutilats de guerra," *Endavant: Òrgan del Moviment Socialista de Catalunya; Federació, democràcia, socialisme*, no. 9, October 1945, no pagination.

Tosquelles, François. "Els límits de l'estructura liberal de la Medicina," *Quaderns d'estudis polítics, econòmics i socials*, no. 11, November 1945, pp. 22–24.

Tosquelles, François; Bonnafé, Lucien; Chaurand, André; Clément, André. "Gestalt-théorie et structures en psychiatrie: La dialectique fond-figure dans la nosologie et la séméiologie," *Annales médico-psychologiques*, vol. 2, June–December, pp. 275–279.

— "Valeur de la théorie de la forme en psychiatrie: La dialectique du moi et du monde et de l'événement morbide," *Annales médico-psychologiques*, vol. 2, June–December 1945, pp. 279–284.

— "L'évolution du béhaviorisme et la notion de structure en psychiatrie," *Annales médico-psychologiques*, vol. 2, June–December 1945, pp. 555–559.

1946

— "L'inconscient et les instincts dans une vue structurale de l'événement psychopathologique," *Annales médico-psychologiques*, January–May 1946, pp. 96–101.

— "Note sur l'originalité du pathologique d'après la psychanalyse et sur la valeur du complexe comme perspective structurale dans l'existence pathologique," *Annales médico-psychologiques*, June–December 1946, pp. 58–63.

Tosquelles, François. "Système réticulo-endothélial et psychiatrie: Quelques résultats du test cancérolytique et du test au bleu de trypan." [Unpublished paper for the Congrès des médecins aliénistes et neurologistes, Geneva/Lausanne, July 22–27, 1946]

— "Le cardiazol dans le diagnostic de l'épilepsie." [Unpublished paper for the Congrès des médecins aliénistes et neurologistes, Geneva/Lausanne, July 22–27, 1946]

1947

— "La psychopathologie à la lumière du matérialisme dialectique," published with the title *Psychopathologie et matérialisme dialectique*, Sophie Legrain (ed). Paris: Éditions d'une, 2019. [Lecture delivered at the École Normale Supérieure as part of the series "Les méthodes de conaissance de l'homme dans la neurologie et la psychiatrie actuelles," February 5, 1947]

1948

— *Le Vécu de la fin du monde dans la folie: Le témoignage de Gérard de Nerval.* Ligné: Éditions de l'AREFPPI, 1986; Grenoble: Jérôme Millón, 2012. [Thesis defended in Paris in 1948]

— "Les conflits humains sont toujours sociaux," *Action: Hebdomadaire de l'indépendance française*, no. 214, November 1948, p. 7.

1949

— "Quelques considérations sur l'opportunité de la leucotomie chimique dans un hôpital psychiatrique rural," in Pierre Adolphe Chatagnon (ed.), *Congrès des médecins aliénistes et neurologistes de France et des pays de langue française: XLVII session, Clermont-Ferrand, 12–18 septembre 1949; Rapports.* Paris: Masson, 1949, pp. 407–410.

1950

— *Trait-d'union: Journal de Saint-Alban; Éditoriaux, articles et notes (1950–1962).* Paris: Éditions d'une, 2016.

— "L'être humain, sexe, violence, amour, langage," 1950. [Unpublished]

— "Organización material del hospital psiquiátrico y finalidad terapéutica," *Journal du premier Congrès Mondiale de Psychiatrie (18–27 septembre 1950)*, no. 3, September 21, 1950, pp. 4–5.

— "Psychothérapie de groupe dans un hôpital psychiatrique," *Journal du premier Congrès mondial de psychiatrie*, no. 7, September 27, 1950, p. 5.

— "Psychopathologie des délires: Discussion des rapports," *L'Évolution psychiatrique*, no. 4, October–December 1950, pp. 556–563.

1951
— "Étude clinique et phénoménologique d'un récit psychanalytique," *L'Évolution psychiatrique*, no. 3, 1951, pp. 405–425.

1952
— "Sur une structure psycho-sociologique typique des conduites amorales en Lozère," in Thorsten Sellin (ed.), *II Congrès international de criminologie, Paris, 10–19 septembre 1950*. Paris: Presses Universitaires de France, 1952, pp. 363–368.

— "Symposium sur la psychothérapie collective: Intervention de Tosquelles," *L'Évolution psychiatrique*, no. 3, September 1952, pp. 535–554 and 572–573.

— "Réponse du Dr Tosquelles au Dr Le Guillant," *L'Évolution psychiatrique*, no. 3, September 1952, pp. 572–573.

— "La société vécue par les malades psychiques," *Misère de la psychiatrie, Esprit*, no. 197, December 1952, pp. 897–904.

1953
Tosquelles, François; Fanon, Frantz. "Sur quelques cas traités par la méthode de Bini," in *Comptes rendus du Congrès des médecins aliénistes et neurologues de France et des pays de langue française (LI session, Pau, 20–26 juillet 1953)*. Paris: Masson, 1953, pp. 363–368.

— "Sur un essai de réadaptation chez une malade avec épilepsie morphéique et troubles de caractère graves," in *Comptes rendus du Congrès des médecins aliénistes et neurologues de France et des pays de langue française (LI session, Pau, 20–26 juillet 1953)*. Paris: Masson, 1953, pp. 539–544.

— "Indications de la thérapeutique de Bini dans le cadre des thérapeutiques institutionnelles," in *Comptes rendus du Congrès des médecins aliénistes et neurologues de France et des pays de langue française (LI session, Pau, 20–26 juillet 1953)*. Paris: Masson, 1953, pp. 545–552.

1954
Tosquelles, François. "Introduction à la sémiologie de l'agitation," *L'Évolution psychiatrique*, no. 1, January–March 1954, pp. 75–97.

1955
— "Analyse d'une psychose aiguë: La sphère de l'existence esthétique selon Kierkegaard," *L'Évolution psychiatrique*, no. 1, January 1955, pp. 159–181.

Tosquelles, François; Milon, Robert; Fargeot, G. "Les problèmes médico-administratifs soulevés par la pratique de l'ergothérapie et de la sociothérapie dans les hôpitaux psychiatriques," *L'Information psychiatrique*, vol. 2, February 1955, pp. 71–104.

Tosquelles, François; Daumézon, George; Paumelle, Philippe. "Le fonctionnement thérapeutique," in *Encyclopédie médico-chirurgicale: Traité de Psychiatrie.* Paris: Masson, 1955.

— "Organisation thérapeutique de l'hôpital psychiatrique: Ergothérapie, sociothérapie," in *Encyclopédie médico-chirurgicale: Traité de Psychiatrie.* Paris: Masson, 1955.

Tosquelles, François; Daumézon, George. "Troubles du comportement: L'agitation," in *Encyclopédie médico-chirurgicale: Traité de psychiatrie.* Paris: Masson, 1955.

1956
Tosquelles, François. "Les tests de personnalité en psychiatrie (discussion du rapport de psychiatrie)." [Unpublished paper for the Congrès des médecins aliénistes et neurologistes de France et des pays de langue française, Bordeaux, August 30–September 4, 1956]

Tosquelles, François; Gentis, Roger; Paillot, Maurice; Bidault, René; Enkin, Marx. "À quoi peut servir la cour de quartier." [Unpublished paper for the Congrès des médecins aliénistes et neurologistes de France et des pays de langue française, Bordeaux, August 30–September 4, 1956]

— "Quelques problèmes sur les services généraux et l'organisation hospitalière thérapeutique." [Unpublished paper for the Congrès des médecins aliénistes et neurologistes de France et des pays de langue française, Bordeaux, August 30–September 4, 1956]

Tosquelles, François. "Un combat douteux," *Esprit*, no. 9, "Demain L'Espagne," September 1956, pp. 428–434.

1957
— "Le manichéisme objectal de Mélanie Klein à la lumière de la psychothérapie des psychoses."

[Unpublished paper for the Société de neuro-psychiatrie de la région lyonnaise, January 20, 1957]

Tosquelles, François; Gentis, Roger. "L'accueil des malades à l'hôpital psychiatrique," *Revue pratique de psychologie de la vie sociales et d'hygiène mentale*, no. 2, 1957, pp. 18–27.

Tosquelles, François; Gentis, Roger; Enkin, Marx; Bonnet, François. "On Group Therapy Within the General Framework of Institutional Therapeutics," in B. Stovkis (ed.), *Group Psychotherapy: II International Congress; Zürich 1957*. Basel and New York: S. Karger, 1959, pp. 133–136.

Tosquelles, François. "Discussion about Dr. Oury's communication," in B. Stovkis (ed.), *Group Psychotherapy: II International Congress; Zürich 1957*. Basel and New York: S. Karger, 1959, pp. 436–437.

— "Intervention sur 'Thérapeutique analytique de groupe,'" *L'Évolution psychiatrique*, no. 2, 1957.

— "La rencontre: Fondement metaphysique," in *Humaniser l'hôpital psychiatrique*. Paris: Les Éditions du Cerf, 1959, pp. 17–32. [Lecture for the study sessions of the Association des aumôniers des hôpitaux psychiatriques, Clamart, 1957]

— "Le psychiatre," in *Humaniser l'hôpital psychiatrique*. Paris: Les Éditions du Cerf, 1959, pp. 107–117. [Lecture for the study sessions of the Association des aumôniers des hôpitaux psychiatriques, Clamart, 1957]

1958

— "Intervention: Congrès de Sèvres," *L'Information psychiatrique*, no. 5, May 1958, pp. 439–441.

— "L'élaboration du contrat entre les comités hospitaliers de Croix-Marine et les administrations des hôpitaux psychiatriques," *Revue pratique de psychologie de la vie sociale et d'hygiène mentale*, no. 3, 1958, pp. 82–92.

Tosquelles, François; Enkin, Marx; Gentis, Roger. "Essai thérapeutique d'une nouvelle préparation d'acides animés libres en neurologie-psychiatrie," *Lyon médical*, no. 37, September 1958, pp. 304–325.

Tosquelles, François. "Le débile profond semi-éducable: Définition. Possibilités. Conditions et limites de son adaptabilité," *Informations sociales*, no. 9–10, October–November 1958, pp. 33–49.

— "Contribution à la recherche des techniques d'éducation des débiles profonds," *Informations sociales*, no. 9–10, October–November 1958, pp. 33–49.

— "L'aménagement de la structure de la rencontre psychothérapeutique en milieu hospitalier psychiatrique," *Pédagogie et psychothérapie institutionnelle*, special issue of the *Revue de psychothérapie institutionnelle*, no. 2–3, 1966, pp. 80–86. [Paper for the Congreso Internacional de Psicoterapia de Barcelona, 1958]

— "Les problèmes des annexes des hôpitaux psychiatriques réservés aux enfants," 1958. [Unpublished text for the Société médicale des hôpitaux psychiatriques de la Seine]

1959

— "Les thérapeutiques de groupe dans le cadre de la thérapeutique institutionnelle," *Acta Psychotherapeutica, Psychosomatica et Orthopaedagogica*, no. 213, 1959.

1960

— "Intervention a la suite du rapport de Nicolas Perrotti intitulé 'Apercus theóriques de la dépersonnalisation,'" *Revue française de psychanalyse*, July–October 1960, pp. 434–448. [XXI Congrès des psychanalystes des langues romanes, Rome, April 7–9, 1960]

— "Présentation de l'année mondiale de la santé mentale," *Revue pratique de psychologie de la vie sociale et d'hygiène mentale*, no. 3, 1960.

— "À propos d'un syndrome d'agitation de type frontal d'un enfant débile profond: Hématome sous-dural," 1960. [Unpublished]

— "Religieux et religieuses au service du malade mental: De l'aspect thérapeutique de la relation malade-religieux hospitaliers," *L'Interdit*, no. 2, 1978, pp. 27–54. [1960]

— "Discussion sur: Stein, Conrad; 'Langage et inconscient'" (1960), in Henri Ey (dir.), *L'Inconscient*. Paris: Desclée de Brouwer, 1966, pp. 153–154. ["Intervención," in Henri Ey (dir.), *El inconsciente (Coloquio de Bonneval)*. Mexico City: Siglo XXI, 1970, pp. 161–163]

1961

— *Fantasme et institution: Groupe de travail de psychothérapie et de sociothérapie institutionnelles* (1961). Paris: Éditions d'une, 2015.

— *Psychothérapie multiréférentielle dans un milieu institutionnel: Groupe de travail de psychothérapie et de sociothérapie institutionnelles* (1961). Paris: Éditions d'une, 2015.

— "Note sur la séméiologie de groupe," *Bulletin technique du personnel soignant de l'hôpital psychiatrique de Saint-Alban*, February 1961, pp. 36–58.

— "Principes et techniques des jeux collectifs notamment chez le débile profond," *Revue Pratique de psychologie de la vie sociale et d'hygiène mentale*, no. 4, October–December 1961, pp. 177–186.

Tosquelles, François; Oury, Jean; Gentis, Roger; Daumézon, Georges (*et al.*). "Les échanges matériels et affectifs dans le travail thérapeutique," *Bulletin technique du personnel soignant de l'hôpital psychiatrique de Saint-Alban*, December 1961, pp. 1–31.

Tosquelles, François. "Au sujet des rapports de Docteurs Bonnafé, Bequart et Muldworf," in Lucien Bonnafé (ed.), *27 opinions sur la psychothérapie*. Paris: Éditions sociales, 1961, pp. 208–226.

1962

Tosquelles, François; Oziol, Lucien; Racine, Yves (*et al.*). *Hygiène mentale des éducateurs et leur efficacité: Conditions techniques et conditions matérielles de leur activité* (1962). Paris: Éditions d'une, 2015.

Tosquelles, François. "Premiers contacts et manipulation d'objets: Rééducation de la main [I]," *Revue pratique de psychologie de la vie sociale et d'hygiène mentale*, no. 1, 1962, pp. 29–35.

— "Évolution des actions de la main et techniques rééducatives [II]," *Revue pratique de psychologie de la vie sociale et d'hygiène mentale*, no. 2, 1962, pp. 83–89.

Tosquelles, François; Gentis, Roger; Racine, Yves. "Le travail thérapeutique," *Bulletin technique du personnel soignant de l'hôpital psychiatrique de Saint-Alban*, February 1962, pp. 29–35. [Roundtable discussion]

Tosquelles, François; Poncin, Claude. "Thérapeutique institutionnelle et psychothérapique de groupe dans les institutions," *Bulletin technique du personnel soignant de l'hôpital psychiatrique de Saint-Alban*, June 1962, pp. 32–37.

Tosquelles, François. "Intervention," *Revue française de psychanalyse*, special issue, vol. XXVIII, 1963, pp. 201–205. [Paper on the report by Pedro Bofill and Pere Folch Mateu titled "Problèmes cliniques et techniques du contre-transfert" presented during the XXIII Congrès des psychanalystes de langues romanes, Barcelona, June 8–11, 1962]

— "Clinique et éclairage psychanalytique dans l'approche de l'apragmatisme sexuel et de la prostitution," 1962. [Unpublished text for the Société de psychanalyse, Marseille]

— "À propos du soi-disant maternage," 1962. [Unpublished]

1963

— "Évolution des actions de la main et techniques rééducatives [III]," *Revue pratique de psychologie de la vie sociale et d'hygiène mentale*, no. 1, 1963, pp. 31–37.

— "L'Apprentissage de la marche," *Revue pratique de psychologie de la vie sociale et d'hygiène mentale*, no. 2, 1963, pp. 81–86.

1964

— "Quelques aperçus sur l'histoire de la psychothérapie" (perspectives sur la psychothérapie institutionnelle), *L'Information psychiatrique*, no. 6, June 1964, pp. 401–416.

— "Psychothérapie de groupe et psychodrame," 1964. [Unpublished]

— "Groupe thérapeutique," June 1964. [Unpublished lecture for the Société française de psychothérapie de groupe]

1965

— *Cours aux éducateurs*. Nîmes: Champ social, 2003. [Texts originally written in 1965–1966]

— "Table ronde avec des parents," "Table ronde avce des professionals," and "Condition et avenir des débiles profonds," *Esprit*, no. 11, "L'Enfance handicapée," November 1965, pp. 824–829, 897–918, 959–969.

— "Éditorial," *Psychothérapie institutionnelle*, no. 1, 1965, p. 1.

— "Introduction au problème du transfert en psychothérapie institutionnelle," *Psychothérapie institutionnelle*, no. 1, 1965, pp. 9–19.

1966

— *Pédagogie & pychothérapie institutionnelles*, special issue of *Pscyhothérapie institutionnelle*, no. 2–3, 1966. [Reproduced with the title *Éducation et psychothérapie institutionnelle*. Mantes-la-ville: Hiatus, 1984; Nîmes: Champ social, 2006]

— *La Pratique du maternage thérapeutique chez les débiles mentaux profonds*. Paris: Jean-Louis Aupetit, 1966. [*Pràctica del maternatge terapèutic en els deficients mentals profunds*. Barcelona: Nova Terra, 1972 / *Maternaje terapéutico con los deficientes mentales profundos*. Barcelona: Nova Terra, 1973]

— "Correspondances," *Recherches*, no. 1, 1966, pp. 123–124. [Letter addressed to the Fédération des groupes d'études et de recherches institutionnelles, as president of the Societé de psychotérapie institutionnelle]

— "Intervention du docteur Tosquelles," *Psychothérapie institutionnelle*, no. 4, 1966, pp. 5–10.

— "À propos de H. S. Sullivan," *Psychothérapie institutionnelle*, no. 6, 1966, pp. 7–12.

— "La psychothérapie institutionnelle: Approches théoriques," *Revue pratique de psychologie de la vie sociale et d'hygiène mentale*, no. 3, 1966, pp. 53–62.

1967

— *Le Travail thérapeutique a l'hôpital psychiatrique.* Paris: Editions du Scarabée, 1967. [Republished with the title *Le Travail thérapeutique en psychiatrie.* Toulouse: Éditions Érès, 2009]

— *Structure et rééducation thérapeutique: Aspects pratiques.* Paris: Éditions Universitaires, 1967. [*Estructura y reeducación terapéutica.* Madrid: Fundamentos, 1973]

— "Sur les difficultés du personnel soignant des débiles mentaux profonds plus ou moins régressifs ou autistiques: Discours sur un discours de Maud Mannoni," *L'Information psychiatrique*, no. 2, 1967, pp. 189–196.

Tosquelles, François; Oury, Jean; Misès, Roger; Sivadon, Paul. "Le rôle thérapeutique spécifique de l'établissement psychiatrique et les psychothérapies institutionnelles [I]," *La Presse médicale*, vol. 1, no. 21, April 1967, pp. 1079–1082.

— "Le rôle thérapeutique spécifique de l'établissement psychiatrique et les psychothérapies institutionnelles [II]," *La Presse médicale*, vol. 2, no. 22, May 1967, pp. 1145–1148.

Tosquelles, François. "Préface," in Bernadette Maurice (ed.), *Recherches pédagogiques: Lecture et latéralisation.* Clarmont d'Alvèrnia: G. de Bussac, 1967.

— "Esquisse d'une problématique analytique dans les soins à donner aux enfants psychotiques en institution," in Maud Mannoni (dir.), *Enfance aliénée I: Enfance aliénée ou Société aliénante?, Recherches*, no. 7, September 1967, pp. 227–252.

1968

Tosquelles, François; Ayme, Jean. "Soins aux psychotiques en institution," in Maud Mannoni (dir.), *Enfance aliénée II: L'enfant, la psychose et l'institution, Recherches*, no. 8, December 1968, pp. 74–79.

Tosquelles, François; Oury, Jean. "L'enfant, la psychose et l'institution," in Maud Mannoni (dir.), *Enfance aliénée II: L'enfant, la psychose et l'institution, Recherches*, no. 8, December 1968, pp. 115–130.

Tosquelles, François. "Considérations sur la formation du psychiatre" (1968), *Perspectives psy*, vol. 52, no. 1, 2013, pp. 7–14.

— "Les institutions sociales et la pathogénie et la pathoplastie des troubles mentaux: Conséquences thérapeutiques." [Unpublished paper for the Congrès de l'Hôpital Psychiatrique de Fan, Dakar, March 1968]

1969

Tosquelles, Francesc; Anglès, Lluís. "El Doctor Francesc Tosquelles, un reusenc universal," *Reus: Semanario de la Ciudad*, April 12, 1969, p. 14.

Tosquelles, François. "Notes sur le traitement des psychoses infantiles," *Confrontations psychiatriques*, no. 3, "Psychoses de l'infant," 1969, pp. 183–203.

— "Que faut-il entendre par psychothérapie institutionnelle?," *L'Information psychiatrique*, no. 4, 1969, pp. 377–384.

1970

— "Interazioni tra attitudine terapeutica e attitudine pedagogica nella struttura istituzionale," *Minerva psychiatrica e psicologica*, no. 13, 1970, pp. 266–284.

— "Preface," *Recherches*, no. 10, "Psychothérapie institutionnelle: Aspects de la vie quotidienne à l'hôpital psychiatrique; La formation des infirmiers," May 1970, pp. 187–192. [Prologue to the doctoral thesis by Catherine Sachot-Poncin, *Les C.E.M.É.A. et le perfectionnement des infirmiers des hôpitaux psychiatriques*]

— "Discussion du rapport: Daumézon, Georges, 'L'apport de la psychanalyse à la séméiologie psychiatrique,'" in Dario De Martis and Fausto Petrella (eds.), *Apport de la psychanalyse à la sémiologie psychiatrique: Rapport de psychiatrie présenté au Congrès de psychiatrie et de neurologie de langue française, LXVIII session, Milan, 7–12 Septembre, 1970.* Paris: Masson, 1970, pp. 428–436.

— "Sémiologie et premiers entretiens en psychiatrie: À propos d'un cas." [Unpublished paper for the I Séminaire de Psychiatrie Communautaire et de Sociothérapie, Milan, 1970]

— "Senso e non senso delle istituzioni psichiatrica." [Unpublished paper for the I Séminaire de Psychiatrie Communautaire et de Sociothérapie, Milan, 1970]

— "Introduction." [Unpublished paper for the roundtable "La problématique du pouvoir dans les communautés thérapeutiques ou dans les collectifs de soins psychiatriques" at the Congrès de l'Association Analytique Internationale, Madrid, September 1970]

— "A propósito del narcicismo en sus relaciones con la formación de la personalidad" (1970), *Clínica y análisis grupal*, vol. 9, no. 36, 1985, pp. 258–272.

1971

— "La problématique du pouvoir dans les collectifs du soins psychiatriques," *La Nef*, no. 42, "L'antipsychiatrie," January–May 1971, pp. 93–102.

— "Critique de la relation duelle dans l'entretien," *L'Information psychologique*, no. 41, 1971, pp. 29–37.

— "Discussion du rapport: Chaigneau H., Chanoit P., Garrabe J., 'Les thérapies institutionnelles,'" in Pierre Warot (ed.), *Comptes rendus du Congrès de psychiatrie et de neurologie de langue française: LXIX session, Caen, 5–10 juillet 1971; Comptes rendus*. Paris: Masson, 1971, pp. 1058–1062.

— "Prólogo," in Maud Mannoni, *El niño retrasado y su madre: Estudio psicoanalítico*. Madrid: Ediciones Fax, 1971.

1973

— "Désir et institution," *Recherches*, no. 11, "Journées d'études de psychothérapie institutionnelle (coloque de Waterloo)," January 1973, pp. 5–22.

— "À propos de la thérapie institutionnelle," *Connexions: Psychosociologie, psychanalyse et sciences humaines*, no. 6, 1973, pp. 9–33.

— "Lettre," *Connexions: Psychosociologie, psychanalyse et sciences humaines*, no. 6, 1973, pp. 133–136.

— "Maestro y amigo," *Revista de psiquiatría de la Facultad de Medicina de Barcelona*, vol. 1, no. 1, 1973, pp. 52–58.

1974

— "Variations polyphoniques autour de la notion de corps social (opérativité et incertitude de la notion du corps institutionnel dans la psychothérapie)," *Psychiatries*, no. 15, May–June 1974, pp. 25–32.

1975

Tosquelles, François; Bonnafé, Lucien; Daumézon, Georges; Oury, Jean. "La résistance: Saint-Alban," *Recherches*, no. 17, "Histoire de la psychiatrie de secteur ou le secteur imposible?," March 1975, pp. 80–95.

Tosquelles, François. "À propos de la réédition de la thèse de Jacques Lacan 'De la psychose paranoïaque et ses rapports avec la personnalité'. Une lettre de François Tosquelles" (June 11, 1975), *Psychiatries*, no. 21, May–June 1975, pp. 93–98.

— "La 'relation' avec l'arriéré profond," *Notre prochain (bulletin trimestriel des asiles John Bost)*, special issue "De l'arriéré au marginal: Accueillir—re-lier—soigner," May 1975, pp. 223–229. [Colloquium, September 20–22, 1974, La Force, Dordogne]

— "Frantz Fanon à Saint-Alban," *L'Information psychiatrique*, vol. 51, no. 10, 1975, pp. 223–229. ["Frantz Fanon en Saint-Alban," *Teoría y crítica de la psicología*, no. 9, 2017, pp. 223–229]

— "Conseils pratiques aux parents," *Réadaptation*, no. 218, 1975, pp. 43–49.

— "Le secteur," 1975. [Unpublished]

1976

— "Préface," in Jean Oury, *Psychiatrie et psychothérapie institutionnelle: Traces et configurations précaires* (1976). Nîmes: Champ Social, 2001, pp. 11–20.

— "Les coupures, les incohérences et la polyphonie dans les institutions pour psychotiques," in Armando Verdiglione (ed.), *Sexualité et pouvoir*. Paris: Payot, 1976, pp. 109–142.

— "Sémiotique et psychanalyse (à propos d'un rêve qui concerne la politique psychiatrique)." [Unpublished paper for the Congrés Politique et psychiatrie, Milan, December 1976]

1977

— *Récital de la chasse aux mots par un Catalan psyschiste devenu pipisiatre françois du cadre* (1977). Paris: Éditions d'une, 2016.

— "Dialogue intérieur sur l'équipe en psychothérapie institutionnelle," *Connexions: Psychosociologie, psychanalyse et sciences humaines*, no. 22, 1977, pp. 25–46.

1978

— "À l'heure de la retraite de Lucien Bonnafé," *L'Information psychiatrique*, no. 8, 1978, pp. 865–868.

— "Préface," in Jean-François Gómez, *Un Éducateur dans les murs: Témoignage sur un métier impossible*. Toulouse: Privat, 1978.

— *Introducción a las XI Jornadas sobre temas de interés psiquiátrico*. Reus: Institut Pere Mata, 1978.

— "A propòsit de les dificultats de la práctica i de l'ensenyament de la psiquiatria: Una orientació que ens ve de lluny; Arnau de Vilanova," *Annals de medicina*, 1978, pp. 1102–1119.

1979

— "Le rôle de l'ethnologie dans l'analyse de l'institution," *L'Évolution psychiatrique*, no. 2, 1979, pp. 337–346.

1980

— "In memoriam sur Georges Daumézon, quelques autres et moi," *L'Information psychiatrique*, no. 5, 1980, pp. 557–588.

— "Institut Pere Mata: Symposium; Interviu al Dr. Tosquelles," *Reus: Semanario de la ciudad*, April 12, 1980, pp. 3–7 and 10.

— "Acting-Out." [Unpublished paper for the Congrès de psychothérapie de groupe, Paris, 1980]

1981

— "Quelques notes encore sur l'hystérie et la simulation ou sur l'homme et la simulation (la psychiatrie, le psychiatre et l'hystérique)," published with the title "Hystérie et simulation," *Spirales: Jounal international de culture*, no 12, February 1982, p. 59. [Conferència per al IV Congrès International de Psychanalyse, "Le Semblant," Milan, January 28–31, 1981]

— "En hommage à André Chaurand," *L'Information psychiatrique*, no. 3, 1981, pp. 401–403.

— "Encore quelques précisions sur la psychothérapie institutionnelle," *Soins psychiatrie*, no. 9, May 1981, pp. 8–20. ["Algunas precisiones sobre la psicoterapia institucional," *Clínica y análisis grupal*, vol. 33–34, 1983]

— "Introduction psychiatrique au débat sur la vie après cinquante ans." [Unpublished paper for the III Rencontres d'été, Biarritz, August 24–26, 1981]

— "À propos de la relation et sa durée dans le domaine de la psychiatrique," *Rencontre: Cahiers du travailleur social*, no. 38, 1981, pp. 13–18.

— "'Le père': Discussion du rapport de M. Patris; 'La fonction paternelle en psychopathologie,'" in Pierre Sizaret (ed.), *Comptes rendues du Congrès de psychiatrie et de neurologie de langue française, LXXIX session, Colmar 28 juin–4 juillet 1981*. Paris: Masson, 1981, pp. 80–88. ["El padre," *Clínica y análisis grupal*, no. 43, 1987, pp. 49–58]

1982

— "Repères d'une pratique de psychothérapie des psychoses infantiles," *Revue internationale de l'enfant*, 1982, pp. 19–33.

— *Seminario sobre los mitos*. Reus: Institut Pere Mata, 1982.

— "Entretiens de Granges," *L'Interdit*, no. 8, 1982, pp. 19–33.

Tosquelles, François; Bassols, Miquel; Calvet, Rosa. "Entrevista a François Tosquelles," *Otium Diagonal*, no. 4–5, 1982, pp. 14–22.

1983

Tosquelles, François; Gárate, Ignacio. "Media hora con ... François Tosquelles," *Clínica y análisis grupal*, no. 33, 1983, pp. 342–354.

Tosquelles, François. "François Tosquelles par lui-même," *L'Âne*, no. 13, 1983, pp. 3–5.

— *Resumen de las conversaciones psiquiátricas del Dr. Tosquelles en el grupo de Reus, a propósito de los grupos familiares de los enfermos*. Reus: Institut Pere Mata, 1983.

— "Réflexions sur le mouvement 'désaliéniste' de la psychothérapie institutionnelle et 'des espaces thérapeuthiques' saisi dans la perspective 'psychanalytique,'" *L'Information psychiatrique*, no. 3, 1983, pp. 425–436.

— *Introducción a las XVI Jornadas sobre Temas de Interés Psiquiátrico, organizadas por el Instituto Pedro Mata, de Reus: Días 28, 29 y 30 de marzo de 1983*. Reus: Institut Pere Mata, 1983.

1984

— "A propósito de los modelos de asistencia en Psiquiatría," *Folia neuropsiquiátrica: Revista de psicología, psiquiatría y ciencias afines*, vol. 19, no. 3, 1984, pp. 253–262.

— "Yves Racine (1928–1983)," *L'Information psychiatrique*, no. 1, 1984, pp. 91–94.

— "Tosquelles: Conjunció d'una 'boja' ironía i el no dogmatisme," *Reus: Setmanari de la ciutat*, May 19, 1984, pp. 8–9.

Tosquelles, François; Barnet, Alex. "François Tosquelles: El psiquiatra que llevó a Freud y Marx al manicomio," *Primera plana*, 1984, pp. 16–23.

1985

Tosquelles, François. "Postface," in René Laffite, *Une journée dans une classe coopérative: Le désir retrouvé* (1985). Vigneux: Matrice, 1997.

— *Funció poètica i psicoteràpia: Una lectura de "In memoriam" de Gabriel Ferrater*. Reus: Institut Pere Mata and Centre de Lectura de Reus, 1985; new revised edition, Barcelona: Arcàdia, 2022; *Función poética y psicoterapia*. Barcelona: Octaedro, 2014.

— "La relación terapèutica," *Folia neuropsiquiátrica*, vol. 20, no. 1, 1985, pp. 65–68.

— "Le travail en équipe," *Les nouvelles du CREAI Midi-Pyrénées*, no. 3, 1985, pp. 23–33. [Text written for the XVII Jornades d'Interès Psiquiàtric, Institut Pere Mata, Reus, April 1–3, 1985]

— "Biographie d'un psychiste," *Traces de faires*, no. 1, 1985, pp. 29–31.

Tosquelles, François; Oury, Jean; Guattari, Félix. *Pratique de l'institutionnel et politique*. Vigneux: Matrice, 1985.

Tosquelles, Francesc; Vilà, Francesc. "Entrevista amb Francesc Tosquelles," *L'Acudit: Publicació de psicoanàlisi*, no. 1, October 1985, pp. 38–45.

1986

Tosquelles, Francesc. "L'autisme." [Unpublished notes for a lecture given at the Alba school, Reus, May 1986]

— "Communication écrite du docteur François Tosquelles," in *Rencontres de Saint-Alban, juin 1986: La psychothérapie institutionnelle*. Saint-Alban-sur-Limagnole: Centre hospitalier François Tosquelles, 1986, pp. 46–52.

— "Les idées en matière de psychiatrie institutionnelle," in *Rencontres de Saint-Alban, juin 1986: La psychothérapie institutionnelle*. Saint-Alban-sur-Limagnole: Centre hospitalier François Tosquelles, 1986, pp. 54–59.

— "Els sentiments, 29 d'abril de 1986," in Josep M. Sánchez Ripollès (ed.), *Algunes conferències inèdites del Doctor François Tosquelles i Llauradó (1912–1994): Escrits periodístics del Doctor Leandre Cervera (1891–1964)*. Tarragona: Universitat Rovira i Virgili, 2000, pp. 44–45.

— "Sessió del 30 d'abril de 1986," in Josep M. Sánchez Ripollès (ed.), *Algunes conferències inèdites del Doctor François Tosquelles i Llauradó (1912–1994): Escrits periodístics del Doctor Leandre Cervera (1891–1964)*. Tarragona: Universitat Rovira i Virgili, 2000, pp. 45–46.

— "Sessió sobre psiquiatria infantil, 5 de maig de 1986," in Josep M. Sánchez Ripollès (ed.), *Algunes conferències inèdites del Doctor François Tosquelles i Llauradó (1912–1994): Escrits periodístics del Doctor Leandre Cervera (1891–1964)*. Tarragona: Universitat Rovira i Virgili, 2000, pp. 27–28.

— "El club, 26 de juny de 1986," in Josep M. Sánchez Ripollès (ed.), *Algunes conferències inèdites del Doctor François Tosquelles i Llauradó (1912–1994): Escrits periodístics del Doctor Leandre Cervera (1891–1964)*. Tarragona: Universitat Rovira i Virgili, 2000, pp. 38–40.

— "Malalts crònics, 6 d'octubre de 1986," in Josep M. Sánchez Ripollès (ed.), *Algunes conferències inèdites del Doctor François Tosquelles i Llauradó (1912–1994): Escrits periodístics del Doctor Leandre Cervera (1891–1964)*. Tarragona: Universitat Rovira i Virgili, 2000, pp. 40–42.

— "Informació obtinguda a través de cassets, 17 de desembre de 1986," in Josep M. Sánchez Ripollès (ed.), *Algunes conferències inèdites del Doctor François Tosquelles i Llauradó (1912–1994): Escrits periodístics del Doctor Leandre Cervera (1891–1964)*. Tarragona: Universitat Rovira i Virgili, 2000, pp. 42–43.

— "Fer un club, 18 de desembre de 1986," in Josep M. Sánchez Ripollès (ed.), *Algunes conferències inèdites del Doctor François Tosquelles i Llauradó (1912–1994): Escrits periodístics del Doctor Leandre Cervera (1891–1964)*. Tarragona: Universitat Rovira i Virgili, 2000, pp. 27–28.

— "El sermó de la muntanya, 19 de desembre de 1986," in Josep M. Sánchez Ripollès (ed.), *Algunes conferències inèdites del Doctor François Tosquelles i Llauradó (1912–1994): Escrits periodístics del Doctor Leandre Cervera (1891–1964)*. Tarragona: Universitat Rovira i Virgili, 2000, pp. 17–21.

1987

— "Transferts et transports," in *Rencontres de Saint-Alban, juin 1987: L'hôpital, le secteur; Transferts et déplacements*. Saint-Alban-sur-Limagnole: Centre hospitalier François Tosquelles, 1987, pp. 114–125.

Tosquelles, François; Guire, Jean; Hamsy, Cécile. "François Tosquelles à France Culture (le 4 novembre 1985)," *L'Interdit*, no. 14, 1987, pp. 54–61.

Tosquelles, Francesc. "Mode d'elaboració i de recollida dels 'trets d'esperit' en la pràctica analítica i en la vida de tots els homes," in *Història de la psicoanàlisi als països catalans*. Perpignan: GAIRPS, 1987, pp. 11–14.

— "L'effervescence sainte-albanaise," *L'Information psychiatrique*, no. 8, 1987, pp. 957–964.

Tosquelles, François; Ellul, Jacques. *La Genèse aujourd'hui*. Le Cellier: Éditions de l'AREFPPI, 1987.

Tosquelles, François; Picard, François. "La guerre d'Espagne," *Vie sociale et traitements*, no. 172, August–September 1987, pp. 35–38.

Tosquelles, François; Gallio, Giovanna; Costantino, Maurizio. "L'École de la liberté," *Per la salute mentale, pratiche, ricerche, culture dell'innovazione*, August 1987, pp. 73–100.

Tosquelles, François. "À propos du moi et de la place de la mouvance sensorimotrice dans le corps vécu et dans les actes d'un chacun," *Les Nouvelles du CREAI Midi-Pyrénées*, no. 4, December 1987, pp. 957–964.

— "Défenses et transferts dans la psychose," in *Journées de Psychothérapie Institutionnelle: Le transfert dans l'institution*, Marseille, November 1987, pp. 15–28.

— "Contribution de la théorie et de la pratique de la psychothérapie institutionnelle à la praxie de la psychiatrie de secteur," *Anais portugueses de saude mental*, no. 3, 1987, pp. 193–195.

— "Reunió amb psiquiatres i psicòlegs, 6 d'abril de 1987," in Josep M. Sánchez Ripollès (ed.), *Algunes conferències inèdites del Doctor François Tosquelles i Llauradó (1912–1994): Escrits periodístics del Doctor Leandre Cervera (1891–1964).* Tarragona: Universitat Rovira i Virgili, 2000, pp. 28–32.

— "Sessió sobre formació, 26 de juny de 1987," in Josep M. Sánchez Ripollès (ed.), *Algunes conferències inèdites del Doctor François Tosquelles i Llauradó (1912–1994): Escrits periodístics del Doctor Leandre Cervera (1891–1964).* Tarragona: Universitat Rovira i Virgili, 2000, pp. 32–34.

— "Seminari per a metges i psicòlegs, 14 de desembre de 1987," in Josep M. Sánchez Ripollès (ed.), *Algunes conferències inèdites del Doctor François Tosquelles i Llauradó (1912–1994): Escrits periodístics del Doctor Leandre Cervera (1891–1964).* Tarragona: Universitat Rovira i Virgili, 2000, pp. 35–38.

— "Què dir? Com dir-ho?, 18 de desembre de 1987," in Josep M. Sánchez Ripollès (ed.), *Algunes conferències inèdites del Doctor François Tosquelles i Llauradó (1912–1994): Escrits periodístics del Doctor Leandre Cervera (1891–1964).* Tarragona: Universitat Rovira i Virgili, 2000, pp. 21–25.

1988

— "L'approche des familles de psychotiques en institution," in *Rencontres de Saint-Alban, juin 1988: La prise en compte des familles de psychotiques et son incidence sur la psychothérapie.* Saint-Alban-sur-Limagnole: Centre hospitalier François Tosquelles, 1988, pp. 296–312.

— "Tosquelles, la psiquiatria com a coneixement," *Revista del Centre de Lectura de Reus,* 1988, p. 4.

— "Ouvertures, priorité et continuité de la perspective psychothérapeutique, dans la délimitation des espaces interhumains organisés pour les diverses tâches psychiatriques," *Communication information (bulletin interne du centre de guidance infantile de Toulouse),* no. 13, November 1988, pp. 1–23.

— "Itinéraires," in *II Journées de psychothérapie institutionnelle,* Marseille, November 25–26, 1988, pp. 130–142.

— "Complexités et métamorphoses des processus psychopathologiques indéfinis: Les pratiques psychiatriques aux prises avec la dimension vagabonde des cheminements humains et avec les retenus instituées." [Unpublished paper for the XVIII Journées Nationales de l'AFPEP, "Le psychiatre, le malade, l'état," Hyères, October 23, 1988]

1989

— "Variations autour du banal et de l'extraordinaire dans la vie quotidienne," in *Rencontres de Saint-Alban, juin 1989: Les effets thérapeutiques des différents actes de la vie quotidienne en institution.* Saint-Alban-sur-Limagnole: Centre hospitalier François Tosquelles, 1989, pp. 201–224.

1990

— *Actualitat de Freud.* Reus: Centre de Lectura, 1990. [Sound recording]

— "La mouvance des groupes dans les espaces institutionnelles," *Empan,* no. 2, 1990, pp. 11–14.

— "Le travail des jours qui passent," in Michel Minard (ed.), *Une psychiatrie en travail.* Sainte-Agne: Éditions Érès, 1990.

— "Intervention," in *IV Journées de psychothérapie institutionnelle: Soins et institution; Vous avez dit psychothérapie,* Marseille, November 30–December 1, 1990, pp. 91–108.

— "Discussion des rapports d'atelier," "Clôture," "Discussion générale," in *Rencontres de Saint-Alban, juin 1990: Où va l'équipe pluridisciplinaire? Intérêts, fonctionnements, éthique.* Saint-Alban-sur-Limagnole: Centre hospitalier François Tosquelles, 1990, pp. 51–59, 65–71, and 71–75.

1991

— "Frantz Fanon et la psychothérapie institutionnelle" (1991), *Sud/Nord,* no. 1, 2007, pp. 71–78. ["Frantz Fanon y la psicoterapia institucional," *Teoría y crítica de la psicologia,* no. 9, 2017, pp. 230–238]

— "Une politique de la folie," *Chimères,* no. 13, 1991, pp. 66–81.

— "Les médiations," *Empan,* no. 4, 1991, pp. 22–26.

— "Naissance et constitution des équipes soignantes," in *Rencontres de Saint-Alban, juin 1991: L'équipe pluridisciplinaire; Pratique et praxis.* Saint-Alban-sur-Limagnole: Centre hospitalier François Tosquelles, 1991, pp. 107–159.

— "Intervention," in *V Journées de psychothérapie institutionnelle: La psychothérapie dans la cité ... Etayage social et/ou approche thérapeutique?,* Marseille, November 15–16, 1991, pp. 125–132.

— "Y'en aura pour tout le monde ... !," in Jiho (ed.), *Petit dictionnaire du social II.* Paris: Éditions Lien Social, 1991.

1992

— *L'Enseignement de la folie* (1992). Paris: Dunod, 2014. [*Las enseñanzas de la locura.* Madrid: Alianza, 2001]

Tosquelles, François; Angosto, Tiburcio. "Entrevista al Dr. Francisco Tosquelles," *Revista Asociación Española Neuropsiquiatría*, vol. 13, no. 46, December 15, 1992, pp. 203–210.

Tosquelles, François. "Xénophobie et psychiatrie" (1992), *Institutions: Revue de psychothérapie institutionnelle*, no. 31, "François Tosquelles: Histoire et transmission," October 2002. ["Xenofobia y psiquiatría," *Topía*, April 2003]

— "De l'histoire et des histoires dans les pratiques psychiatriques," in Michel Minard (dir.), *Histoire et histoires en psychiatrie*. Toulouse: Éditions Érès, 1992, pp. 47–66.

— "Pratiques psychodramatiques et psychiatrie," *Empan*, 1992, pp. 105–109. [Monograph for the VII Jornadas de la Asociación Española de Psicodrama]

— "La santé entre le mutisme insignifiant et le bavardage," *Empan*, no. 7, 1992, pp. 37–46.

— "Mémoire de Félix Guattari," *Lien Social*, no, 181, September 17, 1992, pp. 6–7.

— "Lettre du Docteur François Tosquelles à Pierre Delion" (1992), in Pierre Delion (dir.), *Prendre un enfant autiste par la main*. Paris: Dunod, 2011, pp. 181–192.

— "Intervention," in *VI Journées de psychothérapie institutionnelle: Culture, création et souffrance dans l'existence psychotique*, Marseille, November 27–28, 1992, pp. 189–197.

— "Lleis, violència, fanstames, ètica i moral," in *XXV Jornades d'Interès Psiquiàtric: "Transparència i canvi: Opacitats biosociològiques i processos de canvi en psiquiatria."* Reus: Institut Pere Mata, 1992, pp. 77–130.

— "Penser l'homme et la folie," in *Rencontres de Saint-Alban, juin 1992: Peut-on encore soigner les psychotiques en 1992? Où? Quand? Comment?* Saint-Alban-sur-Limagnole: Centre hospitalier François Tosquelles, 1992, pp. 57–88.

— *Rencontres avec François Tosquelles*. Reus: Institut Pere Mata, 1992.

1993

— "Intervention," in *VII Journées de psychothérapie institutionnelle: Les institutions à l'épreuve du temps*. Marseille, November 19–20, 1993, pp. 38–47.

— "Introducció" and "Comentaris sobre les diferents exposicions," in *XXVI Jornades d'Interès Psiquiàtric: "Emergències de les crisis vitals humanes: Urgències en el seu tractament social, mèdic i psiquiàtric."* Reus: Institut Pere Mata, 1993, pp. 7–9 and 171–178.

1994

— "Actualité de la psychothérapie institutionnelle," in Pierre Delion (ed.), *Actualité de la psychothérapie institutionnelle*. Vigneux: Matrice, 1994, pp. 418–426.

POSTHUMOUS PUBLICATIONS

— "Constellation du verbe," *Sud/Nord*, no. 2, 2001, pp. 37–42.

— *De la personne au groupe: À propos des équipes de soins* (1995). Toulouse: Éditions Érès, 2011.

Tosquelles, François; Tosquellas, Jacques (ed.). *Archives complètes: Chantier I, Sardanes—1928 à 1943*. Cour-Cheverny: Institutions, 2014.

— *Archives complètes: Chantier II, Toros—1943 à 1944*. Cour-Cheverny: Institutions, 2015.

Tosquelles, François. *Trait-d'union, Journal de Saint-Alban (1950–1962)*. Paris: Éditions d'une, 2015.

— *Cours aux infirmiers de Saint-Alban (1943–1945)*. Paris: Éditions d'une, 2018.

— *Psychopathologie et matérialisme dialectique, Conférence à l'École normale supérieure (1947)*. Paris: Éditions d'une, 2019.

FILMOGRAPHY

Film Tosquelles, or *Société lozérienne d'hygiène mentale*, 1958, 40 min.

La nostra sardana, 1964, 110 min.

Le Clos du Nid: Un service pour débiles profonds en Lozère, 41 min., with Maurice Lambilliotte.

Noël de chez nous, 24 min.

En Lozère, 57 min.

Que le blé ne meurt pas, 33 min.

Souvenirs … Souvenirs …, 19 min.

FURTHER READING ON FRANCESC TOSQUELLES

Agay, Cécile. "J'ai visité des femmes enfermées dans leur propre univers," *Les Étoiles*, October 9, 1945, p. 3.

Andreu Domingo, Mariona. "Tosquelles i l'educació a Reus," *Revista del Centre de Lectura de Reus*, 2022, no pagination.

Andreu Domingo, Mariona; Just Masdeu, Rosa. "Entrevista a José García Ibáñez, deixeble de Tosquelles," *Revista del Centre de Lectura de Reus*, 2022, no pagination.

Anguera, Pere. *Menjacapellans, conservadors i revolucionaris*. Reus: Edicions del Centre de Lectura, 1991.

Anguera, Pere; Arnavat, Albert. *A bodes em convides: Estudis d'història social*. Reus: Edicions del Centre de Lectura, 1987.

Anguera Domenjó, Blanca. "La influencia de F. Tosquelles Llauradó (1912–1994) en la institución psiquiátrica francesa," *Revista de historia de la psicología*, vol. 20, no. 3–4, 1999, pp. 397–404.

Aprill, Olivier. *Une avant-garde psychiatrique: Le moment GTPSI (1960–1966)*. Paris: Epel, 2013.

Arveiller, Jean-Paul. "De la rencontre au soin: En hommage à François Tosquelles," *Revue pratique de psychologie de la vie sociale et d'hygiène mentale*, no. 4, 1994, p. 1.

Arveiller, Jacques. "Mon Maître Tosquelles," *L'Évolution psychiatrique*, vol. 60, no. 3, 1995, pp. 665–668.

Aymé, Jean. "Hommage à François Tosquelles," *L'Information psychiatrique*, vol. 700, no. 10, December 1994, pp. 883–901.

Bach Voltas, Cori. "El Dr. Francesc Tosquelles i l'Escola Montsant," *Revista del Centre de Lectura de Reus*, 2022, no pagination.

Bacilio, María E. "Francesc Tosquelles: Guerra y psiquiatría subversiva," *Nexos*, December 20, 2017.

Bakker, Kees. "*Regards sur la folie*: Approches documentaires," *CinémAction*, no. 159, 2016, pp. 156–164.

Balvet, Paul. "L'ambre du musée," *L'Information psychiatrique*, October 1978, pp. 861–864.

Barthes, Roland. "Les Inconnus de la terre," press release for *Les Inconnus de la terre: Une enquête cinématographique*, by Mario Ruspoli. Paris: Argos Films, 1962.

Bassols, Miquel. "Francesc Tosquelles llegeix Gabriel Ferrater, amb Jacques Lacan," *Revista del Centre de Lectura de Reus*, 2022, no pagination.

— "Francesc Tosquelles o la psicoanàlisi a l'inrevés," *Intercambios, papeles de psicoanálisis/Intercanvis, papers de psicoanàlisi*, no. 50, 2023, pp. 81–86.

Battaiellie, Katherine L. *La robe de mariée*. Angulema: Éditions Marguerite Waknine, 2015.

Bazin, Hervé. *La Fin des asiles*. Paris: Grasset, 1959.

— "Le tour d'Europe de la folie," *France-Soir*, April 25, 1959.

Bellet, Henry. "Gérard Vulliamy dans la maison des fous," *Le Monde*, March 17, 2012.

Bellour, Raymond. "Ruspoli au pays des hommes," *Cinéma 63*, no. 76, 1963, pp. 25–27.

Ben Faour, K. "Georges Canguilhem, entre folie et résistance," *Les Chemins de l'art brut à Saint-Alban-sur-Limagnole*. Villeneuve-d'Asq: Lille Métropole Musée d'art moderne, d'art contemporain et d'art brut, 2007, pp. 27–31.

Berti, Gabriela (coord.). *Félix Guattari: Los ecos del pensar entre filosofía, arte y clínica*. Barcelona: Hakabooks.com, 2012.

Berti, Gabriela; Guerra, Carles (*et al.*). *Jornada dedicada a Francesc Tosquelles*. Barcelona: Museu d'Art Contemporani de Barcelona, 2012.

Berton, Mireille. "*Regard sur la folie*: Poétique et politique de la folie et du cinéma," *Décadrages: Cinéma, à travers champs*, no. 18, 2011, pp. 47–68.

Bonnafé, Lucien (*et al.*). *Paul Éluard*. Paris: Éditeurs français réunis, 1972.

Bonnafé, Lucien. *Désaliéner? Folie et Société*. Toulouse: Presses Universitaires du Mirail, 1991.

— "Des cultures originales avec André Chaurand et François Tosquelles," *Empan*, 1992, pp. 19–22.

— "De la Résistance aux Ixocratismes." [Unpublished]

— "Rencontres autour de François Tosquelles," *L'Évolution psychiatrique*, vol. 60, no. 3, 1995.

— "Lettres adressées par Lucien Bonnafé à Paul Bernard," *L'Information psychiatrique*, vol. 79, no. 7, September 2003, pp. 621–626.

Bonnafé, Lucien; Daumézon, Georges. "Perspectives de réforme psychiatrique en France depuis la Libération," in *Comptes rendus de la XLVI session du Congrès des médecins aliénistes et neurologistes de*

France et des pays de langue française. Paris: Masson, 1947, pp. 584–590.

Boulanger, Christophe. *Mots et motifs dans l'œuvre d'Aimable Jayet.* Villeneuve-d'Ascq: École doctorale sciences de l'homme et de la société, 2016. [Doctoral thesis]

Bovier, François. "Regards sur l''impouvoir': Le 'cinéma direct' de Ruspoli, de la terre à l'asile," *Décadrages: Cinéma, à travers champs,* no. 18, 2011, pp. 14–31.

Bruit, Guy; Gauthier-Darley, Michel; Bonnafé, Lucien. "Surréalisme et psychiatrie: La solitude des résistants de fond; Entretien avec Lucien Bonnafé," *Raison présente,* no. 120, 1996, pp. 25–56.

Buqueras i Bach, Francesc Xavier. "Breu semblança del Dr. Francesc Tosquelles i Llauradó (1912–1994)," *Gimbernat: Revista catalana d'història de la medicina i de la ciència,* no. 24, 1995, pp. 79–83.

Cabañas, Kaira M. *Learning from Madness: Brazilian Modernism and Global Contemporary Art.* Chicago: University of Chicago Press, 2019.

Campos i Avillar, Joan. *Del somni d'Irma al somni de Mira: Somnis professionals?* Barcelona: Plexus, 1991.

— "Recuerdos, olvidos y reminiscencias o la SEPTG y 'sus viejas historias,'" *Caleidoscopio histórico de la SEPTG,* 1998.

Canfora, Rosanna. *Patient sujet dans l'institution: Observation et comparaison franco-italiennes; Pratiques de le rencontre anti-institutionnelle entre Basaglia et Tosquelles.* Paris: Université Sorbonne Paris Cité, 2018. [Doctoral thesis]

Canguilhem, Georges. "Ouverture," in Élisabeth Roudinesco (ed.), *Penser la folie: Essais sur Michel Foucault.* Paris: Galilée, 1992, pp. 39–42.

— "Observation à l'hôpital psychiatrique de Saint-Alban (Lozère) (juillet 1944, maquis), M. C. Observation proposée et contrôlée par le Docteur Tosquelles," in Camille Limoges (ed.), *Œuvres complètes: Résistance, philosophie biologique et histoire des sciences (1940–1965),* vol. IV. Paris: Librairie philosophique J. Vrin, 2015, pp. 183–189.

— "Entretien de Georges Canguilhem avec François Bing et Jean-François Braunstein," in Camille Limoges (ed.), *Œuvres complètes: Histoire des sciences, épistémologie, commémorations (1966–1995),* vol. V. Paris: Librairie philosophique J. Vrin, 2018, p. 1283.

Casals, Josep. *Constelación de pasaje: Imagen, experiencia, locura.* Barcelona: Anagrama, 2015.

Castera, Isabelle. "François Tosquelles, psychiatre: Un traducteur de la folie," *Sud-Ouest Dimanche,* August 30, 1992, p. 12.

Cervello, Sophie. "Analyse de film," *L'Information psychiatrique,* vol. 94, no. 4, 2018, p. 317.

Chemla, Patrick. *Le Collectif à venir: Psychiatrie, psychanalyse, psychothérapie institutionnelle.* Toulouse: Éditions Érès, 2018.

Cherki, Alice. *Frantz Fanon, portrait.* Paris: Seuil, 2000.

Chevalier-Fougas, Solène. *Mise en perspective de deux conceptions du soin psychiatrique adulte: La psychothérapie institutionnelle et la réhabilitation psycho-sociale.* Angers: Université d'Angers, faculté de médecine, 2009. [Doctoral thesis]

Clot, Yves. "L'apport de François Tosquelles à la clinique du travail," epilogue to *Travail thérapeutique en psychiatrie.* Toulouse: Éditions Érès, 2009, pp. 143–162.

Coll, Josep; Pané, Josep. *Josep Rovira: Una vida al servei de Catalunya i el socialisme.* Barcelona: Ariel, 1978.

Comelles, Josep Maria. "Catalanisme, salut mental i avantguarda: Les polítiques públiques de salut a Catalunya (1883–1938)," in Montserrat Duch Plana (ed.) *La II República espanyola: Perspectives interdisciplinàries en el seu 75è aniversari.* Tarragona: Publicacions Universitat Rovira i Virgili, 2008, pp. 51–84.

— "Forgotten Paths: Culture and Ethnicity in Catalan Mental Health Policies (1900–1939)," *History of Psychiatry,* vol. 21, no. 4, 2010, pp. 406–423.

Daeninckx, Didier. *Caché dans la maison des fous.* Paris: Gallimard, 2017.

Danchin, Laurent. "Art singulier, art brut, art psychopathologique: Quelques réflexions sur la collection du Dr. Ferdière," in *Psychanalyse, psychiatrie et art-thérapie.* Paris: ATEPP-CEFAT, 1991.

Danchin, Laurent; Roumieux, André. *Artaud et l'asile.* Paris: Séguier, 2015.

Daumézon, Georges; Koechlin, Philippe. "La psychothérapie institutionnelle française contemporaine," *Anais portugueses de psiquiatria,* vol. 4, no. 4, December 1962.

— "Les aliénés pendant la guerre," *Le malade mental: Qu'en avons-nous fait? Présences: Revue trimestrielle du monde des malades,* no. 54, 1956, pp. 65–66

de Kerangal, Maylis; Sorman, Joy. "Saint-Alban, dernière frontière," *Analyse, opinión, critique (AOC),* May 19, 2019.

de la Bretèque, François Amy. "Martin de la Soudière, *Sur les traces de Mario Ruspoli*, En Lozère: Retour sur *Les inconnu de la terre,"* 1895, no. 73, 2014, pp. 222–224.

Delclòs, Isabel Baixeras. "Tosquelles, anada i tornada," *Intercambios, papeles de psicoanàlisis / Intercanvis, papers de psicoanàlisi*, no. 49, 2022, pp. 95–104.

Delion, Pierre. "François Tosquelles ou l'art d'être grand-père," *Empan*, 1992, pp. 35–40.

— "La mort du docteur François Tosquelles: Un pionnier de la psychiatrie institutionnelle," *Le Monde*, October 1, 1994, p. 12.

— "Hommage a François Tosquelles," *L'Information psychiatrique*, no. 10, December 1994.

— "Le moment Tosquelles," *Perspective psy*, vol. 59, no. 1, 2000, pp. 5–9.

— "Contrepoint sur la naissance de la psychiatrie de secteur: Dialogue; Tosquelles et Bonnafé," *Institutions: Revue de la psychothérapie institutionnelle*, no. 31, "François Tosquelles: Histoire et transmission," 2001.

— "L'enseignement de Tosquelles," *Séminaire sur l'autisme et la psychose infantile*. Toulouse: Éditions Érès, 2009, pp. 27–48.

— "François Tosquelles et la décence ordinaire," *Vie sociale et traitements*, no. 2, 2014, pp. 105–108.

— "Tosquelles et Oury, parce que c'était eux ...," *Chimères*, no. 3, 2014, pp. 20–28.

— *La constellation transférentielle*. Toulouse: Érès, 2022.

Desviat, M. "Francesc Tosquelles, política y psiquiatría," *Revista de la Asociación Española de Neuropsiquiatría*, vol. 42, no. 141, pp. 285–292.

Dhainaut, Pierre. "Visages de la folie: Paul Éluard à Saint-Alban," in Mireille Gauzy (*et al.*) (eds.), *L'Invention du lieu: Résistances et création en Gévaudan*. Villeneuve-d'Asq: Lille Métropole Musée d'art moderne, d'art contemporain et d'art brut, 2014.

Didelet, Serge; Oury, Jean. *Celui qui faisait sourire les schizophrènes*. Paris: Champ social, 2017.

Domic, Zorka. "Francesc Tosquelles y la revolución de cada día," *Sansueña*, no. 1, 2019, pp. 145–147.

Dosse, François. *Gilles Deleuze et Félix Guattari: Biographie croisée*. Paris: La Découverte, 2009.

Dreyfus-Armand, Geneviève. *L'exil des républicains espagnols en France: De la guerre civile à la mort de Franco*. Paris: Albin Michel, 1999.

— "Survivre et résister dans les camps: Artistes, intellectuels et activités culturelles," in *Septfonds 1939–1944: Dans l'archipel des camps français*. Perpignan: Le Revenant éditeur, 2019, pp. 293–317.

Drigo Agostinho, Larissa. "Artaud: Desfazer e refazer-se corpo ou como sobreviver ao fim do mundo," *La Deleuziana: Revista online de filosofía*, 2019.

— "Guattari e a psicoterapia institucional," *Ágora: Estudos em Teoria Psicanalítica*, vol. 23, no. 1, 2020.

Dutrenit, Jean-Marc. *Sociologie, travail social et psychiatrie: Le berceau lozérien de la psychothérapie institutionnelle*. Paris: Études vivantes, 1981.

Éluard, Paul. "Le génie sans miroir," *Les feuilles libres*, no. 35, January–February 1924, pp. 301–308.

— "Les sept poèmes d'amour en guerre," a *Œuvres complètes*, vol. 1. Paris: La Pléiade / Gallimard, 1943, pp. 1181–1187.

— *Souvenirs de la maison des fous* (1945). Paris: Seghers, 2011.

Fanon, Frantz; Azoluay, Jacques. "La socialthérapie dans un service d'hommes musulmans: Difficultés méthodologiques," *L'Information psychiatrique*, vol. 30, no. 9, October 1954, pp. 349–361.

Faramelli, Anthony. "The Decolonised Clinic: Fanon with Foucault," *London Journal of Critical Thought*, vol. 1, no. 2, 2017.

Faugeras, Patrick. *L'Ombre portée de François Tosquelles*. Toulouse: Éditions Érès, 2007.

Faugeras, Patrick; Minard, Michel. "Portrait d'un militant, François Tosquelles," *Sud/Nord*, no. 1, 2010, pp. 49–56.

Favereau, Eric; Artières, Phillipe. A series of five articles titled *Une aventure de fous*: "1940, quand le Dr Tosquelles arrive à Saint-Alban," "Quand le Dr Tosquelles combat la faim à Saint-Alban," "Quand le Dr Tosquelles rencontre Éluard à Saint-Alban," "Quand le Dr Tosquelles fonde la Société du Gévaudan," "Quand Saint-Alban pleure le Dr Tosquelles," *Libération*, August 3, 2016.

Fontanals Garcia, David. "Writing in the Apocalypse: The Mental and Experiental Framework of the End of the World," *From the World of Yesterday to the Europe of Tomorrow: On Commitment, Ethics, and Europe in the Works of Stefan Zweig*. Barcelona: Universitat de Barcelona, 2020. [Doctoral thesis]

Forcer, Stephen; Wagstaff, Emma. "Dedication and Friendship in Two Livres d'Artistes: *Parler seul* (Tzara-Miró, 1948–1950) and *Vivantes Cendres, Innommées* (Leiris-Giacometti)," *Nottingham French Studies*, vol. 50, no. 3, 2011, pp. 103–116.

Fortineau, Jacques; Lacour, Michel. "Commentaire sur le texte de François Tosquelles (1968)," *Perspectives psy*, vol. 52, no. 1, 2013, pp. 15–16.

Frey, Nicole. "L'art de soigner de Francesc Tosquelles, psychiatre, psychanalyste, homme de son temps," *Le Coq-héron*, vol. 249, no. 2, 2022, pp. 147–154.

Gaignard, Lise; Molinier, Pascale. "Le travail inestimable," *Travailler*, no. 19, 2008, pp. 9–13.

GAIRPS (ed.). *Història de la psicoanàlisi als Països Catalans*. Perpignan: GAIRPS, 1986.

Gárate Martínez, Ignacio. *Conversations psychanalytiques avec Xavier Audouard, Michel de Certeau, Joël Dor, Maud Mannoni, Octave Mannoni, Ginette Michaud, Francesc Tosquelles*. Paris: Hermann, 2008.

García, German L. "Francesc Tosquelles també lector de Jacques Lacan," *L'Acudit: Publicació de psicoanàlisi*, no. 1, pp. 5–7.

García Ibáñez, José; Labad, Antonio. "Experiència viscuda de les produccions verbals polifòniques: El mètode dels 'cassettes' en la formació professional de l'Institut Pere Mata," in *Història de la psicoanàlisi als Països Catalans*. Perpignan: GAIRPS, 1986, pp. 87–88.

— "Tosquelles i Catalunya," *Nous Horitzons*, no. 137, 1995, pp. 24–28.

García Siso, Andrés. "El Dr. Francesc Tosquelles i Llauradó: Posición del autor dentro de la psiquiatría catalana anterior a la Guerra Civil y la proyección de esta posición en su obra posterior," *Revista de la Asociación Española de Neuropsiquiatría*, no. 13, 1993, pp. 195–202.

Gauchet, Marcel; Swain, Gladys. *La pratique de l'esprit humain: L'institution asilaire et la révolution démocratique*. Paris: Gallimard, 1980.

Gauzy, Louis. "Cinéma et télévision dans l'hôpital psychiatrique," *Bulletin technique du personnel soignant: Hôpital pyschiatrique de Saint-Alban*, August 1958, pp. 30–32.

Gauzy, Mireille. "L'effervescence saint-albanaise," in *Trait d'union: Les chemins de l'art brut à Saint-Alban-sur-Limagnole*. Villeneuve-d'Asq: Lille Métropole Musée d'art moderne, d'art contemporain et d'art brut, 2007, pp. 13–25.

Gauzy, Mireille (*et al.*) (ed.). *L'Invention du lieu—Résistance et création en Guévaudan* (LaM, October 2, 2014–January 11, 2015). Villeneuve-d'Asq: Lille Métropole Musée d'art moderne, d'art contemporain et d'art brut, 2014.

Gaztambide, Daniel José. "'The Possibility of Love': Black Psychoanalysis from Harlem to Algeria," in *A People's History of Psychoanalysis: From Freud to Liberation Psychology*. New York: Lexington Books, 2019, pp. 89–118.

Gence, Maria-Jose; Pineau, Jacques. "Bibliographie indicative d'articles de François Tosquelles," *Empan*, 1992, pp. 19–22.

Gendzier, Irene. *Frantz Fanon: Un estudio crítico*. Mexico City: Serie Popular Era, 1977.

Gentis, Roger. *Les Murs de l'asile*. Paris: François Maspero, 1972.

— "La valeur humaine de la folie," *L'Interdit*, no. 14, June–August 1987, pp. 195–197.

Geroulanos, Stefanos. "Beyond the Normal and the Pathological: Recent Literature on Georges Canguilhem," *Gesnerus*, vol. 66, no. 2, pp. 288–306.

Giménez, Jena; Dizol, Jean-Marie; Forestier, Jean-Claude. "Entretien filmé du Docteur François Tosquelles, réalisé a Reus (Catalogne) à l'occasion du cinquantenaire de Saint-Simon," *Empan*, 1993, pp. 23–29.

Goldstein, Jan Ellen. *Console and Classify: The French Psychiatric Profession in the Nineteenth Century*. New York: Cambridge University Press, 1987.

Gomez, Jean-François. "Traces vivantes de Tosquelles et de quelques autres," *Vie sociale et traitements*, no. 1, 2010, pp. 123–128.

Gómez, Fernando Vicente. "Sobre Tosquelles y sus valores," *Intercambios, papeles de psicoanálisis / Intercanvis, papers de psicoanálisi*, no. 50, 2023, pp. 69–73.

Graff, Séverine. "Mario Ruspoli: Tournages en Lozère," in *Le Cinéma-vérité: Films et controverses*. Rennes: Presses universitaires de Rennes, 2014, pp. 165–188.

Gran Enciclopèdia Catalana. "Francesc Tosquelles i Llauradó," in *Gran Enciclopèdia Catalana*.

Guerra, Carles; Masó Joana (dirs.). *La déconniatrie: Art exil et psychiatrie autour de François Tosquelles*. Toulouse and Barcelona: les Abattoirs Musée—Frac Occitanie Toulouse and Arcàdia, 2021.

— *Tosquelles: Como una máquina de coser en un campo de trigo*. Madrid and Barcelona: Museo Nacional Centro de Arte Reina Sofía, Centre de Cultura Contemporània de Barcelona and Arcàdia, 2022.

Guerra, Carles; Masó, Joana; Rousseau, Valérie; Dioguardi, Edward; Sánchez Urdaneta, Margarita. *Francesc Tosquelles: Avant-Garde Psychiatry, Radical*

Politics, and Art. New York: American Folk Art Museum, 2024.

Harambourg, Lydia. *Gérard Vulliamy*. Paris: Éditions de la RMN-Gran Palais, 2011.

Harbi, Mohammed. "Fanon et le messianisme paysan," *Tumultes*, no. 31, 2008, pp. 11–15.

Henckes, Nicolas. *Le nouveau monde de la psychiatrie française: Les psychiatres, l'Etat et la réforme des hôpitaux psychiatriques de l'après guerre aux années 1970*. Paris: École des hautes etudes en sciences sociales, 2007. [Doctoral thesis]

Hervás i Puyal, Carles. *Sanitat a Catalunya durant la República i la Guerra Civil: Política i organització sanitàries; L'impacte del conflicte bèl·lic*. Barcelona: Institut Universitari d'Història Jaume Vicens i Vives, Universitat Pompeu Fabra, 2005. [Doctoral thesis]

Hortoneda, Patrice. "Un homme dans notre histoire: Hommage à François Tosquelles," *Lien social*, no. 284, December 1994, pp. 5–11.

— "Préface à François Tosquelles," in Jacques Tosquellas (ed.), *Archives complètes: Chantier I, Sardanes—1928 à 1943*. Cour-Cheverny: Institutions, 2014, pp. 16–17.

Huertas, Rafael. *Historia cultural de la psiquiatría: (Re)pensar la locura*. Madrid: Catarata, 2012.

Ibarz, Mercè. "Una lectura d''In memoriam' de Gabriel Ferrater, feta per Francesc Tosquelles," *Avui*, May 12, 1985, p. 6.

— "Encontre històric a Perpinyà de les tendències psicoanalítiques catalanes," *Avui*, May 2, 1986, p. 23.

— "Plorar la República," *El País.cat*, November 13, 2019.

Johnes, Lucile. *Désaliénisme à l'hôpital psychiatrique de Saint-Alban-sur-Limagnole: L'accueil de la folie dans un hôpital public de Lozère de la fin de la deuxième guerre mondiale au début des années 1970*. Montpellier: Université de lettres Paul-Valéry, 2010. [Doctoral thesis]

— "François Tosquelles: De la guerre d'Espagne à Saint-Alban," in Mireille Gauzy (ed.), *L'Invention du lieu, résistances et création en Gévaudan*. Villeneuve-d'Asq: Lille Métropole Musée d'art moderne, d'art contemporain et d'art brut, 2014, pp. 27–33.

Khalfa, Jean. "Soigner les pathologies de la liberté: Fanon psychiatre," *Les Temps modernes*, no. 2, 2015, pp. 229–255.

Koenig, Raphaël. *Art Beyond the Norms: Art of the Insane, Art Brut, and the Avant-Garde from Prinzhorn to Dubuffet* (1922–1949). Cambridge: Harvard University, 2018. [Doctoral thesis]

Krzyzaniak, Patrice. *Georges Daumézon (1912–1979): Un camisard psychiatre et pédagogue; Une contribution singulière aux sciences de l'éducation*. Lille: Université Charles de Gaulle, 2018.

Labad, Antonio. "Théorie et pratique chez Tosquelles," *Institutions: Revue de psychotérapie institutionnelle*, no. 31, October 2002.

— "La psiquiatria pels volts del 1900," in Jordi March (*et al.*) (ed.), *L'Institut Pere Mata de Reus, de Lluís Domènech i Montaner*. Reus: Ajuntament de Reus, 2004, pp. 205–220.

— "Papel de la revista *Club* (1972) en la terapia institucional en el Institut Pere Mata de Reus," in Silvia Esteban Hernández (*et al.*) (eds.), *Historias de la salud mental para un nuevo tiempo*. Madrid: Asociación Española de Neuropsiquiatría, 2015, pp. 117–136.

— "El periódico 'Club' y el libro de actas de la 'Comisión periódico' en el Institut Pere Mata," in Oscar Martínez Azumendi (*et al.*) (eds.), *Psiquiatría y cambio social: Apuntes para una historia reciente*. Madrid: Asociación Española de Neuropsiquiatría, 2019, pp. 57–76.

— "Tosquelles i l'Institut Pere Mata," *Revista del Centre de Lectura de Reus*, 2022, no pagination.

Labad, Antonio; Garcia, Josep; Mallafrè, Joaquim. "Francesc Tosquelles i Llauradó," *Revista del Centre de Lectura de Reus*, no. 11, 1995, pp. 17–18.

Lacan, Jacques. *De la psicosis paranoica en sus relaciones con la personalidad* (1932). Mexico City: Siglo XXI, 2000.

LaSource, Max. *L'Extermination douce: La mort de 40.000 malades mentaux dans les hôpitaux psychiatriques en France, sous le régime de Vichy*. Ligné: Éditions de l'AREFPPI, 1987.

Le Coguic, Elsie. *L'activité intellectuelle et artistique au sein de l'établissement psychiatrique de Saint-Alban-sur-Limagnole de 1914 à 1970*. Paris: Université Paris-Ouest Nanterre-La Defense, 2011. [Master's thesis]

Lecoutey, Carmen. *Soigner l'asile: François Tosquelles et la naissance du mouvement de la psychothérapie institutionnelle en France*. Paris: EHESS, 2004.

Mabin, Dominique; Mabin, Renée. "Art, folie et surréalisme à l'hôpital psychiatrique de Saint-Alban-sur-Limagnole pendant la guerre de 1939–1945," *Mélusine*, March 13, 2015.

Macey, David. *Frantz Fanon: A Biography*. London: Verso Books, 2012.

Markez, Iñaki (*et al.*). "Francesc Tosquelles Llauradó (1912–1994): Del exilio republicano a la psicoterapia institucional," *Intercambios, papeles de psicoanàlisis / Intercanvis, papers de psicoanàlisi*, no. 50, 2023, pp. 45–60.

Martí, Oriol. "Paraules de tancament de la Jornada dedicada a Francesc Tosquelles-Tot parafrasejant a Salvador Espriu," *Intercambios, papeles de psicoanàlisis / Intercanvis, papers de psicoanàlisi*, no. 50, 2023, pp. 101–102.

Martínez Azumendi, Óscar. "La revista *Club* en el contexto de psicoterapia institucional, promovida por Tosquelles, en el Pere Mata (Reus, Tarragona)," in Óscar Martínez Azumendi (*et al.*) (eds.), *Psiquiatría y cambio social: Apuntes para una historia reciente*. Madrid: Asociación Española de Neuropsiquiatría, 2019, pp. 45–56.

Martínez Azumendi, Óscar (*et al.*) (eds.). *Psiquiatría y cambio social: Apuntes para una historia reciente*. Madrid: Asociación Española de Neuropsiquiatría, 2019.

Martínez de Sas, María Teresa; Pagès i Blanch, Pelai. *Diccionari biogràfic del moviment obrer als Països Catalans*. Barcelona: Edicions de la Universitat de Barcelona and Publicacions de l'Abadia de Montserrat, 2000.

Marxen, Eva. "Art, the Clinic, and the Political Exercise of Thinking," *Somatosphere*, January 17, 2020.

Masó, Joana. "Francesc Tosquelles," *Sansueña*, no. 1, 2019, pp. 119–126.

— "Épíleg," in Christian Berst i Oriol Malet, *Un món d'art brut*. Barcelona: Comanegra, 2021.

— "Tosquelles: Filmant el final de la psiquiatria moderna," *El Món d'Ahir*, 2022, pp. 6–13.

— "En mal d'asile," epilogue to Paul Éluard, *Souvenirs de la maison des fous*. Paris: Seghers, 2023.

— "Tosquelles: How Can We Inherit Experiences of Emancipation?," *Los Angeles Review of Books*, no. 39, "Tosquelles Portfolio," 2023, pp. 76–89.

— "Du collectif avec des femmes," *Cahiers du genre*, vol. 73, no. 2, 2022, pp. 233–262. ["The Collective's Women," *Parapraxis*, no. 4, August 2024]

— "Otra cosa que no sé cómo decir: Tosquelles, una historia cultural desde las vanguardias literarias y artísticas," *Culture and History Digital Journal*, vol. 13, no. 1, June 2024.

Mbembe, Achille; Fanon-Mendès-France, Mireille. *Frantz Fanon par les textes de l'époque*. Paris: Les Petits Matins, 2012.

Mendieta, Santiago. *Histoires retrouvées de la guerre d'Espagne*. Villeveyrac: Le Papillon rouge, 2020.

Menéndez Osorio, Fedcrico. "Veinte años de la reforma psiquiátrica: Panorama del estado de la psiquiatría en España de los años 1970 a los 2000; De un pensamiento único a otro," *Revista de la Asociación Española de Neuropsiquiatría*, vol. 25, no. 95, July/September 2005, pp. 69–81.

Michaud, Ginette. *Laborde … un pari nécessaire: De la notion d'institution à la psychothérapie institutionnelle*. Paris: Gauthier-Villars, 1977.

Minard, Michel. "François Tosquelles, l'homme qui faisait feu de tout bois," *Psychiatre Française*, no. 1, March 1995, pp. 127–128.

Minard, Michel; Tosquellas, Jacques. "Entretien avec Jean Ayme," *Sud/Nord*, no. 22, 2007, pp. 119–125.

Miñarro, Anna. "Tosquelles, què en queda a les institucions?," *Intercambios, papeles de psicoanàlisis / Intercanvis, papers de psicoanàlisi*, no. 50, 2023, pp. 43–44.

Mira i López, Emili. *Congrès des médecins aliénistes et neurologistes de France et des pays de langue française: XXXIII session, Barcelone, 21–26 Mai 1929; Comptes rendus*. Paris: Masson, 1929.

— *La psicoanàlisi* (1935). Barcelona: Edicions 62, 1974.

Mira i López, Emili; Strauss, Alfred; de Moragas, Jeroni. "Un any de treball a l'Institut d'Observació Psicològica La Sageta," *Revista catalana de psiquiatria i neurologia*, vol. 1, no. 2, 1937, pp. 230 and following.

Miret Montsó, Josep. "L'exili dels Metges catalans després la Guerra Civil," *Gimbernat*, no. 20, 1993, pp. 213–260.

Molinier, Pascale (dir.). *François Tosquelles et le travail*. Paris: Éditions d'une, 2018.

Montejo Alonso, F. Javier. "En un lugar de La Mancha … Francesc Tosquelles y Max Hodann, creadores de las primeras comunidades terapéuticas durante la Guerra Civil Española," *Intersubjetivo*, vol. 14, no. 1, 2013, pp. 46–66.

Moreau-Ricaud, Michelle. "Una utopía en la encrucijada de la psiquiatría y el psicoanálisis: La psicoterapia institucional," *Clínica i análisis grupal*, vol. 95, no. 27, 2005, pp. 21–36.

Moreu Calvo, Àngel C. "Psicopedagogia i Medicina: El paper dels metges catalans en la primera fonamentació de l'entorn psicopedagògic," *Revista catalana de pedagogia*, no. 2, 2003, pp. 339–367.

Munsó i Cabús, J. (*et al.*). "Congreso y psicoterapia," *Revista de actualidades, artes y letras*, September 13, 1958, p. 16.

Murat, Laure. *La maison du docteur Blanche: Histoire d'un asile et de ses pensionnaires, de Nerval à Maupassant*. Paris: Gallimard, 2013.

Nassib, Sélim. "Tosquelles le 'déconnetier,'" *Libération*, 1992.

Navais i Icart, Joan; Samarra i Sancho, Frederic. "La bandera roja del comunisme dissident: El Bloc Obrer Camperol i el Partit Obrer d'Unificació Marxista," in *Tres banderes i una revolució: Anarcosindicalisme, separatisme i comunisme dissident a Reus*. Reus: Edicions del Centre de Lectura, 2001, pp. 103–156.

Nazif, Perwana. "Filming in and of the Asylum: French Radical Psychiatry on Screen," *MUBI*, July 16, 2024.

Nazif, Perwana (ed.). "Tosquelles Portfolio" (monographic issue), *Los Angeles Review of Books*, no. 39, 2023.

Nerín, Gustau. "Francesc Tosquelles: Un geni freudià, marxista i catalanista," *El Nacional.cat*, May 1, 2018.

Ohayon, Annick. *Psychologie et psychanalyse en France: L'impossible rencontre, 1919–1969*. Paris: La Découverte, 2006.

Olesti i Trillas, Josep. "Un reusenc il·lustre: El doctor Francesc Tosquelles i Llauradó," *Reus: Setmanari de la ciutat*, May 19, 1984, p. 9.

Ou-Rabah, Marie-Rose. *À l'ombre des poiriers: Hélène et François Tosquelles; Un secret de famille*. Saint-Denis: Édilivre, 2010.

Oury, Jean. *Création et schizophrénie*. Paris: Galilée, 1989.

— *L'Aliénation*. Paris: Galilée, 1992.

— *Onze heures du soir à La Borde: Essais sur la psychothérapie institutionnelle*. Paris: Galilée, 1992.

— "Hommage a François Tosquelles," *L'Information psychiatrique*, no. 10, December 1994, pp. 892–898.

— *Les Séminaires de La Borde, 1996–1997*. Nimes: Champ social, 1998.

— *Essai sur la conation esthétique*. Orleans: Éditions Le Pli, 2005.

— *La psychothérapie institutionnelle de Saint-Alban à La Borde*. Paris: Éditions d'une, 2016.

Oury, Jean; Gabarron-Garcia, Florent. "Psychothérapie institutionnelle et Guerre d'Espagne," *Chimères*, no. 72, 2010, pp. 11–20.

Pagès i Blanch, Pelai. "Dirigents i militants del POUM: Un planter divers i plural," *Ebre 38*, no. 5, 2010, pp. 39–66.

Palau, Maria. "Moment Tosquelles," *El Punt Avui*, November 21, 2020.

Palau Centelles, Alba. "La psiquiatria d'arrel humana i d'expressió social de Francesc Tosquelles: Un llegat col·lectiu," *Revista de Catalunya*, no. 320, 2022, pp. 95–103.

Papiau, Danielle. *Psychiatrie, psychanalyse et communisme: Essai de sociobiographie des psychiatres communistes (1924–1985)*. Paris: Université Paris-Nanterre, 2017.

Pardo, Belén. "El baile: La práctica institucional y la formación con Francesc Tosquelles," *Intercambios, papeles de psicoanàlisis / Intercanvis, papers de psicoanàlisi*, no. 50, 2023, pp. 75–79.

Periáñez, M. "El origen de las ideas de Francesc Tosquelles," *Edición digital de la Fundación Andreu Nin*, 2010.

Périlleux, Thomas. "Paysages humains: Clinique de l'oppression, avec Tosquelles et Fanon," *Concordia: International Review of Philosophy*, no. 1, 2017, pp. 37–56.

Planas, Pere Llovet. "Visión breve de la obra de Francesc Tosquelles y su influencia en Catalunya," *Intercambios, papeles de psicoanàlisis / Intercanvis, papers de psicoanàlisi*, no. 49 (2022), pp. 33–43.

Poca Gaya, Josep. *Institut Pere Mata: Cent anys d'història (1896–1996)*. Reus: Institut Pere Mata, 1996.

Polack, Jean-Claude. "François Tosquelles i Fernand Deligny: Psicosis i experiències de l'espai," in *Fernand Deligny: Permetre, traçar, veure*. Barcelona: MACBA, 2009.

Poncin, Claude. *Essai d'analyse structurale appliquée à la psychothérapie institutionnelle*. Nantes: Université de Nantes, 1962–1963. [Doctoral thesis]

Pujol del Pozo, Andreu. "Tosquelles en la història de la medicina," *Revista del Centre de Lectura de Reus*, 2022, no pagination.

Puyuelo, Rémy (*et al.*). "Histoires de rencontres," *Empan*, vol. 45, no. 1, 2002, pp. 111–116.

Quigley, Gabriel. "Tosquelles," *French Politics, Culture & Society*, 2026 (forthcoming monographic issue). [Includes texts by Edward Dioguardi, Éric Fassin, Jean Khalfa, Joana Masó, Marlon Miguel, Gabriel Quigley, Camille Robcis, and Elena Vogman]

Rahmani, Reda; Pacheco, Luis. "A modo de fichas sobre clásicos de la Psiquiatría (XXIX): Francesc Tosquelles Llauradó," *Lmentala*, no. 54, June 2007.

Rappard, Philippe. "François Tosquelles: De la personne au groupe; À propos des équipes de soins," *Che vuoi?*, no. 2, 2003, pp. 205–212.

Rizet, Clément. "Peut-on soigner les institutions aujourd'hui? Hommage à François Tosquelles," *Cliniques méditerranéennes*, vol. 107, no. 1, 2023, pp. 239–250.

Robcis, Camille. "François Tosquelles and the Psychiatric Revolution in Postwar France," *Constellations*, vol. 23, no. 2, 2016, pp. 212–222.

— *Disalienation*. Chicago and London: University of Chicago Press, 2021.

Rochet, Marion. *La vie de l' hôpital psychiatrique de Saint-Alban-sur-Limagnole (Lozère) de septembre 1939 à mai 1945*. Saint-Etienne: Université Jean Monnet, 1993. [Master's thesis]

— "Saint-Alban-sur-Limagnole: Un hôpital psychiatrique dans la guerre," *Information psychiatrique*, 1996, vol. 72, no. 8, pp. 758–765.

Rodrigues, H. B. C. "Um anarquista catalão: Aventuras do freudo-marxismo na França," *Cadernos de psicologia*, no. 7, 1988.

Rodríguez Garzo, Montserrat. *Esquizofrenias y otros hechos de lenguaje: De la clínica analítica del MACBA (2002–2013)*. Madrid: Brumaria, 2015.

— "Què articula la causa artística i el mercat de l'art," *Quadern de les idees, les arts i les lletres*, no. 219, December 2019–January 2020.

Rodríguez Reyes, José. *El departamento de terapias colectivas en el Hospital psiquiátrico de Oviedo*. Oviedo: 1966.

Roudinesco, Elisabeth. *La bataille de cent ans: Histoire de la psychanalyse en France*, vol. 1. Paris: Ramsay, 1982.

— (ed.). *Actualité de Georges Canguilhem: Le normal et le pathologique*. Le Plessis-Robinson: Institut Synthélabo pour le progrès de la connaissance, 1998.

Rousseau, Valérie. "Révéler l'Art Brut: À la recherche d'un musée ideal," *Culture & Musées*, no. 16, 2010, pp. 65–92.

Rouzel, Joseph. "Rencontre avec François Tosquelles," *Lien social*, no. 16, February 1989, pp. 8–10.

— "Le sujet n'est pas handicapé," in Stéphane Pawloff, *L'art d'inventer l'existence dans les pratiques médico-sociales*. Toulouse: Éditions Érès, 2010, pp. 93–102.

Royer, Benjamin. "Collectif et praxis instituantes: Actualité de la publication des Actes du GTPSI," *Vie sociale et traitements*, vol. 125, no. 1, 2015, pp. 90–96.

Ruspoli, Mario. "Remarques sur le cinéma direct, dit: 'Cinéma-vérité,'" *Cinéma 63*, no. 74, 1963.

Ruiz, Valéria Salek (*et al.*). "François Tosquelles, sua história no campo da Reforma Psiquiátrica," *Estudos e pesquisas em psicologia*, vol. 13, no. 3, pp. 855–877.

Ruiz Gaspar, Joaquín. "El Hospital militar de Sariñena," *Os Monegros*, December 15, 2015.

Sadoul, Georges. "Portraits du poète à plusieurs âges de sa vie," *Europe*, July–August 1953, pp. 39–50.

Saint-Jules, Marie. "Une expérience de vente a l'extérieur," *Bulletin technique du personnel soignant: Hôpital pyschiatrique de Saint-Alban*, December 1962, pp. 31–33.

Sallarès, Mireia. "Vida," in Marina Garcés (coord.), *Humanitats en acció*. Barcelona: Raig Verd, 2019.

Schaepelynck, Valentin. "Institution," *Le Télémaque*, vol. 44, no. 2, 2013, pp. 21–34.

— *L'institution renversée: Folie, analyse institutionnelle et champ social*. Paris: Etérotopia, 2018.

Serrano Guerra, Enrique (coord.). *Introducción y compilación de las jornadas "Tosquelles, la paidopsiquiatría y la articulación comunitaria."* Asturias: Servicio de Salud del Principado de Asturias, 2002.

Sidobre, Florian. *L'Hôpital de Saint-Alban-sur-Limagnole de 1939 à 1945: Quand la psychiatrie fait de la résistance*. Montpellier: Université Paul Valéry, 1999. [Master's thesis]

Subirats, Berta. "Imaginar con Tosquelles," *Artnodes*, no. 29, January 2022.

Toda i Bonet, Agnès. "Coneixent una mica més Francesc Tosquelles," *Revista del Centre de Lectura de Reus*, 2022, no pagination.

Tomé Peña, Ricardo. "Ébauche pour une lecture dilatée du contexte intellectuel autour de Francisco Tosquelles Llauradó," in *Coopération, éducation, formation: La pédagogie Freinet face aux défis du XXIe siècle*. Paris: L'Harmattan, 2018.

Torres, Karín Cruz. "Más allá de Tosquelles," *Percurso*, 2023, pp. 9–16.

Tosquellas, Jacques. "Courriers Tosquelles-Balvet," *Sud/Nord*, no. 1, 2004, pp. 171–184.

— "Entretien avec Maurice Despinoy," *Sud/Nord*, no. 22, 2007, pp. 105–114.

— *Francesc Tosquelles: Psychiatre, catalan, marxiste.* Paris: Éditions d'une, 2021.

— "El legado del Dr. Francesc Tosquelles," *Intercambios, papeles de psicoanàlisis / Intercanvis, papers de psicoanàlisi*, no. 50, 2023, pp. 61–68.

Tzara, Tristan. *Parler seul.* Paris: Maeght, 1948–1950.

Vidal Castaño, José Antonio. *Exiliados republicanos en Septfonds* (1939). Madrid: Libros de la Catarata, 2013.

Viger i Rovira, Mercè; Bruguera i Cortada, Miquel. "Francesc Tosquelles i Llauradó," *Galeria de metges catalans.*

Von Bueltzingsloewen, Isabelle. *L'Hécatombe des fous: La famine dans les hôpitaux psychiatriques sous l'Occupation.* Paris: Camps Flammarion, 2009.

Watson, Janell. "Living with Madness: Experimental Asylums in Poststructuralist France," *Cultural Critique*, no. 104, Summer 2004, pp. 137–157.

— "François Tosquelles," *Informes*, no. 4, October 1994.

— "François Tosquelles," *Candé Vie*, no. 26, January 1995.

Zeavin, Hannah. "'We Took Care of the Network,'" *New York Review of Books*, August 17, 2024.

FILM

Les Inconnus de la terre, by Mario Ruspoli, 1961, 39 min.

Regard sur la folie, by Mario Ruspoli, 1962, 53 min.

La Fête prisionnère, by Mario Ruspoli, 1962, 22 min.

La Rue de l'enfer, by Bernard Favre, 1977, 77 min.

Félix Guattari sur un divan, by François Pain, 1986, 20 min.

François Tosquelles: Une politique de la folie, by François Pain, Jean-Claude Polack, and Danielle Sivadon, 1989, 54 min. [Available at https://vimeo.com/167991974]

Entretien filmé du docteur François Tosquelles, by Jean Giménez, Jean-Marie Dizol, and Jean-Claude Forestier, 1992.

Déconnage, by Angela Melitopoulos and Maurizio Lazzarato, 2011, 62 min.

Traces, by Jean-Christophe Montferran, CNRS Images, 2012, 60 min. [Available at https://images.cnrs.fr/video/3740]

Saint-Alban, une révolution psychiatrique, by Sonia Cantalapiedra, Les Films d'un Jour, 2016, 60 min.

Les heures heureuses, by Martin Deyres, Les Films du Tambour de Soie, 2019, 77 min.

Història potencial de Francesc Tosquelles: Catalunya i la por, by Mireia Sallarès, written with Joana Masó, 2021, 135 min.

Oblideu Tosquelles, by Enric Miró, 2022, 110 min.

Tosquelles, Oury, Guattari, by François Pain. [In production]

RADIO

Saint-Alban-sur-Limagnole, broadcast by Claude Hudelot, France Culture, October 28, 1982, 123 min.

François Tosquelles, broadcast by Cécile Hamsy, France Culture, October 4 and 11, 1985, 2 × 60 min.

Saint-Alban-sur-Limagnole: L'esprit d'un lieu, broadcast by Cécile Hamsy, France Culture, September 21 and 28, 1989, 2 × 60 min.

Lucien Bonnafé, broadcast by Patrick Molinier, France Culture, April 12 and 13, 2000, 2 × 28 min.

Saint-Alban, une expérience en psychiatrie, broadcast by Jean Lebrun, France Inter, November 17, 2016, 28 min.

Saint-Alban, lieu d'hospitalité, broadcast by Hélène Delye and François Teste, France Culture, November 23 and 24, 2019, 2 × 28 min.

THEATER

La méningite des poireaux: Ou folies en musique de la donquichottesque existence de François Tosquelles, psychiatre, part 3 of *Trilogie pour interroger nos normes mentales*, by Frédéric Naud and Jeanne Videau, 2017.

OTHER

Rencontre autour de Gabriel Ferrater: "La fonction poétique du langage." Carcassone: Centre Joë Bousquet et son Temps, November 8–10, 2019.

IMAGE SOURCES

—p. 3: Postcard. Aerial view of the Saint-Alban hospital, circa 1960. Source and reproduction: Baldran Collection, Saint-Alban-sur-Limagnole

—pp. 6, 9, 16, 19, 22, 25, 32, 35: Photographs from the Tosquelles family albums, many of which are undated, some taken by Romain Vigouroux. Source: Tosquelles family archives. Photographic reproduction: © Roberto Ruiz

—p. 29: Photomontage *Le méthode hypocritique I*, by Francesc Tosquelles.
Source: Tosquelles family archives
Photographic reproduction: © Roberto Ruiz

—p. 42: Francesc Tosquelles with his daughter Marie-Rose at the Institut Pere Mata, Reus, circa 1936–1937. Source: Hospital Universitari Institut Pere Mata, Reus. Photographic reproduction: © Roberto Ruiz

—p. 43: Copy of Jacques Lacan's thesis, *De la psychose paranoïaque dans ses rapport avec la personnalité*, 1932, Printed by the inpatients at Saint-Alban circa 1960. Source: Hospital Universitari Institut Pere Mata, Reus Photographic reproduction: © Roberto Ruiz

—p. 46: Josep Solanes Vilaprenyó, *Com se surt dels frenocomis: Consideracions sobre unes estadístiques de l'Institut Pere Mata*. Tarragona: Gràfiques Forés, 1935. Source: Hospital Universitari Institut Pere Mata, Reus. Photographic reproduction: © Roberto Ruiz

—p. 48: Man Ray, *L'énigme d'Isidore Ducasse*, 1920/1972, mixed media, 25.5 × 60.5 × 33.5 cm.
© Man Ray Trust, VEGAP, Barcelona, 2021
Source and photographic reproduction: Tate, London

—p. 49: Man Ray, *Hommage à Lautréamont*, 1933/1982, gelatin silver print on paper, 24 × 30 cm.
© Man Ray Trust, VEGAP, Barcelona, 2021
Source: Museo Nacional Centro de Arte Reina Sofía. Photographic reproduction: © Archivo Fotográfico Museo Nacional Centro de Arte Reina Sofía

—p. 50: Cover of the magazine *Estudis*, vol. 3, no. 28, Reus, April 1936. Source and photographic reproduction: Biblioteca de Catalunya, Barcelona

—pp. 51–52: Images of the Institut Pere Mata, Reus, 1930s. Source: Hospital Universitari Institut Pere Mata, Reus, 1930s. Reus. Photographic reproduction: © Roberto Ruiz

—p. 52: (bottom): Excursion with inpatients at the Institut Pere Mata, Reus.
Source and photographic reproduction: Xavier Amorós, Pere Anguera, and Albert Arnavat, *Història gràfica del Reus contemporani I*. Reus: Ajuntament de Reus, 1986. Biblioteca Central Xavier Amorós and Fons Pere Anguera at the Arxiu Municipal de Reus Photographer unknown

—p. 53: Postcards of the Institut Pere Mata, Reus. Source: Centre de la Imatge Mas Iglesias, fons Postal de Reus. Photographs: Photographer unknown

—p. 54: 33è Congrés de neuròlegs i psiquiatres, Reus, 1929. Source and photographic reproduction: Xavier Amorós, Pere Anguera, and Albert Arnavat, *Història gràfica del Reus contemporani I*. Reus: Ajuntament de Reus, 1986. Biblioteca Central Xavier Amorós and Fons Pere Anguera de l'Arxiu Municipal de Reus. Photographer unknown

—pp. 58–59: Farmers at the Institut Pere Mata, Reus. Source: Hospital Universitari Institut Pere Mata, Reus. Photographic reproduction: © Roberto Ruiz

—p. 61: *Cicle de conferències sobre psicopatologia infantil*, Barcelona, 1934.
Source: Biblioteca del Treball de Barcelona. Photographic reproduction: © Institut Escola del Treball de Barcelona

—p. 62: Poster *Companyia general d'autobusos de Barcelona S. A.*, no. 4, Barcelona, 1929.
Source: Biblioteca del Treball de Barcelona. Photographic reproduction: © Institut Escola del Treball de Barcelona

—p. 64: (top) Dr. Alexandre Frias at his office in La Gota de Llet, Reus. Source and photographic reproduction: Centre de la Imatge Mas Iglesias, Col·lecció Arxiu Històric de l'Agrupació Fotogràfica de Reus. Photographer unknown

—p. 64: (bottom): Summer camps during the Republic, 1933 and 1935.Source: Centre de la Imatge Mas Iglesias, Museu de Reus archive. Photographer unknown

—p. 66: Cover of *L'Hora*, no. 20, September 8, 1934. Source and reproduction: CRAI Biblioteca Pavelló de la República at the Universitat de Barcelona, Barcelona

—p. 67: Advertisement for the first issue of *L'Hora*, with a reproduction of *Somni*, by Helios Gómez, December 1930.
©Associació Cultural Helios Gómez, VEGAP, Barcelona, 2021.
Source and reproduction: CRAI Biblioteca Pavelló de la República at the Universitat de Barcelona.

—p. 68: Cover of *La Torxa*, no. 4, 2nd period, February 6, 1937. Source: International Institute of Social History, Amsterdam

—p. 69: (top) Headquarters of the PSUC at the Hotel Colon in the Plaça Catalunya of Barcelona, February 28, 1937. Photograph by Alexander Wheeler Wainman.
© The Estate of Alexander Wheeler Wainman, John Alexander Wainman
Source and photographic reproduction: Wainman Photograph & Archive Fonds (1933–1985)

—p. 69: (bottom) Casal Carles Marx (former Jockey Club), three months after becoming the new headquarters of the PSUC, on the Passeig de Gràcia in Barcelona, January 17, 1937. Photograph by Alexander Wheeler Wainman.
© The Estate of Alexander Wheeler Wainman, John Alexander Wainman
Source and photographic reproduction: Wainman Photograph & Archive Fonds (1933–1985)

—p. 70: Advertisement for the conference by Salvador Dalí and René Crevel in *L'Hora*, no. 43, October 30, 1931.

—p. 92: Francesc Tosquelles and Jaume Sauret at the Septfonds camp, 1939.
Source and photographic reproduction: Tosquelles family archives

—p. 94: (top) Mas del Quer.
Source: Xavier Amorós, Pere Anguera, and Albert Arnavat, *Història gràfica del Reus contemporani*. Reus: Ajuntament de Reus, 1986
Photograph: Photographer unknown

—p. 94: (bottom) The lake at Mas del Quer, circa 1920.
Source: Centre de la Imatge Mas Iglesias, Col·lecció Arxiu Històric de l'Agrupació Fotogràfica de Reus
Photograph: Joaquim Febrer Sánchez

—p. 97: (top) POUM and JCI militiamen heading to the Aragon front, Reus, August 18, 1936.
Source: Xavier Amorós, Pere Anguera, and Albert Arnavat, *Història gràfica del Reus contemporani* Reus: Ajuntament de Reus, 1986. Biblioteca Central Xavier Amorós and Biblioteca Pere Anguera of the Arxiu Municipal de Reus. Photographer unknown

—p. 97: (bottom) POUM militiamen on the train, Grañén (Aragon), September 14, 1936.
© The Estate of Alexander Wheeler Wainman, John Alexander Wainman
Source and photographic reproduction: Wainman Photograph & Archive Fonds (1933–1985)

—p. 98: Servei de Biblioteques del Front (Library Services to the Front), Sariñena substation, on August 13, 1937.
Source and photographic reproduction: Arxiu General de la Diputació de Barcelona
Photograph: Maria Felipa Español (unconfirmed)

—p. 100: Study for *Premonición de Guerra Civil* (*Premonition of Civil War*) by Salvador Dalí, 1935, charcoal, white pencil (chalk), and black ink on paper, 105 × 80 cm.
© Salvador Dalí, Fundació Gala-Salvador Dalí, VEGAP, Barcelona, 2021
Source: Museo Nacional Centro de Arte Reina Sofía
Photograph: © Archivo Fotográfico Museo Nacional Centro de Arte Reina Sofía

—p. 101: (top) *Le Cheval de Troie*, by Gérard Vulliamy, 1936–1937, oil on canvas, 118.5 × 158.5 cm.
© Gérard Vulliamy, VEGAP, Barcelona 2021
Source and photographic reproduction: Col·lecció Claire Sarti

—p. 101: (bottom) *Das Grosse Welttheater*, by Peter Weiss, 1937, oil on canvas, 120 × 160 cm.
© Peter Weiss, VEGAP, Barcelona, 2021
Source: Moderna Museet, Stockholm. Acquired in 1969.
Photographic reproduction: Åsa Lundén, Moderna Museet

—p. 102: Stills from the film *Autour de la fin du monde*, by Eugène Deslaw, 1930, black and white, 15 min.
Source and photographic reproduction: Centre National du Cinéma et de l'Image Animée, Paris

—p. 103: *Portrait de Lily Dubuffet*, by Antonin Artaud, June 22, 1947, drawing on card paper, 67 × 49 cm. © Antonin Artaud, VEGAP, 2021
Source: Adagp. Photographic reproduction: © Jean Bernard, Adagp images

—p. 104: Letter from Francesc Tosquelles, August 25, 1938.
Source: Tosquelles family archives
Photographic reproduction: © Roberto Ruiz

—p. 105: (top) Psychiatric hospital in Almodóvar del Campo during the Civil War, photograph taken in November 1954.
Source: Photograph provided by Javier de la Fuente Martínez, president of the Asociación Cultural de Amigos de la Historia de Almodóvar del Campo. Archivo

General de la Administración de Alcalá de Henares
Photograph: © Sánchez, Almodóvar del Campo

—p. 105: (bottom) Façade of the psychiatric hospital in Almodóvar del Campo during the Civil War, photograph taken in November 1954. There is another photograph of this same building in the same period that allowed for the dating and identification of the photographer. The Ministry of Agriculture constructed this building on lands ceded by the Town Hall of Almodóvar del Campo, between 1934 and 1936. During the war, it was a field hospital and later a psychiatric hospital run by Francesc Tosquelles. We know the images are from 1954 because they show the beginning of the construction of the new Colegio de los Carmelitas Descalzos, which opened in 1955 or 1956.
Source: Photograph provided by Javier de la Fuente Martínez, president of the Asociación Cultural de Amigos de la Historia de Almodóvar del Campo. Archivo General de la Administración de Alcalá de HenaresPhotograph: © Sánchez, Almodóvar del Campo

—p. 109: (left) Portrait of Max Hodann during a trip to Spain, circa 1976.
Source and photographic reproduction: Peter Weiss Archiv, np. 5309-2-8, Akademie der Künste, Berlin
Photograph: Francisco Uriz

—p. 109: (right) Sanatorium for convalescents in Albacete.
Source and photographic reproduction: Peter Weiss Archiv, no. 5309-2-8, Akademia der Künste, Berlin

—p. 110: *Nuit et Jour*, no. 4, January 1944.
Source and photographic reproduction: Bibliothèque National de France

—p. 111: (top) Francesc Tosquelles at the Septfonds camp, 1939–1940.
Source: Tosquelles family archives
Photographic reproduction: © Roberto Ruiz

—p. 111: (bottom) Seal of the infirmary at the Septfonds camp, 1939–1940.
Source: Tosquelles family archives
Photographic reproduction: © Roberto Ruiz

—p. 113: (top) Infirmary at the Septfonds camp, 1939–1940. Source: Musée de la Résistance et du Combattant, fonds Jacques Latu, Montauban
Photographic reproduction: © Pôle Mémoire de Montauban, Musée de la Résistance et du Combattant

—p. 113 (bottom): *Groupe d'hommes à la toilette*, by José Rosé (José Roa), 1939, mixed media on card paper, 52 × 79.5 cm. Source: La Mounière, Maison des Mémoires de Septfonds. Photographic reproduction: © Mairie de Septonds

—p. 114: Letter from the prefect of Lòzere, December 14, 1939.
Source: Archives de Tarn-et-Garonne, Montauban (unconfirmed)

—p. 115: Registry of departures from the Septfonds camp on January 22, 1940.
Source and reproduction: Archives de Tarn-et-Garonne (4M 8 C 114), Montauban

—p. 116 *Revue neurologique*, no. 6, December 1934.
Source and photographic reproduction: Centre de Lectura de Reus

—p. 117: Medical history from the Institut Pere Mata, Reus, 1934–1970.
Source: Hospital Universitari Institut Pere Mata, Reus. © Roberto Ruiz

—p. 152: Théophile Roussel adolescent wing at Le Villaret, 1942.
Source and photographic reproduction: Ponsonnaille family collection, Saint-Alban-sur-Limagnole

—p. 153: Old postcard of the entrance to the Saint-Alban hospital, built in the era of Napoleon III. Photograph taken shortly after the First World War.
Source and photographic reproduction: Baldran collection, Saint-Alban-sur-Limagnole

—pp. 154–155: (top) Front and back of postcard, circa 1940.
Source: Tosquelles family archives
Photographic reproduction: © Roberto Ruiz

—p. 154: (bottom) Elena at Le Villaret, circa 1942.
Source: Tosquelles family archives
Photographic reproduction: © Roberto Ruiz

—p. 155: (bottom) Still from one of the films made by Tosquelles as part of the Société Lozérienne d'Hygiène Mentale, at Saint-Alban, between 1953 and 1958.
Source: Tosquelles family archives
Photographic reproduction: ©Institut Jean Vigo, Cinémathèque euro-regionale, Perpignan

—p. 156: Francesc and Elena Tosquelles, Lucien and Jeanne Bonnafé, and their children, 1943 or 1944.
Source: Tosquelles family archives
Photographic reproduction: © Roberto Ruiz

—p. 157 (top): Group of patients in Garabit (Cantal), 1952. Source: Bonnet family collection, Saint-Alban-sur-Limagnole. Photograph: Jean-Baptiste Metge

p. 157: (bottom): Family group. Source: Tosquelles family archives Photograph: Romain Vigouroux
Photographic reproduction: © Roberto Ruiz

—p. 158: Nurses at Saint-Alban.
Source: Tosquelles family archives
Photographic reproduction: © Roberto Ruiz

—p. 159: Wall newspaper for military clinic no. 3, Manresa, 1937. Source and photographic reproduction: CRAI Biblioteca Pavelló de la República (Universitat de Barcelona)

—p. 160: (left) Poster for the exhibition *Cultura Popular*, Madrid, 1937.
Source and photographic reproduction: Archivo de la Fundación Pablo Iglesias, Madrid

—p. 160: (right, top) *Le Chemin*, December 1948. Saint-Alban: Section Lozérienne de la Ligue d'Higyene Mentale du Centre and Club Paul-Balvet, 1948. Source and photographic reproduction: Archives of the Collection de l'Art Brut, Lausanne

—p. 160: (right, bottom) *Le Chemin*, June–July 1949. Saint-Alban: Section Lozérienne de la Ligue d'Higyene Mentale du Centre and Club Paul-Balvet, 1949. Source and photographic reproduction: Archives of the Collection de l'Art Brut, Lausanne

—p. 161: *Trait d'Union* magazine, Saint-Alban, January 30, 1953.
Source and photographic reproduction: Association Culturelle Saint-Alban, Saint-Alban-sur-Limagnole

—p. 162: Stills from films made by Tosquelles as part of the Société Lozérienne d'Hygiène Mentale, at Saint-Alban, between 1953 and 1958.
Source: Tosquelles family archives
Photographic reproduction: ©Institut Jean Vigo, Cinémathèque euro-regionale, Perpignan

—p. 163: Hervé Bazin, "Le tour d'Europe de la folie," *France-Soir*, April 25, 1959.
Source and photographic reproduction: British Library. Courtesy of *France-Soir*.

—p. 165: Old postcard of the back of the Saint-Alban hospital. Photograph taken shortly after the First World War.
Source and photographic reproduction: Baldran Collection, Saint-Alban-sur-Limagnole

—p. 166: Report from the Mende police station, April 8, 1943.
Source and photographic reproduction: Archives de Tarn-et-Garonne, Montauban (unconfirmed)

—p. 168: Coin used at Saint-Alban hospital, 1934–1936.
Source: Baldran Collection, Saint-Alban-sur-Limagnole
Photographic reproduction: © Roberto Ruiz

—pp. 169–179: Medical and administrative file by Agnès Masson, Mende, 1936.
Source: Baldran Collection, Saint-Alban-sur-Limagnole
Photographic reproduction: © Roberto Ruiz

—p. 180: Reproduction of the article "Pour guérir ses malades, l'aliéniste Agnès Masson les fait danser," *Samedi-soir*, March 22, 1947.

—p. 182: Group of patients on a field trip, Saint-Alban, circa 1950–1955.
Source and photographic reproduction: Baldran Collection, Saint-Alban-sur-Limagnole
Photograph: Photographer unknown

—p. 183: Group of women and children, Saint-Alban, circa 1938–1939.
Source and photographic reproduction: Olivier Balvet. © Balvet family

—p. 185: Jean de Haut (Paul Éluard), *Les Sept Poèmes d'amour et guerre*. Saint-Flour: Bilbiothèque française, 1943.
Source: Baldran Collection, Saint-Alban-sur-Limagnole
Photographic reproduction: © Roberto Ruiz

—p. 186: Paul Éluard, *Poésie et verité*. Neuchâtel: Edition de la Baconnière, collection des Cahiers du Rhône, 1943.
Source: Hospital Universitari Institut Pere Mata, Reus. Photographic reproduction: © Roberto Ruiz

—pp. 188–189: Paul Éluard and Gérard Vulliamy (drawings), *Souvenirs de la maison des fous*. Paris: Pro-França, 1945.
© Gérard Vulliamy, VEGAP, Barcelona, 2022
Source: Baldran Collection, Saint-Alban-sur-Limagnole
Photographic reproduction: © Roberto Ruiz

—p. 190: Photographs of Paul Éluard, Nusch, and Léo Matarasso, Saint-Alban, winter 1943–1944, Photograph: © Jacques Matarasso, Paris
Source and photographic reproduction: Private collection

—p. 191: Text written by a patient at the Saint-Alban hospital, 1943, mixed media, dimensions unknown.
Source: Fonds Gaston Ferdière, Archives cantonales vaudoises (PP1057/3/1/9/01), Chavannes-près-Renens
Photographic reproduction: © Archives cantonales vaudoises

—p. 192: (left) Cécile Vulliamy and Francesc Tosquelles, Saint-Alban, 1945. © Succession Gérard Vulliamy Source and photographic reproduction: Private collection

—p. 192: (right) Cécile Vulliamy with a work by Auguste Forestier, Saint-Alban, 1945.
© Succession Gérard Vulliamy
Source and photographic reproduction: Private collection

—p. 193: Article by Cécile Agay (Cécile Vulliamy) in *Les Étoiles*, October 3, 1945, p. 3.
© Succession Gérard Vulliamy
Source and photographic reproduction: Private collection

—pp. 196–198: Tristan Tzara and Joan Miró, *Parler seul*. Paris: Maeght, 1948–1950.
© Tristan Tzara, VEGAP, 2021 / © Joan Miró, Successió Miró, 2021
Source: Fundació Joan Miró, Barcelona
Photographic reproduction: © Foto Gasull, Fundació Joan Miró

—p. 199: (top) *Portrait de Tristan Tzara*, by Gérard Vulliamy, 1945.
© Gérard Vulliamy, VEGAP, Barcelona, 2021
Source and photographic reproduction: Private collection

—p. 199: (bottom) Letter from Tristan Tzara to Michel Leiris, Saint-Alban, August 20, 1945.
Source and photographic reproduction: Bibliothèque Littéraire Jacques Ducet, Chancellerie des Universités de Paris, Paris. Courtesy of Marie-Thérèse Tzara and Jean Jamin.

—p. 202 (top): Hans Prinzhorn. *Bildnerei der Geisteskranken*. Berlin: Verlag Von Julius Springer, 1922.
Source and photographic reproduction: Staatsbibliothek, Berlin

—p. 202 (bottom): *Untitled* (Dubuisson Album), circa 1899–1915. Album containing 36 pages of drawings in ink, colored pencil, and graphite on paper, collected by Dr. Maxime Dubuisson.
Source: LaM, Lille Metrópole Musée d'art moderne, d'art contemporani et d'art brut, Villeneuve-d'Ascq
Photographic reproduction: © Nicolas Dewitte, LaM

—pp. 204–205: Francesc Tosquelles on the roof of the administrative building at the Saint-Alban hospital, with a boat made by Auguste Forestier, summer 1947.
Photograph: Romain Vigoroux
Source: Tosquelles family archives
Photographic reproduction: © Roberto Ruiz

—p. 207: Page of the album *Auguste For., Fauvel, Antinea, Arnal, Gustav, Fans F., Richard Oui, Guillaume Puj., Germain Crohan, Waedemon, Paul End, Stanislas Lib., Mme Bataille,* made by Jean Dubuffet, circa 1948. It shows a photograph of a figure by Auguste Forestier (photograph 329, figure h.c.).
Source: archives of the Collection de l'Art Brut, Lausanne. Photographic reproduction: Giuseppe Pocetti, Atelier de numérisation, Ville de Lausanne

—pp. 208–209: Page of the album *Auguste For., Fauvel, Antinea, Arnal, Gustav, Fans F., Richard Oui, Guillaume Puj., Germain Crohan, Waedemon, Paul End, Stanislas Lib., Mme Bataille,* made by Jean Dubuffet, circa 1948. It shows a photograph of figures by Auguste Forestier (photographs 780, 782, and 784, of figures cab-281bis, cab-302bis, cab-298bis, cab-387, cab-380bis, cab-385bis, cab-384bis, and cab-381bis).
Source: Archives of the Collection de l'Art Brut, Lausanne. Photographic reproduction: Giuseppe Pocetti, Atelier de numérisation, Ville de Lausanne

—pp. 210–211: Page of the album *Giavarini, Mlle Six, Gaston Duf., Sylvain Lec., Costa, Berthommier, Jardinier du boccage, Inconnu de Sao Paulo, Tripier, Doudin, Vicente, Hill, Albino Braz, Claudio Becattes,* made by Jean Dubuffet, circa 1948. It shows a photograph of embroidery by Marguerite Sirvins (photograph 635, embroidery cab-A446).
Source: Archives of the Collection de l'Art Brut, Lausanne
Photographic reproduction: Giuseppe Pocetti, Atelier de numérisation, Ville de Lausanne

—p. 212: Page of an album made by Jean Dubuffet with photographs of the work of Clément Fraisse, 1930–1931.
Source: Archives of the Collection de l'Art Brut, Lausanne
Photographic reproduction: Wolf Slawny, Claudine Garcia, Atelier de numérisation, Ville de Lausanne

—p. 213: Page of the album *Anonymes, Antinéa, Artaud, Bojnev, Bonamour, Anaïs*, made by Jean Dubuffet, circa 1963. It shows a photograph of *La maladresse sexuelle de Dieu*, by Antonin Artaud (photograph 1234).
Source: Archives of the Collection de l'Art Brut, Lausanne. Photographic reproduction: Atelier de numérisation, Ville de Lausanne

—p. 221: Still from the shooting of the film *Le Moindre Geste*, by Fernand Deligny, Josée Manenti, and Jean-Pierre Daniel, circa 1964.
Source: Any Durand archive
Photograph: © Any Durand

—pp. 222–223: Filmstrip of the *Film Tosquelles*, or *Société Lozérienne d'Hygiène Mental*, 1958.
Source: Tosquelles family archives
Photographic reproduction: © Roberto Ruiz

—p. 224: Poster for the 4th International Congress of Psychotherapy, Barcelona, 1958.
Source and photographic reproduction: Biblioteca de Catalunya, Barcelona

—p. 225: (top) Photographs of the 4th International Congress of Psychotherapy, Barcelona, 1958.
Source: Hospital Universitari Institut Pere Mata, Reus. Photographic reproduction: © Roberto Ruiz

—p. 225: (bottom) Tosquelles and Jacques Lacan during the 4th International Congress of Psychotherapy, Barcelona, 1958.
Source: Revista Freudiana (unconfirmed)

—pp. 226–227: Stills from the films Tosquelles made as part of the Société Lozérienne d'Hygiène Mental, at Saint-Alban, between 1953 and 1958.
Source: Tosquelles family archives
Photographic reproduction: © Institut Jean Vigo, Cinémathèque euro-regionale, Perpignan

—p. 230: Press release by Roland Barthes about the film *La fête prisonnière*, by Mario Ruspoli, Isle-sur-la-Sorge

—pp. 231–238: Stills from the *Film Tosquelles,* or *Société Lozérienne d'Hygiène Mental*, 1958.
Source: Tosquelles family archives
Photographic reproduction: © Institut Jean Vigo, Cinémathèque euro-regionale, Perpignan

—pp. 242–243: Ceremony commemorating the armistice of the First World War, Saint-Alban hospital, 1952.
Source and photographic reproduction: Archive of the Saint-Alban hospital, Saint-Alban-sur-Limagnole

—p. 318: Francesc Tosquelles, circa 1970.
Source: Tosquelles family archives
Photographic reproduction: © Roberto Ruiz

—p. 320: Tosquelles and Jean Oury at the XXI Jornades d'Interès Psiquiàtric, Reus, 1988.
Source: Hospital Universitari Institut Pere Mata, Reus. Photographic reproduction: © Roberto Ruiz

—p. 321: The magazine *Club*, published by the Club Emili Briansó at the Institut Pere Mata, Reus.
Source: Hospital Universitari Institut Pere Mata, Reus. Photographic reproduction: © Roberto Ruiz

—pp. 322–327: Francesc Tosquelles, "Quadres de la paret," diagrams of theoretical and literary references, circa 1970, marker on paper, dimensions unknown.
Source: Hospital Universitari Institut Pere Mata, Reus. Photographic reproduction: © Roberto Ruiz

—pp. 329–335: Cassette recordings of the training and countertransference groups that met at the Institut Pere Mata between 1970 and the early 1990s.
Source: Hospital Universitari Institut Pere Mata, Reus. Photographic reproduction: © Roberto Ruiz

—p. 338: Francesc Tosquelles, *La méthode hypocritique II*, 1941–1944, photomontage, dimensions unknown.
Source: Tosquelles family archives
Photographic reproduction: © Roberto Ruiz

ACKNOWLEDGMENTS

This long journey through the life and writings of Francesc Tosquelles and the intellectual, literary, political, artistic, and historic production of his time, as well as the significant documentary, photographic, and filmic research, was only possible thanks to Jordi Segarra, who, as part of the Fundació Mir-Puig / Fundació Cellex, believed in the need for this research and supported it from the beginning, in 2017. It was also made possible by the work and intelligence of David Fontanals, an essential mainstay of the research project *El llegat oblidat de Francesc Tosquelles*, which I coordinate at the Universitat de Barcelona. For the privilege of being able to get to know and understand the Tosquelles archives, I am indebted to Marie-Rose Ou-Rabah, Germaine Bonnal, Jacques Tosquellas, and Michel Tosquelles, who take care of their father's archives and legacy and have been generous with their time, their words, and their listening. Antonio Labad and Consuelo Centelles offered us the invaluable help of allowing us into the Hospital Universitari Institut Pere Mata de Reus over these past few years, which gave us access to the photographic and documentary memory of Tosquelles's first and last years in Catalonia.

It was with the complicity of the contemporary art world that this book was woven together in different languages and in different places, based on an original idea by Carles Guerra, then, in 2017, the director of the Fundació Antoni Tàpies. This research was carried out with him and the spark of this book was born based on open conversations with other thinkers, artists, and writers, in a volume that dialogues with and accompanies a series of exhibition projects on Francesc Tosquelles that began in 2018. I want to thank Núria Soler of the Fundació Antoni Tàpies in Barcelona for her personal implication in the project, and also Judit Carrera, Jordi Costa, Mònica Ibáñez, Carlota Broggi, and Elisenda Poch, and the CCCB Centre de Cultura Contemporània de Barcelona; as well as Manuel Borja-Villel, Teresa Velázquez, and Alicia Pinteño, and the Museo Nacional Centro de Arte Reina Sofía, Madrid; Valérie Rousseau, Edward Dioguardi, and Margarita Sánchez Urdaneta, and the American Folk Art Museum of New York; Manel Margalef and Museu d'Art Modern de Tarragona; and Annabelle Ténèze, Valentin Rodriguez, and Julien Michel, and Les Abattoirs, Musée – Frac Occitanie Toulouse for their generous commitment to the adventure of bringing Francesc Tosquelles's legacy to life.

Many people have accompanied us throughout this long research process: Sandra Alvarez de Toledo, Yves Baldran, Olivier Balvet, Clara Bardón, Miquel Bassols, Gabriela Berti, Mireille Berton, Marie Bonnafé, Kaira Cabañas, Sonia Cantalapiedra, Jacint Carrera, Josep Maria Comelles, Jordi Cornudella, Manuel Desviat, Martine Deyres, Luis Feduchi, Anne Ferdière, Pedro G. Romero, Evelyne Grossman, Emmanuel Guigon, Carles Hervàs, Guillem Homet, Jean Khalfa, Raphael Koenig, Mireille Larrouy, Sophie Legrain,

Angela Melitopoulos, Jacques-Alain Miller, Pelai Pagès, François Pain, Françoise Petit, Joan Pi, Jean-Claude Polack, Paul B. Preciado, Camille Robcis, Anna Rodríguez, Montserrat Rodríguez Garzo, Roberto Ruiz, Jean-Louis Sadoul, Claire Sarti, Àlex Susanna, Jorge Tizón, Marie-Thérèse Tzara and Jean Jamin, Marie-Claude Vallejo, Elie Vallejo, and Fernando Vicente.

We would like to thank the many organizations, associations, archives, and institutions that, with the complicity of their staff, have sent us documents, photographs, and letters that allowed us to better imagine the landscapes of Francesc Tosquelles: the Sánchez family, Javier de la Fuente, and the Asociación Cultural de Amigos de la Historia de Almodóvar del Campo, who restored the memories of Tosquelles's time spent in Ciudad Real; Luis Alfonso Arcarazo, Gemma Grau, Joaquín Ruiz Gaspar, and the Ayuntamiento de Sariñena, who documented the link between Tosquelles and the Aragon front; Geneviève Dreyfus-Armand, Margot Nicolle, Nadine Sinopoli, and La Mounière Maison des Mémoires de Septfonds, and Laurence Héritier and Musée de la Résistance et du Combattant de Montalban, who allowed us access to the photographic archive of the Republican refugees in the camps; Lourdes Prades and the CRAI Biblioteca Pavelló de la República at the Universitat de Barcelona, who led us in the search for sources within the bibliographic and documentary inheritance from the Second Republic, and the CRAI Biblioteca del Campus de Mundet at the Universitat de Barcelona; Denis Canguilhem, Camille Limoges, Nathalie Queyroux, and the Centre d'Archives en Philosophie, Histoire et Édition des Sciences at the École Normale Supérieure, who reconstructed Georges Canguilhem's time at Saint-Alban; Isabelle Diu and the Bibliothèque Littéraire Jacques Doucet, who gave us access to the correspondence of Tristan Tzara written from Saint-Alban; Teresa Montaner and the Fundació Joan Miró de Barcelona, who helped us come to a better understanding of the various editions of *Parler seul*, by Tristan Tzara and Joan Miró; Sarah Lombardi, Vincent Monod, and the Collection de l'Art Brut Fondation Dubuffet, who welcomed us into the archives and correspondence of Georges Dubuffet; Christophe Boulanger, Sabine Faupin, and LaM Lille Metrópole Musée d'art moderne, d'art contemporain et d'art brut, who allowed us access into the archive of works made at Saint-Alban; Gabriel Gómez Plana and the Associació Cultural Helios Gómez, who authorized us to publish his correspondence with Tosquelles; Pierre Matarasso and Francine Vormesse Matarasso, who helped us to better understand the time Jacques Matarasso spent at Saint-Alban; Séverine Graff and Archives privées de Mario Ruspoli d'Isle-sur-la-Sorge, for the documentation of the filming of Ruspoli's films at Saint-Alban; Michelle Renard and the Collection du Dr Pailhas in Alby, for allowing us access to the collection of Benjamin Pailhas; Frédéric Borgia, Julien Avet, and the Institut Jean Vigo, Cinémathèque de Perpignan, who facilitated our access to the films shot at Saint-Alban; Mireille Gauzy, the Association Culturelle François Tosquelles, and the Archive de l'hôpital de Saint-Alban, who opened the doors of their library to us; the Bonnet and Ponsonnaille families, for the photographs of Saint-Alban during Tosquelles's time; Sophie Le Tétour of the Centre National du Cinéma et de l'Image Animée (CNC), who assisted us in the filmic research about Antonin Artaud; Serge

Alternês and Wainman Photograph & Archive Fonds (1933–1985), who gave us access to the photographic archive of the Civil War; Mercè Costafreda, for telling us about the manuscript by Pere Fort Ferré; Albert Arnavat, who allowed us access to the POUM memorial library in Reus; and Josep Turiel and Imma Marín of the CRAI Biblioteca de Lletres and Neus Jaumot de l'Arxiu Històric at the Universitat de Barcelona, for their unconditional help. We would also like to thank Any Durand and Éditions L'Arachnéen, the Moderna Museet, the Tate, the Museo Nacional Centro de Arte Reina Sofía, and the Akademia der Künste, for permission to use images from their collections.

The documentary contribution from the Centre de la Imatge Mas Iglesias de Reus, facilitated by Marc Ferran and Pep Torrents, was particularly useful.

Other institutions also allowed us into their archives: the archive Lucien Bonnafé, Institut Mémoires de l'Édition Contemporaine, Abbaye d'Ardenne; International Institute of Social History, Amsterdam; Centre Emili Mira; Fons Dr. Emili Mira i López at the Fundació Congrés Català de la Salut Mental; Fons Ramon Sarró and Fons General at the Biblioteca de Catalunya; Biblioteca del Centre de Lectura de Reus; Biblioteca Central Xavier Amorós and Fons Pere Anguera at the Arxiu Municipal de Reus; Ateneu Enciclopèdic Popular, Centre de Documentació Històrica i Social; Arxiu Històric of the Ateneu Barcelonès; Arxiu Nacional de Catalunya; Arxius de l'Institut Psicotècnic, Escola Industrial, and Biblioteca del Treball at the Institut Escola del Treball; Comité Técnico de Ayuda a los Republicanos Españoles at the Biblioteca Nacional de Antropología e Historia de México; Arbetarrörelsens Arkiv och Bibliotek–Swedish Labour Movement's Archives and Library in Huddinge; Fonds Gaston Ferdière, Archives Cantonales Vaudoises; Archives départementales de la Lozère; Arxiu General de la Diputació de Barcelona; Centro Documental de la Memoria Histórica; Archivo Militar de Ávila; Archivo General de la Administración in Alcalá de Henares; Fundación Pablo Iglesias; and Staatsbibliothek in Berlin.

I would like to thank Marta Segarra and Helena González, of the ADHUC–Centre de Recerca Teoria, Gènere, Sexualitat de la Universitat de Barcelona, for all their support that made possible this extensive research, and the editors Montse Ingla and Antoni Munné, for their constant encouragement and assistance in bringing this book into readers' hands.

In addition to their unconditional support and friendship, the work of Sandra Alvarez de Toledo and Anaïs Masson on the French edition of this book, *Tosquelles: Soigner les institutions*, edited by L'Arachnéen and Arcàdia, enriched this text with additional historical and bibliographic information.

This book would not exist if not for conversations with Éric Fassin, Alejandra Riera, and Mireia Sallarès, who have always been there.

I dedicate this book to my father who is no longer with us, with whom I spent so much time talking about the memory of Tosquelles's forgotten experiences and about the difficulty of remembering; to Assumpta and Emília; and to Roser and Emma, for their loving care of Sol while I was writing.

The research project “El llegat oblidat de Francesc Tosquelles” (The forgotten legacy of Francesc Tosquelles) received support from the Fundació Privada Mir-Puig, from 2017 to 2024, under the ADHUC–Centre de Recerca, Teoria, Gènere, Sexualitat at the Universitat de Barcelona.

This book is a companion to the exhibitions around the figure of Francesc Tosquelles that have taken place at Les Abattoirs, Musée – Frac Occitanie Toulouse (2021–2022), the Centre de Cultura Contemporània de Barcelona (CCCB) (2022), the Museo Nacional Centro de Arte Reina Sofía, Madrid (2022–2023), and the American Folk Art Museum in New York (2024), originally curated by Carles Guerra and Joana Masó.

The archives of the Hospital Universitari Institut Pere Mata have been instrumental in carrying out this research.

The Fundació Antoni Tàpies promoted and hosted the project’s first programs in 2018, with the support of the 4Cs: From Conflict to Conviviality through Creativity and Culture.

The Museu d’Art de Tarragona joined the project with an exhibition and a program of activities in 2022.

Fundació Privada
MIR-PUIG

ADHUC
Centre de Recerca
Teoria, Gènere, Sexualitat

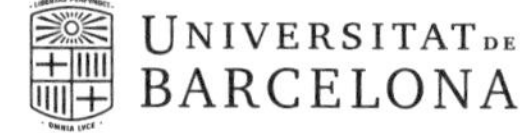

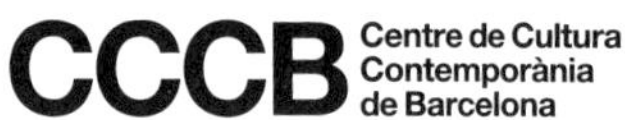

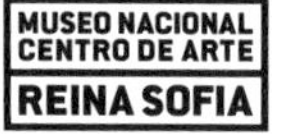

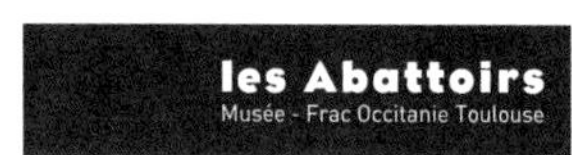

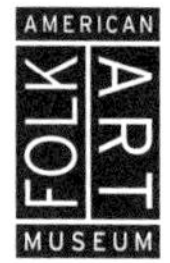

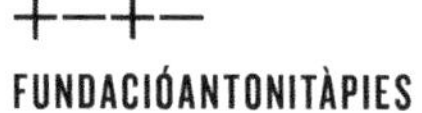

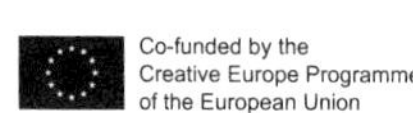

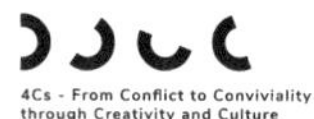

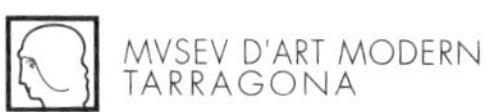

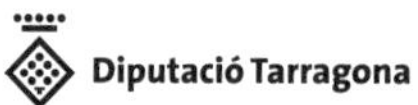

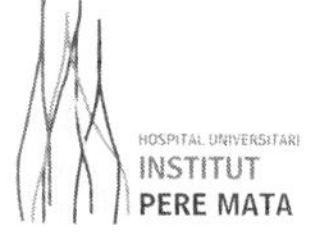

Original title: *Tosquelles: Curar les institucions*

© 2021, 2026 by Joana Masó

All works by Francesc Tosquelles © 2026 by the Estate of Francesc Tosquelles

Translations from the French © 2026 by Robert Hurley

Translations from the Catalan and Spanish © 2026 by Mara Faye Lethem

The short texts by various authors accompanying Joana Masó's essays are reproduced in accordance with the rules governing quotation under the Intellectual Property Code.

All images © their authors / rights holders. For sources and further details, see pp. 387–392 of this volume.

Every effort has been made to identify the rights holders of the works and documents reproduced. Any accidental omission or error should be notified in writing to the publishers and will be corrected in subsequent editions.

David Fontanals created the chronology, as well as the bibliography and filmography, which were checked by Sandra Alvarez de Toledo and Anaïs Masson.

"Social Therapy in a Ward of Muslim Men: Methodological Difficulties," first published 2015, © Éditions La Découverte, Frantz Fanon, *Alienation and Freedom*. English translation © 2018 by Jean Khalfa, Robert J.C. Young, & Steven Corcoran, Bloomsbury Academic, an imprint of Bloomsbury Publishing Plc.

"In Memoriam" © 1968 by Gabriel Ferrater and the Estate of Gabriel Ferrater

Book concept:
Joana Masó and Arcàdia

Images clearance:
Maria Nadal Vallès

Proofreading:
Robert Dewhurst

Original design:
Edicions de l'Eixample, Barcelona